Neuroimaging for the Characterization of Brain Disorders

Neuroimaging for the Characterization of Brain Disorders

Editor: Kathline Swift

AMERICAN
MEDICAL PUBLISHERS
www.americanmedicalpublishers.com

AMERICAN
MEDICAL PUBLISHERS
www.americanmedicalpublishers.com

Cataloging-in-Publication Data

Neuroimaging for the characterization of brain disorders / edited by Kathline Swift.
p. cm.
Includes bibliographical references and index.
ISBN 979-8-88740-308-3
1. Brain--Imaging. 2. Brain--Diseases--Imaging. 3. Brain--Diseases--Diagnosis.
4. Nervous system--Radiography. 5. Nervous system--Imaging. 6. Diagnostic imaging.
I. Swift, Kathline.
RC386.6.D52 N48 2023
616.804 754--dc23

American Medical Publishers,
41 Flatbush Avenue,
1st Floor, New York,
NY 11217, USA

ISBN 979-8-88740-308-3 (Hardback)

Contents

Preface

The purpose of the book is to provide a glimpse into the dynamics and to present opinions and studies of some of the scientists engaged in the development of new ideas in the field from very different standpoints. This book will prove useful to students and researchers owing to its high content quality.

Neuroimaging refers to the utilization of quantitative methods for the study of the structure and function of the central nervous system. It was developed as a non-invasive method to scientifically investigate the healthy human brain. It is widely being used in quantitative investigations for psychiatric illnesses and brain disorders. Various techniques that are used in neuroimaging include computed axial tomography and magnetic resonance imaging, diffuse optical imaging, positron emission tomography, cranial ultrasound. The human brain is a massive, interconnected and complex system. Advanced neuroimaging techniques such as diffusion tensor imaging and functional magnetic resonance imaging allow us to investigate the underlying principles of brain structural and functional architectures. It also enables us to study the pathological changes in a variety of brain disorders. Multi-modal neuroimaging techniques could provide a more thorough understanding of the pathomechanism of brain disorders, which facilitates early diagnosis and helps in assessing prognosis and therapeutic effect. This book elucidates the concepts and innovative models around prospective developments with respect to the characterization of brain disorders. The topics covered herein offer the readers new insights in the field of neuroimaging.

At the end, I would like to appreciate all the efforts made by the authors in completing their chapters professionally. I express my deepest gratitude to all of them for contributing to this book by sharing their valuable works. A special thanks to my family and friends for their constant support in this journey.

Editor

1

Partial Least Square Aided Beamforming Algorithm in Magnetoencephalography Source Imaging

Yegang Hu [1,2,3,4], Chunli Yin [5,6], Jicong Zhang [1,2,3,4] and Yuping Wang [5,6*]*

[1] School of Biological Science and Medical Engineering, Beihang University, Beijing, China, [2] Beijing Advanced Innovation Centre for Big Data-Based Precision Medicine, Beihang University, Beijing, China, [3] Beijing Advanced Innovation Centre for Biomedical Engineering, Beihang University, Beijing, China, [4] Hefei Innovation Research Institute, Beihang University, Hefei, China, [5] Department of Neurology, Xuanwu Hospital, Capital Medical University, Beijing, China, [6] Beijing Key Laboratory of Brain Functional Disease and Neuromodulation, Beijing, China

***Correspondence:**
Jicong Zhang
jicongzhang@buaa.edu.cn
Yuping Wang
wangyuping@xwhosp.org

Beamforming techniques have played a prominent role in source imaging in neuroimaging and in locating epileptogenic zones. However, existing vector-beamformers are sensitive to noise on localization of epileptogenic zones. In this study, partial least square (PLS) was used to aid the minimum variance beamforming approach for source imaging with magnetoencephalography (MEG) arrays, and verified its effectiveness in simulated data and epilepsy data. First, PLS was employed to extract the components of the MEG arrays by maximizing the covariance between a linear combination of the predictors and the class variable. Noise was then removed by reconstructing the MEG arrays based on those components. The minimum variance beamforming method was used to estimate a source model. Simulations with a realistic head model and varying noise levels indicated that the proposed approach can provide higher spatial accuracy than other well-known beamforming methods. For real MEG recordings in 10 patients with temporal lobe epilepsy, the ratios of the number of spikes localized in the surgical excised region to the total number of spikes using the proposed method were higher than that of the dipole fitting method. These localization results using the proposed method are more consistent with the clinical evaluation. The proposed method may provide a new imaging marker for localization of epileptogenic zones.

Keywords: Magnetoencephalography (MEG), beamforming, partial least squares, source imaging, epileptogenic zone, imaging-based marker

INTRODUCTION

Accurate diagnosis of epileptogenic zones has long been a focus of neurology, as it determines whether epilepsy patients can achieve seizure freedom by surgical excision. In recent years, magnetoencephalography (MEG) has been increasingly trusted by clinical epileptologists for preoperative examination (Wennberg and Cheyne, 2014; Nissen et al., 2016). This is because MEG is a non-invasive neuroimaging technique that records brain activity with millisecond temporal resolution and minor signal deterioration from the skull and scalp (Barnes and Hillebrand, 2003; Zumer et al., 2007; Baillet, 2017). Postsynaptic current flow within the dendrites of active neurons produces a weak magnetic field that can be measured by superconducting quantum interference devices (SQUIDS) (Hämäläinen et al., 1993). Because the currents generated by neurons determine the magnitude of the measured fields, these measurements can give information about brain activity on a millisecond time scale. However, the great challenge is to localize the active neurons on the basis of the measured magnetic field. Because the locations of epileptogenic zones estimated using current localization methods are not always accurate, MEG has not been completely accepted by all clinical epileptologists (Englot et al., 2015). In general, the number of sensors is far less than the number of possible current distributions. This inverse problem is an example of what mathematicians call an ill-posed problem (Hadamard and Morse, 1953). Finding the optimal solution of such an underdetermined system of equations often requires specific constraints. In other words, to accurately localize the brain sources of magnetic signals, assumptions must be made about the nature of the neuronal sources.

Many source imaging algorithms for MEG signals have been proposed (Pascual-Marqui et al., 1994; Mattout et al., 2006; Grech et al., 2008; Mäkelä et al., 2018), and each optimizing the solution of the inverse problem under a specific set of assumptions. One type of inverse solution approach is known as "beamforming" (Van Veen et al., 1997; Groß et al., 2001; Sekihara et al., 2002a; Oshino et al., 2007; Zhang and Liu, 2015). Beamforming techniques play a key role in signal processing and neuroimaging. These methods make use of spatial filtering, that is, the MEG signals are decomposed into "beams" based on gain vectors corresponding to specific source-grid points (Diwakar et al., 2011). The most widely used beamforming method, linearly constrained minimum variance (LCMV) beamforming (also called vector beamforming), produces a reliable spatial filter when the weights are chosen to minimize the filter output power subject to a linear constraint. However, the existing vector beamformers for MEG source imaging are sensitive to noise, and poor at localizing sources. The main reason for this problem is that the sensor array geometry is used directly to estimate the covariance matrix. Recently, an iterative spatiotemporal signal decomposition method has been used to modify the vector beamforming technique, and has been successfully applied to source localization for MEG signals (Hu et al., 2017). Although the approach has achieved high spatial accuracy, the correlations of signals from different brain regions are ignored when the components of the MEG arrays are extracted. An improvement would be to use partial least squares (PLS) analysis to make better use of structural information.

PLS analysis originated in the fields of econometrics and chemometrics (Wold et al., 1984; Geladi and Kowalski, 1986). It extracts components in a way that maximizes the covariance between each component and a "class variable." In recent years, this approach has been successfully applied in many fields, including multivariate statistics (Wold et al., 1984), analytical chemistry (Wold et al., 2001), face recognition (Baek and Kim, 2004; Sharma and Jacobs, 2011), and bioinformatics (Boulesteix and Strimmer, 2006). In pattern recognition, the PLS method can be used to extract the principle components with maximum variability and to exploit the class information (Baek and Kim, 2004; Sharma and Jacobs, 2011). PLS has better performance in feature extraction and denoising compared with typical methods, such as principal component analysis (PCA) and linear discrimination analysis (LDA). The principal components extracted by PLS are called "intrinsic components" to indicate that PLS is more representative for biometric signals. In fact, MEG signals are very similar to these biometric signals, and are affected by various noises. If the intrinsic components are found from those MEG signals, these components should be usable to improve the spatial accuracy of source imaging. Thus, in this study we used the PLS method to extract the components of the MEG signals and reconstruct the data matrix in this study. Although recent literatures show that the PLS method has been used in functional neuroimaging (McIntosh and Lobaugh, 2004; Krishnan et al., 2011; Cheung et al., 2016), for purposes such as describing the relationship between brain activity and behavior, these PLS applications are not intended to improve the source imaging method.

The aim of this study was to propose and investigate a new source imaging algorithm with specific applicability to focal epilepsy focus localization. We applied PLS analysis to aid the vector beamforming technique for better performance in source imaging with MEG arrays. First, the MEG arrays were treated as an observation matrix $\boldsymbol{X}$, combined with a class matrix $\boldsymbol{Y}$ of dummy variables that code for brain regions. Second, we employed PLS technique to extract the components of the MEG arrays by maximizing the covariance between a linear combination of the predictors and the class variable. We then reconstructed the sensor arrays based on the components and loadings, and used the vector beamforming technique to estimate the source model. The newly proposed source imaging approach for MEG recordings was first validated on simulated data, and compared with three other well-known beamforming methods, linearly constrained minimum variance (LCMV) (Van Veen et al., 1997), dynamic imaging of coherent sources (DICS) (Groß et al., 2001), and modified LCMV with iterative matrix decomposition (mLCMV) (Hu et al., 2017). Since these methods belong to the beamforming family, the basic assumption in this study is the same as assumption underlying the minimum variance beamforming. We further verify the proposed method in a real dataset that includes the MEG recordings of 10 patients with temporal lobe epilepsy.

METHODS

Partial Least Squares Analysis

PLS analysis is a technique for extracting components and loadings between a set of input variables $\{\boldsymbol{x}_i\}_{i=1}^{M} \in R^N$ and a set of response variables $\{\mathbf{y}_i\}_{i=1}^{M} \in R^L$. As with principal components analysis, PLS generates uncorrelated components that are linear are linear combinations of the original input variables. The difference is that PLS creates the components by modeling the relationship between the input and response variables, while maintaining most of the information in the input variables. The objective criterion is to find a weight vector w_k such that

$$w_k = \arg \max_{\|w\|=1, \|v\|=1} \mathrm{Cov}^2 (Xw,\ Yv) \tag{1}$$

$$\textit{subject to the constraint } w_k^T C w_j = 0$$

where $\|\bullet\|$ denotes the two-norm operator, $1 \leq j \leq k$, and $Cov(\bullet,\ \bullet)$ $Cov(\bullet, \bullet)$ represents the covariance operator, T is the transpose of a vector or matrix, and $C{=}X^T X$. Here, X represents an $M \times N$ matrix of input variables and Y is an $M \times L$ ($M \times L$) matrix made up of corresponding response variables. In general, the column vectors of the data matrices X and Y are normalized before optimization, that is, the mean value is zero and the variance is one.

Next, a well-known iterative algorithm (Lewi, 1995; Rosipal and Trejo, 2001; Hu et al., 2012) is used to optimize formula (1). A description in pseudo-code is shown in **Algorithm 1**:

Algorithm 1: Pseudo-code for partial least squares analysis.

Inputs: Data matrices $X \in R^{M\times N}$, $Y \in R^{M\times L}$
Process:
1. Normalize the matrices X and Y
2. For $i = 1, \ldots, K$
Randomly initialize the loading vector u
Normalize u to length 1: $u = \frac{u}{\|u\|}$, $\hat{u} = 2u$
while $\|\hat{u} - u\| > epsilon$
$\hat{u} = u$
Calculate the weight vector $w : w = X^T u$
Calculate the component vector $t : t = Xw$
Normalize t to length 1: $t = \frac{t}{\|t\|}$
Calculate a temporary vector v: $v = Y^T t$
Calculate a new loading vector u: $u = Yv$
Normalize u to length 1: $u = \frac{u}{\|u\|}$
end
Extract the i-th component t_i and loading vector u_i
Deflate the X, Y matrices:
$X = X - t_i t_i^T X,\ Y = Y - t_i t_i^T Y$
end
3. Obtain the component matrix $T = [t_1, \ldots, t_K]$ and the loading matrix $U = [u_1, \ldots, u_K]$
4. Reconstruct the data matrix $\hat{X} = TU^T$
Outputs: the component matrix T, loading matrix U, reconstructed data matrix $\hat{X}$

Note that the variable K in **Algorithm 1** is determined by the two-norm of the residual matrix of the data matrix X, that is, as long as the norm value is greater than a threshold, the program continues to cycle. In addition to being used for data reconstruction, PLS analysis can also be used effectively for dimensionality reduction, recognition, and regression (Rosipal and Trejo, 2001; Baek and Kim, 2004; Hu et al., 2012).

In feature extraction and pattern classification, PLS is a supervised learning method, and each row in the Y matrix is a class label for each sample. PLS is then used to extract the intrinsic components T and loadings U by using **Algorithm 1**, and the data matrix $\hat{X}$ is reconstructed using these intrinsic components and loadings. The new data matrix $\hat{X}$ is a relatively clean matrix after denoising. This procedure can be considered to improve the spatial accuracy of source imaging. The Y matrix is very important and will be described in Section Source Imaging via Partial Least Squares.

Minimum Variance Beamforming

Beamforming, also called spatial filtering, plays an important role in localizing sources of brain activity from surface recordings. The weights of the spatial filter are usually obtained by minimizing the filter output power (i.e., minimizing the variance). LCMV beamforming optimizes the objective function subject to a linear constraint, and therefore is a type of vector beamforming. The principle of using minimum variance beamforming to solve inverse problems will now be illustrated in detail. For an input variable set $X = [x^{(1)}, x^{(2)}, \ldots, x^{(N)}]$, derived from the MEG sensors, the inverse solution model is given as:

$$X = LD + \varepsilon \tag{2}$$

where $x^{(i)}$ represents an $M \times 1$ vector of the MEG recordings at the i-th time point ($i = 1 \cdots N$), M is the number of MEG sensors, L is the $M \times J$ (lead-field) gain matrix, J is the number of unknown dipole moment parameters, D denotes a $J \times N$ dipole moment matrix for a given time series, N is the number of time points, and ε represents the $M \times N$ noise matrix. We design a spatial filter $W(r_0)$ for the narrowband volume element centered on location r_0, using the following formula:

$$y = W^T (r_0)\, x \tag{3}$$

where $W(r_0)$ is an $M \times 3$ matrix, x represents the input vector of the filter, and y is the output vector. Generally, an ideal narrowband spatial filter needs to satisfy

$$W^T (r_0)\, L(r) = \begin{cases} \mathbf{I}, & r = r_0 \\ 0, & r \neq r_0 \end{cases} \tag{4}$$

where r is the location of a grid point inside the brain, $L(r)$ is the $M \times 3$ (lead-field) gain matrix, and I is the unit matrix. The objective function to be optimized is then posed mathematically as

$$\min_{W(r_0)} tr\left(W^T (r_0)\, C(x)\, W(r_0)\right)$$
$$\textit{subject to}\quad W^T (r_0)\, L(r_0) = I \tag{5}$$

where $tr(\bullet)$ denotes the trace of a matrix, and $C(x)$ is the covariance matrix of random variables based on the row vectors of the data matrix X. A second-order statistic for the sample is used to estimate the population covariance, as illustrated in the study by (Van Veen et al., 1997). The effect of the constraint here is to allow the activity at position r_0 to be passed with unit gain, while inhibiting contributions from all other sources.

An algorithm that minimizes interference (MinInf) is used to optimize the objective function, yielding the optimal solution (Groß and Ioannides, 1999)

$$W^T(r_0) = \left[L^T(r_0)\,C^{-1}(\mathbf{x})\,L(r_0)\right]^{-1} L^T(r_0)\,C^{-1}(\mathbf{x}) \tag{6}$$

where $(\bullet)^{-1}$ denotes the inverse operator. The formula (6) is substituted into the spatial filter, and the variance of the filter output is estimated to be:

$$\hat{Var}(r_0) = tr\left\{\left[L^T(r_0)\,C^{-1}(\mathbf{x})\,L(r_0)\right]^{-1}\right\} \tag{7}$$

The estimated variance is the value of the objective function (5) at its minimum, or it can represent the strength of the activity at grid point r_0. Therefore, if the MEG data matrix $\boldsymbol{X}$ is known, we can calculate the strength of the activity at all grid points in the brain. The position corresponding to the maximum strength is assumed to be the source location.

Source Imaging via Partial Least Squares

The source imaging process includes four parts: head model construction, forward solution, inverse solution, and source display. The aim of this paper is to improve the localization accuracy by optimizing the inverse solution with minimum variance beamforming and PLS analysis. With the selection of the input variables $\boldsymbol{X}$ and the response variables $\boldsymbol{Y}$, the PLS analysis generates multiple variants in different application scenarios. Recent studies (Sekihara et al., 2002b; Brookes et al., 2007; Hu et al., 2017) ignore the correlations between different brain regions when reconstructing the input matrix $\boldsymbol{X}$ in the MEG source imaging. Since PLS is a supervised learning, the first step in using this method is to divide all samples into multiple classes. In the present study, each channel is considered as a sample for the input matrix $\boldsymbol{X}$. All MEG sensors are then classified to integrate the PLS method into brain source imaging. **Figure 1** shows the layout of all the MEG sensors, which are divided into eight brain regions: frontal lobes (left and right), temporal lobes (left and right), parietal lobes (left and right) and occipital lobes (left and right). This classification of brain regions refers to the standard brain regions provided by Elekta Neuromag MEG. Thus, the full set of samples is divided into eight classes according to the distribution of brain regions of the sensors. The $\boldsymbol{Y}$ matrix is then generated according to these classes.

The MEG recordings were acquired inside a magnetically shielded room, with 306 channels in total, using a helmet-shaped whole-head system (VectorView, Elekta Neuromag Oy, Finland) comprising 102 locations in triplets. The system included one magnetometer and two orthogonal planar gradiometers. To compute the forward solution, we used a realistically-shaped single-shell approximation for constructing a volume conduction model based on the implementation from Nolte (2003). The anatomical MRI scans of the second patient in Section Experimental Results in Epilepsy Data were used to produce a realistic head shape in all simulated data.

Next, we consider a set of N-dimensional samples $\boldsymbol{X}_{M\times N}$, where M represents the total number of MEG channels (306), and N represents the width of the time series (600). The $\boldsymbol{Y}$ matrix represents the labels for supervised learning. The $\boldsymbol{Y}$ matrix in this study directly refers to the definition of the $\boldsymbol{Y}$ matrix in the existing PLS methods that are used for dimensionality reduction and feature extraction (Baek and Kim, 2004; Sharma and Jacobs, 2011). For the PLS analysis, according to the input matrix $\boldsymbol{X}$, we define an $M \times C$ class membership matrix $\boldsymbol{Y}$ to be

$$\boldsymbol{Y} = \begin{bmatrix} \boldsymbol{1}_{n_1} & \boldsymbol{0}_{n_1} & \cdots & \boldsymbol{0}_{n_1} \\ \boldsymbol{0}_{n_2} & \boldsymbol{1}_{n_2} & \cdots & \boldsymbol{0}_{n_2} \\ \vdots & \vdots & \ddots & \vdots \\ \boldsymbol{0}_{n_C} & \boldsymbol{0}_{n_C} & \cdots & \boldsymbol{1}_{n_C} \end{bmatrix} \tag{8}$$

where n_i is the number of samples in the i-th class (i.e., the number of sensors in the i-th brain region), C is the number of classes (i.e., 8), $\boldsymbol{1}_{n_i}$ denotes an $n_i \times 1$ vector of all ones, $\boldsymbol{0}_{n_i}$ denotes an $n_i \times 1$ vector of all zeros, and $M = \sum_{i=1}^{C} n_i$. A "1" in the $\boldsymbol{Y}$ matrix means that the sensor belongs to the corresponding class, while "0" means that the sensor does not belongs to this class.

In the inverse solution, under the condition that the MEG sensor array $\boldsymbol{X}$ and the corresponding class matrix $\boldsymbol{Y}$ are known, the component matrix $\boldsymbol{T}$ and the loading matrix $\boldsymbol{U}$ are extracted using **Algorithm 1**, and the sensor array is reconstructed, denoted as $\hat{\boldsymbol{X}}$. The reconstructed sensor array is applied to estimate the covariance matrix in formula (5), and the optimal solutions of formula (6) and (7) are obtained by optimizing the objective function (5). Using formula (7), we calculate the maximum strength and the location in the brain, which is the sought-for source. Finally, the computed source can be displayed in an individual MRI scan using an established individual head model. To clearly convey the MEG source imaging procedure, the steps are summarized in the algorithm flow chart shown in **Figure 2**. In the following section, we verify the feasibility of the algorithm using two different simulation sources. Three primary toolboxes, Matlab R2014a (The MathWorks Inc., Natick, MA, USA), SPM8 (Litvak et al., 2011), and FieldTrip (Oostenveld et al., 2011), are used jointly for the MEG data analysis. All source imaging algorithms are implemented based on the ft_sourceanalysis function in the FieldTrip toolkit. All parameters are optimized based on this toolkit, and the parameters of the pLCMV and mLCMV methods are the same as that of the LCMV method.

RESULTS

Simulated Data Generation

In view of a simulation source with explicit ground truth, we first performed experiments on simulated MEG data as follows. Source imaging is often used to find the source of event-related fields within the brain based on a task, and to locate epileptic foci. The waveforms of event-related fields and epileptiform waves are often very close to the sinc function, which is an aperiodic attenuation signal. The mathematical expression of the sinc function is described as:

$$S(t) = \frac{\sin(\pi(t+\tau))}{\pi(t+\tau)} \tag{9}$$

where τ is the translation width of the function. To show that the proposed localization algorithm can also be applied

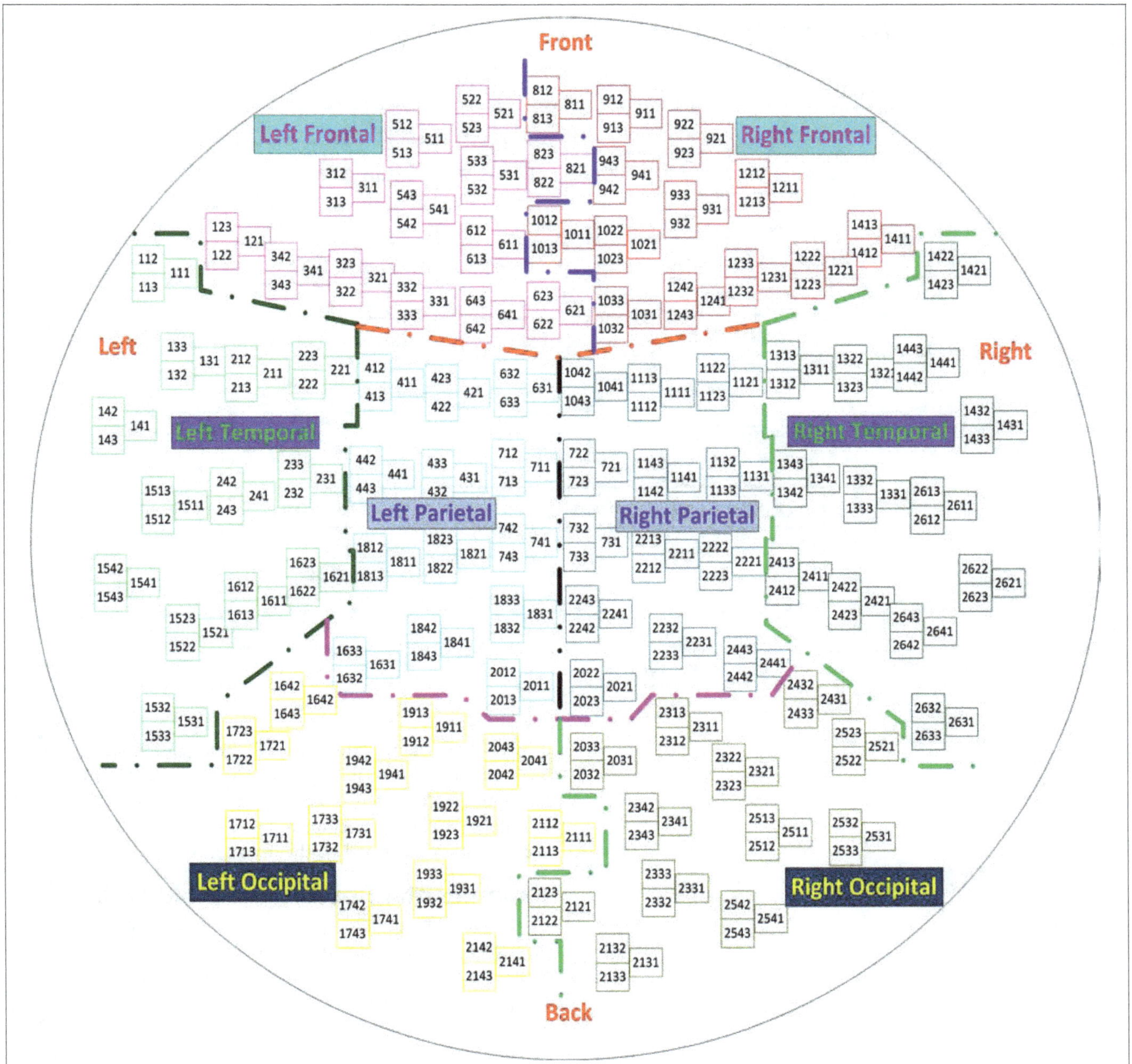

FIGURE 1 | Layout of the sensor elements. The helmet-shaped sensor array is flattened into a plane, and the 306 sensor channels are divided into eight brain regions: frontal lobes (left and right), temporal lobes (left and right), parietal lobes (left and right), and occipital lobes (left and right).

with contaminated signals, Gaussian noise was added to the time-course of the real signal. The simulated data was then generated by a sinc function plus the Gaussian noise. The noise intensity was divided into 12 levels, from weak to strong, to allow observation of the robustness of the proposed localization method. The signal-to-noise ratio (SNR) was used to quantify different noise levels, as defined in the following formula:

$$SNR_{dB} = 10\ \log_{10}\left(\frac{P_A}{P_B}\right) = 10\ \log_{10}\left(\frac{\|\boldsymbol{A}\|_F^2}{\|\boldsymbol{B}\|_F^2}\right) \tag{10}$$

where P_A denotes the power of the synthetic sensor signals $\boldsymbol{A}$, $P_{\boldsymbol{B}}$ is the power of the background noise, and $\|\bullet\|_F$ represents the Frobenius norm of a matrix or vector. For each level of noise, 100 Gaussian noise samples were generated randomly. The mean of these SNR values are shown in **Figure 3**. These SNR values decrease from a maximum of 6.990 to a minimum of 0.043 with the changes in the noise level.

In this study, the time duration of all the simulated MEG data is 600 ms, and the sampling rate is 1,000 Hz. The planar gradiometers were used to localize the sources. The source space

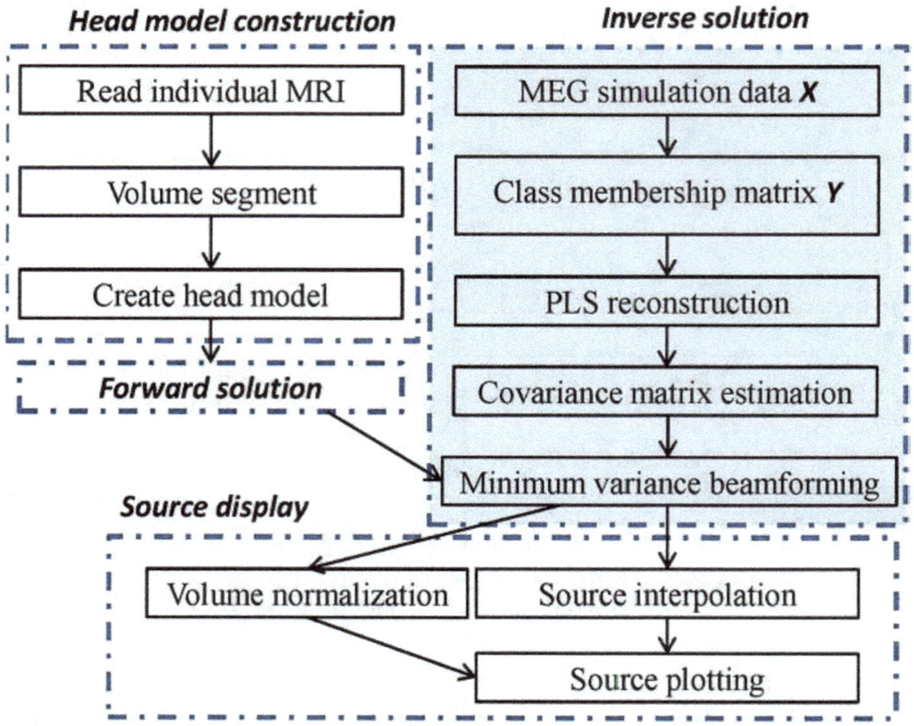

FIGURE 2 | The flow chart of source imaging consists of four parts. Head model construction, forward solution, inverse solution, and source display, in which the inverse solution is modified by PLS analysis and minimum variance beamforming.

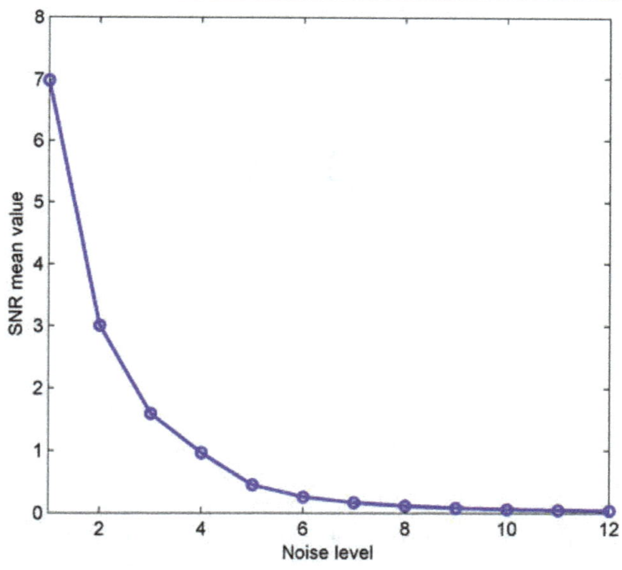

FIGURE 3 | The mean signal-to-noise ratio of the simulation is given for 12 different noise levels. Fifty noise samples were generated at each level; the x-axis represents the noise level and the y-axis represents the mean value.

was based on a subject's realistic head shape, which was modeled as a single shell based on a magnetic resonance imaging scan. For a realistic head model, the brain space was partitioned into a three-dimensional grid with millimeter resolution, including 3,704 points in total. Each point could be regarded as a source location. The MEG sensor arrays were implemented through the ft_dipolesimulation function in the Fieldtrip toolbox, based on the previously described synthetic signals for the location.

Experimental Results in Simulated Data

In this section, we first verify the source imaging algorithm through the experiments based on simulated data, generated by a sinc function plus Gaussian noise. The proposed method is compared with three well-known beamforming methods: linearly constrained minimum variance (LCMV) (Van Veen et al., 1997), dynamic imaging of coherent sources (DICS) (Groß et al., 2001), and modified LCMV with iterative matrix decomposition (mLCMV) (Hu et al., 2017). Because the new method combines PLS with beamforming, pLCMV is regarded as an acronym of the new method. Spatial accuracy is used to evaluate the results of source imaging, with the evaluation index defined as:

$$Location\ error = \sqrt{\left\| \gamma - \hat{\gamma} \right\|_2} \tag{11}$$

where $\|\bullet\|_2$ represents the two-norm operator, γ is the spatial location of the real source, and $\hat{\gamma}$ is the spatial location of the source estimated by the localization algorithm. A smaller location error corresponds to a higher spatial accuracy.

We chose six sources to construct the simulations. The spatial locations of the six sources were represented in the Neuromag coordinate system as {(−29, 11, 38), (67, 11, 30), (59, 43, 70), (59,

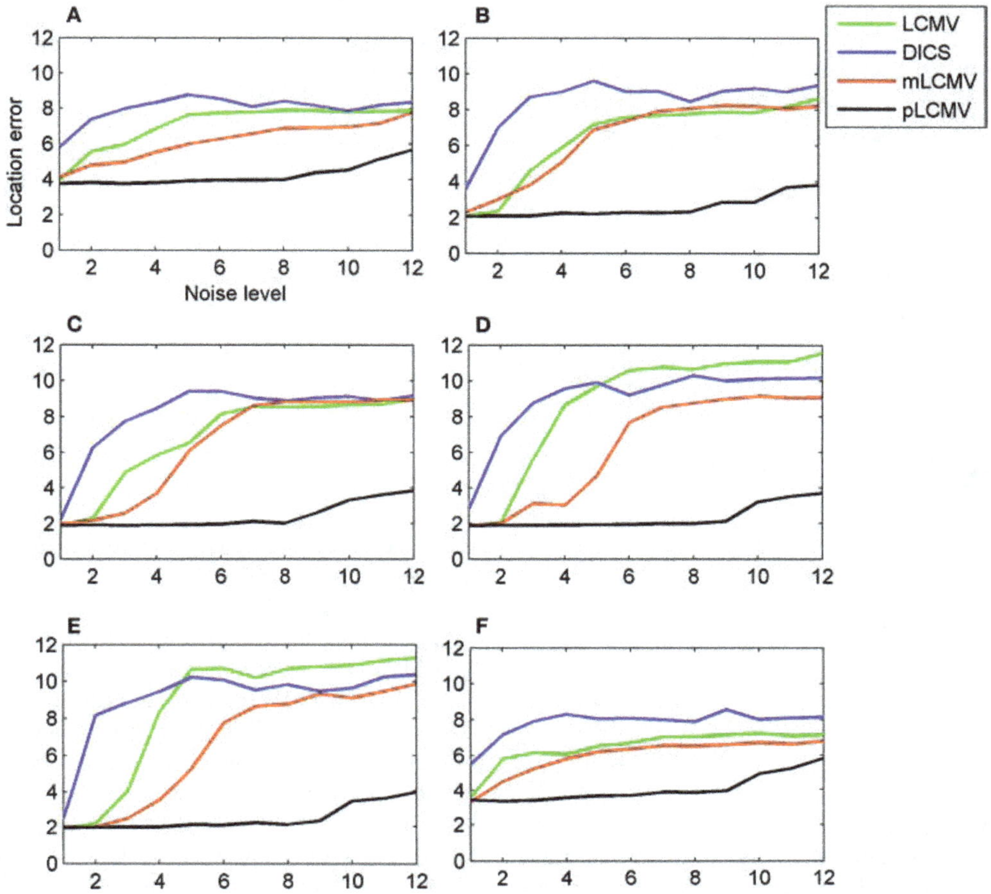

FIGURE 4 | For a simulated data generated by an aperiodic signal (sinc) plus the Gaussian noise, the spatial accuracy of the proposed approach (pLCMV) was compared with that of the other three approaches (DICS, LCMV, mLCMV). The x-axis of each plot represents the noise level, and the y-axis represents the location error. Each plot shows a comparison of the localization results of the four approaches based on simulated data generated for six different locations of the brain. The six locations were the left mesial temporal lobe **(A)**, right lateral temporal lobe **(B)**, right frontal lobe **(C)**, right occipital lobe **(D)**, right parietal lobe **(E)**, and right mesial temporal lobe **(F)**. Plots **(A)** and **(F)** represent deep sources; the rest represent shallow sources.

−53, 54), (67, −29, 86), (35, 11, 38)} mm. The six locations were in the left mesial temporal lobe, right lateral temporal lobe, right frontal lobe, right occipital lobe, right parietal lobe, and right mesial temporal lobe. The first and last were deep sources, the rest were shallow sources. **Figure 4** shows that the localization results using the proposed method (pLCMV) were obviously better than those obtained from the other three methods (LCMV, DICS, and mLCMV). The spatial accuracies on the localization results using the four methods became lower as SNR value became smaller. The spatial accuracies of the three alternative methods (LCMV, mLCMV, DICS) were very similar with the increase of noise. Thus, the proposed method had the highest spatial accuracy, and that the spatial accuracy was affected little by the noise level.

Although the **six** locations covered the major regions of the brain, these locations cannot represent all possible grid points in the brain. To obtain more representative results, 309 locations were selected from the 3,704 points of the grid, by starting from the **first** point and using a step length of 12. As in the previous set of experiments, the real signal (a sinc signal) and Gaussian noise were used to generate 309 simulations for these 309 locations. For these simulations, the location errors of the **four** localization methods (LCMV, DICS, mLCMV, pLCMV) were calculated. **Figure 5** shows the mean value and standard deviation of the spatial accuracy of source localization for the 309 simulations generated using the sinc function. The localization results for the mLCMV method were better than those for DCIS and LCMV, and the difference in source localization between LCMV and DICS was not obvious. Also, the spatial accuracies on the localization results using the **four** methods became lower as SNR value became smaller, and the proposed method had the highest spatial accuracy.

Experimental Results in Epilepsy Data

By adding a Gaussian noise to the source signal, the experimental results show that the proposed method was effective and had the highest spatial accuracy in simulated MEG data. However, an actual MEG signal is often disturbed by noise of many complex origins, such as breathing, heart beats, eye movements, small movements of the facial muscles and so on. In the following experiments, we further verify the proposed method in a real

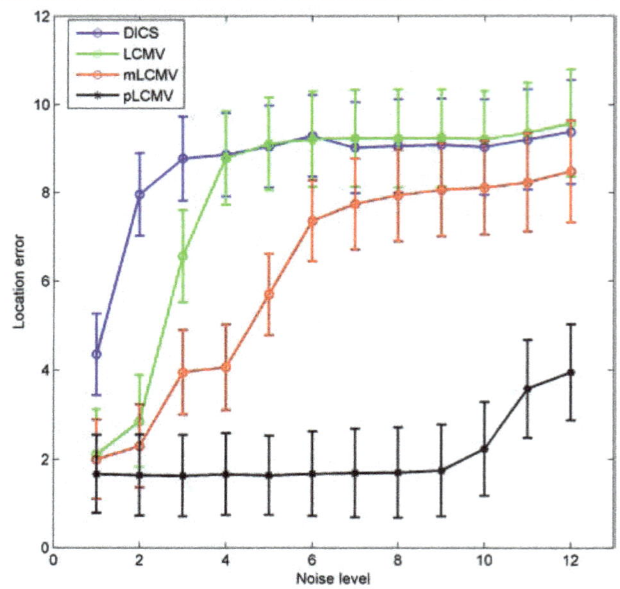

FIGURE 5 | Comparison of the spatial accuracy of the four methods. The x-axis of each plot represents the noise level, and the y-axis represents the mean value ± standard deviation of the location error, based on 309 simulations. Each simulation was generated by a sinc function and Gaussian noise.

MEG dataset with focal temporal lobe epilepsy (TLE). A total of 10 patients with medically refractory TLE were obtained retrospectively. All clinical characteristics of the patients are described in **Table 1**. These patients were diagnosed as focal unilateral TLE by a comprehensive preoperative assessment, including seizure history and semiology, neurological examination, 3-Tesla magnetic resonance imaging (MRI), scalp electroencephalography, invasive electroencephalography. All patients were from Xuanwu hospital in Beijing and underwent anterior temporal lobectomy including hippocampus (Schaller and Cabrilo, 2016). The results of at least **1** year follow-up indicated that these patients achieved seizure free status (Engel class IA). Written informed consent was obtained from each participant. The study was performed under a protocol approved by the medical ethics committee of Xuanwu Hospital of Capital Medical University.

MRI indicates magnetic resonance imaging; M, male; F, female; LT, left temporal; RT, right temporal; LHS, left hippocampal sclerosis; RHS, right hippocampal sclerosis; HRH, hyper T2 in right hippocampus; HLC, hyper T2 in left temporal cortex; ARH, atrophy in right hippocampus; BHS, bilateral hippocampal sclerosis; FCD, focal cortical dysplasia; HS, hippocampal sclerosis.

The epileptic spikes were visually marked by **two** experienced clinical epileptologists in the MEG signals. The MEG data with a spike was localized using the proposed method and the dipole fitting. The dipole fitting method here is performed using the software provided by the MEG and is widely recognized in clinical epilepsy localization. **One** spike in this study yields a localization result. The localization results of all epilepsy patients

TABLE 1 | Clinical characteristics of the patients.

Patient no.	Age (years)	Seizure duration (years)	MRI	Spike number	Preoperative assessment	Pathology
1	16–20	8	HLC	45	LT	FCD
2	16–20	9	RHS	37	RT	FCD, HS
3	20–25	17	LHS	23	LT	FCD, HS
4	26–30	5	LHS	18	LT	FCD, HS
5	26–30	14	Normal	42	RT	FCD
6	20–25	14	HRH	38	RT	FCD, HS
7	30–35	11	Normal	46	RT	FCD
8	20–25	20	LHS	32	LT	FCD, HS
9	30–35	17	ARH	27	RT	FCD
10	36–40	16	Normal	25	RT	FCD

were checked by the clinical epileptologists. We counted the number of those spikes in the resection region for source localization results. **Figure 6** shows a comparison of localization results obtained for patients with TLE using the proposed method (pLCMV) with those obtained using the dipole fitting, LCMV, DICS, and mLCMV methods. The ratios of the number of spikes counted in the resection region to the total number of spikes in each patient are shown in **Figure 6**. The localization results of most spikes should appear in the surgical resection region based on preoperative assessments, pathological findings, and postoperative follow-up results. **Figure 6** shows that the dipole fitting method is not always effective for finding epileptogenic zones, especially in the 6th and 10th patients. The ratios of the number of spikes localized in the surgical excised region to the total number of spikes using the proposed method were highest compared with those ratios of that using the other **four** methods: dipole fitting, LCMV, DICS, and mLCMV. The analysis of variance (ANOVA) was used to further compare the mean difference of the **five** groups of localization results. **Figure 7** shows significance test of mean difference of the **five** groups using ANOVA. The localization results for the mLCMV method were better than those for dipole fitting, DCIS, and LCMV, and the difference in source localization between dipole fitting and DICS was not obvious. The localization results using the proposed method in these patients are more consistent with the clinical evaluation. The proposed method may provide a new imaging marker for localization of epileptogenic zones.

DISCUSSION AND CONCLUSIONS

MEG is a non-invasive type of preoperative examination and therefore plays an indispensable role in the localization of epileptogenic foci in epilepsy patients. Because the locations of epileptogenic zones estimated using the current localization methods are not always accurate, MEG examination results are sometimes questioned by clinical epileptologists (Englot et al., 2015). A number of source imaging algorithms for MEG recordings have been proposed and successfully applied for several purposes, such as localization of epileptic foci (Bast et al.,

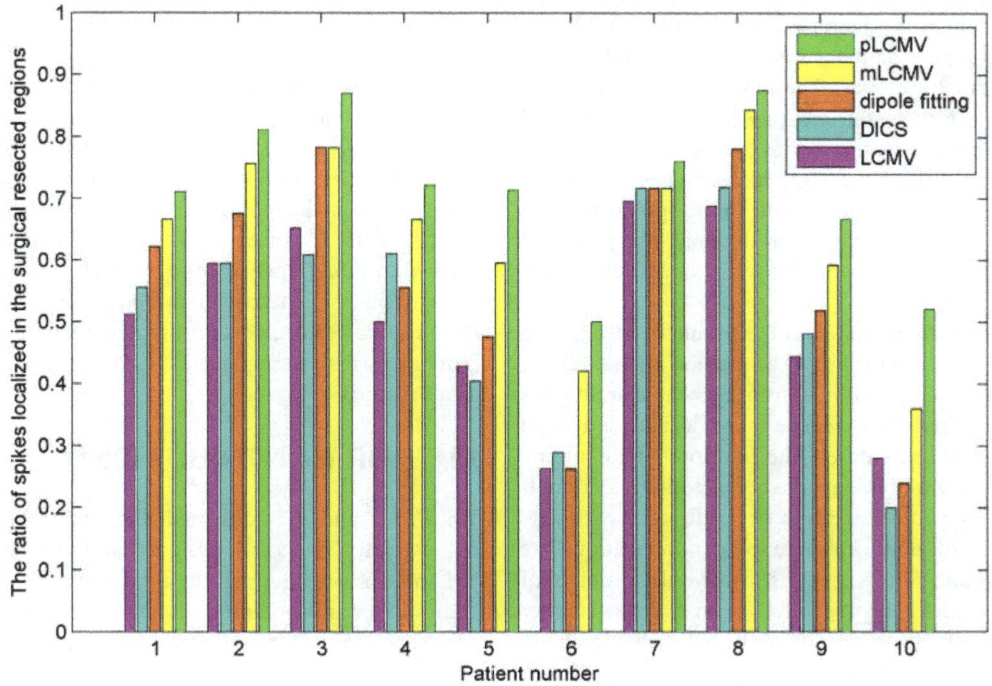

FIGURE 6 | Comparison of localization results obtained for patients with TLE using the proposed method (pLCMV) to those obtained using dipole fitting, LCMV, DICS, and mLCMV methods. The x-axis represents the patient number, and the y-axes represent the ratios of the number of spikes localized in the surgical resected region to the total number of spikes.

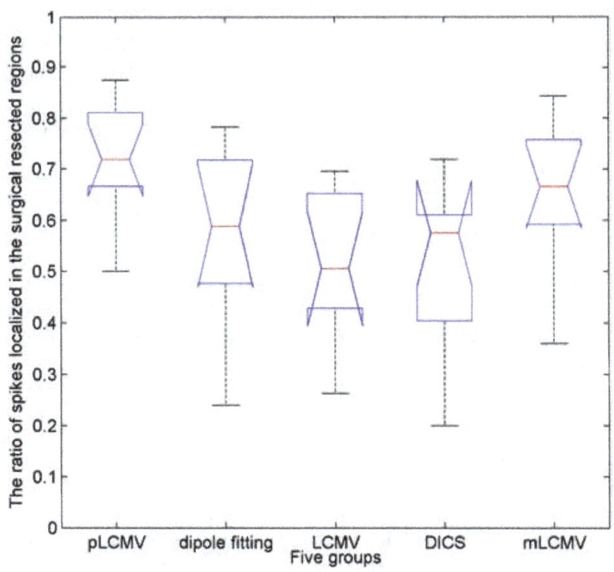

FIGURE 7 | Significance test of mean difference of the five groups of localization results using analysis of variance (ANOVA). The x-axis represents the five groups, and the y-axes represent the ratios of the number of spikes localized in the surgical resected region to the total number of spikes.

2004; Sutherling et al., 2008; Englot et al., 2015). In this work, PLS analysis was used in combination with minimum variance beamforming to reconstruct sensor arrays and locate sources. As is widely known, beamforming techniques play an important role in source imaging. LCMV is a typical representative of time domain beamforming, and DICS is a representative of frequency domain beamforming. These two methods have achieved effective localization results and have been successfully applied in many fields (Hoogenboom et al., 2006; Van Essen et al., 2013). The most recent literature shows that a modified LCMV (mLCMV) source imaging algorithm has been proposed, and has achieved good spatial accuracy in deep source imaging (Hu et al., 2017). Therefore, to test the effectiveness of the proposed algorithm (pLCMV), we compared it to LCMV, DICS, and mLCMV. The single-shell approximation technique was used as a forward method to construct a volume conduction model in this study. A proper head volume conductor in the forward method is helpful to improve the spatial accuracy of source imaging. Many improved forward models have been proposed for accurate source analysis and connectivity measures (Vorwerk et al., 2014; Neugebauer et al., 2017). Taking into account the cerebrospinal fluid and distinguishing between gray and white matter are effective in head volume conductor modeling. The improved forward models should be combined with the proposed method in future study, and may significantly improve the spatial accuracy of source imaging.

In conclusion, we designed a new method that combines partial least squares analysis of MEG arrays with minimum variance beamforming to localize brain activity in simulated data and epilepsy data. Compared to that obtained using DICS, LCMV, and mLCMV, the spatial accuracy obtained using the proposed method (pLCMV) was highest, and the location error fluctuated little with increases in noise. For simulations generated using a sinc function plus Gaussian noise, the proposed method had the highest spatial accuracy. The spatial accuracies on the localization results using the four methods became lower as SNR value became smaller. We further verified the proposed method in a real dataset that includes the MEG recordings of 10 patients with TLE. The localization results using the proposed method are more consistent with the clinical evaluation. The proposed method may provide a new imaging marker for localization of epileptogenic zones.

We do not hypothesize that the sources should be localized in only one brain area, because the proposed method is to search for the epileptogenic zones or the sources from the whole brain. This study focuses on the discussion of single source localization based on simulated data and real dataset. The position corresponding to the maximum strength is assumed to be the source location. If we choose the top 5 or 10% maximum strength, we may be able to solve the situation of multiple source spikes or activation. The application background of this study is to solve the problem of MEG localization of the epileptogenic zone in epilepsy surgery candidates. Usually, a large proportion of those patients (epilepsy surgery candidates) have single source (Englot et al., 2015; Nissen et al., 2016). At present, most epileptic experts believe that only one source is localized from a spike with MEG recordings (Englot et al., 2015). In addition, multiple sources can also be localized by single source localization for epileptic patients with multiple lesions. Therefore, the proposed method does not highlight the assumption of single source localization in this study. We will continue to study the multiple sources localization in future research.

Limitations

In order to implement the PLS method, the array of sensors was divided into eight classes according to the standard brain regions provided by Elekta Neuromag MEG in this study. The $\boldsymbol{Y}$ matrix is then generated according to these classes. In fact, it is not necessary to divide all sensors into 8 classes. It is possible that 4, 12, or even 16 classes could be used to localize the sources using the PLS method. In future work, we can examine the effect of different class numbers on the spatial accuracy of source imaging. Since adjacent sensors may be divided into two different classes, this may be a challenge for PLS method to extract the components of MEG data. In future work, the proposed method should be verified in more types of epilepsy, such as frontal lobe epilepsy, insular epilepsy, and occipital lobe epilepsy. We also hope that the effective performance of the new method can be verified in more realistic scenarios, such as locating brain tumor lesions and locating functional areas.

AUTHOR CONTRIBUTIONS

YH, YW, and JZ: designed the research; YH: wrote the manuscript; YH and JZ: designed and implemented algorithm; YH and CY: prepared figures and tables; CY and YW: collected clinical data and preliminarily analyzed the MEG data; JZ and YW: supervised study and revised the manuscript.

FUNDING

This work was supported by the National Key Research and Development Program of China (Grant Number: 2016YFF0201002), the Natural Science Foundation of China (Grant Numbers: 61301005, 61572055), the project of the Brain Functional Disease and Neuromodulation of Beijing Key Laboratory, Hefei Innovation Research Institute, Beihang University, Project of The Thousand Talents Plan for Young Professionals, and The Thousand Talents Plan Workstation between Beihang University and Jiangsu Yuwell Medical Equipment and Supply Co. Ltd.

REFERENCES

Baek, J., and Kim, M. (2004). Face recognition using partial least squares components. *Pattern Recog.* 37, 1303–1306. doi: 10.1016/j.patcog.2003.10.014

Baillet, S. (2017). Magnetoencephalography for brain electrophysiology and imaging. *Nat. Neurosci.* 20, 327–339. doi: 10.1038/nn.4504

Barnes, G. R., and Hillebrand, A. (2003). Statistical flattening of MEG beamformer images. *Hum. Brain Mapp.* 18, 1–12. doi: 10.1002/hbm.10072

Bast, T., Oezkan, O., Rona, S., Stippich, C., Seitz, A., Rupp, A., et al. (2004). EEG and MEG source analysis of single and averaged interictal spikes reveals intrinsic epileptogenicity in focal cortical dysplasia. *Epilepsia* 45, 621–631. doi: 10.1111/j.0013-9580.2004.56503.x

Boulesteix, A. L., and Strimmer, K. (2006). Partial least squares: a versatile tool for the analysis of high-dimensional genomic data. *Brief. Bioinform.* 8, 32–44. doi: 10.1093/bib/bbl016

Brookes, M. J., Stevenson, C. M., Barnes, G. R., Hillebrand, A., Simpson, M. I., Francis, S.T., et al. (2007). Beamformer reconstruction of correlated sources using a modified source model. *Neuroimage* 34, 1454–1465. doi: 10.1016/j.neuroimage.2006.11.012

Cheung, M. J., Kovačević, N., Fatima, Z., Mišić, B., and McIntosh, A. R. (2016). [MEG] PLS: a pipeline for MEG data analysis and partial least squares statistics. *Neuroimage* 124, 181–193. doi: 10.1016/j.neuroimage.2015.08.045

Diwakar, M., Huang, M. X., Srinivasan, R., Harrington, D. L., Robb, A., Angeles, A., et al. (2011). Dual-core beamformer for obtaining highly correlated neuronal networks in MEG. *Neuroimage* 54, 253–263. doi: 10.1016/j.neuroimage.2010.07.023

Englot, D. J., Nagarajan, S. S., Imber, B. S., Raygor, K. P., Honma, S. M., Mizuiri, D., et al. (2015). Epileptogenic zone localization using magnetoencephalography predicts seizure freedom in epilepsy surgery. *Epilepsia* 56, 949–958. doi: 10.1111/epi.13002

Geladi, P., and Kowalski, B.R. (1986). Partial least-squares regression: a tutorial. *Anal. Chim. Acta* 185, 1–17. doi: 10.1016/0003-2670(86)80028-9

Grech, R., Cassar, T., Muscat, J., Camilleri, K. P., Fabri, S. G., Zervakis, M., et al. (2008). Review on solving the inverse problem in EEG source analysis. *J. Neuroeng. Rehabil.* 5:25. doi: 10.1186/1743-0003-5-25

Groß, J., and Ioannides, A. (1999). Linear transformations of data space in MEG. *Phys. Med. Biol.* 44, 2081–2097.

Groß, J., Kujala, J., Hämäläinen, M., Timmermann, L., Schnitzler, A., and Salmelin, R. (2001). Dynamic imaging of coherent sources: studying neural interactions in the human brain. *Proc. Natl. Acad. Sci. U.S.A.* 98, 694–699. doi: 10.1073/pnas.98.2.694

Hadamard, J., and Morse, P. M. (1953). Lectures on Cauchy's problem in linear partial differential equations. *Phys. Today* 6:18. doi: 10.1063/1.3061337

Hämäläinen, M., Hari, R., Ilmoniemi, R. J., Knuutila, J., and Lounasmaa, O.V. (1993). Magnetoencephalography—theory, instrumentation, and applications to noninvasive studies of the working human brain. *Rev. Mod. Phys.* 65, 413–460. doi: 10.1103/RevModPhys.65.413

Hoogenboom, N., Schoffelen, J. M., Oostenveld, R., Parkes, L. M., and Fries, P. (2006). Localizing human visual gamma-band activity in frequency, time and space. *Neuroimage* 29, 764–773. doi: 10.1016/j.neuroimage.2005.08.043

Hu, Y., Lin, Y., Yang, B., Tang, G., Liu, T., Wang, Y., et al. (2017). Deep source localization with magnetoencephalography based on sensor array decomposition and beamforming. *Sensors* 17:E1860. doi: 10.3390/s17081860

Hu, Y. G., Ren, C. X., Yao, Y. F., and Li, W. Y. (2012). "Face recognition using nonlinear partial least squares in reproducing kernel hilbert space", in *Chinese Conference on Pattern Recognition* (Beijing: Springer), 316–323.

Krishnan, A., Williams, L. J., McIntosh, A. R., and Abdi, H. (2011). Partial Least Squares (PLS) methods for neuroimaging: a tutorial and review. *Neuroimage* 56, 455–475. doi: 10.1016/j.neuroimage.2010.07.034

Lewi, P. J. (1995). Pattern recognition, reflections from a chemometric point of view. *Chemometr. Intell. Lab. Sys.* 28, 23–33. doi: 10.1016/0169-7439(95)80037-A

Litvak, V., Mattout, J., Kiebel, S., Phillips, C., Henson, R., Kilner, J., et al. (2011). EEG and MEG data analysis in SPM8. *Comput. Intell. Neurosci.* 2011:852961. doi: 10.1155/2011/852961

Mäkelä, N., Stenroos, M., Sarvas, J., and Ilmoniemi, R.J. (2018). Truncated RAP-MUSIC (TRAP-MUSIC) for MEG and EEG source localization. *Neuroimage* 167, 73–83. doi: 10.1016/j.neuroimage.2017.11.013

Mattout, J., Phillips, C., Penny, W. D., Rugg, M. D., and Friston, K. J. (2006). MEG source localization under multiple constraints: an extended Bayesian framework. *Neuroimage* 30, 753–767. doi: 10.1016/j.neuroimage.2005.10.037

McIntosh, A. R., and Lobaugh, N. J. (2004). Partial least squares analysis of neuroimaging data: applications and advances. *Neuroimage* 23, S250–S263. doi: 10.1016/j.neuroimage.2004.05.018

Neugebauer, F., Möddel, G., Rampp, S., Burger, M., and Wolters, C. H. (2017). The effect of head model simplification on beamformer source localization. *Front. Neurosci.* 11:625. doi: 10.3389/fnins.2017.00625

Nissen, I., Stam, C., Citroen, J., Reijneveld, J., and Hillebrand, A. (2016). Preoperative evaluation using magnetoencephalography: experience in 382 epilepsy patients. *Epilepsy Res.* 124, 23–33. doi: 10.1016/j.eplepsyres.2016.05.002

Nolte, G. (2003). The magnetic lead field theorem in the quasi-static approximation and its use for magnetoencephalography forward calculation in realistic volume conductors. *Phys. Med. Biol.* 48, 3637–3652. doi: 10.1088/0031-9155/48/22/002

Oostenveld, R., Fries, P., Maris, E., and Schoffelen, J. M. (2011). FieldTrip: open source software for advanced analysis of MEG, EEG, and invasive electrophysiological data. *Comput. Intell. Neurosci.* 2011:156869. doi: 10.1155/2011/156869

Oshino, S., Kato, A., Wakayama, A., Taniguchi, M., Hirata, M., and Yoshimine, T. (2007). Magnetoencephalographic analysis of cortical oscillatory activity in patients with brain tumors: synthetic aperture magnetometry (SAM) functional imaging of delta band activity. *Neuroimage* 34, 957–964. doi: 10.1016/j.neuroimage.2006.08.054

Pascual-Marqui, R. D., Michel, C. M., and Lehmann, D. (1994). Low resolution electromagnetic tomography: a new method for localizing electrical activity in the brain. *Int. J. Psychophysiol.* 18, 49–65. doi: 10.1016/0167-8760(84)90014-X

Rosipal, R., and Trejo, L. J. (2001). Kernel partial least squares regression in reproducing kernel hilbert space. *J. Mach. Learn. Res.* 2, 97–123. doi: 10.1162/15324430260185556

Schaller, K., and Cabrilo, I. (2016). Anterior temporal lobectomy. *Acta Neurochir.* 158, 161–166. doi: 10.1007/s00701-015-2640-0

Sekihara, K., Nagarajan, S. S., Poeppel, D., and Marantz, A. (2002a). Performance of an MEG adaptive-beamformer technique in the presence of correlated neural activities: effects on signal intensity and time-course estimates. *IEEE Trans. Biomed. Eng.* 49, 1534–1546. doi: 10.1109/TBME.2002.805485

Sekihara, K., Nagarajan, S. S., Poeppel, D., Marantz, A., and Miyashita, Y. (2002b). Application of an MEG eigenspace beamformer to reconstructing spatio-temporal activities of neural sources. *Hum. Brain Mapp.* 15, 199–215. doi: 10.1002/hbm.10019

Sharma, A., and Jacobs, D. W. (2011). "Bypassing synthesis: PLS for face recognition with pose, low-resolution and sketch," in 2011 *IEEE Conference on Computer Vision and Pattern Recognition (CVPR)*(Colorado Springs, CO: IEEE), 593-600.

Sutherling, W., Mamelak, A., Thyerlei, D., Maleeva, T., Minazad, Y., Philpott, L., et al. (2008). Influence of magnetic source imaging for planning intracranial EEG in epilepsy. *Neurology* 71, 990–996. doi: 10.1212/01.wnl.0000326591.29858.1a

Van Essen, D. C., Smith, S. M., Barch, D. M., Behrens, T. E., Yacoub, E., Ugurbil, K., et al. (2013). The WU-Minn human connectome project: an overview. *Neuroimage* 80, 62–79. doi: 10.1016/j.neuroimage.2013.05.041

Van Veen, B. D., Van Drongelen, W., Yuchtman, M., and Suzuki, A. (1997). Localization of brain electrical activity via linearly constrained minimum variance spatial filtering. *IEEE Trans. Biomed. Eng.* 44, 867–880. doi: 10.1109/10.623056

Vorwerk, J., Cho, J. H., Rampp, S., Hamer, H., Knösche, T. R., and Wolters, C. H. (2014). A guideline for head volume conductor modeling in EEG and MEG. *Neuroimage* 100, 590–607. doi: 10.1016/j.neuroimage.2014.06.040

Wennberg, R., and Cheyne, D. (2014). Reliability of MEG source imaging of anterior temporal spikes: analysis of an intracranially characterized spike focus. *Clin. Neurophysiol.* 125, 903–918. doi: 10.1016/j.clinph.2013.08.032

Wold, S., Ruhe, A., Wold, H., and Dunn, W. J. (1984). The collinearity problem in linear regression. the partial least squares (PLS) approach to generalized inverses. SIAM. *J. Sci. Stat. Comp.* 5, 735–743.

Wold, S., Sjöström, M., and Eriksson, L. (2001). PLS-regression: a basic tool of chemometrics. *Chemometr. Intell. Lab. Sys.* 58, 109–130. doi: 10.1016/S0169-7439(01)00155-1

Zhang, J., and Liu, C. (2015). On linearly constrained minimum variance beamforming. *J. Mach. Learn. Res.* 16, 2099–2145. Available Online at: http://www.jmlr.org/papers/volume16/zhang15b/zhang15b.pdf

Zumer, J., Attias, H., Sekihara, K., and Nagarajan, S. (2007). A probabilistic algorithm integrating source localization and noise suppression for MEG and EEG data. *Neuroimage* 37:102. doi: 10.1016/j.neuroimage.2007.04.054

2

Structural and Functional Brain Connectivity Changes Between People with Abdominal and Non-Abdominal Obesity and their Association with Behaviors of Eating Disorders

Bo-yong Park[1,2], Mi Ji Lee[3], Mansu Kim[1,2], Se-Hong Kim[4] and Hyunjin Park[2,5]*

[1] Department of Electrical and Computer Engineering, Sungkyunkwan University, Suwon, South Korea, [2] Center for Neuroscience Imaging Research, Institute for Basic Science, Suwon, South Korea, [3] Departments of Neurology, Samsung Medical Center, Sungkyunkwan University School of Medicine, Seoul, South Korea, [4] Department of Family Medicine, St. Vincent's Hospital, Catholic University College of Medicine, Suwon, South Korea, [5] School of Electronic and Electrical Engineering, Sungkyunkwan University, Suwon, South Korea

***Correspondence:**
Hyunjin Park
hyunjinp@skku.edu

Abdominal obesity is important for understanding obesity, which is a worldwide medical problem. We explored structural and functional brain differences in people with abdominal and non-abdominal obesity by using multimodal neuroimaging and up-to-date analysis methods. A total of 274 overweight people, whose body mass index exceeded 25, were enrolled in this study. Participants were divided into abdominal and non-abdominal obesity groups using a waist–hip ratio threshold of 0.9 for males and 0.85 for females. Structural and functional brain differences were assessed with diffusion tensor imaging and resting-state functional magnetic resonance imaging. Centrality measures were computed from structural fiber tractography, and static and dynamic functional connectivity matrices. Significant inter-group differences in structural and functional connectivity were found using degree centrality (DC) values. The associations between the DC values of the identified regions/networks and behaviors of eating disorder scores were explored. The highest association was achieved by combining DC values of the cerebral peduncle, anterior corona radiata, posterior corona radiata (from structural connectivity), frontoparietal network (from static connectivity), and executive control network (from dynamic connectivity) compared to the use of structural or functional connectivity only. Our results demonstrated the effectiveness of multimodal imaging data and found brain regions or networks that may be responsible for behaviors of eating disorders in people with abdominal obesity.

Keywords: abdominal obesity, multimodal imaging analysis, probabilistic fiber tractography, static and dynamic connectivity analysis, eating disorder behaviors

INTRODUCTION

Obesity is a worldwide medical problem that is responsible for inducing insulin resistance, type 2 diabetes, cardiovascular diseases, and some cancers (Raji et al., 2010; Malik et al., 2013; Val-Laillet et al., 2015). However, medical complications are not always manifested in people with obesity. A recent study showed that abdominal obesity was associated with increased risk for cardiovascular disease and mortality, while non-abdominal obesity had fewer adverse effects overall, and in some instances it even elicited protective effects (Zhang et al., 2008). In this context, the concept of metabolically healthy obesity has been extensively accepted (Stefan et al., 2013). In addition, previous studies suggested that abdominal obesity differs from non-abdominal obesity (Folsom et al., 1993, 2000; Bujalska et al., 1997; Després and Lemieux, 2006; Després et al., 2008). People with abdominal obesity have been shown to be at a higher risk for the metabolic syndrome, which is linked to diabetes and cardiovascular disease (Folsom et al., 2000; Després and Lemieux, 2006; Després et al., 2008). Folsom et al. (1993, 2000) found that abdominal obesity was a better biomarker for predicting mortality than non-abdominal obesity, and Bujalska et al. (1997) demonstrated that the risk of diabetes was better quantified with the waist-hip ratio (WHR), a measure of abdominal obesity, than with the body mass index (BMI), a measure of general obesity. These studies collectively provided a rationale for distinguishing abdominal obesity from non-abdominal obesity. Thus, identifying differences between abdominal and non-abdominal obesity may provide additional information for the better understanding of the diverse characteristics of obesity.

Obesity is a heterogeneous disease with a multifactorial etiology, including the eating behavior, and genetic and other environmental factors (Brownell and Wadden, 1991; McLaughlin, 2012). Binge eating behavior is believed to be genetically determined and is an important factor in obesity (Bulik et al., 2003; Carnell et al., 2011). However, only few prior studies have reported an association between dietary patterns and abdominal obesity (Azadbakht and Esmaillzadeh, 2011; Zhang et al., 2015). Correspondingly, the elucidation of the mechanisms based on which adverse eating behaviors may differentially affect the brain of the people with abdominal and non-abdominal obesity is largely unknown, and thus constitutes one of the aims of this study.

Recent studies reported that abdominal obesity is linked to altered reward and cognitive systems (Hollmann et al., 2012; Yates et al., 2012; Yau et al., 2012; Val-Laillet et al., 2015; Gaudio et al., 2017; Olivo et al., 2017), which regulate the appetite response (Hollmann et al., 2012; Val-Laillet et al., 2015). It has been shown that the altered reward and cognitive processes are highly associated with errant eating behaviors (Hollmann et al., 2012; Yates et al., 2012; Yau et al., 2012; Val-Laillet et al., 2015). In addition to brain function alterations, structural abnormalities were identified in people with abdominal obesity, such as altered fractional anisotropy and volume changes in white matter (Jagust et al., 2005; Gaudio et al., 2017; Olivo et al., 2017). These studies collectively suggest that abdominal obesity is possibly related to both brain structure and function. They also motivated us to consider multimodal neuroimaging to explore the differences between people with abdominal and non-abdominal obesity.

Many neuroimaging studies have used connectivity analysis to quantify brain structure and function (Bullmore and Sporns, 2009; Rubinov and Sporns, 2010). Connectivity analysis measures the connectedness among brain regions or networks. In this study, we performed connectivity analysis based on graph theory that requires graph nodes (i.e., brain regions or networks) and edges (i.e., neuronal fibers or correlation of time series data between nodes) based on many approaches (Bullmore and Sporns, 2009; Rubinov and Sporns, 2010). Connectivity analysis assesses the entire brain as a complex interconnected network, and many studies have successfully used connectivity analysis to explore Alzheimer's disease, attention deficit/hyperactivity disorders, and schizophrenia (Seo et al., 2013; Damaraju et al., 2014; Park et al., 2016a).

Recently, neuroimaging methods, including magnetic resonance imaging (MRI) and positron emission tomography, have been used to non-invasively link obesity with brain structure and function (Tataranni et al., 1999; Jagust et al., 2005; Hollmann et al., 2012; Lips et al., 2014; Val-Laillet et al., 2015). However, almost all of the neuroimaging studies compared people with obesity to those with healthy weights (Jagust et al., 2005; Hollmann et al., 2012; Val-Laillet et al., 2015). Studies exploring the brain structure and function of people with abdominal and non-abdominal obesity are lacking, even though the two groups may have distinct brain structures and functions. To fill this gap, we aimed to compare structural and functional brain connectivity between abdominal and non-abdominal obesity groups by applying network analysis using diffusion tensor imaging (DTI) and resting-state functional MRI (rs-fMRI). Motivated by the recent findings of functional network changes and their associations with eating behaviors in people with obesity (Park et al., 2016b), we aimed to associate identified neuroimaging findings of abdominal obesity with eating behaviors.

MATERIALS AND METHODS

Imaging Data and Participants

T1-weighted structural data, DTI, and rs-fMRI data were obtained from the openly accessible Nathan Kline Institute-Rockland Sample (NKI-RS) database (Nooner et al., 2012). All imaging data were scanned with a 3T Siemens Magnetom Trio Tim scanner. The scanning parameters for the T1-weighted structural data acquisitions were as follows: repetition time (TR) = 1,900 ms, echo time (TE) = 2.52 ms, flip angle = 9°, field-of-view (FOV) = 250 mm × 250 mm, 1 mm^3 voxel resolution, and 176 slices. The DTI parameters were as follows: TR = 2,400 ms, TE = 85 ms, flip angle = 90°, FOV = 212 mm × 180 mm, 2 mm^3 voxel resolution, 64 slices, b-value = 1,500 s/mm^2, and gradient = 137. The rs-fMRI parameters were as follows: TR = 645 ms, TE = 30 ms, flip angle = 60°, FOV = 222 mm × 222 mm, 3 mm^3 voxel resolution, 40 slices, and 900 volumes. Of the 650 total participants, participants with a BMI of 25 or greater and those with full demographic information and eating disorder examination questionnaire (EDE-Q) scores were considered in this study. Participants with severe head motion were excluded (see the Section "Preprocessing of Rs-fMRI Data"). The selected 274 participants were divided into abdominal and non-abdominal obesity groups based on WHR. Participants with a WHR larger than 0.9 for males and 0.85 for females were classified in the abdominal obesity group, and the remaining participants were classified in the non-abdominal obesity group (World Health Organization, 2008). Detailed demographics are reported in **Table 1**. The Institutional Review Board (IRB) of Sungkyunkwan University approved this retrospective study. Our study was performed in full accordance with local IRB guidelines and informed consent was obtained from all participants.

Tractography and Connectivity Analysis of DTI Data

Probabilistic tractography of DTI data was performed using the FSL software (Jenkinson et al., 2012). The original DTI data were corrected for distortions due to eddy currents and head motion. DTI data were reconstructed based on the corresponding gradient table using the FDT toolbox. The diffusion parameters were computed with the Bedpostx toolbox, and probabilistic tractography was performed with the ProbtrackX toolbox in FSL (Jenkinson et al., 2012). Specifically, fibers were repeatedly sampled 5,000 times based on diffusion parameters that originated from the seed region and a probabilistic distribution of neuronal fibers was constructed. The probability of fibers connecting two brain regions was computed based on a probabilistic distribution of neuronal fibers, and the value was entered into a matrix called the fiber probability matrix. The nodes of the fiber probability matrix (i.e., brain regions) were defined by the ICBM DTI-81 atlas. A weighted and directed network model was applied to the fiber probability matrix and degree centrality (DC) values were computed. DC values were defined in a directed network model as the sum of in-degree and out-degree values that, respectively, included the column and row sums of the edge weights connected to the given node in the matrix (Rubinov and Sporns, 2010). DC values represent the importance of the node (Bullmore and Sporns, 2009; Rubinov and Sporns, 2010). DC values were used to identify brain regions that differed significantly between people with abdominal and non-abdominal obesity. The group differences in DC values between people with abdominal and non-abdominal obesity were assessed using permutation tests followed by false discovery rate (FDR) procedure to avoid multiple comparisons issues (Benjamini and Hochberg, 1995; Chen et al., 2013; Smith et al., 2013). We randomly assigned participants to either the abdominal or non-abdominal obesity group 5,000 times and created a null distribution of differences in DC values. If the differences in DC values of a region did not belong to the 95% of the null distribution, the region was considered significant. The p-values were further corrected using FDR ($p < 0.05$, corrected) (Benjamini and Hochberg, 1995). The overall processing flow of the DTI data is represented in the DTI part of **Figure 1**.

TABLE 1 | Participant demographics.

Parameter		Abdominal obesity (n = 152)	Non-abdominal obesity (n = 122)	P-value
Age		54.94 (17.23)	40.84 (19.09)	<0.001
Sex (Male:Female)		69:83	47:75	0.2527*
BMI		31.37 (5.01)	29.84 (4.40)	0.0086
WHR	Male	0.98 (0.06)	0.84 (0.04)	<0.001
	Female	0.91 (0.05)	0.79 (0.05)	<0.001
EDE-Q-R		1.44 (1.40)	1.67 (1.56)	0.2053
EDE-Q-E		0.35 (0.69)	0.46 (0.86)	0.2495
EDE-Q-S		1.85 (1.41)	1.87 (1.50)	0.8925
EDE-Q-W		1.54 (1.19)	1.58 (1.31)	0.7843

**Chi-square test. BMI, body mass index; WHR, waist–hip ratio; EDE-Q-R, eating disorder examination questionnaire restraint; EDE-Q-E, eating disorder examination questionnaire eating concern; EDE-Q-S, eating disorder examination questionnaire shape concern; EDE-Q-W, eating disorder examination questionnaire weight concern.*

Preprocessing of Rs-fMRI Data

Rs-fMRI data were preprocessed using the AFNI and FSL software (Cox, 1996; Jenkinson et al., 2012). The volumes of the first 10 s were discarded to adjust for the hemodynamic response delay. The frame-wise displacement (FD) between fMRI time series volumes was calculated and the volumes whose FDs exceeded 0.5 mm were eliminated (Power et al., 2012). We excluded participants who had more than 10% of the time series volumes removed. Volumes were adjusted for head motion and slice timing. The skull was removed, and the intensity was normalized with the mean value of 10,000 across 4D volumes. Rs-fMRI data were registered onto the T1-weighted structural data, followed by a subsequent registration onto the Montreal Neurological Institute (MNI) brain template. From the registered rs-fMRI data, nuisance variables of cerebrospinal fluid, white matter, head motion, cardiac, and large-vein-related artifacts were removed using the FMRIB's ICA-based X-noiseifier (FIX) software (Salimi-Khorshidi et al., 2014). The first step of ICA-FIX performed a single independent component analysis (ICA) on an individual rs-fMRI data. From the decomposed independent components (ICs), a large number of temporal and spatial features were calculated. The calculated features were then input into a multilevel classifier, and signal and noise ICs were distinguished using the pretrained data by the Human Connectome Project (Salimi-Khorshidi et al., 2014). The noise ICs were regressed out from the rs-fMRI time series. A bandpass filter with a frequency between 0.009 and 0.08 and spatial smoothing with a full-width-at-half-maximum of 6 mm were applied.

Group ICA

The rs-fMRI data from all participants were temporally concatenated, and group ICA was performed using the FSL MELODIC software (Beckmann et al., 2005; Jenkinson et al., 2012). The ICA produces spatial ICs by using probabilistic principal component analysis (Beckmann and Smith, 2004; Beckmann et al., 2005; Minka, 2000; Smith et al., 2012). The generated ICs were classified into signal or noise components according to two criteria. First, the ICs were compared with known resting state networks (RSNs) by using a cross-correlation, and those lower than 0.2 were considered as noise (Smith et al., 2009). Second, signal and noise components were classified by visual inspection considering the spatial and temporal characteristics (Kelly et al., 2010; Griffanti et al., 2017). Signal components showed a large spatial overlap with gray matter and a low overlap with white matter, cerebrospinal fluid, and blood

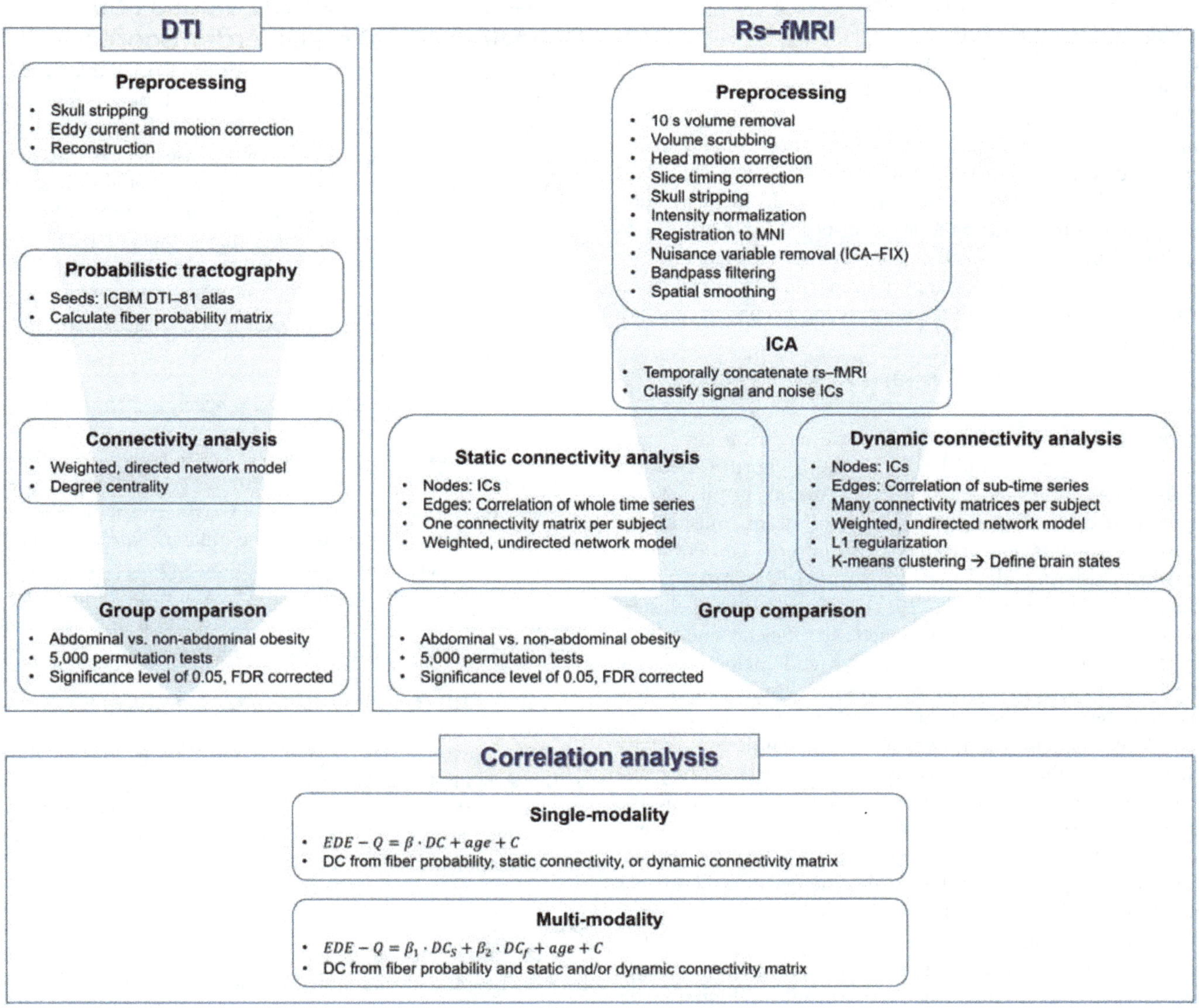

FIGURE 1 | Flowchart of processing steps adopted in this analysis.

vessels. The time series of the signal components was a regular wave without notable spikes, and had a power spectrum of at least one low-frequency peak between 0.01 and 0.1 Hz (Kelly et al., 2010; Griffanti et al., 2017).

Static and Dynamic Connectivity Analyses of fMRI Data

The static and dynamic connectivity analyses with weighted and undirected network models were performed to quantify the functional characteristics of rs-fMRI. Graph nodes were defined as functionally interpretable ICs, and graph edges were defined as the Pearson correlation of time series between two nodes. For the static connectivity analysis, a connectivity matrix was constructed by computing the Pearson correlation of the entire time series between nodes, which yielded one connectivity matrix for each participant. A soft thresholding approach was adopted to avoid binarizing edge weights with the use of Equation 1.

$$w_{ij} = \left(\frac{r_{ij} + 1}{2}\right)^{\beta} \quad (1)$$

where r_{ij} is the correlation coefficient between nodes i and j (Mumford et al., 2010; Schwarz and McGonigle, 2011). β was set to six to conform to an unsigned network (Mumford et al., 2010). The elements of the soft thresholded matrix were converted to z-values using the Fisher's r-to-z transformation. DC values were extracted from the z-transformed matrix by summing the edge weights connected to the given node in the column direction of the matrix and were then used to compare groups. The differences in DC values between people with abdominal and non-abdominal obesity were assessed based on 5,000 permutations, and the p-values were corrected using FDR ($p < 0.05$, corrected).

The dynamic connectivity analysis used a sliding window technique (Allen et al., 2012; Damaraju et al., 2014). A window size of 172 TRs (111 s) and a stride of 1 TR (0.645 s) were used to capture the lowest frequency (0.009 Hz) of the data (Hutchison et al., 2013; Damaraju et al., 2014). A rectangular window was convolved with a Gaussian kernel of size three. Finally, many dynamic connectivity matrices (mean of 770.45 and a standard deviation [SD] of 26.14) were constructed. L1 regularization was applied to the matrices to avoid ill-posed problems due to the limited information on the short time series segments. The regularization parameter λ was optimized with a cross-validation framework by maximizing the following log-likelihood function (Equation 2).

$$\log \det\theta - tr(S\theta) - \lambda \,||\theta||_1 \quad (2)$$

where θ is the precision matrix, S is the empirical covariance matrix, tr is the trace, and $||.||_1$ is the L1 norm (Friedman et al., 2008; Allen et al., 2012; Damaraju et al., 2014). Regularized dynamic connectivity matrices were concatenated across participants and grouped into several clusters by a K-means clustering algorithm to define brain states (Allen et al., 2012; Damaraju et al., 2014). The number of clusters was determined using the silhouette coefficient and elbow method (Allen et al., 2012; Kodinariya and Makwana, 2013; Damaraju et al., 2014). The most common number of clusters was considered as the optimal number and was used for group-level clustering of the concatenated dynamic connectivity matrices. Using the determined number of clusters, participant-level states were defined by applying the K-means clustering algorithm for each participant. We started with the participant-level cluster that explained the largest variance, and we matched it with the group-level state that yielded the maximum Pearson's correlation (Park et al., 2018). We repeated the process for the subsequent participant-level cluster with the largest variance explained excluding the clusters that had already been processed. This allowed us to map each participant-level state with a corresponding group-level state. The dynamic connectivity matrices of each state were averaged, and DC values were extracted from the mean state matrices for each participant. The brain networks with significant differences in DC values between people with abdominal and non-abdominal obesity were assessed based on the 5,000 permutations followed by FDR at a significance level of 0.05. The overall rs-fMRI processing steps are summarized in the rs-fMRI part of **Figure 1**.

Representative Brain States

Group-level states were defined from the dynamic connectivity analysis, and each state was associated with brain networks by computing the hubness of nodes for each state. For each group-level state, the betweenness centrality (BC) values of all nodes were calculated and normalized by dividing them with the mean value. Nodes with normalized BC values higher than 1.5 were defined as hub nodes, and were considered as a representative network for the state (Seo et al., 2013).

Correlation Between DC Values and Behaviors of Eating Disorder Scores

DC values of the brain regions or networks that yielded significant group-wise differences in structural or functional connectivity between abdominal and non-abdominal obesity were correlated with behaviors of eating disorders assessed with the EDE-Q (Fairburn and Beglin, 1994; Mond et al., 2004). The EDE-Q assessment contained four subscales of restraint (EDE-Q-R), eating concern (EDE-Q-E), shape concern (EDE-Q-S), and weight concern (EDE-Q-W), which were based on the self-reported questionnaire (Fairburn and Beglin, 1994; Mond et al., 2004). A multiple linear regression model was constructed in accordance to Equation 3.

$$EDE{-}Q = \beta \cdot DC + age + C \quad (3)$$

where DC is the DC value of the brain region or network identified in the structural or functional connectivity analysis, β is the regression coefficient, and C is a constant. Age was added as a covariate to adjust for the difference between people with abdominal and non-abdominal obesity groups. A regression model was also constructed with DC values of brain regions and networks identified in both the structural and functional connectivity analyses in accordance to Equation 4.

$$EDE{-}Q = \beta_1 \cdot DC_s + \beta_2 \cdot DC_f + age + C \quad (4)$$

where DC_s denotes the DC values of the brain regions identified in the structural connectivity analysis, and DC_f indicates the DC values of the brain networks identified in the functional connectivity analysis. The correlation analysis is summarized in the correlation analysis part of **Figure 1**.

Statistics

The structural and functional group differences in DC values between people with abdominal and non-abdominal obesity were assessed using permutation tests followed by FDR. Participants were randomly assigned to the abdominal and non-abdominal obesity groups 5,000 times, and a null distribution was created. A brain region or network with DC values outside the 95% of the null distribution was considered to be associated with significant differences between the abdominal and non-abdominal obesity groups. The p-values were further corrected using the FDR approach suggested by Benjamini and Hochberg ($p < 0.05$, corrected) (Benjamini and Hochberg, 1995). The representative networks of group-level states in the dynamic connectivity analysis were defined using normalized BC values that were higher than 1.5. Correlation between DC values and EDE-Q scores were computed using a multiple linear regression model. The quality of the correlation was quantified using R^2 and p-values. The DC values of the identified brain regions or networks were correlated with four EDE-Q scores. The correlation results were corrected for the identified brain regions/networks, and for the four EDE-Q scores with FDR (Benjamini and Hochberg, 1995). All statistical analyses were performed in MATLAB (Mathworks Inc., Natick, MA, United States).

RESULTS

Nodes for Connectivity Analysis

The structural characteristics of the brain were quantified with a fiber probability matrix. The nodes of the fiber probability matrix were defined by the ICBM DTI-81 atlas (**Figure 2A**). Functional characteristics of the brain were quantified with rs-fMRI. Group ICA was performed to define brain networks. Twenty spatial ICs that explained 94.1% of the variance were automatically generated and four ICs were eliminated as noise components. The 16 functionally interpretable ICs (mean correlation with RSNs of $r = 0.48$, with an SD of 0.14) were considered to be graph nodes (**Figure 2A**). ICs 1–3 constitute the visual network (VN), ICs 4 and 5 constitute the default mode network (DMN), ICs 6–8 constitute the executive control network (ECN), ICs 9 and 10 constitute the frontoparietal network (FPN), ICs 11 and 12 constitute the sensorimotor network (SMN), ICs 13 and 14 constitute the auditory network (AN), IC 15 denotes the basal ganglia (BG) with part of the ECN, and IC 16 is the cerebellum.

Differences in Structural and Functional Connectivity

We compared the structural brain differences between people with abdominal and non-abdominal obesity using the probabilistic fiber tractography approach derived from DTI. DC values, which represent the importance of a given node, were calculated from the fiber probability matrix. DC values were used to identify significant differences between groups. The pontine crossing tract, fornix, corticospinal tract, medial lemniscus, inferior and superior cerebellar peduncles, cerebral peduncle, internal capsule, anterior, superior, and posterior corona radiata, thalamic radiation, sagittal stratum, superior longitudinal fasciculus, and superior fronto-occipital fasciculus, showed significant between group differences ($p < 0.05$, permutation followed by FDR correction) (**Supplementary Table S1**).

The inter-group differences in the static and dynamic connectivity analyses were performed by using the 16 ICs as the graph nodes. One connectivity matrix was constructed for each participant for the static connectivity analysis. DC values were computed from the connectivity matrix and VN (ICs #1–3), DMN (IC #5), ECN (IC #6), FPN (ICs #9 and 10), and SMN (ICs #11 and 12), yielded significant differences in DC values between people with abdominal and non-abdominal obesity groups (**Supplementary Table S2**, $p < 0.05$, permutation followed by FDR correction). For the dynamic connectivity analysis, many connectivity matrices (mean of 770.45 and SD of 26.14) were constructed, and the matrices were grouped into nine clusters (i.e., brain states) using a K-means clustering algorithm (**Figure 3**). For each group-level state, the hubness of any node was computed, and if the given node satisfied the hub node criterion, it was considered as a representative network for the state (Seo et al., 2013). The ECN (IC #8, normalized BC 1.51) in state 3, ECN (IC #7, normalized BC 1.57), and FPN (IC #10, normalized BC 1.56) in state 5, DMN (IC #5, normalized BC 1.77), FPN (IC #9, normalized BC 1.63), and SMN (IC #11, normalized BC 1.63) in state 6, two ECNs (ICs #6 and 8, normalized BCs 1.81 and 1.52, respectively), AN (IC #14, normalized BC 1.79), and cerebellum (IC #16, normalized BC 1.51) in state 7, DMN (IC #4, normalized BC 1.52), ECN (IC #6, normalized BC 1.57), SMN (IC #11, normalized BC 1.57), AN (IC #13, normalized BC 1.63), and cerebellum (IC #16, normalized BC 1.55) in state 8, and AN (IC #14, normalized BC 1.54) in state 9, were identified as the representative networks (**Figure 4**). The connectivity matrices were clustered and averaged to yield a mean state matrix for each brain state. DC values were extracted from the mean state matrices, and the groups were then compared. VN (IC #2), DMN (IC #5), ECN (IC #6), FPN (ICs #9 and 10), and SMN (ICs #11 and 12), showed significant ($p < 0.05$, permutation followed by FDR correction) inter-group differences in DC values, and the results for each state were reported in the **Supplementary Table S3**.

Correlation Between DC Values and Behaviors of Eating Disorder Scores

We calculated the correlation between the DC values of the identified brain regions from structural connectivity analysis or brain networks from the functional connectivity analysis and EDE-Q scores. The correlation between neuroimaging findings and the behaviors of eating disorders was explored as an eating disorder that was reported to be associated with abdominal obesity (Dallman et al., 2003; Gluck et al., 2004; Daubenmier et al., 2011; Succurro et al., 2015).

When only the estimated DC values from the structural connectivity analysis were used, the right cerebral peduncle, the right anterior, and posterior corona radiata were significantly correlated with EDE-Q scores (**Figure 2B** and **Table 2**, $p < 0.05$, FDR corrected). In the case of the static connectivity analysis, FPN (IC #9) yielded significant correlations with EDE-Q-S and W scores (**Figure 2B** and **Table 2**, $p < 0.05$, FDR corrected). In the case of the dynamic connectivity analysis, no networks showed significant correlation with EDE-Q scores at the significance level of 0.05. When we relaxed the significance level to 0.1, ECN (IC #8) in state 5 was correlated with the EDE-Q-S score (**Figure 2B** and **Table 2**, $p < 0.1$, FDR corrected).

We performed further correlation analysis that combined the DC values identified from the single-modal results. We considered various combinations of the following DC values: the right cerebral peduncle and right anterior and posterior corona radiata from structural connectivity analysis, FPN (IC #9) from the static functional connectivity analysis, and the ECN (IC #8) in state 5 from the dynamic functional connectivity analysis (**Table 3**). Our results showed that EDE-Q scores elicited the highest correlations with the DC values that combined the identified brain regions and networks from the structural connectivity, static functional connectivity, and dynamic functional connectivity analyses, followed by the structural connectivity and dynamic functional connectivity analyses, the structural connectivity and static functional connectivity analyses, structural connectivity analysis only, static and dynamic functional connectivity analyses, static functional connectivity analysis only, and the dynamic functional connectivity analysis only.

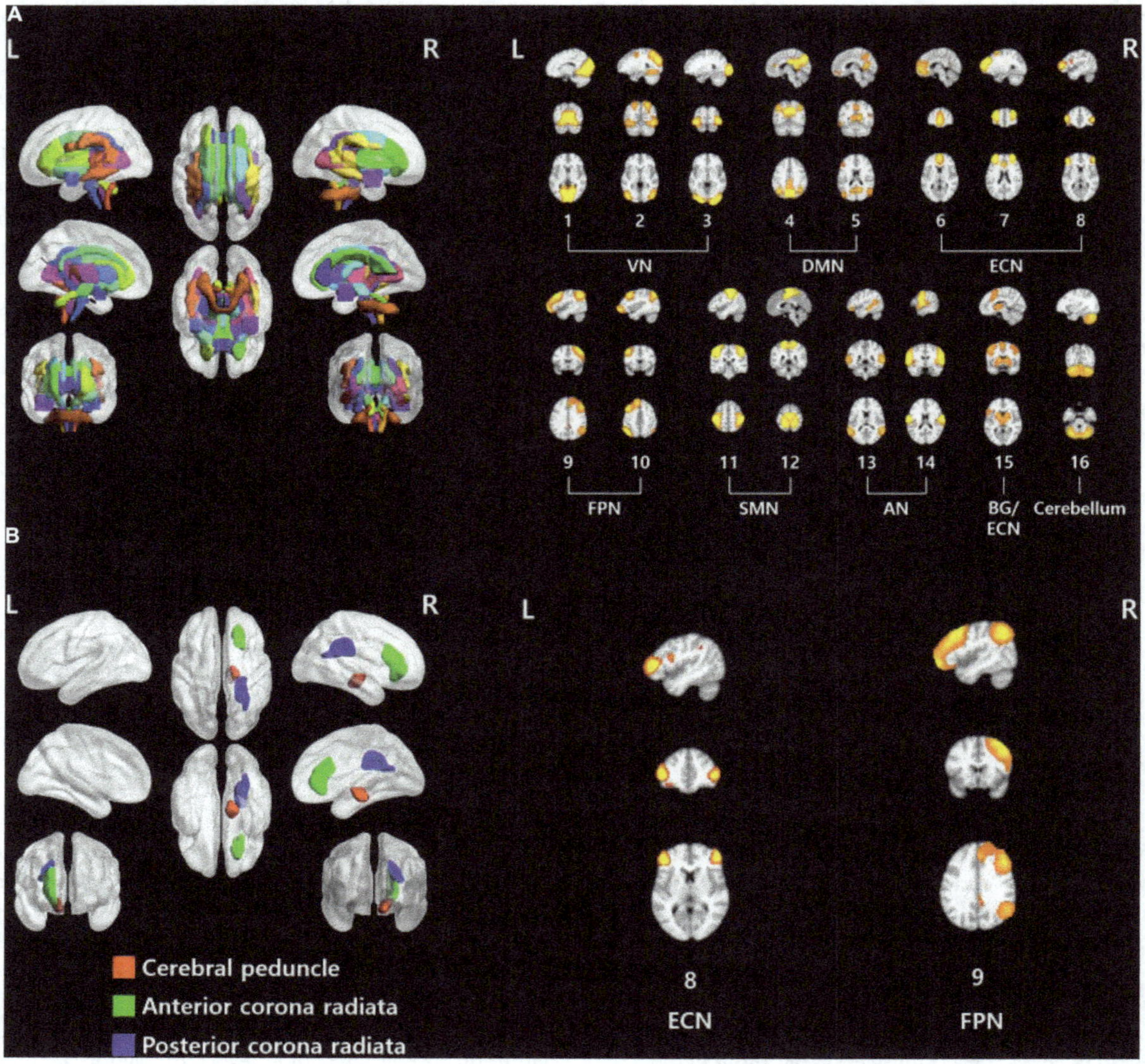

FIGURE 2 | (A) ROIs used in this study. (Left) ICBM DTI-81 atlas and (right) 16 functionally interpretable ICs. **(B)** Brain regions and networks that showed significant associations with EDE-Q scores. VN, visual network; DMN, default mode network; ECN, executive control network; FPN, frontoparietal network; SMN, sensorimotor network; AN, auditory network; BG, basal ganglia.

DISCUSSION

We explored the differences in structural and functional connectivity in brain regions and networks related to the behaviors of eating disorders between people with abdominal and non-abdominal obesity with the use of DTI and rs-fMRI. Probabilistic fiber tractography and static and dynamic connectivity analyses were used to quantify the characteristics of brain regions and networks. The DC values of several brain regions and networks showed significant inter-group differences. We further explored the relationship between structural and functional connectivity and key behaviors of eating disorders, and significant correlations were found. Our results indicated that altered brain structure and function in people with abdominal and non-abdominal obesity were associated with eating disorders behaviors.

We found that the functional connectivity in FPN and ECN showed significant inter-group differences between people with abdominal and non-abdominal obesity. Furthermore, significant associations with key behaviors of eating disorders were observed. The FPN and ECN mainly contain the dorsolateral prefrontal cortex which controls cognitive functions, such as planning, working memory, and inhibition (Le et al., 2007; Stice et al., 2008; Davids et al., 2010). Some considered obesity as a type of psychological disease related to deranged eating behaviors, which results from a dysfunctional fronto-striatal circuitry (Volkow et al., 2009). Previous studies observed that the impaired inhibitory control in people with obesity suggesting the lateral prefrontal cortex is an important region of the fronto-striatal circuit that controls the regulation of eating behaviors (DelParigi et al., 2004; Wang et al., 2004; Le et al., 2006). One study showed that altered activity in the dorsolateral prefrontal cortex broke

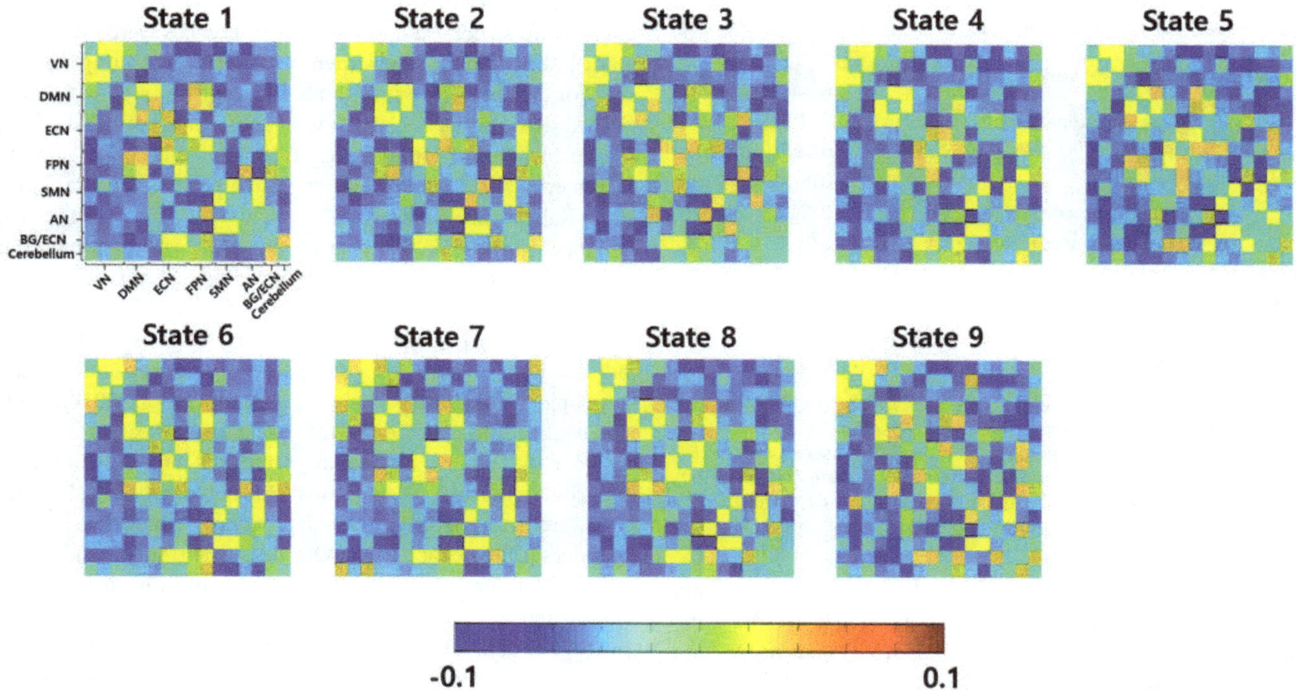

FIGURE 3 | Nine group-level brain states. VN, visual network; DMN, default mode network; ECN, executive control network; FPN, frontoparietal network; SMN, sensorimotor network; AN, auditory network; BG, basal ganglia.

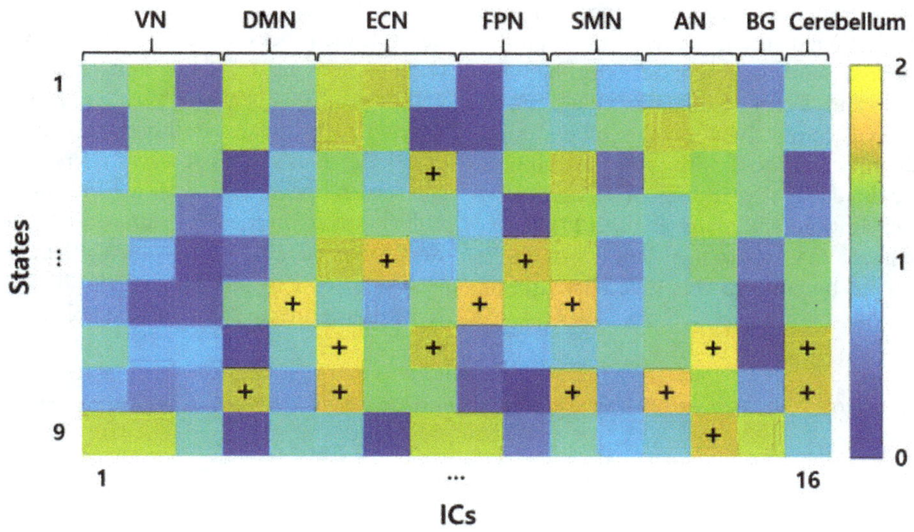

FIGURE 4 | Representative networks of each group-level states. Elements of the matrix represent the hubness of BC. Representative networks are marked with the symbols "+." VN, visual network; DMN, default mode network; ECN, executive control network; FPN, frontoparietal network; SMN, sensorimotor network; AN, auditory network; BG, basal ganglia; ICs, independent components.

the balance between the reward and cognitive systems and led to errant eating behaviors (Val-Laillet et al., 2015). In addition, previous studies found an imbalance in the prefrontal and limbic brain circuits that support aspects of cognition- and reward-related eating behaviors (Carnell et al., 2011; Brooks et al., 2013; Vainik et al., 2013). In summary, it is possible that lack of regulatory influences from the dorsolateral prefrontal cortex in people with obesity might cause a psychological dependence on food and overeating (Wang et al., 2004).

One possible interpretation of our findings on differences between people with abdominal and non-abdominal obesity is that insulin levels may influence brain function during rest in brain networks that control reward and food regulation. Abdominal obesity is known to be strongly related to insulin

TABLE 2 | Brain regions and networks that yielded significant correlations between the DC values of the identified regions/networks and the EDE-Q scores.

Information	Region/Network	EDE-Q	R^2	*P*-value
DTI	Right cerebral peduncle	E	0.0377	0.0109
		S	0.0324	0.0153
		W	0.0530	0.0025
	Right anterior corona radiata	R	0.0323	0.0468
	Right posterior corona radiata	R	0.0288	0.0407
		S	0.0283	0.0407
fMRI: Static	FPN (IC #9)	S	0.0270	0.0491
		W	0.0363	0.0268
fMRI: Dynamic	ECN (IC #8) in state 5	S	0.0285	0.0794

The significance of the dynamic connectivity analysis was 0.1. P-values were corrected using FDR. DC, degree centrality; EDE-Q-R, eating disorder examination questionnaire restraint; EDE-Q-E, eating disorder examination questionnaire eating concern; EDE-Q-S, eating disorder examination questionnaire shape concern; EDE-Q-W, eating disorder examination questionnaire weight concern; FPN, frontoparietal network; ECN, executive control network.

resistance, and it has been recognized as a key determinant of the metabolic syndrome (Carr et al., 2004; Després and Lemieux, 2006). A previous study reported that individuals who were resistant to insulin showed an increase of functional connectivity in the reward network, but a reduction in cognitive control networks (Kullmann et al., 2012). In addition, altered brain activity in the frontoparietal executive system was found in metabolic syndrome patients (Hoth et al., 2011). Interestingly, a study that utilized intranasal insulin administration reported altered brain activity in cognitive brain regions and altered functional connectivity between the hippocampal region and DMN (Kullmann et al., 2017). The change of functional connectivity in the hippocampal region was significantly correlated with visceral adipose tissue and the change in subjective feeling of hunger after intranasal insulin administration (Kullmann et al., 2017). These studies collectively suggest that abdominal obesity may be indirectly related to altered function in cognitive related brain areas.

In addition to functional connectivity differences, the inter-group structural connectivity differences were observed in many brain regions (**Supplementary Table S1**). Among them, the anterior and posterior corona radiata and the cerebral peduncle yielded significant associations with behaviors of eating disorders. The corona radiata is part of the limbic-thalamo-cortical circuitry that is critical for reward and cognitive processes (Catani et al., 2002; Kalivas and Volkow, 2005; Olivo et al., 2017). The corona radiata is a key region that projects thalamic information onto the prefrontal cortex, and the alteration in this region is shown to be associated with cognitive dysfunction and central taste disorders (Shott et al., 2015; Olivo et al., 2017). Previous studies found that fractional anisotropy in corona radiata showed abnormalities in people with anorexia nervosa (Gaudio et al., 2017), and it was significantly related to the behaviors of eating disorders (Olivo et al., 2017). They also reported that altered white matter integrity in corona radiata was associated with dysfunctions in reward and cognitive related processes, which led to eating disorders (Olivo et al., 2017). Our results and these studies were consistent in that altered structural connectivity in corona radiata was related to the behaviors of eating disorders. In addition to the corona radiata, we found significant inter-group structural connectivity differences in the cerebral peduncle and associations with the behaviors of eating disorders. The cerebral peduncle is included in the corticospinal tracts that contain large fiber tracts (Ramnani, 2006; Koyama et al., 2013). The fiber tracts of the cerebral peduncle primarily originate from the prefrontal cortex in the human (Ramnani, 2006). The prefrontal cortex controls the process of reward, inhibitory control, and executive decision making (Holland and Gallagher, 2004; Kringelbach and Rolls, 2004; Petrovich et al., 2007). It is an important region that modulates an individual's eating behavior (van Vugt, 2009). Previous studies observed altered white matter integrity of the cerebral peduncle, including the cortico-spinal and cortico-bulbar tracts in people with obesity (Civardi et al., 2004; Karlsson et al., 2013; Ryan and Walther, 2014; van Bloemendaal et al., 2016; Papageorgiou et al., 2017). Taken together, the structural connectivity in the cerebral peduncle, which is strongly

TABLE 3 | Correlation analysis between DC values of both the brain regions and networks that showed a good correlation in the first step and EDE-Q scores.

Information	EDE-Q							
	R		E		S		W	
	R^2	*P*-value	R^2	*P*-value	R^2	*P*-value	R^2	*P*-value
Only DTI	***0.0453***	***0.0139***	***0.0530***	***0.0054***	***0.0602***	***0.0022***	***0.0765***	***<0.001***
Only fMRI: Static	0.0130	0.1691	0.0113	0.2132	***0.0270***	***0.0245***	***0.0363***	***0.0067***
Only fMRI: Dynamic	0.0072	0.3777	0.0118	0.2005	***0.0285***	***0.0198***	0.0174	0.0921
fMRI: Static and dynamic	0.0183	0.1725	0.0195	0.1490	***0.0566***	***0.0013***	***0.0589***	***<0.001***
DTI and fMRI: Static	***0.0516***	***0.0139***	***0.0567***	***0.0077***	***0.0759***	***<0.001***	***0.1105***	***<0.001***
DTI and fMRI: Dynamic	***0.0497***	***0.0174***	***0.0609***	***0.0046***	***0.0868***	***<0.001***	***0.0953***	***<0.001***
DTI and fMRI: Static and dynamic	***0.0576***	***0.0140***	***0.0662***	***0.0053***	***0.1087***	***<0.001***	***0.1294***	***<0.001***

P-values were corrected using FDR. Significant results (p < 0.05) are reported in bold italics. DC, degree centrality; EDE-Q-R, eating disorder examination questionnaire restraint; EDE-Q-E, eating disorder examination questionnaire eating concern; EDE-Q-S, eating disorder examination questionnaire shape concern; EDE-Q-W, eating disorder examination questionnaire weight concern.

connected to the prefrontal cortex, may be indirectly related to eating behaviors in people with obesity. However, the cerebral peduncle contains fiber tracts that originate from the motor, temporal, and parietal cortices, as well as the prefrontal cortex (Ramnani, 2006). Thus, additional experiments are required to elucidate the relationship between structural connectivity in the cerebral peduncle and eating behaviors in more detail.

In the correlation analyses conducted herein, we found that the DC values computed from multimodality imaging data (i.e., both DTI and rs-fMRI) explained the behaviors of eating disorders with higher R^2 values compared to those from single-modality imaging data (i.e., DTI or rs-fMRI alone) (**Table 3**). This result may be attributed to the heterogeneity of obesity associated with eating behaviors, genetic factors, or insulin resistance (Brownell and Wadden, 1991; McLaughlin, 2012). Using only structural or functional characteristics of the brain may not provide sufficient information to quantify the diverse aspects of obesity. The results indicate that multimodality imaging data provides complementary information to understand the links between the brain and behaviors of eating disorders. In this study, both static and dynamic functional connectivity analyses were considered, and the dynamic connectivity results correlated better with behaviors of eating disorders. Unlike the static connectivity analysis, many connectivity matrices that reflect the temporal dynamics of the brain states were constructed in the dynamic connectivity analysis. The additional information may better link changes in the brain structure and function to behaviors associated with eating disorders. Our study suggested that using the structural and functional information and using dynamic, rather than static, connectivity analysis could best explain the elicited behaviors of eating disorders.

Our study has a few limitations. Although we associated brain states derived from dynamic connectivity analysis with representative brain networks, we could not match the brain states with specific cognitive conditions owing to validation difficulties. In future studies, we will collect various clinical scores to correlate cognitive conditions with brain states. In this study, we used WHR instead of other direct measures of abdominal obesity, such as visceral fat from abdominal MRI and body fat measures from bioelectrical impedance analyses. The NKI-RS database did not provide such measures, and we were thus limited to the use of WHR.

In this study, we found significant brain structural and functional differences between people with abdominal and non-abdominal obesity and strong associations between the connectivity values and EDE-Q scores in the cerebral peduncle, anterior and posterior corona radiata, ECN, and FPN. When both the structural and dynamic functional connectivity were used, the relationships between brain connectivity and the behaviors of the eating disorders were strengthened, thus indicating that multimodal imaging data is more effective than single-modal imaging data. Our reported results are expected to provide more evidence on the mechanisms associated with abdominal obesity and behaviors of eating disorders.

AUTHOR CONTRIBUTIONS

BP and HP wrote the manuscript. MK aided the experiments. ML and SK aided the clinical interpretation. HP is the guarantor of this work, and as such, had full access to all the data in the study and takes responsibility for the integrity of the data and the accuracy of the data analyses.

FUNDING

This work was supported by the Institute for Basic Science (Grant No. IBS-R015-D1), the NRF (National Research Foundation of Korea) (Grant Nos. NRF-2016H1A2A1907833, NRF-2016R1A2B4008545, NRF-2017R1A2B2009086, and NRF-2017R1A2B4007254), and the Ministry of Science and ICT of Korea under the ITRC program (IITP-2018-0-01798).

REFERENCES

Allen, E. A., Damaraju, E., Plis, S. M., Erhardt, E. B., Eichele, T., and Calhoun, V. D. (2012). Tracking whole-brain connectivity dynamics in the resting state. *Cereb. Cortex* 24, 663–676. doi: 10.1093/cercor/bhs352

Azadbakht, L., and Esmaillzadeh, A. (2011). Dietary diversity score is related to obesity and abdominal adiposity among Iranian female youth. *Public Health Nutr.* 14, 62–69. doi: 10.1017/S1368980010000522

Beckmann, C. F., DeLuca, M., Devlin, J. T., and Smith, S. M. (2005). Investigations into resting-state connectivity using independent component analysis. *Philos. Trans. R. Soc. B* 360, 1001–1013. doi: 10.1098/rstb.2005.1634

Beckmann, C. F., and Smith, S. M. (2004). Probabilistic independent component analysis for functional magnetic resonance imaging. *IEEE Trans. Med. Imaging* 23, 137–152.

Benjamini, Y., and Hochberg, Y. (1995). Controlling the false discovery rate?: a practical and powerful approach to multiple testing. *J. R. Stat. Soc.* 57, 289–300.

Brooks, S. J., Cedernaes, J., and Schiöth, H. B. (2013). Increased prefrontal and parahippocampal activation with reduced dorsolateral prefrontal and insular cortex activation to food images in obesity: a meta-analysis of fMRI studies. *PLoS One* 8:e60393. doi: 10.1371/journal.pone.0060393

Brownell, K. D., and Wadden, T. A. (1991). The heterogeneity of obesity: fitting treatments to individuals. *Behav. Ther.* 22, 153–177. doi: 10.1016/j.beth.2016.11.009

Bujalska, I. J., Kumar, S., and Stewart, P. M. (1997). Does central obesity reflect "Cushing's disease of the omentum"? *Lancet* 349, 1210–1213. doi: 10.1016/S0140-6736(96)11222-8

Bulik, C. M., Sullivan, P. F., and Kendler, K. S. (2003). Genetic and environmental contributions to obesity and binge eating. *Int. J. Eat. Disord.* 33, 293–298. doi: 10.1002/eat.10140

Bullmore, E., and Sporns, O. (2009). Complex brain networks: graph theoretical analysis of structural and functional systems. *Nat. Neurosci.* 10, 186–198. doi: 10.1038/nrn2575

Carnell, S., Gibson, C., Benson, L., Ochner, C. N., and Geliebter, A. (2011). Neuroimaging and obesity: current knowledge and future directions. *Obes. Rev.* 13, 1–14. doi: 10.1111/j.1467-789X.2011.00927.x

Carr, D. B., Utzschneider, K. M., Hull, R. L., Kodama, K., Retzlaff, B. M., Brunzell, J. D., et al. (2004). Intra-abdominal fat is a major determinant of the national cholesterol education program adult treatment panel III criteria for the metabolic syndrome. *Diabetes Metab. Res. Rev.* 53, 2087–2094. doi: 10.2337/diabetes.53.8.2087

Catani, M., Howard, R. J., Pajevic, S., and Jones, D. K. (2002). Virtual *in Vivo* interactive dissection of white matter fasciculi in the human brain. *Neuroimage* 17, 77–94. doi: 10.1006/nimg.2002.1136

Chen, C., Witte, M., Heemsbergen, W., and Herk, M. V. (2013). Multiple comparisons permutation test for image based data mining in radiotherapy. *Radiat. Oncol.* 8:293. doi: 10.1186/1748-717X-8-293

Civardi, C., Vicentini, R., Grugni, G., and Cantello, R. (2004). Corticospinal physiology in patients with prader-willi syndrome. *Arch. Neurol.* 61, 1585–1589.

Cox, R. W. (1996). AFNI?: software for analysis and visualization of functional magnetic resonance neuroimages. *Comput. Biomed. Res.* 29, 162–173. doi: 10.1006/cbmr.1996.0014

Dallman, M. F., Pecoraro, N., Akana, S. F., Fleur, S. E., Gomez, F., Houshyar, H., et al. (2003). Chronic stress and obesity: a new view of "comfort food. *Proc. Natl. Acad. Sci. U.S.A* 100, 11696–11701.

Damaraju, E., Allen, E. A., Belger, A., Ford, J. M., McEwen, S., Mathalon, D. H., et al. (2014). Dynamic functional connectivity analysis reveals transient states of dysconnectivity in schizophrenia. *NeuroImage Clin.* 5, 298–308. doi: 10.1016/j.nicl.2014.07.003

Daubenmier, J., Kristeller, J., Hecht, F. M., Maninger, N., Kuwata, M., Jhaveri, K., et al. (2011). Mindfulness intervention for stress eating to reduce cortisol and abdominal fat among overweight and obese women?: an exploratory randomized controlled study. *J. Obes.* 2011:651936. doi: 10.1155/2011/651936

Davids, S., Lauffer, H., Thoms, K., Jagdhuhn, M., Hirschfeld, H., Domin, M., et al. (2010). Increased dorsolateral prefrontal cortex activation in obese children during observation of food stimuli. *Int. J. Obes.* 34, 94–104. doi: 10.1038/ijo.2009.193

DelParigi, A., Chen, K., Salbe, A. D., Hill, J. O., Wing, R. R., Reiman, E. M., et al. (2004). Persistence of abnormal neural responses to a meal in postobese individuals. *Int. J. Obes.* 28, 370–377. doi: 10.1038/sj.ijo.0802558

Després, J.-P., and Lemieux, I. (2006). Abdominal obesity and metabolic syndrome. *Nature* 444, 881–887. doi: 10.1038/nature05488

Després, J. P., Lemieux, I., Bergeron, J., Pibarot, P., Mathieu, P., Larose, E., et al. (2008). Abdominal obesity and the metabolic syndrome: contribution to global cardiometabolic risk. *Arterioscler. Thromb. Vasc. Biol.* 28, 1039–1049. doi: 10.1161/ATVBAHA.107.159228

Fairburn, C., and Beglin, S. (1994). Assessment of eating disorders: interview or self- report questionnaire? *Int. J. Eat. Disord.* 16, 363–370.

Folsom, A. R., Kaye, S. A., Sellers, T. A., Hong, C.-P., Cerhan, J. R., Potter, J. D., et al. (1993). Body fat distribution and 5-year risk of death in older women. *JAMA J. Am. Med. Assoc.* 269, 483–487. doi: 10.1001/jama.1993.03500040049035

Folsom, A. R., Kushi, L. H., Anderson, K. E., Mink, P. J., Olson, J. E., Hong, C.-P., et al. (2000). Associations of general and abdominal obesity with multiple health outcomes in older women. *Arch. Intern. Med.* 160, 2117–2128. doi: 10.1001/archinte.160.14.2117

Friedman, J., Hastie, T., and Tibshirani, R. (2008). Sparse inverse covariance estimation with the graphical lasso. *Biostatistics* 9, 432–441. doi: 10.1093/biostatistics/kxm045

Gaudio, S., Quattrocchi, C. C., Piervincenzi, C., Zobel, B. B., Montecchi, F. R., Dakanalis, A., et al. (2017). White matter abnormalities in treatment-naive adolescents at the earliest stages of Anorexia Nervosa: a diffusion tensor imaging study. *Psychiatry Res. Neuroimaging* 266, 138–145. doi: 10.1016/j.pscychresns.2017.06.011

Gluck, M. E., Geliebter, A., and Lorence, M. (2004). Cortisol stress response is positively correlated with central obesity in obese women with binge eating disorder (BED) before and after cognitive-behavioral treatment. *Ann. N. Y. Acad. Sci.* 1032, 202–207. doi: 10.1196/annals.1314.021

Griffanti, L., Douaud, G., Bijsterbosch, J., Evangelisti, S., Alfaro-Almagro, F., Glasser, M. F., et al. (2017). Hand classification of fMRI ICA noise components. *Neuroimage* 154, 188–205. doi: 10.1016/j.neuroimage.2016.12.036

Holland, P. C., and Gallagher, M. (2004). Amygdala-frontal interactions and reward expectancy. *Curr. Opin. Neurobiol.* 14, 148–155. doi: 10.1016/j.conb.2004.03.007

Hollmann, M., Hellrung, L., Pleger, B., Schlögl, H., Kabisch, S., Stumvoll, M., et al. (2012). Neural correlates of the volitional regulation of the desire for food. *Int. J. Obes.* 36, 648–655. doi: 10.1038/ijo.2011.125

Hoth, K. F., Gonzales, M. M., Tarumi, T., Miles, S. C., Tanaka, H., and Haley, A. P. (2011). Functional MR imaging evidence of altered functional activation in metabolic syndrome. *Am. J. Neuroradiol.* 32, 541–547. doi: 10.3174/ajnr.A2315

Hutchison, R. M., Womelsdorf, T., Allen, E. A., Bandettini, P. A., Calhoun, V. D., Corbetta, M., et al. (2013). Dynamic functional connectivity: promise, issues, and interpretations. *Neuroimage* 80, 360–378. doi: 10.1016/j.neuroimage.2013.05.079

Jagust, W., Harvey, D., Mungas, D., and Haan, M. (2005). Central obesity and the aging brain. *Arch. Neurol.* 62, 1545–1548. doi: 10.1001/archneur.62.10.1545

Jenkinson, M., Beckmann, C. F., Behrens, T. E. J., Woolrich, M. W., and Smith, S. M. (2012). Fsl. *Neuroimage* 62, 782–790. doi: 10.1016/j.neuroimage.2011.09.015

Kalivas, P. W., and Volkow, N. D. (2005). The neural basis of addiction:a pathology of motivation and choice. *Am. J. Psychiatry* 162, 1403–1413. doi: 10.1176/appi.ajp.162.8.1403

Karlsson, H. K., Tuulari, J. J., Hirvonen, J., Lepomäki, V., Parkkola, R., Hiltunen, J., et al. (2013). Obesity is associated with white matter atrophy: a combined diffusion tensor imaging and voxel-based morphometric study. *Obesity* 21, 2530–2537. doi: 10.1002/oby.20386

Kelly, R. E. J., Alexopoulos, G. S., Wang, Z., Gunning, F. M., Murphy, C. F., Morimoto, S. S., et al. (2010). Visual inspection of independent components: defining a procedure. *J. Neurosci. Methods* 189, 233–245. doi: 10.1016/j.jneumeth.2010.03.028.Visual

Kodinariya, T. M., and Makwana, P. R. (2013). Review on determining number of cluster in K-means clustering. *Int. J. Adv. Res. Comput. Sci. Manag. Stud.* 1, 90–95.

Koyama, T., Tsuji, M., Nishimura, H., Miyake, H., Ohmura, T., and Domen, K. (2013). Diffusion tensor imaging for intracerebral hemorrhage outcome prediction: comparison using data from the corona radiata/internal capsule and the cerebral peduncle. *J. Stroke Cerebrovasc. Dis.* 22, 72–79. doi: 10.1016/j.jstrokecerebrovasdis.2011.06.014

Kringelbach, M. L., and Rolls, E. T. (2004). The functional neuroanatomy of the human orbitofrontal cortex: evidence from neuroimaging and neuropsychology. *Prog. Neurobiol.* 72, 341–372. doi: 10.1016/j.pneurobio.2004.03.006

Kullmann, S., Heni, M., Veit, R., Ketterer, C., Schick, F., Häring, H. U., et al. (2012). The obese brain: association of body mass index and insulin sensitivity with resting state network functional connectivity. *Hum. Brain Mapp.* 33, 1052–1061. doi: 10.1002/hbm.21268

Kullmann, S., Heni, M., Veit, R., Scheffler, K., Machann, J., Häring, H. U., et al. (2017). Intranasal insulin enhances brain functional connectivity mediating the relationship between adiposity and subjective feeling of hunger. *Sci. Rep.* 7, 1–10. doi: 10.1038/s41598-017-01907-w

Le, D. S. N. T., Pannacciulli, N., Chen, K., Del Parigi, A., Salbe, A. D., Reiman, E. M., et al. (2006). Less activation of the left dorsolateral prefrontal cortex in response to a meal: a feature of obesity. *Am. J. Clin. Nutr.* 84, 725–731.

Le, D. S. N. T., Pannacciulli, N., Chen, K., Salbe, A. D., Hill, J. O., Wing, R. R., et al. (2007). Less activation in the left dorsolateral prefrontal cortex in the reanalysis of the response to a meal in obese than in lean women and its association with successful weight loss. *Am. J. Clin. Nutr.* 86, 573–579.

Lips, M. A., Wijngaarden, M. A., Van Der Grond, J., Van Buchem, M. A., De Groot, G. H., Rombouts, S. A., et al. (2014). Resting-state functional connectivity of brain regions involved in cognitive control, motivation, and reward is enhanced in obese females. *Am. J. Clin. Nutr.* 100, 524–531. doi: 10.3945/ajcn.113.080671

Malik, V. S., Willett, W. C., and Hu, F. B. (2013). Global obesity: trends, risk factors and policy implications. *Nat. Rev. Endocrinol.* 9, 13–27. doi: 10.1038/nrendo.2012.199

McLaughlin, T. (2012). Metabolic heterogeneity of obesity: role of adipose tissue. *Int. J. Obes. Suppl.* 2, S8–S10. doi: 10.1038/ijosup.2012.3

Minka, T. P. (2000). *Automatic Choice of Dimensionality for PCA*. Cambridge, MA: MIT Media Laboratory.

Mond, J. M., Hay, P. J., Rodgers, B., Owen, C., and Beumont, P. J. V. (2004). Validity of the Eating Disorder Examination Questionnaire (EDE-Q) in screening for eating disorders in community samples. *Behav. Res. Ther.* 42, 551–567. doi: 10.1016/S0005-7967(03)00161-X

Mumford, J. A., Horvath, S., Oldham, M. C., Langfelder, P., Geschwind, D. H., and Poldrack, R. A. (2010). Detecting network modules in fMRI time series: a weighted network analysis approach. *Neuroimage* 52, 1465–1476. doi: 10.1016/j.neuroimage.2010.05.047

Nooner, K. B., Colcombe, S. J., Tobe, R. H., Mennes, M., Benedict, M. M., Moreno, A. L., et al. (2012). The NKI-rockland sample: a model for accelerating the pace of discovery science in psychiatry. *Front. Neurosci.* 6:152. doi: 10.3389/fnins.2012.00152

Olivo, G., Wiemerslage, L., Swenne, I., Zhukowsky, C., Salonen-Ros, H., Larsson, E. M., et al. (2017). Limbic-thalamo-cortical projections and reward-related circuitry integrity affects eating behavior: a longitudinal DTI study in adolescents with restrictive eating disorders. *PLoS One* 12:e0172129. doi: 10.1371/journal.pone.0172129

Papageorgiou, I., Astrakas, L. G., Xydis, V., Alexiou, G. A., Bargiotas, P., Tzarouchi, L., et al. (2017). Abnormalities of brain neural circuits related to obesity: a diffusion tensor imaging study. *Magn. Reson. Imaging* 37, 116–121. doi: 10.1016/j.mri.2016.11.018

Park, B., Kim, M., Lee, J., and Park, H. (2016a). Connectivity analysis and feature classification in attention deficit hyperactivity disorder sub-types: a task functional magnetic resonance imaging study. *Brain Topogr.* 29, 429–439. doi: 10.1007/s10548-015-0463-1

Park, B., Moon, T., and Park, H. (2018). Dynamic functional connectivity analysis reveals improved association between brain networks and eating behaviors compared to static analysis. *Behav. Brain Res.* 337, 114–121. doi: 10.1016/j.bbr.2017.10.001

Park, B., Seo, J., and Park, H. (2016b). Functional brain networks associated with eating behaviors in obesity. *Sci. Rep.* 6:23891. doi: 10.1038/srep23891

Petrovich, G. D., Ross, C. A., Holland, P. C., and Gallagher, M. (2007). Medial prefrontal cortex is necessary for an appetitive contextual conditioned stimulus to promote eating in sated rats. *J. Neurosci.* 27, 6436–6441. doi: 10.1523/JNEUROSCI.5001-06.2007

Power, J. D., Barnes, K. A., Snyder, A. Z., Schlaggar, B. L., and Petersen, S. E. (2012). Spurious but systematic correlations in functional connectivity MRI networks arise from subject motion. *Neuroimage* 59, 2142–2154. doi: 10.1016/j.neuroimage.2011.10.018

Raji, C. A., Ho, A. J., Parikshak, N., Becker, J. T., Lopez, O. L., Kuller, L. H., et al. (2010). Brain structure and obesity. *Hum. Brain Mapp.* 31, 353–364. doi: 10.1002/hbm.20870.Brain

Ramnani, N. (2006). The primate cortico-cerebellar system: anatomy and function. *Nat. Rev. Neurosci.* 7, 511–522. doi: 10.1038/nrn1953

Rubinov, M., and Sporns, O. (2010). Complex network measures of brain connectivity: uses and interpretations. *Neuroimage* 52, 1059–1069. doi: 10.1016/j.neuroimage.2009.10.003

Ryan, L., and Walther, K. (2014). White matter integrity in older females is altered by increased body fat. *Obesity* 22, 2039–2046. doi: 10.1002/oby.20815

Salimi-Khorshidi, G., Douaud, G., Beckmann, C. F., Glasser, M. F., Griffanti, L., and Smith, S. M. (2014). Automatic denoising of functional MRI data: Combining independent component analysis and hierarchical fusion of classifiers. *Neuroimage* 90, 449–468. doi: 10.1016/j.neuroimage.2013.11.046

Schwarz, A. J., and McGonigle, J. (2011). Negative edges and soft thresholding in complex network analysis of resting state functional connectivity data. *Neuroimage* 55, 1132–1146. doi: 10.1016/j.neuroimage.2010.12.047

Seo, E. H., Lee, D. Y., Lee, J.-M., Park, J.-S., Sohn, B. K., Lee, D. S., et al. (2013). Whole-brain functional networks in cognitively normal, mild cognitive impairment, and Alzheimer's disease. *PLoS One* 8:e53922. doi: 10.1371/journal.pone.0053922

Shott, M. E., Cornier, M.-A., Mittal, V. A., Pryor, T. L., Orr, J. M., Brown, M. S., et al. (2015). Orbitofrontal cortex volume and brain reward response in obesity. *Int. J. Obes.* 39, 214–221. doi: 10.1038/ijo.2014.121

Smith, S. M., Fox, P. T., Miller, K. L., Glahn, D. C., Fox, P. M., Mackay, C. E., et al. (2009). Correspondence of the brain's functional architecture during activation and rest. *Proc. Natl. Acad. Sci. U.S.A.* 106, 13040–13045. doi: 10.1073/pnas.0905267106

Smith, S. M., Miller, K. L., Moeller, S., Xu, J., Auerbach, E. J., Woolrich, M. W., et al. (2012). Temporally-independent functional modes of spontaneous brain activity. *Proc. Natl. Acad. Sci. U.S.A.* 109, 3131–3136. doi: 10.1073/pnas.1121329109

Smith, S. M., Vidaurre, D., Beckmann, C. F., Glasser, M. F., Jenkinson, M., Miller, K. L., et al. (2013). Functional connectomics from resting-state fMRI. *Trends Cogn. Sci.* 17, 666–682. doi: 10.1016/j.tics.2013.09.016

Stefan, N., Häring, H.-U., Hu, F. B., and Schulze, M. B. (2013). Metabolically healthy obesity: epidemiology, mechanisms, and clinical implications. *Lancet Diabetes Endocrinol.* 1, 152–162. doi: 10.1016/S2213-8587(13)70062-7

Stice, E., Spoor, S., Bohon, C., Veldhuizen, M., and Small, D. (2008). Relation of reward from food intake and anticipated food intake to obesity: a functional magnetic resonance imaging study. *J. Abnorm. Psychol.* 117, 924–935. doi: 10.1037/a0013600.Relation

Succurro, E., Segura-garcia, C., Ruffo, M., Caroleo, M., Rania, M., Aloi, M., et al. (2015). Obese patients with a binge eating disorder have an unfavorable metabolic and inflammatory profile. *Medicine* 94, 1–7. doi: 10.1097/MD.0000000000002098

Tataranni, P. A., Gautier, J.-F., Chen, K., Uecker, A., Bandy, D., Salbe, A. D., et al. (1999). Neuroanatomical correlates of hunger and satiation in humans using positron emission tomography. *Proc. Natl. Acad. Sci. U.S.A.* 96, 4569–4574. doi: 10.1073/pnas.96.8.4569

Vainik, U., Dagher, A., Dubé, L., and Fellows, L. K. (2013). Neurobehavioural correlates of body mass index and eating behaviours in adults: a systematic review. *Neurosci. Biobehav. Rev.* 37, 279–299. doi: 10.1016/j.neubiorev.2012.11.008

Val-Laillet, D., Aarts, E., Weber, B., Ferrari, M., Quaresima, V., Stoeckel, L. E., et al. (2015). Neuroimaging and neuromodulation approaches to study eating behavior and prevent and treat eating disorders and obesity. *NeuroImage Clin.* 8, 1–31. doi: 10.1016/j.nicl.2015.03.016

van Bloemendaal, L., Ijzerman, R. G., ten Kulve, J. S., Barkhof, F., Diamant, M., Veltman, D. J., et al. (2016). Alterations in white matter volume and integrity in obesity and type 2 diabetes. *Metab. Brain Dis.* 31, 621–629. doi: 10.1007/s11011-016-9792-3

van Vugt, D. A. (2009). Brain imaging studies of appetite in the context of obesity and the menstrual cycle. *Hum. Reprod. Update* 16, 276–292. doi: 10.1093/humupd/dmp051

Volkow, N. D., Fowler, J. S., Wang, G. J., Baler, R., and Telang, F. (2009). Imaging dopamine's role in drug abuse and addiction. *Neuropharmacology* 56, 3–8. doi: 10.1016/j.neuropharm.2008.05.022

Wang, G. J., Volkow, N. D., Telang, F., Jayne, M., Ma, J., Rao, M., et al. (2004). Exposure to appetitive food stimuli markedly activates the human brain. *Neuroimage* 21, 1790–1797. doi: 10.1016/j.neuroimage.2003.11.026

World Health Organization (2008). *Waist Circumference and Waist-Hip Ratio: Report of a WHO Expert Consultation*. Geneva: World Health Organization.

Yates, K. F., Sweat, V., Yau, P. L., Turchiano, M. M., and Convit, A. (2012). Impact of metabolic syndrome on cognition and brain. *Arterioscler. Thromb. Vasc. Biol.* 32, 2060–2067. doi: 10.1161/ATVBAHA.112.252759

Yau, P. L. P. L., Castro, M. G., Tagani, A., Tsui, W. H., and Convit, A. (2012). Obesity and metabolic syndrome and functional and structural brain impairments in adolescence. *Pediatrics* 130, e856–e864. doi: 10.1542/peds.2012-0324

Zhang, C., Rexrode, K. M., van Dam, R. M., Li, T. Y., and Hu, F. B. (2008). Abdominal obesity and the risk of all-cause, cardiovascular, and cancer mortality: sixteen years of follow-up in US women. *Circulation* 117, 1658–1667. doi: 10.1161/CIRCULATIONAHA.107.739714

Zhang, J. G., Wang, Z. H., Wang, H. J., Du, W. W., Su, C., Zhang, J., et al. (2015). Dietary patterns and their associations with general obesity and abdominal obesity among young Chinese women. *Eur. J. Clin. Nutr.* 69, 1009–1014. doi: 10.1038/ejcn.2015.8

3

Disrupted Balance of Long- and Short-Range Functional Connectivity Density in Type 2 Diabetes Mellitus: A Resting-State fMRI Study

Daihong Liu[1,2†], Lihua Chen[3†], Shanshan Duan[4], Xuntao Yin[1], Wu Yang[5], Yanshu Shi[1], Jiuquan Zhang[6,7]* and Jian Wang[1]*

[1] Department of Radiology, Southwest Hospital, Third Military Medical University (Army Medical University), Chongqing, China, [2] Department of Imaging Diagnosis, Lanzhou General Hospital of Chinese PLA Lanzhou Command (PLA No. 940 Hospital), Lanzhou, China, [3] Department of Radiology, PLA No. 904 Hospital, Wuxi, China, [4] Department of Endocrinology, Southwest Hospital, Third Military Medical University (Army Medical University), Chongqing, China, [5] Medical Company, The Chinese People's Liberation Army No.31610 Troop, Zhoushan, China, [6] Department of Radiology, Chongqing University Cancer Hospital & Chongqing Cancer Institute & Chongqing Cancer Hospital, Chongqing, China, [7] Key Laboratory for Biorheological Science and Technology of Ministry of Education (Chongqing University), Chongqing University Cancer Hospital & Chongqing Cancer Institute & Chongqing Cancer Hospital, Chongqing, China

***Correspondence:**
Jiuquan Zhang
zhangjq_radiol@foxmail.com
Jian Wang
wangjian_811@yahoo.com

[†] These authors have contributed equally to this work

Previous studies have shown that type 2 diabetes mellitus (T2DM) can accelerate the rate of cognitive decline in patients. As an organ with high energy consumption, the brain network balances between lower energy consumption and higher information transmission efficiency. However, T2DM may modify the proportion of short- and long-range connections to adapt to the inadequate energy supply and to respond to various cognitive tasks under the energy pressure caused by homeostasis alterations in brain glucose metabolism. On the basis of the above theories, this study determined the abnormal functional connections of the brain in 32 T2DM patients compared with 32 healthy control (HC) subjects using long- and short-range functional connectivity density (FCD) analyses with resting-state fMRI data. The cognitive function level in these patients was also evaluated by neuropsychological tests. Moreover, the characteristics of abnormal FCD and their relationships with cognitive impairment were investigated in T2DM patients. Compared with the HC group, T2DM patients exhibited decreased long-range FCD in the left calcarine and left lingual gyrus and increased short-range FCD in the right angular gyrus and medial part of the left superior frontal gyrus ($p < 0.05$, Gaussian random-field theory corrected). In T2DM patients, the FCD z scores of the medial part of the left superior frontal gyrus were negatively correlated with the time cost in part B of the Trail Making Test ($\rho = -0.422$, $p = 0.018$). In addition, the FCD z scores of the right angular gyrus were negatively correlated with the long-term delayed recall scores of the Auditory Verbal Learning Test ($\rho = -0.356$, $p = 0.049$) and the forward scores of the Digital Span Test ($\rho = -0.373$, $p = 0.039$). T2DM patients exhibited aberrant long-range and short-range FCD patterns, which may suggest brain network reorganization at the expense of losing the integration of long-range FCD to adapt to the deficiency in energy supply. These changes may be associated with cognitive decline in T2DM patients.

Keywords: type 2 diabetes mellitus, cognitive impairment, resting-state functional MRI, functional connectivity density, functional connectivity

INTRODUCTION

Type 2 diabetes mellitus (T2DM) is characterized by disordered glucose metabolism and the number of affected individuals increased rapidly from 415 million in 2015 to 425 million in 2017 according to the 8th edition of Diabetes Atlas published by the International Diabetes Federation. A growing number of publications have demonstrated that T2DM accelerates the speed of cognitive decline which could be up to twice as fast as normal aging (Koekkoek et al., 2015). However, the brain dysfunction and cognitive impairment associated with T2DM have not been fully investigated. As the brain has high energy consumption, it is vulnerable to the fluctuations in plasma glucose levels caused by T2DM. Therefore, a better understanding of the characteristics of brain dysfunction on the background of impaired energy homeostasis may enable early diagnosis and treatment.

Type 2 diabetes mellitus is associated with reduced glucose metabolism in the brain, which may result in putative reorganization of long- and short-range functional connections. The development of normal brain functional networks is characterized by a "local to distant" organization (Fair et al., 2009). Brain regions with short-range functional connections are often specialized for modular information processing and operate with lower time- and energy-cost. By contrast, long-range functional connections allow integrative information processing across distributed brain systems with higher time- and energy-cost (Sepulcre et al., 2010). The balance of long- and short-range functional connections is critical for the efficiency of cortical information communication and energy-cost (Sepulcre et al., 2010). However, T2DM patients are reported to have reduced brain glucose metabolism which is correlated with poor performance on executive and memory function tests (Garcia-Casares et al., 2014). Thus, impaired glucose homeostasis may disrupt the established balance of long- and short-range functional connections for the economical trade-off between cost and efficiency in T2DM patients (Bullmore and Sporns, 2012). As the alterations in glucose metabolism are coupled with alterations in blood-oxygen level-dependent signals, functional magnetic resonance imaging (fMRI) is advantageous in mapping the reorganization of long- and short-range functional connections (Sepulcre et al., 2010; Magistretti and Allaman, 2015).

Resting-state fMRI has been widely used to determine the aberrations in brain function in T2DM patients. On the one hand, T2DM patients exhibited altered amplitude of low frequency fluctuation in the middle temporal gyrus, lingual gyrus, postcentral gyrus and occipital lobe in functional segregation studies (Xia et al., 2013; Cui et al., 2014). On the other hand, T2DM patients showed aberrant local synchronization in the lingual gyrus, fusiform gyrus, and frontal lobe (Cui et al., 2014; Liu et al., 2016) and disrupted functional connectivity anchoring in the posterior cingulate cortex (Chen et al., 2014) or within the default mode network, frontal parietal network and sensorimotor network (Chen et al., 2015) in functional integration studies. As an approach for functional integration, the analysis of long- and short-range functional connections facilitates the investigation of brain dysfunction in patients with schizophrenia (Guo et al., 2015), minimal hepatic encephalopathy (Qi et al., 2015), non-alcoholic cirrhosis after liver transplantation (Zhang et al., 2015a), end-stage renal disease (Zhang et al., 2015b) and conduct disorder (Lu et al., 2017). Previous studies have also suggested that T2DM patients may suffer from cognition decline linked to alterations in long- and short-range brain functional synchronization and functional connectivity strength (Liu et al., 2016, 2017). In addition to the aforementioned neuroimaging indicators, the functional connectivity density (FCD), which quantifies the number of functional connections between a given voxel and the remaining voxels in the entire brain, is a graph theoretical indicator to analyze the complex brain networks (Tomasi et al., 2016). However, a map of the long- and short-range functional connections assessed using FCD remains to be delineated in T2DM patients. Furthermore, the similar definitions of FCD and degree of centrality suggest that the brain regions with aberrant FCD may play pivotal roles in global information communication (Zuo et al., 2012). Therefore, they can be considered as seed regions to calculate their functional connectivity with the whole brain as in a previous study (Cui et al., 2016) and the pattern of the changed FCD can be characterized.

In the present study, we assume that the cognitive impairment in T2DM patients may be associated with disruption of the balance between long- and short-range FCD. We first investigated the changed long- and short-range FCD pattern in T2DM patients, and then calculated the functional connectivity of the identified brain regions with the whole brain. Finally, we examined the relationships between these neuroimaging changes and cognition decline. This study may contribute to understanding the reorganization of brain functional architecture accompanying cognitive decline in T2DM patients.

MATERIALS AND METHODS

Subjects

This study recruited 32 T2DM patients from inpatients and communities and 32 healthy controls (HC) from communities during December 2013 and November 2016. The T2DM group and HC group were matched for age, sex, education, and body mass index (BMI). T2DM diagnosis conformed to the criteria published by the World Health Organization in 1999 (Alberti and Zimmet, 1998). Subjects in the two groups were included according to the following criteria: (1) 45 years $\leq$ age $\leq$ 70 years; (2) education $\geq$6 years; (3) right-handedness; (4) normal general cognitive level defined by a Mini-Mental State Examination (MMSE) score $\geq$25; (5) T2DM duration of patients at least 1 year. Key exclusion criteria for both groups were as follows: (1) brain structural abnormalities including trauma, stroke, tumor, or white matter changes with a rating score $\geq$2 (Wahlund et al., 2001); (2) neurological or psychiatric diseases including major depression, dementia, schizophrenia and epilepsy; (3) pregnancy, extremity disability, and the loss of audition or vision; (4) contraindications for MRI examination. T2DM patients with diabetic foot, retinopathy, nephropathy and other complications were also excluded. The Medical Research Ethics Committee of the Southwest Hospital (Chongqing, China) approved the study protocol in accordance with the recommendations of the declaration of Helsinki for investigation of human participants. All participants provided written informed consent after being informed of the study details.

Clinical Evaluation

All subjects underwent clinical evaluation with a standardized protocol. Demographic information included age, sex and education. The physical data included handedness, height, weight, and resting arm arterial blood pressure. BMI was calculated according to height and weight [(weight in kg)/(height in m)^2]. Medical history and current medications were also recorded. The dates of T2DM diagnoses were recorded to compute the disease duration. After an overnight abrosia, venous blood samples were collected by venipuncture for the evaluation of biometric measurements, including glucose parameters, lipid parameters, renal function parameters, thyroid function parameters, and homocysteine (listed in **Table 1**). Fasting insulin and plasma glucose were used to calculate the updated homeostasis model assessment of insulin resistance (HOMA2-IR) index with HOMA2 Calculator v2.2.3 software[1].

Cognitive Assessment

Cognitive assessments were performed before MRI scanning. A battery of neuropsychological tests in a fixed order was used to assess the general cognitive level and major cognitive domains. The general cognitive level was evaluated by the MMSE and Montreal Cognitive Assessment (MoCA) tests. The executive function and psychomotor speed were evaluated by the Trail Making Test (TMT, including parts A and B) (Bowie and Harvey, 2006). Mental flexibility was evaluated by the Verbal Fluency Test (VFT) (Diamond, 2013). Working memory was evaluated with the Digital Span Test (DST, including forward and backward) (Diamond, 2013). Episodic memory was evaluated by the Auditory Verbal Learning Test (AVLT, including immediate recall, short-term delayed recall, long-term delayed recall, long-term delayed recognition and total score) (Zhao et al., 2015). In addition, depression was evaluated with the Hamilton Depression Rating Scale-24 item (HAMD) to exclude cases with major depression. The test battery was administered by a trained neuropsychologist blinded to the grouping situation. It took approximately 60 min/subject to complete all the tests.

MRI Scan Protocol

MRI scanning was carried out with a 3.0-T MR scanner (Trio, Siemens Medical, Erlangen, Germany) using a 12-channel head coil on the same day as the clinical evaluation and cognitive assessment. Subjects were awake with their eyes closed and were relaxed during the scan. They were scanned in the supine and head-first position, with earplugs to alleviate the noise and cushions to restrict head motion. The T2-weighted images and fluid attenuated inversion recovery (FLAIR) images were acquired for radiological evaluation. The scan parameters were as follows: T1-weighted structural images were acquired using volumetric 3D magnetization prepared by rapid-acquisition gradient-echo (MP-RAGE) sequence for radiological evaluation and the anatomical segmentation and spatial normalization in preprocessing. The scan parameters were as follows: TR = 1900 ms, TE = 2.52 ms, FA = 9°, FOV = 256 × 256 mm^2, slices = 176, thickness = 1 mm, matrix = 256 × 256 and voxel size = 1 × 1 × 1 mm^3, sagittally scanned and lasted 4 min and 26 s. Resting-state functional images were collected using an echo planar imaging (EPI) sequence for functional processing: TR = 2000 ms, TE = 30 ms, FA = 90°, FOV = 192 × 192 mm^2, slices = 36, thickness = 3 mm, matrix = 64 × 64 and voxel size = 3 × 3 × 3 mm^3, 240 volumes, transversely scanned and lasted 8 min and 8 s.

[1] http://www.dtu.ox.ac.uk/homacalculator/

TABLE 1 | Demographic and clinical data of all included subjects.

	T2DM	HC	*p*-value
Age (years)	58.09 ± 7.26	56.88 ± 5.01	0.437
Sex (male:female)	19:13	18:14	0.800[a]
Education (years)	9.00 (9.00, 12.00)	12.00 (9.00, 12.00)	0.122[b]
T2DM duration (years)	10.00 (4.00, 12.50)	–	–
BMI (kg/m^2)	24.40 ± 2.73	23.89 ± 4.40	0.585
Systolic blood pressure (mmHg)	131.91 ± 17.23	133.72 ± 17.43	0.677
Diastolic blood pressure (mmHg)	82.00 ± 8.99	79.66 ± 10.06	0.330
HbA_{1c} (%)	8.30 ± 1.88	5.62 ± 0.39	<0.001
HbA_{1c} (mmol/mol)	67.25 ± 20.59	38.00 ± 4.28	<0.001
Fasting plasma glucose (mmol/L)	7.59 ± 2.82	5.25 ± 0.45	<0.001
Fasting insulin (mIU/L)	14.86 (9.66, 25.02)	12.85 (9.04, 17.35)	0.272[b]
Fasting C-peptide (ng/ml)	1.89 ± 1.08	2.34 ± 1.04	0.106
HOMA2-IR	0.29 (0.20, 0.53)	0.25 (0.17, 0.33)	0.124[b]
Total cholesterol (mmol/L)	5.01 ± 1.13	5.02 ± 0.98	0.955
Triglyceride (mmol/L)	1.64 (1.27, 3.00)	1.31 (0.89, 1.56)	0.018[b]
HDL cholesterol (mmol/L)	1.04 ± 0.23	1.39 ± 0.33	<0.001
LDL cholesterol (mmol/L)	3.21 ± 0.92	3.22 ± 0.75	0.944
Homocysteine (μmol/L)	16.01 ± 10.85	10.80 ± 4.47	0.260
Blood urea nitrogen (mmol/L)	6.08 ± 2.36	5.67 ± 1.23	0.392
Serum creatine (μmol/L)	73.38 ± 28.57	78.31 ± 16.20	0.399
Cystatin C (mg/L)	0.71 (0.63, 0.88)	0.79 (0.69, 0.86)	0.151[b]
Uric acid (μmol/L)	302.38 ± 76.77	325.88 ± 73.25	0.215
Free triiodothyronine, FT3 (pmol/L)	4.22 ± 0.86	5.05 ± 0.57	<0.001
Free thyroxine, FT4 (pmol/L)	15.09 ± 2.03	16.38 ± 2.02	0.014
Thyroid stimulating hormone, TSH (mIU/L)	1.96 ± 1.12	2.33 ± 1.42	0.251

$p < 0.05$ indicates statistically significant. [a]The Chi-square test for dichotomous data. [b]The Mann-Whitney U-test for non-normally distributed data [median (QR)]. Two sample t-test for normally distributed continuous data (means ± SD).

MRI Data Processing

Two radiologists with at least 5-year work experience reviewed the T1-weighted, T2-weighted and FLAIR images to identify brain structural abnormalities and to rate white matter changes. None of the subjects met the exclusion criteria. The structural and functional images underwent preprocessing with a standard protocol in Graph Theoretical Network Analysis Toolbox version 1.2.1 (GRETNA V1.2.1) (Wang et al., 2015) as follows: (1) The DICOM data were transformed into NIfTI format. (2) The first 10 volumes of individual functional images were then removed for magnetization equilibrium. (3) Next, slice timing was performed to correct the temporal offsets between slices. (4) Realignment was performed to make each part of the brain across volumes in the same position. (5) Spatial normalization was performed to warp individual functional images to standard Montreal Neurological Institute (MNI) space derived from T1 images segmentation. (6) Detrend was applied to reduce the systematic drift in the signal. (7) The data were bandpass filtered (0.01–0.08 Hz) to reduce the effects of low frequency drift and physiological noises at high-frequency band. (8) Covariate regression was applied to remove the confounding variables, including head motion profiles, the cerebrospinal fluid signal, the white matter signals and the global signal.

Voxel-based degree analysis was conducted within a gray matter mask on the basis of preprocessed images. The connectional threshold of FCD was set at 0.3 (Tomasi et al., 2016). It has been proven that 75 mm approximately reflects the true physical distance of connections between regions (He et al., 2007). Therefore, the sum of functional connectivity between a given voxel and other voxels beyond the sphere radius of 75 mm were defined as long-range FCD, whereas the sum of functional connectivity between a given voxel and other voxels within the sphere radius of 75 mm were defined as short-range FCD (Guo et al., 2015). Taking the sign into consideration, the FCD can be classified into four categories: long-range positive/negative FCD (lpFCD and lnFCD) and short-range positive/negative FCD (spFCD and snFCD). Spatial smoothing with 4 mm full-width half-maximum was used to improve the signal-to-noise ratio of FCD maps (Tomasi and Volkow, 2010). The brain regions with aberrant FCD obtained from the subsequent two-sample *t*-test were saved as seeds for the functional connectivity calculation. The functional connectivity calculation was performed with Resting-State fMRI Data Analysis Toolkit version 1.8 (REST V1.8) software on the basis of preprocessed images. To facilitate the statistical analyses, Fisher transformation (*r*-to-*z* transformation) was applied to normalize the distribution of *Pearson* correlation coefficient values of functional connectivity.

Statistical Analyses

Numeric data analysis was conducted with SPSS software (version 20.0; IBM Corp., Armonk, NY, United States). Firstly, the *Kolmogorov-Smirnov* test was applied to confirm normal distribution of the data. According to the results, the two-sample *t*-test was applied to normally distributed continuous data, whereas the *Mann-Whitney U*-test was applied to non-normally distributed data comparisons between the T2DM group and HC group. The inter-group comparison of dichotomous data (sex) was performed using the *Chi-square* test. Values of $p < 0.05$ were considered statistically significant.

Functional connectivity density and functional connectivity maps analyses were conducted with the Statistical Analysis module of Data Processing & Analysis of Brain Imaging version 2.3 (DPABI V2.3). Firstly, the one-sample *t*-test was performed to confirm the FCD and functional connectivity distribution pattern with the base of "0" in each group. The two-sample *t*-test was then performed to compare the differences in FCD between the T2DM group and HC group, with age, sex, education, BMI, Power framewise displacement for head motion (Power et al., 2013) and the blood biometric measurements that showed significant differences (with the exception of glycemic measurements) entered as covariates. The resulting maps were multiple comparisons corrected with the Gaussian random-field theory (voxel $p = 0.01$, cluster $p < 0.05$). Z scores of T2DM patients were extracted from significantly changed brain regions according to the inter-group FCD comparison. Finally, *Pearson* correlation analyses were conducted to investigate the relationships among the changed FCD, neuropsychological test scores and clinical data after adjustment for age, sex, education, BMI and the blood biometric measurements that showed significant differences (with the exception of glycemic measurements) using SPSS software.

RESULTS

Demographic and Clinical Data Comparisons

The T2DM patients were not significantly different to the HC group in terms of age, sex, education, BMI, blood pressure, fasting insulin, fasting C-peptide, HOMA2-IR, total cholesterol, low-density lipoprotein (LDL) cholesterol, homocysteine, blood urea nitrogen, serum creatine, cystatin C, uric acid, and thyroid stimulating hormone ($p > 0.05$). As expected, the levels of HbA_{1c} and fasting plasma glucose were elevated in T2DM patients. In addition, higher triglyceride and lower high-density lipoprotein (HDL) cholesterol, free triiodothyronine (FT3) and free thyroxine (FT4) levels were observed in T2DM patients ($p < 0.05$, **Table 1**).

Neuropsychological Tests Comparisons

The T2DM patients scored lower in the MMSE, MoCA, DST forward, and AVLT (including short-term delayed recall, long-term delayed recall, long-term delayed recognition and total score) tests, and took longer to finish the TMT-B test ($p < 0.05$). There were no significant inter-group differences in the other neuropsychological tests (**Table 2**).

FCD and Functional Connectivity Analyses

The one-sample *t*-test suggested that both the HC and T2DM groups exhibited higher long-range FCD than the mean brain

TABLE 2 | Comparisons of neuropsychological test performance between the T2DM group and HC group.

	T2DM	HC	*p*-value
General cognition			
MMSE	28.00 (27.00, 29.00)	29.00 (28.00, 29.75)	0.044[a]
MoCA	22.88 ± 2.64	24.78 ± 2.35	0.003
Executive function and psychomotor speed			
TMT-A	76.31 ± 45.42	61.31 ± 35.33	0.145
TMT-B	173.53 ± 85.23	132.59 ± 61.58	0.033
Mental flexibility			
VFT	39.75 ± 6.49	42.63 ± 6.30	0.077
Working memory			
DST forward	8.84 ± 1.25	9.63 ± 1.66	0.038
DST backward	4.00 (3.00, 4.00)	4.00 (3.00, 4.00)	0.657[a]
Episodic memory			
AVLT immediate recall	6.50 ± 1.51	7.18 ± 1.23	0.052
AVLT short-term delayed recall	6.41 ± 3.20	8.13 ± 2.14	0.014
AVLT long-term delayed recall	4.72 ± 3.59	7.00 ± 2.09	0.003
AVLT long-term delayed recognition	10.13 ± 3.60	11.72 ± 2.22	0.038
AVLT total score	27.75 ± 9.56	34.03 ± 6.11	0.003

$p < 0.05$ indicates statistically significant. [a]The Mann-Whitney U-test for non-normally distributed data [median (QR)]. Two sample t-test for normally distributed continuous data (means ± SD).

level primarily in the bilateral posterior cingulate gyri and precuneus, and lower long-range FCD than the mean brain level primarily in the bilateral temporal lobes and frontal lobes; higher short-range FCD primarily in the bilateral calcarine, angular gyri, and frontal lobes, and lower short-range FCD primarily in the bilateral middle cingulate gyri and temporal lobes were also observed (**Figure 1**). Taking the identified brain areas as seed regions, they showed positive and negative correlations with comprehensive areas of the rest of the brain. That is, the seed regions exhibited functional connectivity throughout the brain (**Figure 2**).

Compared with the HC group, T2DM patients showed significantly decreased long-range FCD including lnFCD in the left lingual gyrus and lpFCD in the left calcarine extending to the left lingual gyrus after multiple comparisons correction. In addition, T2DM patients showed increased short-range FCD including snFCD in the medial part of the left superior frontal gyrus and spFCD in the right angular gyrus after multiple comparisons correction (**Table 3** and **Figure 3**). T2DM patients also showed aberrant functional connectivity anchoring in these identified brain regions. However, these results did not survive multiple comparisons correction.

Correlation Analyses

In T2DM patients, the z scores of FCD in the medial part of the left superior frontal gyrus were negatively correlated with the time cost of the TMT-B test ($r = -0.422$, $p = 0.018$; **Figure 4A**). In addition, the z scores of FCD in the right angular gyrus were negatively correlated with the scores of AVLT long-term delayed recall ($r = -0.356$, $p = 0.049$; **Figure 4B**) and DST forward ($r = -0.373$, $p = 0.039$; **Figure 4C**). No correlations were observed among the aberrant neuroimaging indicators, blood biometric measurements and other neuropsychological tests.

DISCUSSION

Previous research proposed that brain networks may negotiate a trade-off between the energy-cost and information propagation efficiency (Bullmore and Sporns, 2012). As the disturbance in glucose metabolism may affect the brain energy homeostasis in T2DM, the present study investigated the disruption in the balance between the long- and short-range FCD. We found that T2DM patients showed decreased long-range FCD in the left calcarine and lingual gyrus and increased short-range FCD in the left superior frontal gyrus and right angular gyrus. These changes were significantly associated with performance on neuropsychological tests in T2DM patients. Our findings may update the insight into T2DM-related brain dysfunction.

The brain regions which exhibited aberrant FCD were reported to be abnormal in previous studies, which suggest that they are susceptible to T2DM. A meta-analysis demonstrated that the superior frontal gyrus and lingual gyrus are robust brain regions with altered resting-state brain activity (Xia et al., 2017). The frontal lobe is involved in executive function and attention that underlies advanced cognition (Xia et al., 2017). Together with occipital regions, the lingual gyrus was considered a brain region involved in vision-related information processing and visual memory encoding (Cui et al., 2016). The lingual gyrus was reported to have a reduced degree of centrality in T2DM patients (Cui et al., 2016), which was similar to that found in the present study. Our previous study also demonstrated aberrant functional connectivity anchoring in the angular gyrus that may serve as a neuroimaging marker for T2DM-related cognitive decline (Liu et al., 2016). With regard to the calcarine, decreased regional homogeneity and amplitude of low frequency fluctuations were observed in T2DM patients, which were associated with cognitive performance (Cui et al., 2014; Peng et al., 2016). In addition to the aforementioned studies, the present study also identified these abnormal brain regions with high centrality due to the similar definition of FCD and degree of centrality (Zuo et al., 2012). According to the computational modeling of neural dynamics, the cerebral cortex with a high degree of centrality plays a pivotal role in global information integration and intermodular communication, which are vulnerable to attack by disease (Bullmore and Sporns, 2012).

The disruption in the balance between long- and short-range FCD may suggest a shift from the costly metabolic connection to an economic connection. Previous studies have reported alterations in long- and short-range functional connectivity strength (Liu et al., 2017), and local and remote brain activity synchronization in T2DM patients (Liu et al., 2016). The present study further suggests that T2DM patients have more short-range connections and fewer long-range connections. There

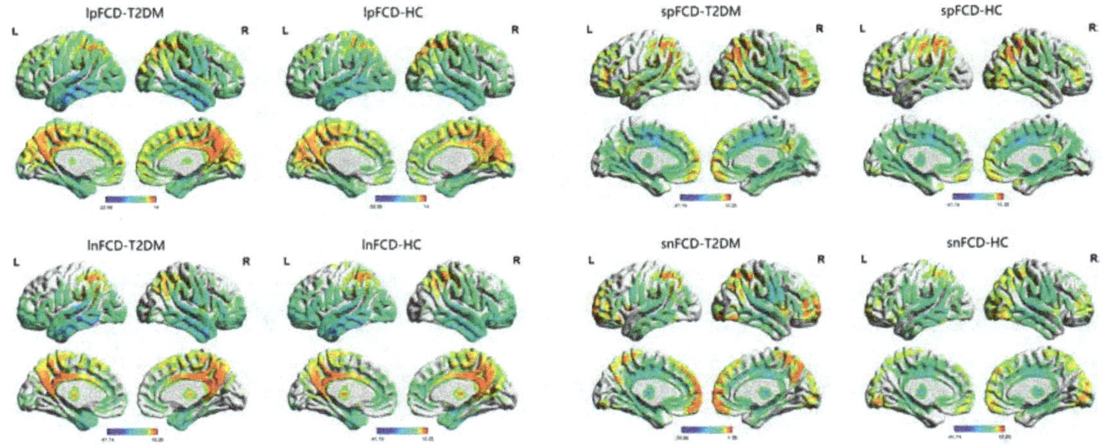

FIGURE 1 | The distribution of FCD in the T2DM group and HC group. Color scale denotes the *t*-value. L, left; R, right.

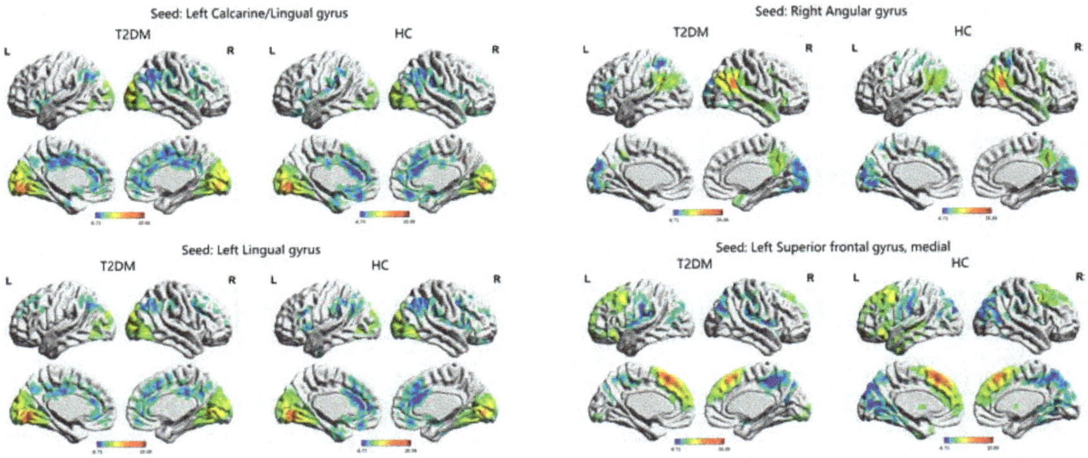

FIGURE 2 | The distribution of functional connectivity of each seed region in the T2DM group and HC group. Color scale denotes the *t*-value. L, left; R, right.

TABLE 3 | Brain regions with significant differences in FCD between the T2DM group and HC group.

		Brodmann	Peak MNI coordinates			*T*-values	Voxels	Cluster size
		Area	X	Y	Z			(mm^3)
lpFCD	Left Calcarine/Lingual gyrus	17/18	−3	−90	0	−4.0559	36	972
lnFCD	Left Lingual gyrus	18	−9	−78	−6	−4.122	41	1107
spFCD	Right Angular gyrus	39/40	54	−51	33	3.8163	44	1188
snFCD	Left Superior frontal gyrus, medial	8	−3	30	51	4.4059	39	1053

MNI, Montreal Neurological Institute; Gaussian random-field theory corrected (voxel $p = 0.01$, cluster $p < 0.05$).

is evidence that the energy-cost of a node increases with the number of connections, and that the energy-cost of a connection increases with length (Sepulcre et al., 2010; Bullmore and Sporns, 2012). Moreover, it was proposed that brain regions with high energy-cost such as hubs and long-distance connections may be sensitive to metabolic distress, and they may reconfigure to achieve variable cognitive demands via the negotiation between connection cost and topological properties of the networks (Kitzbichler et al., 2011; Bullmore and Sporns, 2012). This process of negotiating continues across milliseconds to decades (Bullmore and Sporns, 2012). As with the reduced proportion of long connections in Alzheimer's disease (Yao et al., 2010), the decreased long-range FCD in T2DM patients may be associated with diminished integrative capacity. We can therefore speculate that the high-cost components in T2DM patients including hubs with high-degree and long-distance connections may be selectively attacked. Furthermore, according to recent findings, the decreased long-range FCD may be prejudicial to the diversity

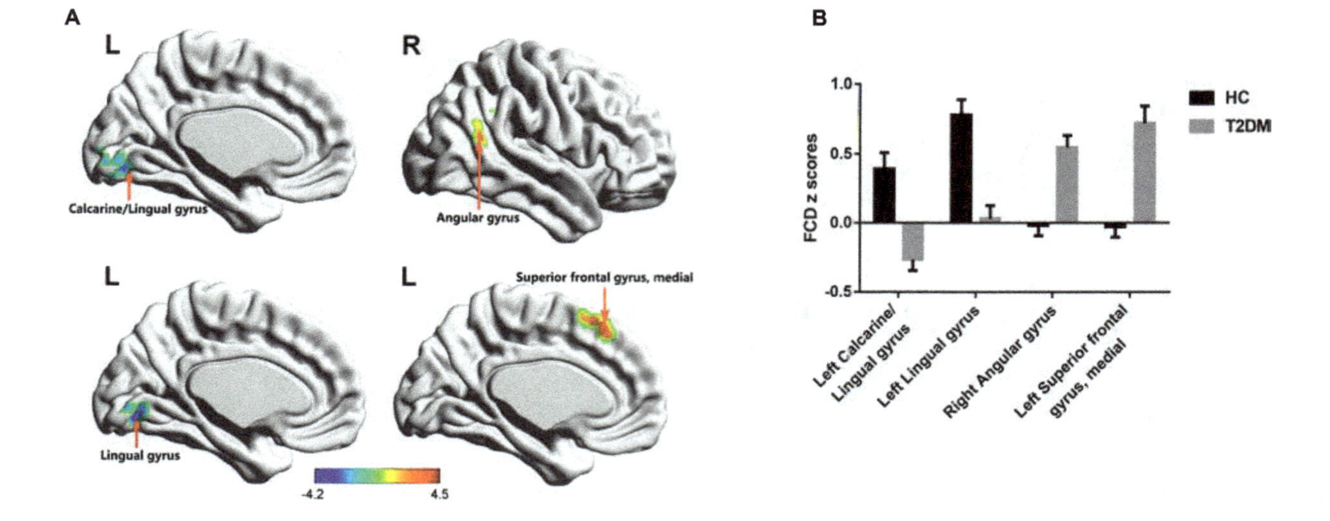

FIGURE 3 | FCD maps of inter-group comparisons. **(A)** The distribution of brain regions with changed FCD in the T2DM group. **(B)** The comparison of FCD z scores between the T2DM group and HC group. Gaussian random-field theory corrected (voxel $p = 0.01$, cluster $p < 0.05$). Color scale denotes the *t*-value. Error bars define the standard error of the mean. L, left; R, right.

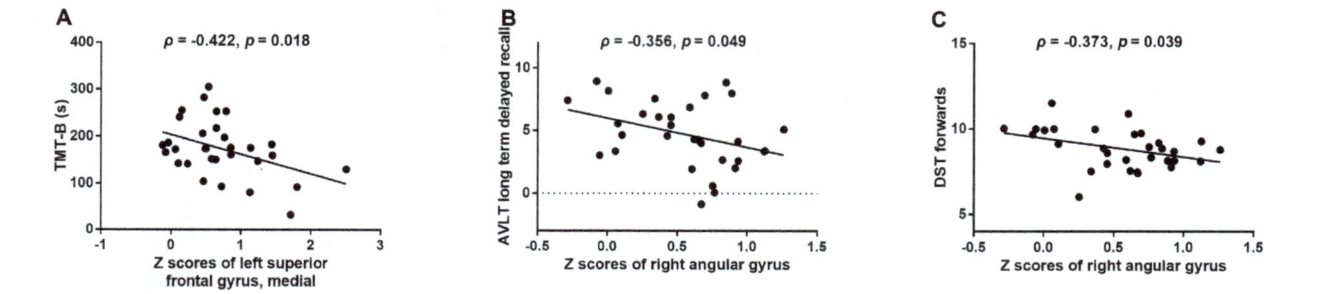

FIGURE 4 | The relationships between changed FCD and aberrant neuropsychological tests in the T2DM group. **(A)** Z scores of FCD in the medial part of the left superior frontal gyrus vs. scores of the TMT-B test. **(B)** Z scores of FCD in the right angular gyrus vs. scores of the AVLT long-term delayed recall. **(C)** Z scores of FCD in the right angular gyrus vs. scores of the DST forward.

of inputs and outputs in brain areas (Betzel and Bassett, 2018).

Our findings also suggest that the reconfiguration of long- and short-range FCD was associated with the neurocognitive outcomes in T2DM patients. On the one hand, T2DM patients with higher z scores in the right angular gyrus scored lower in the AVLT long-term delayed recall and DST forward tests. This situation is partly similar to patients with autism spectrum disorders whose short-range functional overconnectivity was reported to be positively associated with symptom severity (Keown et al., 2013). The brain regions with preferential short-range connections may be characterized by low energy-cost and high clustering coefficients, but a long path length which have low information propagation efficiency through the network (Sepulcre et al., 2010). On the other hand, the short-range functional overconnectivity of the medial part of the left superior frontal gyrus may play a compensatory role in the better performance of T2DM patients in the TMT-B test. The brain network of children was found to communicate more efficiently due to more short-range interactions and the small world property of the brain network was comparable to that of adults (Fair et al., 2009). A possible explanation for this might be that the reconfigured brain network shares the characteristics of those in children to maintain normal cognitive function. However, the discrepant neurocognitive outcomes of increased short-range FCD require further clarification.

There are several notable limitations in this study. First, this was a cross-sectional study; therefore, the progress of supposed neural compensation cannot be captured and interpretation of the findings should be taken with caution, especially in terms of causality. Second, the functional connections were calculated on the assumption that the time series of distinct brain regions is constant over time. However, this is not ideal for reflecting the dynamic nature of brain activity (Hutchison et al., 2013). Third, the relatively small sample of subjects may restrict the statistical power. Longitudinal studies with a larger sample size to investigate the dynamic connectome may better characterize the diabetic brain and update the neuroimaging evidence of cognitive decline in T2DM patients. Moreover, we conducted global signal regression in the present study to denoise the artifactual fMRI signal, however, it may result in spurious anticorrelations and the global signal fluctuations could reflect true neural variance (Power et al., 2017). Strategies of isolating and removing global artifactual variance while preserving potential global variance may end the controversy on global signal regression in the future.

CONCLUSION

In the present study, long- and short-range FCD were used to determine distance information in the brain network of T2DM patients. We found that T2DM patients exhibited increased short-range FCD and decreased long-range FCD which may suggest a trade-off between energy-cost and network efficiency at the expense of losing cognitive function. These findings may improve our understanding and provide potential neuroimaging markers for T2DM brain dysfunction.

AUTHOR CONTRIBUTIONS

DL contributed to the experiments, data analysis, and writing of the manuscript. LC contributed to the data analysis and revised the manuscript. SD contributed to data collection. XY contributed to the data analysis. WY contributed to the statistical analysis. YS contributed to the manuscript revision. JZ and JW are the guarantors of this study and had complete access to all data in the study. All authors accept responsibility for the integrity of the data and the accuracy of the data analysis.

FUNDING

The study was supported by the National Natural Science Foundation of China (81471647) and the National Key R&D Program of China (No. 2016YFC0107101).

ACKNOWLEDGMENTS

The authors thank all volunteers who participated in the study and the staff of the Department of Laboratory Medicine and Department of Nuclear Medicine at the Southwest Hospital of the Third Military Medical University (Army Medical University) in Chongqing, China for their selfless and valuable assistance.

REFERENCES

Alberti, K. G., and Zimmet, P. Z. (1998). Definition, diagnosis and classification of diabetes mellitus and its complications. Part 1: diagnosis and classification of diabetes mellitus provisional report of a WHO consultation. *Diabet. Med.* 15, 539–553.

Betzel, R. F., and Bassett, D. S. (2018). Specificity and robustness of long-distance connections in weighted, interareal connectomes. *Proc. Natl. Acad. Sci. U.S.A.* 115, E4880–E4889. doi: 10.1073/pnas.1720186115

Bowie, C. R., and Harvey, P. D. (2006). Administration and interpretation of the trail making test. *Nat. Protoc.* 1, 2277–2281. doi: 10.1038/nprot.2006.390

Bullmore, E., and Sporns, O. (2012). The economy of brain network organization. *Nat. Rev. Neurosci.* 13, 336–349. doi: 10.1038/nrn3214

Chen, Y., Liu, Z., Zhang, J., Tian, G., Li, L., Zhang, S., et al. (2015). Selectively disrupted functional connectivity networks in type 2 diabetes mellitus. *Front. Aging Neurosci.* 7:233. doi: 10.3389/fnagi.2015.00233

Chen, Y. C., Jiao, Y., Cui, Y., Shang, S. A., Ding, J., Feng, Y., et al. (2014). Aberrant brain functional connectivity related to insulin resistance in type 2 diabetes: a resting-state fMRI study. *Diabetes Care* 37, 1689–1696. doi: 10.2337/dc13-2127

Cui, Y., Jiao, Y., Chen, Y. C., Wang, K., Gao, B., Wen, S., et al. (2014). Altered spontaneous brain activity in type 2 diabetes: a resting-state functional MRI study. *Diabetes Metab. Res. Rev.* 63, 749–760. doi: 10.2337/db13-0519

Cui, Y., Li, S. F., Gu, H., Hu, Y. Z., Liang, X., Lu, C. Q., et al. (2016). Disrupted brain connectivity patterns in patients with type 2 diabetes. *AJNR Am. J. Neuroradiol.* 37, 2115–2122. doi: 10.3174/ajnr.A4858

Diamond, A. (2013). Executive functions. *Annu. Rev. Psychol.* 64, 135–168. doi: 10.1146/annurev-psych-113011-143750

Fair, D. A., Cohen, A. L., Power, J. D., Dosenbach, N. U., Church, J. A., Miezin, F. M., et al. (2009). Functional brain networks develop from a "local to distributed" organization. *PLoS Comput. Biol.* 5:e1000381. doi: 10.1371/journal.pcbi.1000381

Garcia-Casares, N., Jorge, R. E., Garcia-Arnes, J. A., Acion, L., Berthier, M. L., Gonzalez-Alegre, P., et al. (2014). Cognitive dysfunctions in middle-aged type 2 diabetic patients and neuroimaging correlations: a cross-sectional study. *J. Alzheimers. Dis.* 42, 1337–1346. doi: 10.3233/JAD-140702

Guo, W., Liu, F., Xiao, C., Liu, J., Yu, M., Zhang, Z., et al. (2015). Increased short-range and long-range functional connectivity in first-episode, medication-naive schizophrenia at rest. *Schizophr. Res.* 166, 144–150. doi: 10.1016/j.schres.2015.04.034

He, Y., Chen, Z. J., and Evans, A. C. (2007). Small-world anatomical networks in the human brain revealed by cortical thickness from MRI. *Cereb. Cortex* 17, 2407–2419. doi: 10.1093/cercor/bhl149

Hutchison, R. M., Womelsdorf, T., Allen, E. A., Bandettini, P. A., Calhoun, V. D., Corbetta, M., et al. (2013). Dynamic functional connectivity: promise, issues, and interpretations. *Neuroimage* 80, 360–378. doi: 10.1016/j.neuroimage.2013.05.079

Keown, C. L., Shih, P., Nair, A., Peterson, N., Mulvey, M. E., and Muller, R. A. (2013). Local functional overconnectivity in posterior brain regions is associated with symptom severity in autism spectrum disorders. *Cell Rep.* 5, 567–572. doi: 10.1016/j.celrep.2013.10.003

Kitzbichler, M. G., Henson, R. N., Smith, M. L., Nathan, P. J., and Bullmore, E. T. (2011). Cognitive effort drives workspace configuration of human brain functional networks. *J. Neurosci.* 31, 8259–8270. doi: 10.1523/jneurosci.0440-11.2011

Koekkoek, P. S., Kappelle, L. J., van den Berg, E., Rutten, G. E., and Biessels, G. J. (2015). Cognitive function in patients with diabetes mellitus: guidance for daily care. *Lancet Neurol.* 14, 329–340. doi: 10.1016/S1474-4422(14)70249-2

Liu, D., Duan, S., Zhang, J., Zhou, C., Liang, M., Yin, X., et al. (2016). Aberrant brain regional homogeneity and functional connectivity in middle-aged T2DM patients: a resting-state functional MRI study. *Front. Hum. Neurosci.* 10:490. doi: 10.3389/fnhum.2016.00490

Liu, L., Li, W., Zhang, Y., Qin, W., Lu, S., and Zhang, Q. (2017). Weaker functional connectivity strength in patients with type 2 diabetes mellitus. *Front. Neurosci.* 11:390. doi: 10.3389/fnins.2017.00390

Lu, F. M., Zhou, J. S., Wang, X. P., Xiang, Y. T., and Yuan, Z. (2017). Short- and long-range functional connectivity density alterations in adolescents with pure conduct disorder at resting-state. *Neuroscience* 351, 96–107. doi: 10.1016/j.neuroscience.2017.03.040

Magistretti, P. J., and Allaman, I. (2015). A cellular perspective on brain energy metabolism and functional imaging. *Neuron* 86, 883–901. doi: 10.1016/j.neuron.2015.03.035

Peng, J., Qu, H., Peng, J., Luo, T. Y., Lv, F. J., Chen, L., et al. (2016). Abnormal spontaneous brain activity in type 2 diabetes with and without microangiopathy revealed by regional homogeneity. *Eur. J. Radiol.* 85, 607–615. doi: 10.1016/j.ejrad.2015.12.024

Power, J. D., Barnes, K. A., Snyder, A. Z., Schlaggar, B. L., and Petersen, S. E. (2013). Steps toward optimizing motion artifact removal in functional connectivity

MRI; a reply to Carp. *Neuroimage* 76, 439–441. doi: 10.1016/j.neuroimage.2012.03.017

Power, J. D., Plitt, M., Laumann, T. O., and Martin, A. (2017). Sources and implications of whole-brain fMRI signals in humans. *Neuroimage* 146, 609–625. doi: 10.1016/j.neuroimage.2016.09.038

Qi, R., Zhang, L. J., Chen, H. J., Zhong, J., Luo, S., Ke, J., et al. (2015). Role of local and distant functional connectivity density in the development of minimal hepatic encephalopathy. *Sci. Rep.* 5:13720. doi: 10.1038/srep13720

Sepulcre, J., Liu, H., Talukdar, T., Martincorena, I., Yeo, B. T., and Buckner, R. L. (2010). The organization of local and distant functional connectivity in the human brain. *PLoS Comput. Biol.* 6:e1000808. doi: 10.1371/journal.pcbi.1000808

Tomasi, D., Shokri-Kojori, E., and Volkow, N. D. (2016). High-resolution functional connectivity density: hub locations, sensitivity, specificity, reproducibility, and reliability. *Cereb. Cortex* 26, 3249–3259. doi: 10.1093/cercor/bhv171

Tomasi, D., and Volkow, N. D. (2010). Functional connectivity density mapping. *Proc. Natl. Acad. Sci. U.S.A.* 107, 9885–9890. doi: 10.1073/pnas.1001414107

Wahlund, L. O., Barkhof, F., Fazekas, F., Bronge, L., Augustin, M., Sjogren, M., et al. (2001). A new rating scale for age-related white matter changes applicable to MRI and CT. *Stroke* 32, 1318–1322. doi: 10.1161/01.STR.32.6.1318

Wang, J., Wang, X., Xia, M., Liao, X., Evans, A., and He, Y. (2015). GRETNA: a graph theoretical network analysis toolbox for imaging connectomics. *Front. Hum. Neurosci.* 9:386. doi: 10.3389/fnhum.2015.00386

Xia, W., Chen, Y. C., and Ma, J. (2017). Resting-state brain anomalies in type 2 diabetes: a meta-analysis. *Front. Aging Neurosci.* 9:14. doi: 10.3389/fnagi.2017.00014

Xia, W., Wang, S., Sun, Z., Bai, F., Zhou, Y., Yang, Y., et al. (2013). Altered baseline brain activity in type 2 diabetes: a resting-state fMRI study. *Psychoneuroendocrinology* 38, 2493–2501. doi: 10.1016/j.psyneuen.2013.05.012

Yao, Z., Zhang, Y., Lin, L., Zhou, Y., Xu, C., and Jiang, T. (2010). Abnormal cortical networks in mild cognitive impairment and Alzheimer's disease. *PLoS Comput. Biol.* 6:e1001006. doi: 10.1371/journal.pcbi.1001006

Zhang, X. D., Cheng, Y., Poon, C. S., Qi, R., Xu, Q., Chen, H. J., et al. (2015a). Long- and short-range functional connectivity density alteration in non-alcoholic cirrhotic patients one month after liver transplantation: a resting-state fMRI study. *Brain Res.* 1620, 177–187. doi: 10.1016/j.brainres.2015.04.046

Zhang, X. D., Wen, J. Q., Xu, Q., Qi, R., Chen, H. J., Kong, X., et al. (2015b). Altered long- and short-range functional connectivity in the patients with end-stage renal disease: a resting-state functional MRI study. *Metab. Brain Dis.* 30, 1175–1186. doi: 10.1007/s11011-015-9683-z

Zhao, Q., Guo, Q., Liang, X., Chen, M., Zhou, Y., Ding, D., et al. (2015). Auditory verbal learning test is superior to rey-osterrieth complex figure memory for predicting mild cognitive impairment to Alzheimer's disease. *Curr. Alzheimer Res.* 12, 520–526. doi: 10.2174/1567205012666150530202729

Zuo, X. N., Ehmke, R., Mennes, M., Imperati, D., Castellanos, F. X., Sporns, O., et al. (2012). Network centrality in the human functional connectome. *Cereb. Cortex* 22, 1862–1875. doi: 10.1093/cercor/bhr269

4

Increased Functional Connectivity Between Medulla and Inferior Parietal Cortex in Medication-Free Major Depressive Disorder

Lizhu Luo[1†], Kunhua Wu[2†], Yi Lu[3†], Shan Gao[1,4], Xiangchao Kong[1], Fengmei Lu[1], Fengchun Wu[5,6], Huawang Wu[5,6] and Jiaojian Wang[1*]*

[1] The Clinical Hospital of Chengdu Brain Science Institute, MOE Key Laboratory for Neuroinformation, University of Electronic Science and Technology of China, Chengdu, China, [2] Department of MRI, The First People's Hospital of Yunnan Province, The Affiliated Hospital of Kunming University of Science and Technology, Kunming, China, [3] The Department of Medical Imaging, The First Affiliated Hospital of Kunming Medical University, Kunming, China, [4] School of Foreign Languages, University of Electronic Science and Technology of China, Chengdu, China, [5] The Affiliated Brain Hospital of Guangzhou Medical University (Guangzhou Huiai Hospital), Guangzhou, China, [6] Guangdong Engineering Technology Research Center for Translational Medicine of Mental Disorders, Guangzhou, China

***Correspondence:**
Huawang Wu
huawangwu@126.com
Jiaojian Wang
jiaojianwang@gmail.com

† These authors have contributed equally to this work

Emerging evidence has documented the abnormalities of primary brain functions in major depressive disorder (MDD). The brainstem has shown to play an important role in regulating basic functions of the human brain, but little is known about its role in MDD, especially the roles of its subregions. To uncover this, the present study adopted resting-state functional magnetic resonance imaging with fine-grained brainstem atlas in 23 medication-free MDD patients and 34 matched healthy controls (HC). The analysis revealed significantly increased functional connectivity of the medulla, one of the brainstem subregions, with the inferior parietal cortex (IPC) in MDD patients. A positive correlation was further identified between the increased medulla-IPC functional connectivity and Hamilton anxiety scores. Functional characterization of the medulla and IPC using a meta-analysis revealed that both regions primarily participated in action execution and inhibition. Our findings suggest that increased medulla-IPC functional connectivity may be related to over-activity or abnormal control of negative emotions in MDD, which provides a new insight for the neurobiology of MDD.

Keywords: major depressive disorder, resting-state functional connectivity, brainstem, subregions, medulla, inferior parietal cortex

INTRODUCTION

Major depressive disorder (MDD) is mainly characterized with sustained negative affect and diminished positive affect. Neuroimaging studies, especially those using resting-state functional magnetic resonance imaging (rs-fMRI), have revealed that MDD is a disease with aberrant interactions of brain networks (Buchanan et al., 2014; Mulders et al., 2015; Smith, 2015; Wu et al., 2016; Kang et al., 2017; Sun et al., 2018; Wang C. et al., 2018). Using resting-state functional connectivity (RSFC) analyses, abnormalities in cortical networks including the default mode network (DMN), central executive network (CEN), and salience network (SN) have been well delineated (Mulders et al., 2015; Wang J. et al., 2018). Moreover, recent studies have demonstrated that the functional connectivities in frontostriatal and limbic circuits could be effective indicators to subdivide MDD into four biotypes, which in turn also serve as good predictors of treatment response in MDD (Drysdale et al., 2017; Wager and Woo, 2017). Although the high-order functional network abnormalities have been well studied, basic functions related brain areas including the brainstem in MDD remain largely unknown.

The brainstem, together with limbic and cortical areas, compose a vertical-integrative and interconnected hierarchical system that is critical in emotion as well as kinds of cognition (Geva and Feldman, 2008; Abe et al., 2010; Lee et al., 2015; Nishijo et al., 2018). Brainstem lesions could have a crucial impact on higher-level functions of cortical regions, such as attention, executive function and self-regulation (Geva and Feldman, 2008; Nishijo et al., 2018). The brainstem is called "the emotional brainstem" due to its critical role in human emotions by integrating its subregions into three major networks involving in emotional sensory, motor and modulatory (Venkatraman et al., 2017). Moreover, the brainstem is a primary source of neurotransmitter innervations such as serotonergic and dopaminergic ones that are critically associated with a wide range of brain functions, and their dysregulations of fronto-limbic circuits and the hypothalamic-pituitary-adrenal (HPA) axis in MDD have been reported (Aihara et al., 2007; Song et al., 2014; Han et al., 2017). These findings point to a key role of the brainstem in the pathophysiology of MDD.

However, the brainstem anatomically includes three parts, from top to bottom namely the midbrain, the pons, and the medulla oblongata. Most previous studies emphasized the critical role of upper brainstem including midbrain and pons with its connection to cortical networks through serotonergic, dopaminergic, and noradrenergic neurotransmission in the pathophysiology of depression (Nye et al., 2013; Hahn et al., 2014; Smith, 2015; Numasawa et al., 2017; Wagner et al., 2017; Post and Warden, 2018). Unlike the midbrain and pons, the medulla is a more primitive location controlling low-level autonomic functions such as breathing, blood pressure and heart rate (Smythies, 2011) and was one part of the human central homeostatic network (CHN) (Edlow et al., 2016). Therefore, to identify aberrant interconnections between brainstem subregions and cortical networks at fine-grained level may contribute to a better understanding of the mechanism of onset of MDD.

In the present study, we investigated the functional connectivity pattern alterations of brainstem subregions using rs-fMRI in a group of 23 medication-free MDD patients and 34 gender-, age-, and education level-matched healthy controls (HC). We first defined three subregions of brainstem, namely the midbrain, pons and medulla separately using a recently developed brainstem atlas (Iglesias et al., 2015). Then, whole brain RSFC analyses were performed to identify the changed functional connectivity patterns for each brainstem subregion in MDD patients. According to previous findings on disrupted functional connectivity of brainstem and its subregions in depression (Smith, 2015; Wagner et al., 2017), we hypothesized that there might be also dysfunctions within the functional network based on the three subregions of brainstem in medication-free MDD patients.

MATERIALS AND METHODS

Subjects

Twenty three medication-free, right-handed MDD patients and 34 age-, gender-, and educational level- matched healthy controls (18–46 years) were recruited from the Affiliated Brain Hospital of Guangzhou Medical University (**Table 1**). The diagnosis of MDD used the Structured Clinical Interview based on DSM-IV criteria (SCID) and the Chinese version of 24-item Hamilton Depression Rating Scale (HDRS). Hamilton Anxiety scale (HAMA) was also used to assess their anxiety level. Additionally, HCs were screened with no Axis I Disorders based on the SCID non-patient edition. All the HCs reported no history of psychiatric illness for all biological relatives within three generations. Both MDD and HC groups reported no lifetime history of head injury, seizures, serious medical or surgical illness, as well as substance abuse, and were free of MRI contraindications. This study was approved by the local Ethics Committee of the Affiliated Brain Hospital of Guangzhou Medical University with written informed consent from all subjects and was carried out in accordance with their recommendations. All subjects gave written informed consent in accordance with the Declaration of Helsinki.

Resting-State fMRI Data Acquisition

Resting-state fMRI data were acquired on a 3 Tesla MR imaging system (Philips Medical Systems, Best, Netherlands) with an eight-channel SENSE head coil in the Affiliated Brain Hospital of Guangzhou Medical University, Guangzhou, China, using a gradient-echo echo-planar imaging (GRE-EPI) sequence sensitive to blood oxygenation level-dependent (BOLD) contrast. Before scanning, tight and comfortable foam paddings and earplugs were used to reduce head moving and noise in the scanner separately. During the scanning, subjects were instructed to close their eyes but not to sleep. The acquisition parameters were as follows: repetition time (TR) = 2000 ms, echo time (TE) = 30 ms, flip angle (FA) = 90°, matrix = 64 × 64, field of

TABLE 1 | Demographics and clinical characteristics of the subjects used in the present study.

Subjects	MDD	HC	*p*-value
Number of subjects	23	34	
Gender (male: female)	9/14	15/19	0.7083
Age (mean ± *SD*)	30.48 ± 7.13	29.71 ± 7.09	0.6888
Years of education (mean ± *SD*)	13.35 ± 3.89	14.18 ± 2.17	0.3072
HDRS scores (mean ± *SD*)	34.30 ± 7.58		
HAMA scores (mean ± *SD*)	24.36 ± 8.63		
Age of onset (years)	27 ± 7.44		
Duration of illness (months)	43.04 ± 58.18		
Episodes (n, patients)			
First	17		
Recurrence	6		
Family history cf MDD (n, patients)	5		

Pearson's chi-squared test was used for gender comparison. Two-sample t-tests were used for age and education comparisons. HDRS, hamilton depression rating scale; HAMA, hamilton anxiety scale.

view (FOV) = 220 × 220 mm^2, 33 axial slices, slice thickness = 4 mm, inter-slice gap = 0.6 mm, 240 volumes.

Resting-State fMRI Data Preprocessing

The resting-state fMRI data were preprocessed using Statistical Parametric Mapping (SPM8[1]) software and DPARSF (version 2.3[2]). It was started with discard of the first 10 volumes, slice timing, realignment based on the first volume for head motion correction, and followed by normalization based on MNI space template with 3 mm cubic voxel resolution, smoothing with a Gaussian kernel of 6 mm full-width at half maximum (FWHM), as well as regression of six motion parameters, white matter, and cerebrospinal fluid signals, and finally ended by filter with a temporal band-path of 0.01–0.1 Hz. After realignment, data with head-movement exceeded 1.5 mm of translation or 1.5 degrees of rotation in any direction was discarded. Moreover, "scrubbing" method was also used to eliminate the bad images based on the pre-set criteria (frame displacement, FD < 0.5), but no frame was deleted (FD < 0.3). Given the whole-brain signal regression exaggerates anti-correlation and to ensure the reliability of the obtained results, the global signal was not regressed (Wang et al., 2017a,b).

Definition of Brainstem Subregions

The bilateral brainstem subregions were defined based on a recent brainstem atlas which was constructed using Bayesian segmentation approach in MRI (Iglesias et al., 2015). In this atlas, brainstem was symmetrically segmented into 4 subregions in each hemisphere, namely the midbrain, pons, medulla oblongata, and superior cerebellar peduncle. Given the superior cerebellar peduncle is too small and the smoothing effects of fMRI images, we did not include the superior cerebellar peduncle in our current study (**Figure 1**).

Functional Connectivity Analyses

To identify the changed functional connectivity patterns of the brainstem subregions between MDD and HC, the whole brain functional connectivity analysis of each brainstem subregion was performed. We first extracted the mean time series of the brainstem subregions. Next, the functional connectivity was measured using Pearson's correlations between the averaged time series of the brainstem subregions and voxels in the rest of the brain and Fisher's z transformation was applied to normalize the functional connectivity maps. Two-sample *t*-tests (gender, age, and education as covariates) were performed to determine areas with significantly different functional connectivity to the brainstem subregions between MDD and the healthy controls. The significance was determined by a cluster-level Monte Carlo simulation (5000 times) using the updated Alphasim correction with corrected threshold of $p < 0.05$ (cluster-forming threshold at voxel-level $p < 0.001$), and minimum cluster size of 47 voxels.

[1] http://www.fil.ion.ucl.ac.uk/spm

[2] www.restfmri.net/forum/DPARSF

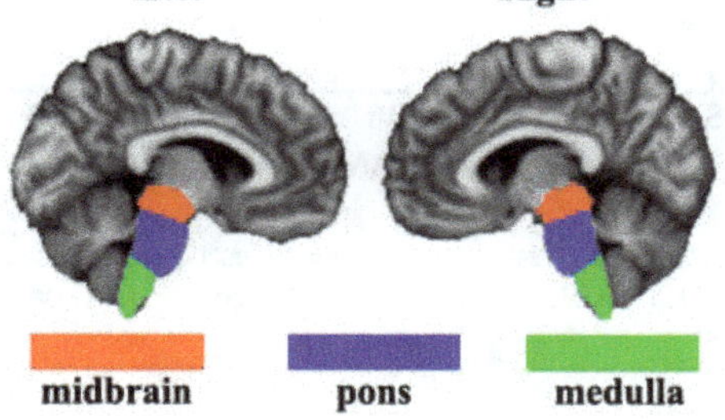

FIGURE 1 | The definition of brainstem subregions based on a recent brainstem atlas which was constructed using Bayesian segmentation approach in MRI. Three subregions including midbrain, pons, and medulla were used in the present study.

Functional Characterization With BrainMap Database

To determine the functional roles of the brain regions showing changed functional connectivity, BrainMap database[3] was used to characterize the behavior of these areas. The behavioral domains were determined by examining which types of tasks were significantly associated with these areas. Functional characterization of these areas was determined using forward inferences (Bzdok et al., 2013). The significance was established using a binomial test with $p < 0.05$ false discovery rate (FDR) corrected for multiple comparisons.

Correlation Analyses

To determine the relationships between resting-state functional connection and HDRS, HAMA scores, correlation analyses were performed in MDD patients. The threshold of significance was set at $p < 0.05$.

RESULTS

Demographics and Clinical Characteristics

The demographics and clinical characteristics of the subjects were shown in **Table 1**. No significant differences of gender ($p = 0.81$), age ($p = 0.92$), or education level ($p = 0.17$) were observed between MDD and HC groups.

Disrupted Functional Connectivity of Brainstem Subregions

The whole brain functional connectivity analysis was performed for each brainstem subregion, and only increased functional connectivity between left medulla and right inferior parietal cortex (IPC) was found in the MDD group compared with the HC group (**Figure 2**).

[3] www.brainmap.org

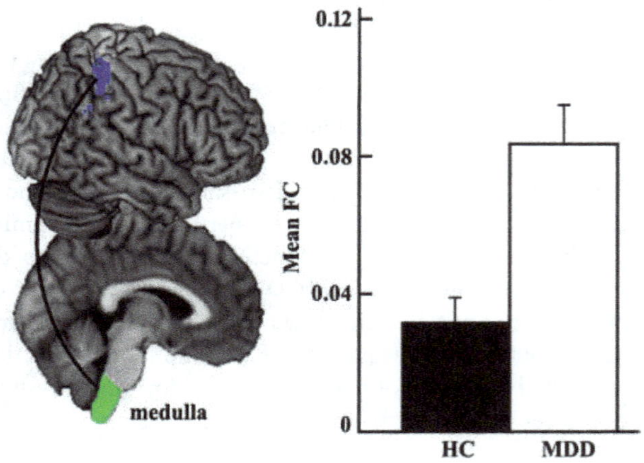

FIGURE 2 | Increased functional connectivity between left medulla and right inferior parietal cortex (IPC) in MDD patients compared to healthy controls using two-sample *t*-test.

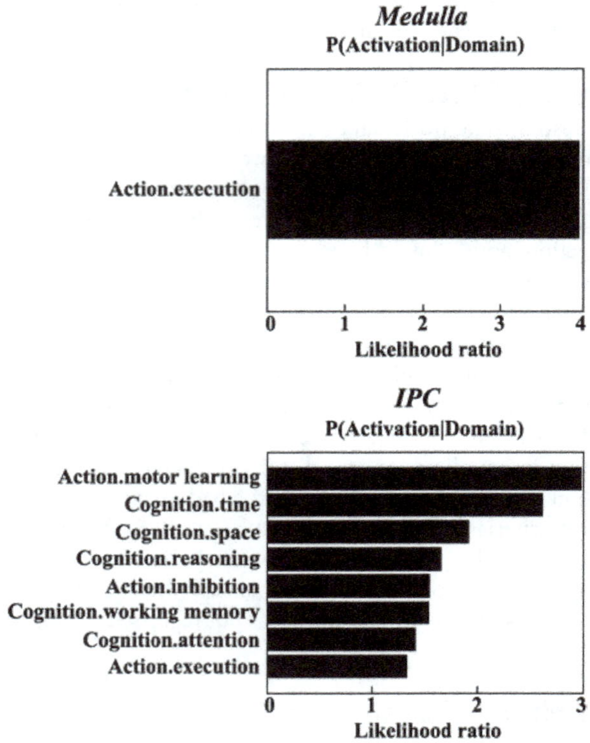

FIGURE 3 | Functional characterization identified a significant association of the left medulla with action execution, and significant associations of right IPC with motor learning, execution, inhibition, and cognition of time, space, reasoning, working memory, as well as attention.

Functional Characterization Using Meta-Analysis

The meta-analysis on functional characterization of the left medulla was significantly involved in action execution, while that of right IPC was significantly associated with motor learning, execution, inhibition, and cognition of time, space, as well as reasoning. Moreover, functional characterization of IPC also identified its association with working memory and attention (**Figure 3**).

Correlations With Clinical Characteristics

Given the normal distribution of both HDRS and HAMA scores in patient group shown by Shapiro-Wilks test (both *ps* > 0.2), Pearson correlations were used to determine the associations between the functional connectivity and scales. The result showed a significant association between the mean RSFC of left medulla – right IPC and HAMA scores ($r = 0.518, p = 0.014$) (**Figure 4**), but not with HDRS ($r = 0.183, p = 0.403$) in MDD patients.

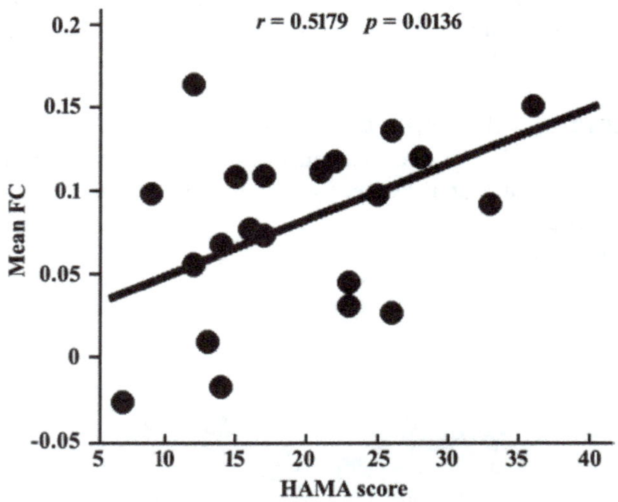

FIGURE 4 | Positive correlation between mean resting-state functional connection of left medulla-right IPC and HAMA scores in MDD patients.

DISCUSSION

In the present study, we investigated the functional connectivity patterns of brainstem subregions in medication-free MDD patients. Compared to healthy controls, we found increased functional connectivity between the left medulla and right inferior parietal cortex/lobule (IPC/IPL) in MDD. The changed functional connectivity showed significantly positive correlation with HAMA scores, suggesting higher functional connectivity between the left medulla and right IPC associates higher anxiety.

The increased functional connectivity between left medulla to cortical IPC/IPL in MDD patients was found. Previous studies found the associations between medulla and depression whereas they mostly focused on cardiovascular (Geraldes et al., 2016; Tsai et al., 2016) or central respiratory depression (Kashiwagi et al., 2011). However, increasing studies have indicated the important role of the interconnection from the medulla to limbic system including the amygdala, hippocampus, hypothalamus, insula, etc., involved in higher-level functions, such as mood control (Smythies, 2011), and conditioned fear expression

(Vianna et al., 2008), response (Yoshida et al., 2014) as well as extinction (Rosa et al., 2014). A recent review demonstrated that almost all levels of the brainstem are involved in emotion, including regions in the medulla such as nucleus of the tractus solitaries in ascending emotional sensory network, rostral ventrolateral medullary nuclei and dorsal motor nucleus of the vagus nerve in descending emotional motor network, and caudal raphe nuclei in both descending and modulatory network (Venkatraman et al., 2017). Therefore, the medulla may also be an indispensable part of depressive disorder based network.

We found the role of the left medulla in depression through its connection to the right IPC/IPL. The IPL is a critical node in an integrative multiple networks such as DMN (Wang et al., 2012, 2016, 2017c; Guo et al., 2013; Mulders et al., 2015), CEN (Ellard et al., 2018), and the cognitive control network (CCN) (Crane et al., 2016; Stange et al., 2017), playing an important role in emotion, cognition and behavior. For example, previous studies showed a causal role of IPL with its transcranial magnetic stimulation (TMS) in enhanced processing of fearful body expressions (Engelen et al., 2015). IPL is also activated during self-face processing, and the intensity increased with subject age (Morita et al., 2018). Thus the dysfunction of IPL was obviously and frequently reported in MDD, such as increased fractional amplitude of low-frequency fluctuation (fALFF) values (Yamamura et al., 2016) and lower ReHo values (Lai and Wu, 2016) of the IPL, and decreased functional connectivity between the cerebellar and IPL, with the treatment-resistant depression (TRD) group decreased more than the sensitive (Guo et al., 2013). MDD also exhibited higher connectivity between the dorsal agranular insula and IPL compared with HCs (Wang C. et al., 2018). Even in the subclinical depression participants, positive correlations were observed between left IPL activity and happy attentional biases, suggesting an active coping attempt (Dedovic et al., 2016). Moreover, antidepressant drug treatment would lead to decreased activation in IPL, suggesting a restored deactivation of the DMN (Delaveau et al., 2011). The right IPL was indicated to be involved in interoception, execution, attention, action inhibition, social and spatial cognition, etc., and more implicated in visuospatial attention processing than the left one (Wang et al., 2016). Therefore, the impaired connection between the left medulla and right IPL may be associated with the neuropathology of MDD.

Indeed, this is confirmed by the functional characterization using meta-analysis, which showed medulla and IPC in motor learning, execution, inhibition, and cognition. The increased functional connectivity between both regions may indicate the dysfunctions of these fields in MDD patients, especially cognition such as working memory and attention. These deficits have been frequently reported in previous studies in MDD patients (Mulders et al., 2015; Wang J. et al., 2018). Our functional characterization findings provide further evidence for the important role of the connection between the medulla and IPC in the pathology of MDD.

We also found significant positive associations between HAMA scores and functional connectivity of left medulla and right IPC, indicating that down-regulation of their functional connectivity may decrease anxiety symptoms of MDD. Previous studies found increased ALFF in the right IPL (Yuan et al., 2018) and enhanced functional connectivity between periaqueductal gray and IPL (Arnold Anteraper et al., 2014) in social anxiety disorder (SAD) patients as compared to healthy controls. Also, the activation of IPL may differentiate the comorbid MDD and anxiety (MDD + Anx) patients to MDD patients to some extent in cognitive tasks such as Go/No-Go task (Crane et al., 2016). Research also demonstrated the important role of cognitive behavioural therapy (CBT) in SAD mainly via the brain activations of emotional response to and regulation of social criticism which both include IPL activation (Goldin et al., 2014). Even though the RSFC study found the biotypes for depression, it also overlapped with generalized anxiety disorder (GAD) at a very high proportion (Drysdale et al., 2017; Wager and Woo, 2017). Therefore, the present correlation finding may suggest anxiety-related symptoms in depression and provide a potential neural marker of distinguishing the depression and anxiety.

There are some limitations in the present study. First, only 23 MDD patients were used to investigate changes of the functional connectivity patterns of brainstem subregions. Therefore, the validity of the findings should be further tested in a larger sample. Second, as shown by **Table 1**, there is a wide range of the course of disease for MDD patients, which may have some impact on the results of functional connectivity. Third, the exact roles of the increased functional connectivity between medulla and IPC playing in depression needs to be further examined by task-related fMRI studies.

CONCLUSION

The present study examined the abnormality of functional connectivity patterns of brainstem subregions and revealed increased functional connection between left medulla and right IPC in MDD patients compared to healthy controls. This finding indicates the functional abnormality in the early primary automatic functional system in MDD patients, which may facilitate the future early diagnosis for MDD.

AUTHOR CONTRIBUTIONS

JW and HW designed and supervised the study. HW and FW collected the data. LL, KW, YL, SG, XK, and FL analyzed the data. LL, KW, YL, HW, and JW drafted the manuscript. All authors discussed the results and commented on the manuscript.

FUNDING

This work was financially supported in part by grants from the National Natural Science Foundation of China (31800961; 31600880), Sichuan Science and Technology Program (2018JY0361), China Postdoctoral Science Foundation (2018M633336), the Shenzhen Basic Research Project (JCYJ2017081802123707), Chinese Fundamental

Research Funding for Central Universities (ZYGX2015002), Interdisciplinary Development Project of University of Electronic Science and Technology of China (Y03111023901014007), Early Career Funding in Social Science (Y03001023601039010), Science and Technology Program of Guangzhou (201807010064).

REFERENCES

Abe, O., Yamasue, H., Kasai, K., Yamada, H., Aoki, S., Inoue, H., et al. (2010). Voxel-based analyses of gray/white matter volume and diffusion tensor data in major depression. *Psychiatry Res.* 181, 64–70. doi: 10.1016/j.pscychresns.2009.07.007

Aihara, M., Ida, I., Yuuki, N., Oshima, A., Kumano, H., Takahashi, K., et al. (2007). HPA axis dysfunction in unmedicated major depressive disorder and its normalization by pharmacotherapy correlates with alteration of neural activity in prefrontal cortex and limbic/paralimbic regions. *Psychiatry Res.* 155, 245–256. doi: 10.1016/j.pscychresns.2006.11.002

Arnold Anteraper, S., Triantafyllou, C., Sawyer, A. T., Hofmann, S. G., Gabrieli, J. D., and Whitfield-Gabrieli, S. (2014). Hyper-connectivity of subcortical resting-state networks in social anxiety disorder. *Brain Connect.* 4, 81–90. doi: 10.1089/brain.2013.0180

Buchanan, A., Wang, X., and Gollan, J. K. (2014). Resting-state functional connectivity in women with major depressive disorder. *J. Psychiatr. Res.* 59, 38–44. doi: 10.1016/j.jpsychires.2014.09.002

Bzdok, D., Laird, A. R., Zilles, K., Fox, P. T., and Eickhoff, S. B. (2013). An investigation of the structural, connectional, and functional subspecialization in the human amygdala. *Hum. Brain Mapp.* 34, 3247–3266. doi: 10.1002/hbm.22138

Crane, N. A., Jenkins, L. M., Dion, C., Meyers, K. K., Weldon, A. L., Gabriel, L. B., et al. (2016). Comorbid anxiety increases cognitive control activation in major depressive disorder. *Depress. Anxiety* 33, 967–977. doi: 10.1002/da.22541

Dedovic, K., Giebl, S., Duchesne, A., Lue, S. D., Andrews, J., Efanov, S., et al. (2016). Psychological, endocrine, and neural correlates of attentional bias in subclinical depression. *Anxiety Stress Coping* 29, 479–496. doi: 10.1080/10615806.2015.1101457

Delaveau, P., Jabourian, M., Lemogne, C., Guionnet, S., Bergouignan, L., and Fossati, P. (2011). Brain effects of antidepressants in major depression: a meta-analysis of emotional processing studies. *J. Affect. Disord.* 130, 66–74. doi: 10.1016/j.jad.2010.09.032

Drysdale, A. T., Grosenick, L., Downar, J., Dunlop, K., Mansouri, F., Meng, Y., et al. (2017). Erratum: resting-state connectivity biomarkers define neurophysiological subtypes of depression. *Nat. Med.* 23:264. doi: 10.1038/nm0217-264d

Edlow, B. L., McNab, J. A., Witzel, T., and Kinney, H. C. (2016). The structural connectome of the human central homeostatic network. *Brain Connect.* 6, 187–200. doi: 10.1089/brain.2015.0378

Ellard, K. K., Zimmerman, J. P., Kaur, N., Van Dijk, K. R. A., Roffman, J. L., Nierenberg, A. A., et al. (2018). Functional connectivity between anterior insula and key nodes of frontoparietal executive control and salience networks distinguish bipolar depression from unipolar depression and healthy control subjects. *Biol. Psychiatry Cogn. Neurosci. Neuroimaging* 3, 473–484. doi: 10.1016/j.bpsc.2018.01.013

Engelen, T., de Graaf, T. A., Sack, A. T., and de Gelder, B. (2015). A causal role for inferior parietal lobule in emotion body perception. *Cortex* 73, 195–202. doi: 10.1016/j.cortex.2015.08.013

Geraldes, V., Goncalves-Rosa, N., Tavares, C., Paton, J. F. R., and Rocha, I. (2016). Reversing gene expression in cardiovascular target organs following chronic depression of the paraventricular nucleus of hypothalamus and rostral ventrolateral medulla in spontaneous hypertensive rats. *Brain Res.* 1646, 109–115. doi: 10.1016/j.brainres.2016.05.041

Geva, R., and Feldman, R. (2008). A neurobiological model for the effects of early brainstem functioning on the development of behavior and emotion regulation in infants: implications for prenatal and perinatal risk. *J. Child Psychol. Psychiatry* 49, 1031–1041. doi: 10.1111/j.1469-7610.2008.01918.x

Goldin, P. R., Ziv, M., Jazaieri, H., Weeks, J., Heimberg, R. G., and Gross, J. J. (2014). Impact of cognitive-behavioral therapy for social anxiety disorder on the neural bases of emotional reactivity to and regulation of social evaluation. *Behav. Res. Ther.* 62, 97–106. doi: 10.1016/j.brat.2014.08.005

Guo, W., Liu, F., Xue, Z., Gao, K., Liu, Z., Xiao, C., et al. (2013). Abnormal resting-state cerebellar-cerebral functional connectivity in treatment-resistant depression and treatment sensitive depression. *Prog. Neuropsychopharmacol. Biol. Psychiatry* 44, 51–57. doi: 10.1016/j.pnpbp.2013.01.010

Hahn, A., Haeusler, D., Kraus, C., Hoflich, A. S., Kranz, G. S., Baldinger, P., et al. (2014). Attenuated serotonin transporter association between dorsal raphe and ventral striatum in major depression. *Hum. Brain Mapp.* 35, 3857–3866. doi: 10.1002/hbm.22442

Han, K. M., Kim, D., Sim, Y., Kang, J., Kim, A., Won, E., et al. (2017). Alterations in the brainstem volume of patients with major depressive disorder and their relationship with antidepressant treatment. *J. Affect. Disord.* 208, 68–75. doi: 10.1016/j.jad.2016.08.066

Iglesias, J. E., Van Leemput, K., Bhatt, P., Casillas, C., Dutt, S., Schuff, N., et al. (2015). Bayesian segmentation of brainstem structures in MRI. *Neuroimage* 113, 184–195. doi: 10.1016/j.neuroimage.2015.02.065

Kang, S. G., Na, K. S., Choi, J. W., Kim, J. H., Son, Y. D., and Lee, Y. J. (2017). Resting-state functional connectivity of the amygdala in suicide attempters with major depressive disorder. *Prog. Neuropsychopharmacol. Biol. Psychiatry* 77, 222–227. doi: 10.1016/j.pnpbp.2017.04.029

Kashiwagi, M., Osaka, Y., Onimaru, H., and Takeda, J. (2011). Optical imaging of propofol-induced central respiratory depression in medulla-spinal cord preparations from newborn rats. *Clin. Exp. Pharmacol. Physiol.* 38, 186–191. doi: 10.1111/j.1440-1681.2011.05480.x

Lai, C. H., and Wu, Y. T. (2016). The alterations in regional homogeneity of parieto-cingulate and temporo-cerebellum regions of first-episode medication-naive depression patients. *Brain imaging Behav.* 10, 187–194. doi: 10.1007/s11682-015-9381-9

Lee, J. H., Ryan, J., Andreescu, C., Aizenstein, H., and Lim, H. K. (2015). Brainstem morphological changes in Alzheimer's disease. *Neuroreport* 26, 411–415. doi: 10.1097/WNR.0000000000000362

Morita, T., Saito, D. N., Ban, M., Shimada, K., Okamoto, Y., Kosaka, H., et al. (2018). Self-Face recognition begins to share active region in right inferior parietal lobule with proprioceptive Illusion during adolescence. *Cereb. Cortex* 28, 1532–1548. doi: 10.1093/cercor/bhy027

Mulders, P. C., van Eijndhoven, P. F., Schene, A. H., Beckmann, C. F., and Tendolkar, I. (2015). Resting-state functional connectivity in major depressive disorder: a review. *Neurosci. Biobehav. Rev.* 56, 330–344. doi: 10.1016/j.neubiorev.2015.07.014

Nishijo, H., Rafal, R., and Tamietto, M. (2018). Editorial: limbic-brainstem roles in perception. Cognition, Emotion, and Behavior. *Front. Neurosci.* 12:395. doi: 10.3389/fnins.2018.00395

Numasawa, Y., Hattori, T., Ishiai, S., Kobayashi, Z., Kamata, T., Kotera, M., et al. (2017). Depressive disorder may be associated with raphe nuclei lesions in patients with brainstem infarction. *J. Affect. Disord.* 213, 191–198. doi: 10.1016/j.jad.2017.02.005

Nye, J. A., Purselle, D., Plisson, C., Voll, R. J., Stehouwer, J. S., Votaw, J. R., et al. (2013). Decreased brainstem and putamen SERT binding potential in depressed suicide attempters using [11C]-ZIENT PET imaging. *Depress. Anxiety* 30, 902–907. doi: 10.1002/da.22049

Post, R. J., and Warden, M. R. (2018). Melancholy, anhedonia, apathy: the search for separable behaviors and neural circuits in depression. *Curr. Opin. Neurobiol.* 49, 192–200. doi: 10.1016/j.conb.2018.02.018

Rosa, J., Myskiw, J. C., Furini, C. R., Sapiras, G. G., and Izquierdo, I. (2014). Fear extinction can be made state-dependent on peripheral epinephrine: role of norepinephrine in the nucleus tractus solitarius. *Neurobiol. Learn. Mem.* 113, 55–61. doi: 10.1016/j.nlm.2013.09.018

Smith, D. F. (2015). Systematic review of an emerging trend in china: resting-state functional connectivity in major depressive disorder. *J. Neuropsychiatry Clin. Neurosci.* 27, 104–111. doi: 10.1176/appi.neuropsych.13110343

Smythies, J. (2011). The neural control of mood: the possible role of the adrenergic system in the medulla. *Conscious. Cogn.* 20, 489–493. doi: 10.1016/j.concog.2010.10.014

Song, Y. J., Korgaonkar, M. S., Armstrong, L. V., Eagles, S., Williams, L. M., and Grieve, S. M. (2014). Tractography of the brainstem in major depressive disorder using diffusion tensor imaging. *PLoS One* 9:e84825. doi: 10.1371/journal.pone.0084825

Stange, J. P., Bessette, K. L., Jenkins, L. M., Peters, A. T., Feldhaus, C., Crane, N. A., et al. (2017). Attenuated intrinsic connectivity within cognitive control network among individuals with remitted depression: temporal stability and association with negative cognitive styles. *Hum. Brain Mapp.* 38, 2939–2954. doi: 10.1002/hbm.23564

Sun, H., Luo, L., Yuan, X., Zhang, L., He, Y., Yao, S., et al. (2018). Regional homogeneity and functional connectivity patterns in major depressive disorder, cognitive vulnerability to depression and healthy subjects. *J. Affect. Disord.* 235, 229–235. doi: 10.1016/j.jad.2018.04.061

Tsai, C. Y., Li, F. C., Wu, C. H., Chang, A. Y., and Chan, S. H. (2016). Sumoylation of IkB attenuates NF-kB-induced nitrosative stress at rostral ventrolateral medulla and cardiovascular depression in experimental brain death. *J. Biomed. Sci.* 23:65.

Venkatraman, A., Edlow, B. L., and Immordino-Yang, M. H. (2017). The brainstem in emotion: a review. *Front. Neuroanat.* 11:15. doi: 10.3389/fnana.2017.00015

Vianna, D. M., Allen, C., and Carrive, P. (2008). Cardiovascular and behavioral responses to conditioned fear after medullary raphe neuronal blockade. *Neuroscience* 153, 1344–1353. doi: 10.1016/j.neuroscience.2008.03.033

Wager, T. D., and Woo, C.-W. (2017). Imaging biomarkers and biotypes for depression. *Nat. Med.* 23, 16–17. doi: 10.1038/nm.4264

Wagner, G., de la Cruz, F., Kohler, S., and Bar, K. J. (2017). Treatment associated changes of functional connectivity of midbrain/brainstem nuclei in major depressive disorder. *Sci. Rep.* 7:8675. doi: 10.1038/s41598-017-09077-5

Wang, C., Wu, H., Chen, F., Xu, J., Li, H., Li, H., et al. (2018). Disrupted functional connectivity patterns of the insula subregions in drug-free major depressive disorder. *J. Affect. Disord.* 234, 297–304. doi: 10.1016/j.jad.2017.12.033

Wang, J., Fan, L., Zhang, Y., Liu, Y., Jiang, D., Zhang, Y., et al. (2012). Tractography-based parcellation of the human left inferior parietal lobule. *Neuroimage* 63, 641–652. doi: 10.1016/j.neuroimage.2012.07.045

Wang, J., Wei, Q., Bai, T., Zhou, X., Sun, H., Becker, B., et al. (2017a). Electroconvulsive therapy selectively enhanced feedforward connectivity from fusiform face area to amygdala in major depressive disorder. *Soc. Cogn. Affect. Neurosci.* 12, 1983–1992. doi: 10.1093/scan/nsx100

Wang, J., Wei, Q., Wang, L., Zhang, H., Bai, T., Cheng, L., et al. (2018). Functional reorganization of intra- and internetwork connectivity in major depressive disorder after electroconvulsive therapy. *Hum. Brain Mapp.* 39, 1403–1411. doi: 10.1002/hbm.23928

Wang, J., Wei, Q., Yuan, X., Jiang, X., Xu, J., Zhou, X., et al. (2017b). Local functional connectivity density is closely associated with the response of electroconvulsive therapy in major depressive disorder. *J. Affect. Disord.* 225, 658–664. doi: 10.1016/j.jad.2017.09.001

Wang, J., Xie, S., Guo, X., Becker, B., Fox, P. T., Eickhoff, S. B., et al. (2017c). Correspondent functional topography of the human left inferior parietal lobule at rest and under task revealed using resting-state fMRI and coactivation based parcellation. *Hum. Brain Mapp.* 38, 1659–1675. doi: 10.1002/hbm.23488

Wang, J., Zhang, J., Rong, M., Wei, X., Zheng, D., Fox, P. T., et al. (2016). Functional topography of the right inferior parietal lobule structured by anatomical connectivity profiles. *Hum. Brain Mapp.* 37, 4316–4332. doi: 10.1002/hbm.23311

Wu, H., Sun, H., Xu, J., Wu, Y., Wang, C., Xiao, J., et al. (2016). Changed hub and corresponding functional connectivity of subgenual anterior cingulate cortex in major depressive disorder. *Front. Neuroanat.* 10:120. doi: 10.3389/fnana.2016.00120

Yamamura, T., Okamoto, Y., Okada, G., Takaishi, Y., Takamura, M., Mantani, A., et al. (2016). Association of thalamic hyperactivity with treatment-resistant depression and poor response in early treatment for major depression: a resting-state fMRI study using fractional amplitude of low-frequency fluctuations. *Transl. Psychiatry* 6:e754. doi: 10.1038/tp.2016.18

Yoshida, M., Takayanagi, Y., and Onaka, T. (2014). The medial amygdala-medullary PrRP-synthesizing neuron pathway mediates neuroendocrine responses to contextual conditioned fear in male rodents. *Endocrinology* 155, 2996–3004. doi: 10.1210/en.2013-1411

Yuan, C., Zhu, H., Ren, Z., Yuan, M., Gao, M., Zhang, Y., et al. (2018). Precuneus-related regional and network functional deficits in social anxiety disorder: a resting-state functional MRI study. *Compr. Psychiatry* 82, 22–29. doi: 10.1016/j.comppsych.2017.12.002

5

The Abnormality of Topological Asymmetry in Hemispheric Brain Anatomical Networks in Bipolar Disorder

*Bin Wang[1], Ting Li[1], Mengni Zhou[1], Shuo Zhao[2], Yan Niu[1], Xin Wang[1], Ting Yan[3], Rui Cao[1], Jie Xiang[1] and Dandan Li[1]**

[1] College of Information and Computer, Taiyuan University of Technology, Taiyuan, China, [2] Faculty of Human Health Science, Graduate School of Medicine, Kyoto University, Kyoto, Japan, [3] Translational Medicine Research Center, Shanxi Medical University, Taiyuan, China

Correspondence:
Dandan Li
lidandan@tyut.edu.cn

Convergent evidences have demonstrated a variety of regional abnormalities of asymmetry in bipolar disorder (BD). However, little is known about the alterations in hemispheric topological asymmetries. In this study, we used diffusion tensor imaging to construct the hemispheric brain anatomical network of 49 patients with BD and 61 matched normal controls. Graph theory was then applied to quantify topological properties of the hemispheric networks. Although small-world properties were preserved in the hemispheric networks of BD, the degrees of the asymmetry in global efficiency, characteristic path length, and small-world property were significantly decreased. More changes in topological properties of the right hemisphere than those of left hemisphere were found in patients compared with normal controls. Consistent with such changes, the nodal efficiency in patients with BD also showed less rightward asymmetry mainly in the frontal, occipital, parietal, and temporal lobes. In contrast to leftward asymmetry, significant rightward asymmetry was found in supplementary motor area of BD, and attributed to more deficits in nodal efficiency of the left hemisphere. Finally, these asymmetry score of nodal efficiency in the inferior parietal lobule and rolandic operculum were significantly associated with symptom severity of BD. Our results suggested that abnormal hemispheric asymmetries in brain anatomical networks were associated with aberrant neurodevelopment, and providing insights into the potential neural biomarkers of BD by measuring the topological asymmetry in hemispheric brain anatomical networks.

Keywords: bipolar disorder, diffusion tensor imaging, graph theory, hemispheric asymmetry, structural connectivity

INTRODUCTION

The human brain is structurally and functionally asymmetrical or lateralized (Watkins et al., 2001; Toga and Thompson, 2003). Even subtle perturbations to anatomical asymmetries between two hemispheres, such as gray matter volume (Sigalovsky et al., 2006), cortical thickness (Rimol et al., 2010), or white matter (WM) integrity (Park et al., 2004), can cause disturbances in cognitive and emotion processes. Studies have shown that aberrant brain region asymmetries are highly correlated with disturbed functions such as executive function (Yin et al., 2013), emotion (Schulte et al., 2012), and language (O'Donoghue et al., 2017). Hence, abnormal anatomical asymmetries have been observed in a variety of neurological and psychiatric disorders, including schizophrenia (Highley et al., 1999), depression (Kwon et al., 1996), attention-deficit hyperactivity disorder (Miller et al., 2006), and Bipolar disorder (BD) (Beyer et al., 2005; Bruno et al., 2008). As one of the most distinct syndromes in psychiatry, BD is mainly characterized as episodic elevations in emotion and disturbances in cognition (Belmaker, 2004; Saunders and Goodwin, 2010). Convergent studies on BD have showed abnormal asymmetries in WM (Bruno et al., 2008; Kafantaris et al., 2009; Wessa et al., 2009; Mahon et al., 2013), for example, less WM volume within the left frontal lobes, the rightward WM in orbital frontal. These results indicated that the alteration in WM asymmetries have been proposed as a key factor in the manifestation of BD symptoms.

As an imaging method, diffusion tensor imaging (DTI) can reconstruct the major WM tracts faithfully (Dae-Jin et al., 2013) and has been proved to be a promising tool for assessing WM abnormalities. Recently, using the DTI tractography and graph theory, connectome studies demonstrated abnormal topological properties in BD (Leow et al., 2013; Forde et al., 2015; Collin et al., 2016, 2017; Spielberg et al., 2016; O'Donoghue et al., 2017). The patients with BD showed decrease in global integration (longer characteristic path length, smaller global efficiency), increase in functional segregation (larger clustering coefficient and local efficiency), and loss of small-world property (the balance between local integration and functional segregation) (Leow et al., 2013; Forde et al., 2015; Collin et al., 2016; Spielberg et al., 2016; O'Donoghue et al., 2017). These studies have mainly focused on the WM topological properties in whole network rather than hemispheric network. Analyzing the hemispheric anatomical networks and further determination of the status of the anatomical network asymmetries might benefit the understanding of the underlying nature of alteration in the brain of BD, and potentially help to elucidate the etiology of the disorder. However, the hemispheric asymmetries of anatomical network in patients with BD were remained unclear.

In present study, we adopted the DTI deterministic tractography method and graph theory to investigate the abnormality of hemispheric asymmetries in brain anatomical networks in BD. In particular, we focused on global graph measures, including small-world property, global and local efficiency, and regional parameters to evaluate (1) the abnormal hemispheric asymmetries in brain anatomical networks in patients with BD and (2) whether the abnormal hemispheric asymmetries in network organization were related to clinical features of BD.

MATERIALS AND METHODS

Subjects

Data were selected from the UCLA Consortium for Neuropsychiatric Phenomics LA5c Study, and the study was approved by the UCLA Institutional Review Board. The data were obtained via a public database, openfMRI (Poldrack and Gorgolewski, 2015). About 49 BD patients and 61 age- and gender-matched normal subjects were selected for further analyzing. All subjects were right-handed. There are more details available in openfMRI[1] (ds000030). The detailed demographics and clinical features of the patients with BD and normal controls are described in **Table 1**. Patient symptoms were evaluated using the 17-item Hamilton Depression Rating Scale (HAMD) (Hamilton, 1960) and the Young Mania Rating Scale (YMRS) (Young et al., 1978).

Data Acquisition and Preprocessing

Structural MRI data were acquired on 3T Siemens Trio scanners located at the Ahmanson-Lovelace Brain Mapping Center (Siemens version syngo MRB15) and the Staglin Center for Cognitive Neuroscience (Siemens version syngo MRB17) at UCLA. A high-resolution 3D echoplanar imaging was acquired with the following parameters: TR = 1.9 s, TE = 2.26 ms, FOV = 250 mm, matrix = 256 × 256, sagittal plane, slice thickness = 1 mm, 176 slices. Diffusion weighted imaging (DWI) data were collected using an echo-planar sequence with parameters: 64 directions, 2 mm slices, TR/TE = 9000/93 ms, 1 average, 96 × 96 matrix, 90° flip angle, axial slices, $b = 1000$ s/mm^2.

This study used the MATLAB toolbox named PANDA to perform data preprocessing and the construction of the brain network (Cui et al., 2013). Specifically, data preprocessing approaches included correction for simple head movements and eddy current distortions using affine transformation to the b0 image (Jenkinson et al., 2002). After data preprocessing, the seven independent components of the diffusion tensor were estimated and from which fractional anisotropy (FA, a DTI measurement) was calculated. Subsequently, the deterministic fiber tracking algorithms were used to reconstruct fiber paths (Mori et al., 1999). The fiber tracking procedure started from the deep WM regions and terminated if two consecutive moving directions had a crossing angle above 35° or the FA was out of the threshold range (0.1~1).

Network Construction and Analysis

In this study, the method of constructing the WM network was described in Gong et al. (Gong et al., 2009). Based on the automated anatomical labeling (AAL) parcellation scheme (Tzouriomazoyer et al., 2002), the brain was divided into 90 regions (45 in each hemisphere). Each region was defined as one node in the anatomical network. A linear transformation was applied locally within each subject's DTI image correlated with the T1-weighted image to coregister them to the b0 image with DTI space followed by applying a nonlinear transformation to map to the ICBM152 T1 template [Montreal Neurological Institute (MNI)]. Then, the subject-specific AAL mask was weaved from the MNI space to the DTI native space with the corresponding inverse transformation, such that separate labeling values were maintained via nearest-neighbor interpolation (Gong et al., 2009; Cui et al., 2013). The FA between

[1] https://www.openfmri.org/

TABLE 1 | Demographic and clinical characteristics[a].

Characteristic	Group (patients/controls = 49/61)		Statistical test	
	Patients with BD	Normal controls		
Age (years)	22–50(32.3 ± 9.0)	21–49(33.1 ± 9.2)	$t_{108} = -1.218$	$P = 0.226^b$
Male/Female	28/21	32/29	$\chi_1^2 = 0.909$	$P = 0.340^c$
Education (years)	11–19(14.6 ± 2.0)	12–19(15.2 ± 1.5)	$t_{108} = -2.080$	$P = 0.040^b$
Duration of illness (months)	0–24(2.1 ± 5.2)	N/A		
Medication dose (mg/day)	0–6210(784.8 ± 1035.3)			
Handscore[d]	0.75–1(0.93 ± 0.1)	0.80–1(0.93 ± 0.1)		
YMRS_score[e]	0–41(11.9 ± 11.0)	N/A		
HAMD[e]	0–32 (12.0 ± 8.4)	N/A		

[a]Unless otherwise indicated, data are expressed as a range of minimum–maximum (mean ± SD). [b]The P-value was obtained using a two-sample two-tailed t-test. [c]The P-value was obtained using a two-tail Pearson's χ^2 test. [d]The Handscore described the handedness of subjects. It was obtained using a formula (Right − Left)/(Right ± Left). [e]The score of Young Mania Rating Scale (YMRS_score) and the 17-item Hamilton Depression Rating Scale (HAMD) was used to assess the symptom severity of patients with BD.

two regions was defined as the network edge (Shu et al., 2011; Bai et al., 2012). Prior to constructing the network, the connection between these two regions was adopted if the fiber number (FN) between the two regions was larger than 3 (Shu et al., 2011). It was helpful to reduce the influence of pseudo-connections owing to possible noise effects on whole-brain tractography. For each subject, we eliminated the inter-hemispheric connections and then obtained two weighted 45 × 45 hemispheric brain networks, one for the left hemisphere and the other for the right hemisphere.

The network architecture was then investigated at both global and regional levels for the constructed WM networks. The small-world property suggests the architecture of networks with higher local clustering and equivalent characteristic path length compared with the random network (Watts and Strogatz, 1998). In this work, eight network properties were used to analyze the topological organization of the WM networks. The clustering coefficient (C_p) of a network is thus the average of clustering coefficients across nodes and is a measure of functional segregation. The characteristic path length (L_p) of a network is the average shortest path length between all pairs of nodes in the network and is the most commonly used measure of global integration. The normalized clustering coefficients (γ), $\gamma = C_p/C_{rand}$ and the normalized characteristic path length (λ), $\lambda = L_p/L_{rand}$, C_{rand} and L_{rand} represent indices derived from matched random networks (100 matched random networks were selected). The small-world property of a network can be characterized by both γ and λ, indicating a balance between integration and segregation. In a small-world network, the C_p is significantly higher than that of random networks (γ greater than 1), while the L_p is comparable to random networks (λ close to 1). The global efficiency (E_g), reflecting the efficiency of whole network information transmission (integration), is the inverse relation of L_p. The local efficiency (E_{loc}), reflected the efficiency of the network segregation. Regional properties were described in terms of nodal efficiency, $E_{nodal}(i)$ (Achard and Bullmore, 2007). It measures the information transmission ability of node i in the network. A node with high $E_{nodal}(i)$ indicates great interconnectivity with other regions in the network. The detailed descriptions of these graph theory parameters can be found in a previous work (Bullmore and Sporns, 2009; Rubinov and Sporns, 2010). The graph theory analysis was performed with GRETNA[2] software.

Asymmetry Score

The degree of hemispheric network asymmetry was estimated by the asymmetry score (Iturriamedina et al., 2011; Ratnarajah et al., 2013) using the following formulation: $AS(X) = 100 \times [X(R) - X(L)]/[X(R) + X(L)]$, where X(R) and X(L) represent the network properties of the right and left hemisphere, respectively. The asymmetry score AS(X) helps us look at the differences between the right and left hemisphere. Notably, a positive value of AS(X) represents a rightward asymmetry, while a negative value of AS(X) indicates a leftward asymmetry.

Statistical Analysis

All statistical analyses were performed using SPSS 19 software (SPSS, Inc., Chicago, IL, United States). To determine whether there was any significant group difference in age and education, this work performed the separate two-tailed t-tests to analyze data. We used a χ^2 test to analyze the gender data. To assess the group differences in hemispheric network properties, we used a general linear model (GLM) that was performed with hemisphere as a within-subject factor, group as a between-subject factor, and a group-by-hemisphere interaction. Studies have shown that hemispheric asymmetries are related to age (Cabeza, 2002; Dolcos et al., 2002) and gender (McGlone, 1980; Good et al., 2001). Hence, we set the age, gender, and age-by-gender interaction as covariates in the GLM. Further *post hoc* tests, including two-sample t-test for group differences and paired t-test for hemisphere differences, were used if any difference survived a threshold of $P < 0.05$. To determine whether the *AS* of the network properties within each group was significantly different from zero, one-sample t-test was performed on the asymmetry score. Meanwhile, a univariate analysis with covariance of age,

[2]http://www.nitrc.org/projects/gretna/

gender, and age-by-gender interaction was performed on the *AS* to assess group differences. The threshold of $P < 0.05$ was considered to be significant for global properties. In particular, for the regional properties, the Bonferroni-correction was performed on that threshold ($P < 0.05$).

This work also studied the relationships between the hemispheric asymmetry scores and symptom severity of patients with BD. Considering age, gender, and age-by-gender as the covariates, we used both Pearson and Spearman correlation to analyze the relationship between network properties and BD symptom severity. Pearson is used to measure the linear relationship between two consecutive variables. Spearman does not require the distribution of primitive variables and belongs to a non-parametric statistical method. It was unnecessary to correct multiple comparisons because the aforementioned analyses were exploratory in nature. Hence, a significant relationship was considered at an uncorrected *P*-value of 0.05.

RESULTS

Global Properties of Hemispheric Networks

Group and Hemispheric Differences

As shown in **Figure 1**, all four hemispheric brain anatomical networks (2 hemispheres × 2 groups) exhibited prominent features of small-world property, as expressed by a larger γ ($\gamma > 1$) and a smaller λ ($\lambda \approx 1$). Statistical analysis results showed significantly topological changes in the global properties in both groups and hemispheres. Except for local efficiency E_{loc} ($F_{1,106} = 2.372$, $P = 0.127$), the rest of the six network properties exhibited significant group differences between normal controls and patients with BD. There was a reduced global integration (decreased global efficiency and increased characteristic path length) and increased small-world property in patients with BD. Furthermore, we observed a significant group-by-hemisphere interaction on global efficiency E_g ($F_{1,106} = 9.311$, $P = 0.003$), the characteristic path length L_p ($F_{1,106} = 7.323$, $P = 0.008$), the normalized clustering coefficients γ ($F_{1,106} = 30.107$, $P < 0.001$) and the small-world property σ ($F_{1,106} = 32.163$, $P < 0.001$). *Post hoc* analysis indicated that this interaction resulted from a significant rightward trend in global integration ($P = 0.001$) and a significant leftward trend in the characteristic path length ($P = 0.003$), the normalized clustering coefficients ($P < 0.001$), and small-world architecture ($P < 0.001$) in normal controls and a symmetrical trend in patients with BD.

Asymmetry Score

The asymmetry score was helpful for us to evaluate the differences between the right and left hemisphere for the network properties. Additionally, the group differences in asymmetry scores would directly reflect the abnormal of hemispheric lateralization of topological organization in BD, and supplemented the result of the group-by-hemisphere interaction. **Table 2** summarizes the statistical analysis results of the asymmetry scores of the global network properties for the two groups. Significant differences in hemispheric asymmetry were only observed in normal controls and disappeared in patients with BD. Normal controls showed more globally efficient in the right hemisphere than the left hemisphere [AS(E_g), $t_{52} = 3.852$, $P < 0.001$]. Additionally, the characteristic path length [AS(L_p), $t_{52} = -3.852$, $P < 0.001$], the normalized clustering coefficients [AS(γ), $t_{52} = -6.447$, $P < 0.001$], and the small-world property [AS(σ), $t_{52} = -6.578$, $P < 0.001$] showed leftward hemispheric asymmetries in normal controls. When comparing the asymmetry scores between two groups, we observed significant group differences in asymmetry scores of E_g ($F_{1,106} = 8.268$, $P = 0.005$), L_p ($F_{1,106} = 8.268$, $P = 0.005$), γ ($F_{1,106} = 33.684$, $P < 0.001$), and σ ($F_{1,106} = 35.657$, $P < 0.001$), which agreed with the significant group-by-hemisphere interaction on E_g, L_p, γ, and σ revealed by the GLM model. This result indicated that the rightward asymmetries of global integration and leftward asymmetries of small-world feature were observed only in normal controls but disappeared in patients with BD.

Regional Properties of the Hemispheric Networks

Hemispheric and Group Differences

The statistical results of nodal efficiency differences are summarized in **Figure 2**. Using Bonferroni-correction, we observed five regions exhibited significant hemispheric differences ($P < 0.05$) (**Figure 2A**). Among these five brain regions, regions with significant leftward advantage in nodal efficiency mainly included the anterior cingulate gyrus (ACG) and the inferior parietal lobule (IPL), whereas regions with significant rightward nodal efficiency were predominantly located at the supramarginal gyrus (SMG), the angular gyrus (ANG), and the rolandic operculum (ROL). Moreover, regions with significant group differences (BD < CN, $P < 0.05$, Bonferroni-corrected) in nodal efficiency included the amygdala (AMYG), IPL, putamen (PUT), and temporal pole (middle) (TPOmid) (**Figure 2B**). The PUT region could not be marked in **Figure 2B**. Furthermore, we found significant group-by-hemisphere interactions in the ROL ($F_{1,106} = 12.930$, $P < 0.001$), the lingual gyrus (LING) ($F_{1,106} = 19.011$, $P < 0.001$), the superior occipital gyrus (SOG) ($F_{1,106} = 21.221$, $P < 0.001$), the IPL ($F_{1,106} = 36.225$, $P < 0.001$), the SMG ($F_{1,106} = 21.617$, $P < 0.001$), the inferior temporal gyrus (ITG) ($F_{1,106} = 15.900$, $P < 0.001$), and the ACG ($F_{1,106} = 10.547$, $P = 0.002$, **Figure 2C**). *Post hoc* analysis indicated that these interaction effects resulted from significantly reduced rightward hemispheric asymmetry in nodal efficiency in patients with BD (**Figure 3**). Specially, we revealed significant group-by-hemisphere interaction in the supplementary motor area (SMA) ($F_{1,106} = 34.907$, $P < 0.001$). *Post hoc* analysis showed that this interaction in SMA was attributed to significantly rightward hemispheric asymmetry in nodal efficiency in patients with BD (**Figure 3**).

Asymmetry Score

The asymmetry score of nodal efficiency indicated that the region was leftward or rightward in each group subject. Consistent with the prior GLM hemispheric results, both groups exhibited significant hemispheric asymmetry ($P < 0.05$, Bonferroni-corrected) in nodal efficiency. For the normal controls shown

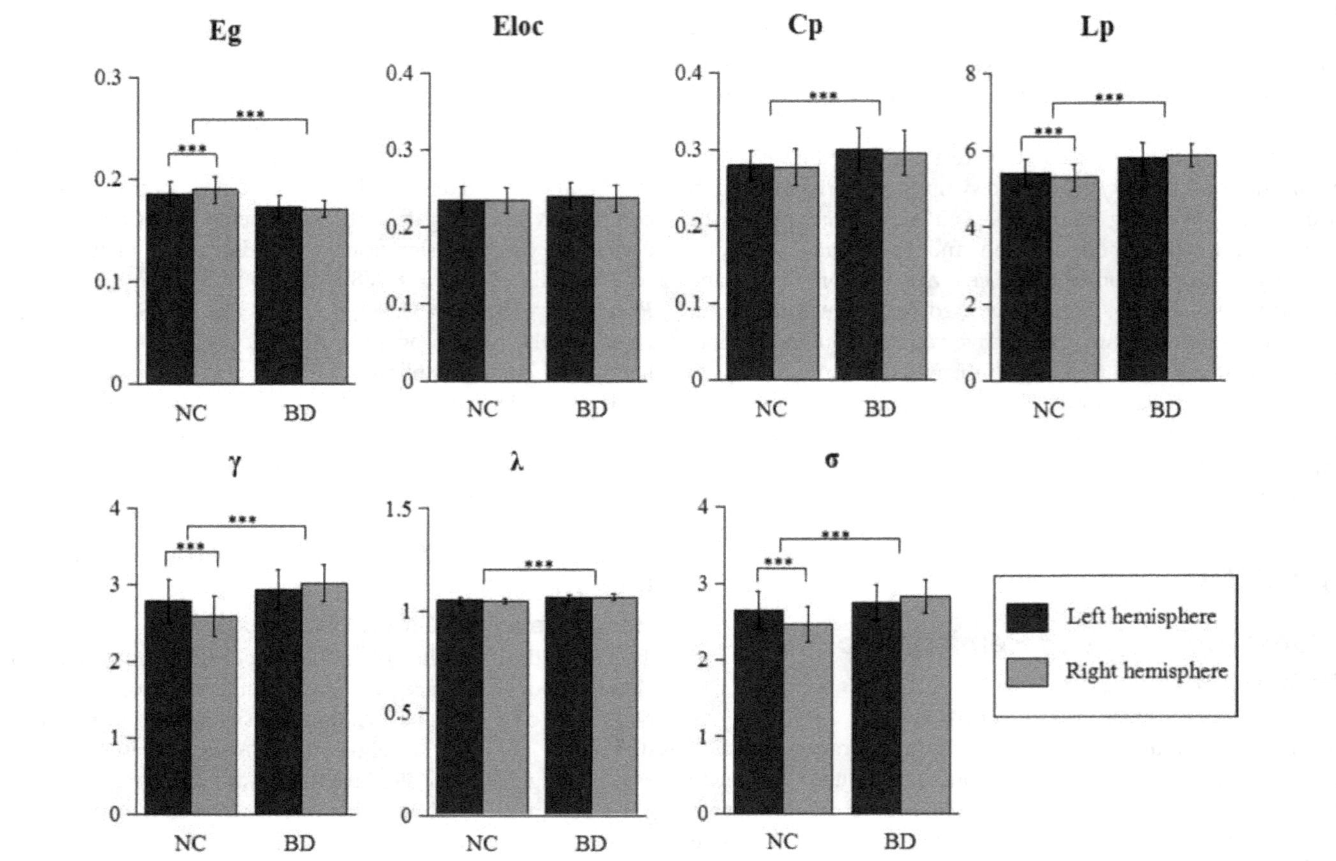

FIGURE 1 | Further statistical analysis of network properties. Bars represent mean ± SD. Each horizontal line and associated number represent the *P*-value of a *t*-test (paired *t*-test for hemispheric difference at each group and two-sample *t*-test for group difference). Significant differences are marked with asterisk (***$P < 0.001$). BD, bipolar disorder; NC, normal control.

TABLE 2 | Group differences on the asymmetry scores of the network properties.

Properties	Patients with BD t_{48} (*P*-value)	NC subjects t_{60} (*P*-value)	BD versus NC $F_{1,106}$ (*P*-value)
AS(E_g)	−0.201(0.842)	3.852(**< 0.001**)	8.268(**0.005**)
AS(E_{loc})	−0.756(0.453)	0.078(0.938)	0.048(0.827)
AS(C_p)	−0.719(0.476)	−0.591(0.557)	0.001(0.998)
AS(L_p)	1.118(0.269)	−3.852(**< 0.001**)	8.268(**0.005**)
AS(γ)	0.916(0.061)	−6.447(**< 0.001**)	33.684(**< 0.001**)
AS(λ)	0.693(0.491)	−1.624(0.110)	1.649(0.202)
AS(σ)	1.899(0.064)	−6.578(**< 0.001**)	35.657(**< 0.001**)

A one-sample two-tailed t-test was used to evaluate the statistical results within each group. The between-group differences were computed via a univariate ANCOVA, and the effects of age, gender, and age by-gender interaction were controlled for all of these analyses. A negative t-value within each group shows a leftward asymmetry and vice versa. The significant effect (P < 0.05) of network property was expressed in bold. BD, bipolar disorder; NC, normal control.

in **Figure 4A**, the nodal efficiency with rightward asymmetry covered the inferior occipital gyrus (IOG), the orbitofrontal gyrus, the middle part (ORBmid), Cuneus (CUN), and ANG, SMG, SOG, and ROL. In contrast, the leftward asymmetric nodes were mainly located at the superior frontal gyrus, medial part (SFGmed), SMA, and Heschl (HES). For patients with BD shown in **Figure 4B**, the regions with significant leftward asymmetries in nodal efficiency involved the ITG, LING, SFGmed, ACG, middle occipital gyrus (MOG), HES, and IPL regions. Regions with significant rightward asymmetries in nodal efficiency were located at the ANG, Pallidium (PAL), CAL, and SMA. Additionally, the group differences in asymmetry score can find the reasons resulted from group-by-hemisphere interaction. When comparing the group differences in the asymmetry score, significant differences ($P < 0.05$, Bonferroni-corrected) were observed in the SMG, SOG, ROL, ITG, LING, IPL, ACG, and SMA. Specifically, patient with BD showed significant less rightward asymmetry in the ROL, SOG, and SMG, and more leftward asymmetry in the IPL, ACG, ITG, and LING, which were attributed to significantly more reductions nodal

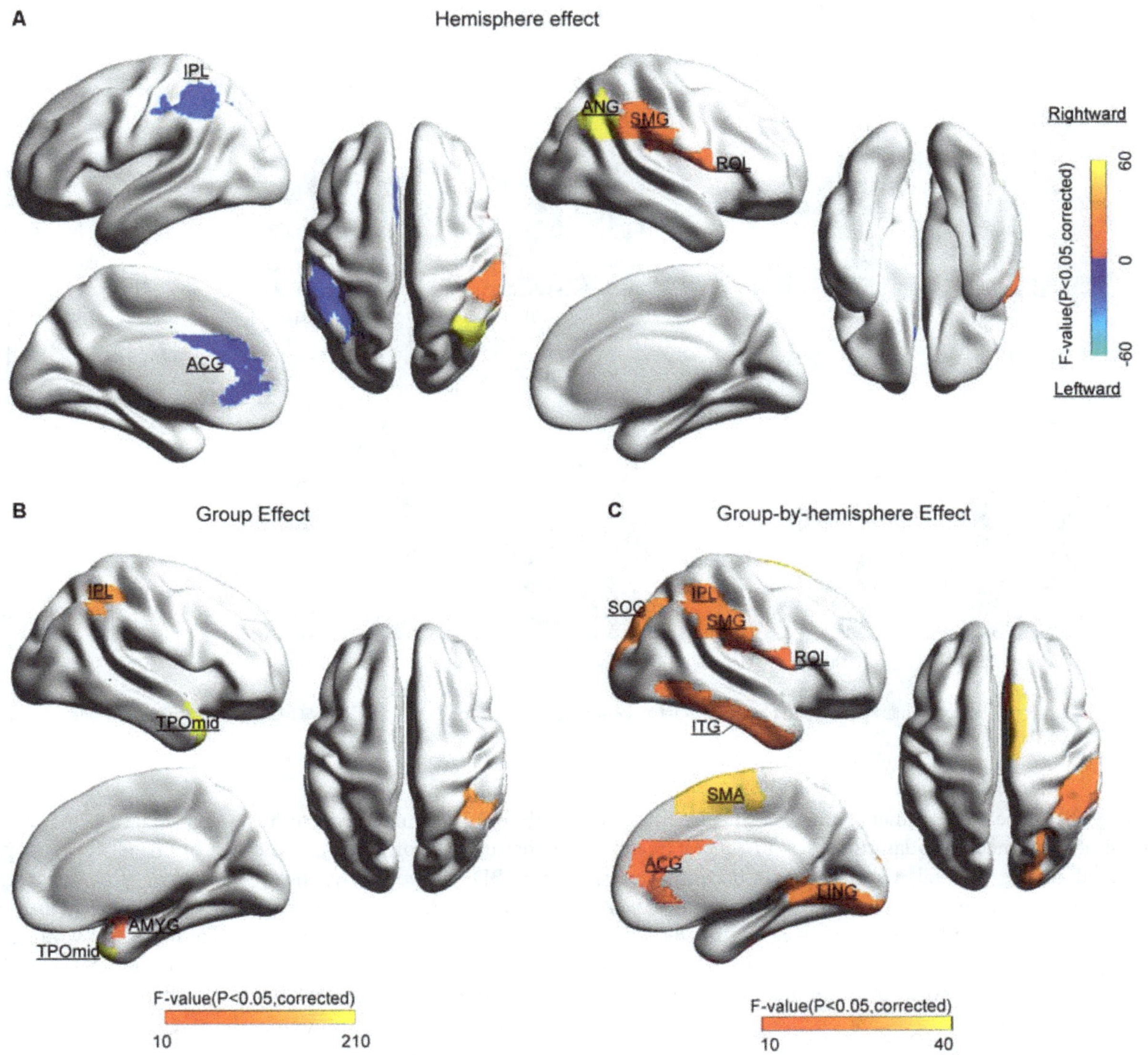

FIGURE 2 | Cortical regions with significant differences **(A)** hemispheric difference, **(B)** group difference, and **(C)** group-by-hemispheric interaction on the nodal efficiency. The color bar denotes *F*-values. Significant difference was identified with a threshold value of $P < 0.05$ (Bonferroni-corrected). Significantly different regions were overlaid on surface maps provided by BrainNet Viewer software (Xia et al., 2013).

efficiency in right hemispheric. Only nodal efficiency of SMA in left hemisphere significantly reduced in patients with BD when compared with normal controls, and resulting in reversed hemispheric asymmetry.

Relationship Between Hemispheric Asymmetry and BD Symptom Severity

Interestingly, we found the asymmetry scores of regional properties were correlated with BD symptom severity no matter using the Pearson or Spearman method. As shown in **Figure 5**, the nodal efficiency in ROL showed a significant and positive correlation with YMRS [AS(ROL), Pearson: $r = 0.24$, $P = 0.05$; Spearman: $r = 0.29$, $P = 0.02$], and the nodal efficiency in IPL showed a significant and negative correlation with YMRS [AS(IPL), Pearson: $r = -0.31$, $P = 0.02$; Spearman: $r = -0.25$, $P = 0.04$].

DISCUSSION

This current study employed DTI tractography and graph theory to examine the hemispheric asymmetries in brain WM networks in patients with BD. The hemispheric networks of patients were observed to have abnormal small-world property and reduced in global integration. Significant group-by-hemisphere interaction was revealed in the global efficiency, characteristic path length, and small-world property, which was attributed to significantly reduced global integration and increased small-word characteristic of right hemisphere in patients with BD

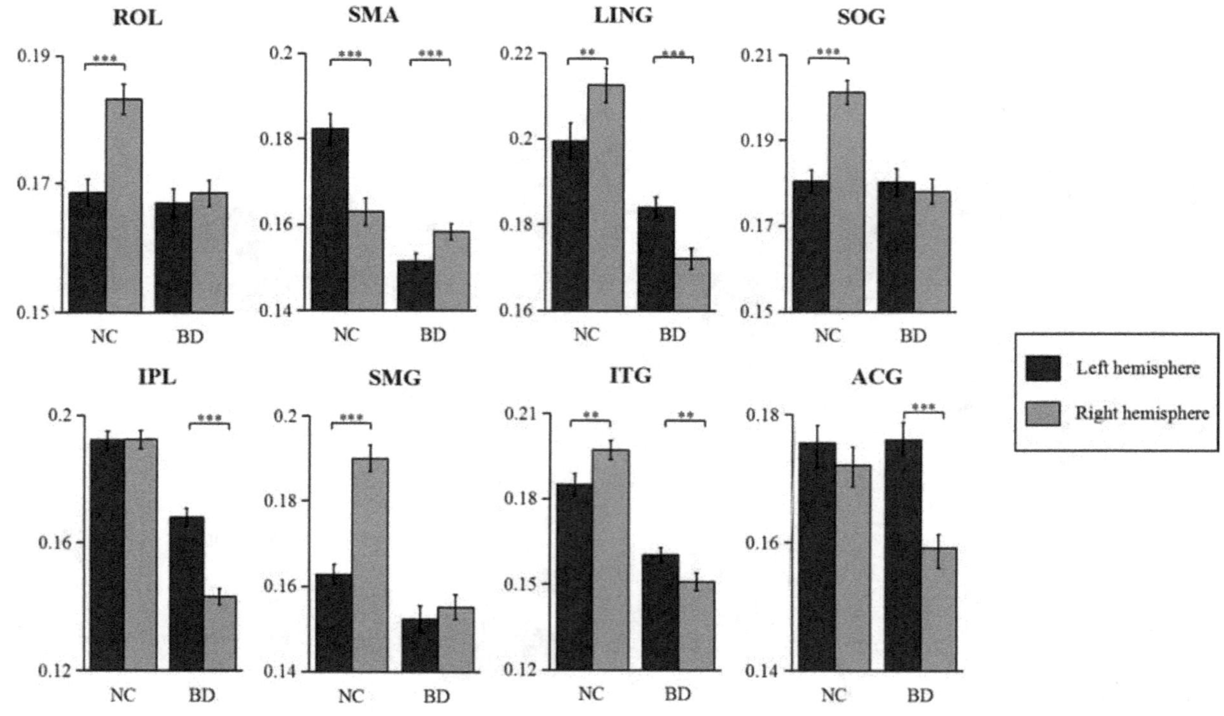

FIGURE 3 | The nodal efficiency of normal controls and bipolar disorder in several regions including PUT, ROL, and SFGdor. Error bar indicates standard error. $^{***}P < 0.001$, $^{**}P < 0.01$.

compared with those in normal controls. Specifically, we found atypical asymmetric nodal efficiency in several regions mostly located at the parietal, temporal, and occipital areas. Furthermore, we revealed that the network properties were significantly correlated with symptom severity in BD. Our findings might provide a potential neural biomarkers of that the altered hemispheric asymmetries in brain anatomical networks for clinical presentation of BD.

Hemisphere-Related Differences in Small-World Properties

In present work, hemispheric anatomical networks were used to evaluate the abnormal topological properties in patients with BD. Consistent with previous studies on whole-brain anatomical networks (Puetz et al., 2016; O'Donoghue et al., 2017), the hemispheric networks of both normal controls and BD patients preserved significant small-world property, that was significantly more clustered than random networks and had approximately the same characteristic path length as random networks (Watts and Strogatz, 1998). Moreover, we observed significant group differences in topological properties between normal controls and patients with BD. The smaller global efficiency, longer path length, and larger small-world property were shown in patients with BD compared with normal controls, suggesting a deficit in global integration (Munarini, 2013). Consistently, previous studies on whole-brain networks (Collin et al., 2016; Spielberg et al., 2016; Roberts et al., 2018) also showed smaller global efficiency and longer characteristic path length in patients with BD. Overall, these results suggested that the deficits in global integration were common in brain networks in patients with BD. Importantly, these abnormal global integrations were hemisphere-independent, which might be mainly due to the deficits of intra-hemispheric connections. Contemporary theories suggest that the complex clinical presentation of BD can be described as an aberration in the efficiency of information exchange between separate neural networks in the human brain (Vargas et al., 2013). Along this notion, our findings suggested the hemisphere-independent anatomical network with significantly smaller global efficiency and longer characteristic path length provides evidence for the hemispheric anatomical networks in patients with BD as a disconnection syndrome (Dae-Jin et al., 2013; Collin et al., 2016), especially for the right hemisphere.

The currently observed rightward asymmetry in global efficiency for normal controls suggests that the right hemisphere is intra-connected in a better integrated way, allowing for more efficient communication at the hemispheric level. Consistently, rightward asymmetry in network efficiency has been reported in healthy adults(Iturria-Medina et al., 2008; Sun et al., 2015). Interestingly, such rightward advantage in global integration in normal controls was absent in patients with BD. Instead, a roughly symmetrical pattern of global integration at the global level was found. The absence of rightward asymmetry in global integration was mainly due to the decrease of global integration in right hemisphere. According to lateralization of brain cognation theories, such absence of rightward asymmetry in global integration might underlie the BD dysfunctions in attention, visuospatial abilities (Cullen et al., 2016), and emotion

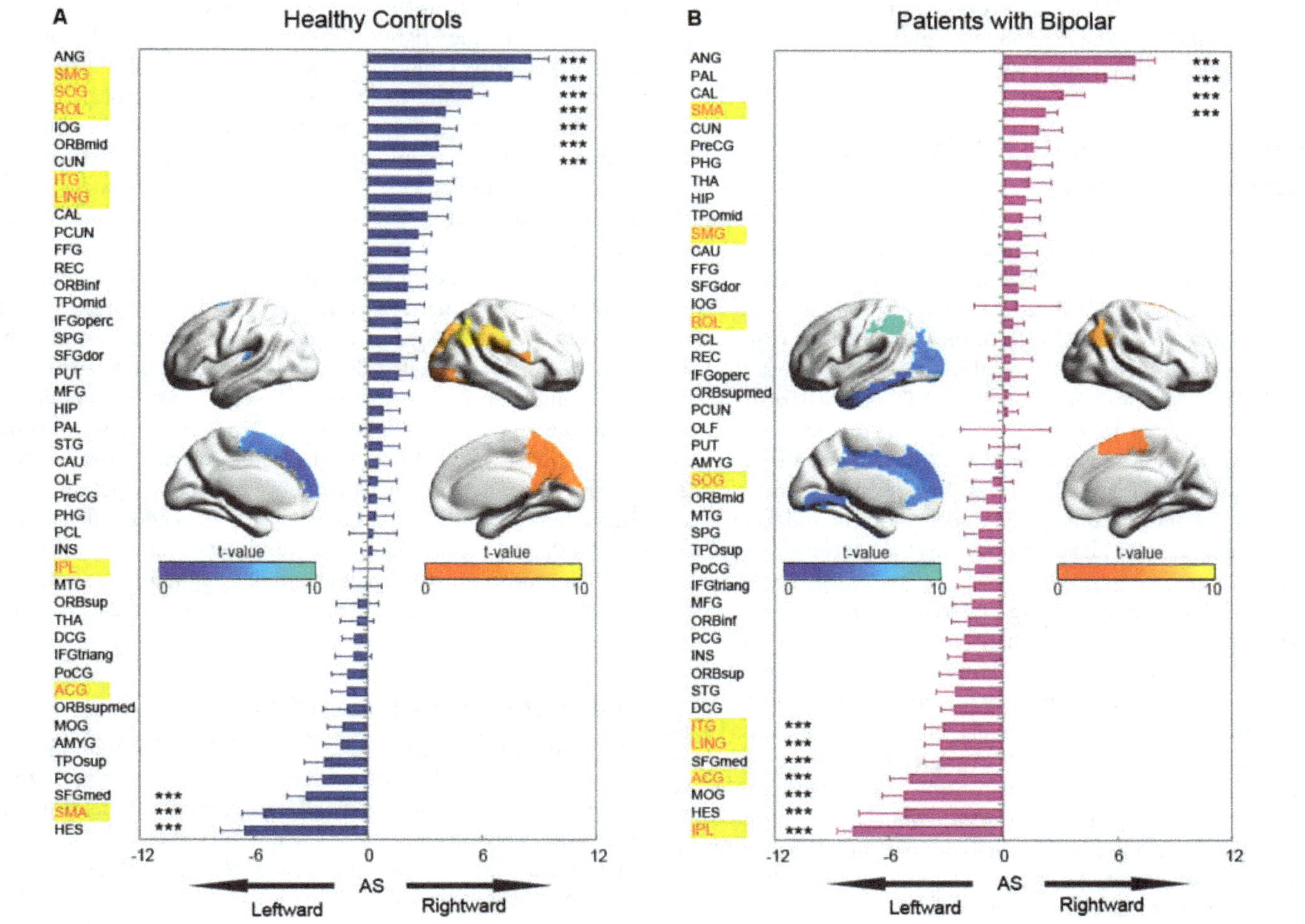

FIGURE 4 | The asymmetry scores of nodal efficiency for the hemispheric network with 45 nodes. Each bar indicates the mean asymmetry scores (AS). Error bars represent standard error. For both groups of **(A)** normal controls and **(B)** patients with BD, regions with significant AS are marked with asterisk (***$P < 0.001$, Bonferroni-corrected). All the regions in each group were ascending sorted according to the statistical *t*-values. Similarly, the color bar indicated the statistical *t*-values. The spatial distributions of cortical regions with significant AS in both groups were also presented with BrainNet Viewer software (Xia et al., 2013). Cortical regions with significant group difference were presented with yellow background.

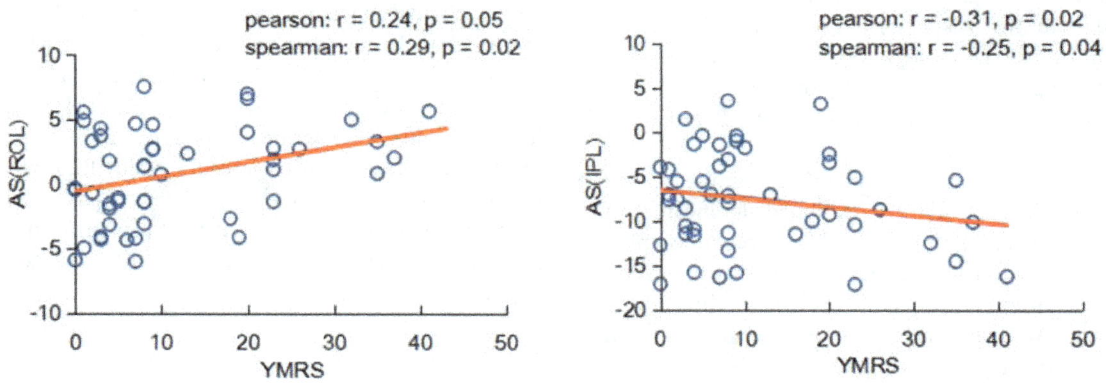

FIGURE 5 | Partial correlation coefficients between the nodal asymmetry scores and clinical features of patients with BD.

regulation (Schwartz et al., 1975), which are considered to be dominantly processed in the right hemisphere. The decreased global integration in the right hemisphere was supported by the WM destruction in BD, specifically in the cingulum, corpus callosum, and superior longitudinal fasciculus (Ho et al., 2017). Our findings extend earlier work and provide network evidence that patients with BD have abnormal asymmetries in hemispheric networks and deficits in global integration in the functional networks of the right hemisphere.

Hemisphere-Related Differences in Nodal Properties

Compared with normal controls, patients with BD exhibited reduced nodal efficiency in several regions (including the AMYG, the IPL, the PUT, and the TPOmid). Previous DTI studies (Rosso et al., 2007; Passarotti et al., 2012) also reported that patients with BD exhibited degenerated WM connectivity in these regions. For example, the disturbed anatomical connectivity (decreased FA) in the AMYG (Mcintosh et al., 2008) and TPOmid (Barnea-Goraly et al., 2009) may represent the reduction of nodal efficiency observed in this study. Haller et al. (2011) found that the gray matter of the PUT in patients with BD was significantly smaller than that in normal controls. The aberrations in nodal efficiency provided regional evidence to underline the neurobiological basis of BD.

In addition to the group differences in nodal efficiency, significant group-by-hemisphere interactions were found in ROL, SMG, ITG, SOG, and LING, attributing to significantly reduced hemispheric asymmetry in patients with BD compared with normal controls. The nodal efficiency of patients with BD showed more decreased in right hemisphere than left hemisphere relative to normal controls. Consistently, previous studies on BD revealed disrupted connectivity in the right hemisphere including ROL (Gernsbacher and Kaschak, 2003) and SMG (Wang et al., 2016), ITG, SOG, and LING (Green, 2006; Bearden et al., 2015). The right ROL and SMG regions were demonstrated involving emotional regulation (Silani et al., 2013). Considering one of significant symptoms of patients with BD was emotional regulation (Pavuluri et al., 2006, 2007), the reduction of nodal efficiency in these regions were proposed to associate with the impaired in emotional regulation in BD (Pavuluri et al., 2007). Moreover, it has been demonstrated that the right SOG, ITG, and LING regions were as associated with the visuospatial processing (Green, 2006; Bearden et al., 2015). The reduction of nodal efficiency in these occipital and temporal regions might be associated with the deficits in visuospatial functions (Green, 2006; Bearden et al., 2015).

Moreover, we also found that attention cognitive function regions including the ACG and IPL exhibited significant group-by-hemisphere interaction and group differences in asymmetry score. Because the nodal efficiency of right hemisphere in BD patients showed more reduction than those in left hemisphere, the ACG and IPL exhibited significant leftward hemispheric asymmetry. Consistently, previous studies have reported decreased connectivity in these two regions in patients with BD. For example, significantly decreased connectivity was found in the right ACG (Anand et al., 2009; Wang et al., 2009). Barnea-Goraly et al. (2009) reported that adolescents with BD had lower FA values than normal controls in the IPL region. Moreover, studies have showed that alterations in two regions are closely to the brain function in patients with BD. Patients with BD was demonstrated with decrease activation in the right ACG relative to normal controls during response inhibition task (Passarotti et al., 2010). The gray matter volume in the right parietal cortical regions correlated positively with the better inhibitory control in BD patients (Haldane et al., 2008). We further proposed that the abnormal asymmetries of nodal efficiency in patients with BD were associated with abnormal attention or inhibition function.

Interestingly, the patients with BD exhibited the significant rightward hemispheric asymmetry only in the SMA region, whereas a reversed asymmetry (leftward) in normal controls. The SMA region was revealed significant difference between the BD group and normal controls (Khadka et al., 2013). In addition, convergent studies (Caligiuri et al., 2003, 2004) have reported that patients with BD exhibited greater activities in right SMA during motor performance than those in left SMA. These results suggested that abnormalities in asymmetries of nodal efficiency in SMA influenced processing of motor function in BD (Puri et al., 2010; Rashid et al., 2014). These findings might provide potential neural biomarkers of the altered asymmetries in nodal efficiency for clinical presentation of BD.

Relationship Between Regional Asymmetries and BD Symptom Severity

An interesting finding of the current study was that within patients with BD, the topological properties in hemispheric networks were related to BD symptom severity. We found that nodal efficiency was associated with the YMRS, which reflected the severity of the current manic episode; a higher YMRS resulted in a more severe episode. A positive relationship between the asymmetry score of nodal efficiency in the ROL and the YMRS was revealed, indicating that the more connectivity in the right ROL, the more severe symptoms of BD. Recently, Gao et al. (2017) found that connectivity in the right ROL was positively associated with the classification of BD. Moreover, a negative relationship between the asymmetry score of nodal efficiency in the IPL and YMRS was observed. We suggested that the negative correlation might result from significantly decreased connectivity in the right IPL. That is, the larger YMRS score the less connected communication in the right IPL region. Similarly, Barnea-Goraly et al. (2009) reported that adolescents with BD had lower FA values than normal subjects in inferior parietal region. Our observation suggested that abnormal properties of hemispheric asymmetries may underlie the dysfunctions existed in patients with BD.

CONCLUSION

Using the DTI deterministic tractography method and graph theory, the current work evaluated the hemispheric effects on brain anatomical networks in patients with BD. The results revealed abnormalities in hemispheric asymmetries in patients with BD compared with those in normal controls. For the global network properties, the hemispheric asymmetry in global efficiency was significantly decreased and small-world property was significantly increased. Compared with normal controls, the nodal efficiency of patients also showed decreased rightward asymmetry mainly in the frontal, occipital, parietal, and temporal lobes. Exceptionally, the SMA region in patients with BD showed increased rightward asymmetries, attributing to a significantly reduction of the efficiency in left SMA. The asymmetry score of nodal efficiencies in the IPL and ROL exhibited correlations with clinical features of BD. These observations highlight that the altered hemispheric asymmetries in brain anatomical networks and the potential of brain hemispheric network measures as neural biomarkers for clinical presentation of BD. Our findings suggested that abnormal asymmetries in properties of hemispheric networks may underlie the dysfunctions in emotion and attention in patients with BD.

The research of this paper still has some limitations. In this study, the subjects was chosen from one site with small number of BD patient, limiting the statistical results of hemispheric effects and may bring about the type I error on brain network and region alterations. In order to evaluate accurately alteration in hemispheric asymmetry in patients with BD, the subjects with large number or from multi-site will be considered in the future work. Additionally, studies have reported that both gender and age are potential factors linked to brain asymmetry. Hence, we will further examine gender and age effects on hemispheric asymmetries in brain anatomical networks in BD.

AUTHOR CONTRIBUTIONS

BW completed the entire study of the experiment and writing. TL, MZ, SZ, YN, and XW revised the manuscript. TY, RC, and JX provided advice and guidance. DL provided the research ideas.

FUNDING

This work was supported by the National Natural Science Foundation of China (Grant Nos. 61503272, 61503273, 61873178, and 61741212), the project funded by the China Postdoctoral Science Foundation (Grant No. 2016 M601287), the Shanxi Provincial Foundation for Returned Scholars, China (Grant No. 2016-037), the Scientific Research Foundation for Returned Overseas Chinese Scholars (Grant No. 20151098-2), the Key Research and Development Project in Shanxi (Grant No. 201603D111014).

REFERENCES

Achard, S., and Bullmore, E. (2007). Efficiency and cost of economical brain functional networks. *PLoS Comput. Biol.* 3:e17. doi: 10.1371/journal.pcbi.0030017

Anand, A., Li, Y., Wang, Y., Lowe, M. J., and Dzemidzic, M. (2009). Resting state corticolimbic connectivity abnormalities in unmedicated bipolar disorder and unipolar depression. *Psychiatry Res.* 171, 189–198. doi: 10.1016/j.pscychresns.2008.03.012

Bai, F., Shu, N., Yuan, Y., Shi, Y., Yu, H., Wu, D., et al. (2012). Topologically convergent and divergent structural connectivity patterns between patients with remitted geriatric depression and amnestic mild cognitive impairment. *J. Neurosci.* 32, 4307–4318. doi: 10.1523/JNEUROSCI.5061-11.2012

Barnea-Goraly, N., Chang, K. D., Karchemskiy, A., Howe, M. E., and Reiss, A. L. (2009). Limbic and corpus callosum aberrations in adolescents with bipolar disorder: a tract-based spatial statistics analysis. *Biol. Psychiatry* 66, 238–244. doi: 10.1016/j.biopsych.2009.02.025

Bearden, C. E., Hoffman, K. M., and Cannon, T. D. (2015). The neuropsychology and neuroanatomy of bipolar affective disorder: a critical review. *Bipolar Disord.* 3, 106–150. doi: 10.1034/j.1399-5618.2001.030302.x

Belmaker, R. H. (2004). Bipolar disorder (invited review). *New Engl. J. Med.* 351, 476–486. doi: 10.1056/NEJMra035354

Beyer, J. L., Taylor, W. D., Macfall, J. R., Kuchibhatla, M., Payne, M. E., Provenzale, J. M., et al. (2005). Cortical white matter microstructural abnormalities in bipolar disorder. *Neuropsychopharmacology* 30, 2225–2229. doi: 10.1038/sj.npp.1300802

Bruno, S., Cercignani, M., and Ron, M. A. (2008). White matter abnormalities in bipolar disorder: a voxel-based diffusion tensor imaging study. *Bipolar Disord.* 10, 460–468. doi: 10.1111/j.1399-5618.2007.00552.x

Bullmore, E., and Sporns, O. (2009). Complex brain networks: graph theoretical analysis of structural and functional systems. *Nat. Rev. Neurosci.* 10, 186–198. doi: 10.1038/nrn2575

Cabeza, R. (2002). Hemispheric asymmetry reduction in older adults: the harold model. *Psychol. Aging* 17, 85–100. doi: 10.1037/0882-7974.17.1.85

Caligiuri, M. P., Brown, G. G., Meloy, M., Eyler, L. T., Kindermann, S. S., Eberson, S., et al. (2004). A functional magnetic resonance imaging study of cortical asymmetry in bipolar disorder. *Bipolar Disord.* 6, 183–196. doi: 10.1111/j.1399-5618.2004.00116.x

Caligiuri, M. P., Brown, G. G., Meloy, M. J., Eberson, S. C., Kindermann, S. S., Frank, L. R., et al. (2003). An fMRI study of affective state and medication on cortical and subcortical brain regions during motor performance in bipolar disorder. *Psychiatry Res.* 123, 171–182. doi: 10.1016/S0925-4927(03)00075-1

Collin, G., Scholtens, L. H., Kahn, R. S., Mhj, H., and van den Heuvel, M. P. (2017). Affected anatomical rich club and structural-functional coupling in young offspring of schizophrenia and bipolar disorder patients. *Biol. Psychiatry* 82, 746–755. doi: 10.1016/j.biopsych.2017.06.013

Collin, G., van den Heuvel, M. P., Abramovic, L., Vreeker, A., de Reus, M. A., van Haren, N. E., et al. (2016). Brain network analysis reveals affected connectome structure in bipolar I disorder. *Hum. Brain Mapp.* 37, 122–134. doi: 10.1002/hbm.23017

Cui, Z., Zhong, S., Xu, P., He, Y., and Gong, G. (2013). PANDA: a pipeline toolbox for analyzing brain diffusion images. *Front. Hum. Neurosci.* 7:42. doi: 10.3389/fnhum.2013.00042

Cullen, B., Ward, J., Graham, N. A., Deary, I. J., Pell, J. P., Smith, D. J., et al. (2016). Prevalence and correlates of cognitive impairment in euthymic adults with bipolar disorder: a systematic review. *J. Affect. Disord.* 205, 165–181. doi: 10.1016/j.jad.2016.06.063

Dae-Jin, K., Bolbecker, A. R., Josselyn, H., Olga, R., Olaf, S., Hetrick, W. P., et al. (2013). Disturbed resting state EEG synchronization in bipolar disorder: a graph-theoretic analysis. *Neuroimage Clin.* 2, 414–423. doi: 10.1016/j.nicl.2013.03.007

Dolcos, F., Rice, H. J., and Cabeza, R. (2002). Hemispheric asymmetry and aging: right hemisphere decline or asymmetry reduction. *Neurosci. Biobehav. Rev.* 26, 819–825. doi: 10.1016/S0149-7634(02)00068-4

Forde, N. J., O'Donoghue, S., Scanlon, C., Emsell, L., Chaddock, C., Leemans, A., et al. (2015). Structural brain network analysis in families multiply affected with bipolar I disorder. *Psychiatry Res.* 234, 44–51. doi: 10.1016/j.pscychresns.2015.08.004

Gao, S., Osuch, E. A., Wammes, M., Theberge, J., Jiang, T. Z., Calhoun, V. D., et al. (2017). Discriminating bipolar disorder from major depression based on kernel SVM using functional independent components. *Paper Presented at the IEEE International Workshop on Machine Learning for Signal Processing*, Aalborg. doi: 10.1109/MLSP.2017.8168110

Gernsbacher, M. A., and Kaschak, M. P. (2003). Neuroimaging studies of language production and comprehension. *Annu. Rev. Psychol.* 54, 91–114. doi: 10.1146/annurev.psych.54.101601.145128

Gong, G., He, Y., Concha, L., Lebel, C., Gross, D. W., Evans, A. C., et al. (2009). Mapping anatomical connectivity patterns of human cerebral cortex using in vivo diffusion tensor imaging tractography. *Cereb. Cortex* 19, 524–536. doi: 10.1093/cercor/bhn102

Good, C. D., Johnsrude, I., Ashburner, J., Henson, R. N., Friston, K. J., and Frackowiak, R. S. (2001). Cerebral asymmetry and the effects of sex and handedness on brain structure: a voxel-based morphometric analysis of 465 normal adult human brains. *Neuroimage* 14, 685–700. doi: 10.1006/nimg.2001.0857

Green, M. F. (2006). Cognitive impairment and functional outcome in schizophrenia and bipolar disorder. *J. Clin. Psychiatry* 67(Suppl. 9), 3–8; discussion 36–42. doi: 10.4088/JCP.1006e12

Haldane, M., Cunningham, G., Androutsos, C., and Frangou, S. (2008). Structural brain correlates of response inhibition in bipolar disorder I. *J. Psychopharmacol.* 22, 138–143. doi: 10.1177/0269881107082955

Haller, S., Xekardaki, A., Delaloye, C., Canuto, A., Lövblad, K. O., Gold, G., et al. (2011). Combined analysis of grey matter voxel-based morphometry and white matter tract-based spatial statistics in late-life bipolar disorder. *J. Psychiatry Neurosci.* 36, 391–401. doi: 10.1503/jpn.100140

Hamilton, M. (1960). A rating scale for depression. *J. Neurol Neurosurg. Psychiatry* 23, 56–62. doi: 10.1136/jnnp.23.1.56

Highley, J. R., Mcdonald, B., Walker, M. A., Esiri, M. M., and Crow, T. J. (1999). Schizophrenia and temporal lobe asymmetry. A post-mortem stereological study of tissue volume. *Br. J. Psychiatry* 175, 127–134. doi: 10.1192/bjp.175.2.127

Ho, N. F., Li, Z., Ji, F., Wang, M., Kuswanto, C. N., Sum, M. Y., et al. (2017). Hemispheric lateralization abnormalities of the white matter microstructure in patients with schizophrenia and bipolar disorder. *J. Psychiatry Neurosci.* 42, 242–251. doi: 10.1503/jpn.160090

Iturriamedina, Y., Pérez, F. A., Morris, D. M., Canalesrodríguez, E. J., Haroon, H. A., García, P. L., et al. (2011). Brain hemispheric structural efficiency and interconnectivity rightward asymmetry in human and nonhuman primates. *Cereb. Cortex* 21, 56–67. doi: 10.1093/cercor/bhq058

Iturria-Medina, Y., Sotero, R. C., Canales-Rodríguez, E. J., Alemán-Gómez, Y., and Melie-García, L. (2008). Studying the human brain anatomical network via diffusion-weighted MRI and graph theory. *Neuroimage* 40, 1064–1076. doi: 10.1016/j.neuroimage.2007.10.060

Jenkinson, M., Bannister, P., Brady, M., and Smith, S. (2002). Improved optimization for the robust and accurate linear registration and motion correction of brain images. *Neuroimage* 17, 825–841. doi: 10.1006/nimg.2002.1132

Kafantaris, V., Kingsley, P., Ardekani, B., Saito, E., Lencz, T., Lim, K., et al. (2009). Lower orbital frontal white matter integrity in adolescents with bipolar I disorder. *J. Am. Acad. Child Adolesc. Psychiatry* 48, 79–86. doi: 10.1097/CHI.0b013e3181900421

Khadka, S., Meda, S. A., Stevens, M. C., Glahn, D. C., Calhoun, V. D., Sweeney, J. A., et al. (2013). Is aberrant functional connectivity a psychosis endophenotype? A resting state functional magnetic resonance imaging study. *Biol. Psychiatry* 74, 458–466. doi: 10.1016/j.biopsych.2013.04.024

Kwon, J. S., Youn, T., and Jung, H. Y. (1996). Right hemisphere abnormalities in major depression: quantitative electroencephalographic findings before and after treatment. *J. Affect. Disord.* 40, 169–173. doi: 10.1016/0165-0327(96)00057-2

Leow, A., Ajilore, O., Zhan, L., Arienzo, D., Gadelkarim, J., Zhang, A., et al. (2013). Impaired inter-hemispheric integration in bipolar disorder revealed using brain network analyses. *Biol. Psychiatry* 73, 183–193. doi: 10.1016/j.biopsych.2012.09.014

Mahon, K., Burdick, K. E., Ikuta, T., Braga, R. J., Gruner, P., Malhotra, A. K., et al. (2013). Abnormal temporal lobe white matter as a biomarker for genetic risk of bipolar disorder. *Biol. Psychiatry* 73, 177–182. doi: 10.1016/j.biopsych.2012.07.033

McGlone, J. (1980). Sex differences in human brain asymmetry: a critical survey. *Behav. Brain Sci.* 3, 215–227. doi: 10.1017/S0140525X00004398

Mcintosh, A. M., Muñoz, M. S., Lymer, G. K., Mckirdy, J., Hall, J., Sussmann, J. E., et al. (2008). White matter tractography in bipolar disorder and schizophrenia. *Biol. Psychiatry* 64, 1088–1092. doi: 10.1016/j.biopsych.2008.07.026

Miller, S. R., Miller, C. J., Bloom, J. S., Hynd, G. W., and Craggs, J. G. (2006). Right hemisphere brain morphology, attention-deficit hyperactivity disorder (ADHD) subtype, and social comprehension. *J. Child Neurol.* 21, 139–144. doi: 10.1177/08830738060210021901

Mori, S., Crain, B. J., Chacko, V. P., and van Zijl, P. C. (1999). Three-dimensional tracking of axonal projections in the brain by magnetic resonance imaging. *Ann. Neurol.* 45, 265–269. doi: 10.1002/1531-8249(199902)45:2<265::AID-ANA21>3.0.CO;2-3

Munarini, G. (2013). Presentazione articolo: complex network measures of brain connectivity uses and interpretations. *Paper Presented at the Corso Psicologia Matematica*, Cattolica.

O'Donoghue, S., Kilmartin, L., O'Hora, D., Emsell, L., Langan, C., Mcinerney, S., et al. (2017). Anatomical integration and rich-club connectivity in euthymic bipolar disorder. *Psychol. Med.* 47, 1609–1623. doi: 10.1017/S0033291717000058

Park, H., Westin, C., Kubicki, M., Maier, S. E., Niznikiewicz, M., Baer, A., et al. (2004). White matter hemisphere asymmetries in healthy subjects and in schizophrenia: a diffusion tensor MRI study. *Neuroimage* 23, 213–223. doi: 10.1016/j.neuroimage.2004.04.036

Passarotti, A. M., Ellis, J., Wegbreit, E., Stevens, M. C., and Pavuluri, M. N. (2012). Reduced functional connectivity of prefrontal regions and amygdala within affect and working memory networks in pediatric bipolar disorder. *Brain Connect.* 2, 320–334. doi: 10.1089/brain.2012.0089

Passarotti, A. M., Sweeney, J. A., and Pavuluri, M. N. (2010). Neural correlates of response inhibition in pediatric bipolar disorder and attention deficit hyperactivity disorder. *Psychiatry Res.* 181, 36–43. doi: 10.1016/j.pscychresns.2009.07.002

Pavuluri, M. N., O'Connor, M. M., Harral, E., and Sweeney, J. A. (2007). Affective neural circuitry during facial emotion processing in pediatric bipolar disorder. *Biol. Psychiatry* 62, 158–167. doi: 10.1016/j.biopsych.2006.07.011

Pavuluri, M. N., Schenkel, L. S., Aryal, S., Harral, E. M., Hill, S. K., Herbener, E. S., et al. (2006). Neurocognitive function in unmedicated manic and medicated euthymic pediatric bipolar patients. *Am. J. Psychiatry* 163, 286–293. doi: 10.1176/appi.ajp.163.2.286

Poldrack, R. A., and Gorgolewski, K. J. (2015). OpenfMRI: open sharing of task fMRI data. *Neuroimage* 144(Pt B), 259–261. doi: 10.1016/j.neuroimage.2015.05.073

Puetz, V. B., Parker, D., Kohn, N., Dahmen, B., Verma, R., and Konrad, K. (2016). Altered brain network integrity after childhood maltreatment: a structural connectomic DTI-study. *Hum. Brain Mapp.* 38, 855–868. doi: 10.1002/hbm.23423

Puri, B. K., Agour, M., Gunatilake, K. D., Fernando, K. A., Gurusinghe, A. I., and Treasaden, I. H. (2010). Reduction in left supplementary motor area grey matter in adult female fibromyalgia sufferers with marked fatigue and without affective disorder: a pilot controlled 3-T magnetic resonance imaging voxel-based morphometry study. *J. Int. Med. Res.* 38, 1468–1472. doi: 10.1177/147323001003800429

Rashid, B., Damaraju, E., Pearlson, G. D., and Calhoun, V. D. (2014). Dynamic connectivity states estimated from resting fMRI Identify differences among Schizophrenia, bipolar disorder, and healthy control subjects. *Front. Hum. Neurosci.* 8:897. doi: 10.3389/fnhum.2014.00897

Ratnarajah, N., Rifkin-Graboi, A., Fortier, M. V., Chong, Y. S., Kwek, K., Saw, S. M., et al. (2013). Structural connectivity asymmetry in the neonatal brain. *Neuroimage* 75, 187–194. doi: 10.1016/j.neuroimage.2013.02.052

Rimol, L. M., Hartberg, C. B., Nesvåg, R., Fennemanotestine, C., Hagler, D. J., Pung, C. J., et al. (2010). Cortical thickness and subcortical volumes in schizophrenia and bipolar disorder. *Biol. Psychiatry* 117, 41–50. doi: 10.1016/j.biopsych.2010.03.036

Roberts, G., Perry, A., Lord, A., Frankland, A., Leung, V., Holmespreston, E., et al. (2018). Structural dysconnectivity of key cognitive and emotional hubs in young people at high genetic risk for bipolar disorder. *Mol. Psychiatry* 23, 413–421. doi: 10.1038/mp.2016.216

Rosso, I. M., Killgore, W. D., Cintron, C. M., Gruber, S. A., Tohen, M., and Yurgelun-Todd, D. A. (2007). Reduced amygdala volumes in first-episode bipolar disorder and correlation with cerebral white matter. *Biol. Psychiatry* 61, 743–749. doi: 10.1016/j.biopsych.2006.07.035

Rubinov, M., and Sporns, O. (2010). Complex network measures of brain connectivity: uses and interpretations. *Neuroimage* 52, 1059–1069. doi: 10.1016/j.neuroimage.2009.10.003

Saunders, K. E. A., and Goodwin, G. M. (2010). The course of bipolar disorder. *Adv. Psychiatr. Treat.* 16, 318–328. doi: 10.1192/apt.bp.107.004903

Schulte, T., Mülleroehring, E. M., Sullivan, E. V., and Pfefferbaum, A. (2012). White matter fiber compromise contributes differentially to attention and emotion processing impairment in alcoholism, HIV-infection, and their comorbidity. *Neuropsychologia* 50, 2812–2822. doi: 10.1016/j.neuropsychologia.2012.07.042

Schwartz, G. E., Davidson, R. J., and Maer, F. (1975). Right hemisphere lateralization for emotion in the human brain: interactions with cognition. *Science* 190, 286–288. doi: 10.1126/science.1179210

Shu, N., Liu, Y., Li, K., Duan, Y., Wang, J., Yu, C., et al. (2011). Diffusion tensor tractography reveals disrupted topological efficiency in white matter structural networks in multiple sclerosis. *Cereb. Cortex* 21, 2565–2577. doi: 10.1093/cercor/bhr039

Sigalovsky, I. S., Fischl, B., and Melcher, J. R. (2006). Mapping an intrinsic MR property of gray matter in auditory cortex of living humans: a possible marker for primary cortex and hemispheric differences. *Neuroimage* 32, 1524–1537. doi: 10.1016/j.neuroimage.2006.05.023

Silani, G., Lamm, C., Ruff, C. C., and Singer, T. (2013). Right supramarginal gyrus is crucial to overcome emotional egocentricity bias in social judgments. *J. Neurosci.* 33, 15466–15476. doi: 10.1523/JNEUROSCI.1488-13.2013

Spielberg, J. M., Beall, E. B., Hulvershorn, L. A., Altinay, M., Karne, H., and Anand, A. (2016). Resting state brain network disturbances related to hypomania & depression in medication-free bipolar disorder. *Neuropsychopharmacology* 41, 3016–3024. doi: 10.1038/npp.2016.112

Sun, Y., Chen, Y., Collinson, S. L., Bezerianos, A., and Sim, K. (2015). Reduced hemispheric asymmetry of brain anatomical networks is linked to schizophrenia: a connectome study. *Cereb. Cortex* 27, 602–615. doi: 10.1093/cercor/bhv255

Toga, A. W., and Thompson, P. M. (2003). Mapping brain asymmetry. *Nat. Rev. Neurosci.* 4, 37–48. doi: 10.1038/nrn1009

Tzouriomazoyer, N., Landeau, B., Papathanassiou, D., Crivello, F., Etard, O., Delcroix, N., et al. (2002). Automated anatomical labeling of activations in SPM using a macroscopic anatomical parcellation of the MNI MRI single-subject brain. *Neuroimage* 15, 273–289. doi: 10.1006/nimg.2001.0978

Vargas, C., López-Jaramillo, C., and Vieta, E. (2013). A systematic literature review of resting state network—functional MRI in bipolar disorder. *J. Affect. Disord.* 150, 727–735. doi: 10.1016/j.jad.2013.05.083

Wang, F., Kalmar, J. H., He, Y., Jackowski, M., Chepenik, L. G., Edmiston, E. E., et al. (2009). Functional and structural connectivity between the perigenual anterior cingulate and amygdala in bipolar disorder. *Biol. Psychiatry* 66, 516–521. doi: 10.1016/j.biopsych.2009.03.023

Wang, Y., Zhong, S., Jia, Y., Sun, Y., Wang, B., Liu, T., et al. (2016). Disrupted resting-state functional connectivity in nonmedicated bipolar disorder. *Radiology* 280, 529–536. doi: 10.1148/radiol.2016151641

Watkins, K. E., Paus, T., Lerch, J. P., Zijdenbos, A., Collins, D. L., Neelin, P., et al. (2001). Structural asymmetries in the human brain: a voxel-based statistical analysis of 142 MRI scans. *Cereb. Cortex* 11, 868–877. doi: 10.1093/cercor/11.9.868

Watts, D. J., and Strogatz, S. H. (1998). Collectivedynamics of 'small-world' networks. *Nature* 393, 440–442. doi: 10.1038/30918

Wessa, M., Houenou, J., Leboyer, M., Chanraud, S., Poupon, C., Martinot, J. L., et al. (2009). Microstructural white matter changes in euthymic bipolar patients: a whole-brain diffusion tensor imaging study. *Bipolar Disord.* 11, 504–514. doi: 10.1111/j.1399-5618.2009.00718.x

Xia, M., Wang, J., and He, Y. (2013). BrainNet Viewer: a network visualization tool for human brain connectomics. *PLoS One* 8:e68910. doi: 10.1371/journal.pone.0068910

Yin, X., Han, Y., Ge, H., Xu, W., Huang, R., Zhang, D., et al. (2013). Inferior frontal white matter asymmetry correlates with executive control of attention. *Hum. Brain Mapp.* 34, 796–813. doi: 10.1002/hbm.21477

Young, R. C., Biggs, J. T., Ziegler, V. E., and Meyer, D. A. (1978). A rating scale for mania: reliability, validity and sensitivity. *Br. J. Psychiatry* 133, 429–435. doi: 10.1192/bjp.133.5.429

6

Gradual Disturbances of the Amplitude of Low-Frequency Fluctuations (ALFF) and Fractional ALFF in Alzheimer Spectrum

Liu Yang[1†], Yan Yan[2†], Yonghao Wang[2], Xiaochen Hu[3], Jie Lu[4], Piu Chan[1,5,6], Tianyi Yan[2] and Ying Han[1,5,6,7*]*

[1] Department of Neurology, Xuanwu Hospital, Capital Medical University, Beijing, China, [2] School of Life Science, Beijing Institute of Technology, Beijing, China, [3] Department of Psychiatry and Psychotherapy, Medical Faculty, University of Cologne, Cologne, Germany, [4] Department of Radiology, Xuanwu Hospital, Capital Medical University, Beijing, China, [5] Beijing Institute of Geriatrics, Beijing, China, [6] National Clinical Research Center for Geriatric Disorders, Eeijing, China, [7] Center of Alzheimer's Disease, Beijing Institute for Brain Disorders, Beijing, China

Correspondence:
Tianyi Yan
yantianyi@bit.edu.cn
Ying Han
hanying@xwh.ccmu.edu.cn

†These authors have contributed equally to this work

Background: Alzheimer's disease (AD) is a common neurodegenerative disease in which the brain undergoes alterations for decades before symptoms become obvious. Subjective cognitive decline (SCD) have self-complain of persistent decline in cognitive function especially in memory but perform normally on standard neuropsychological tests. SCD with the presence of AD pathology is the transitional stage 2 of Alzheimer's continuum, earlier than the prodromal stage, mild cognitive impairment (MCI), which seems to be the best target to research AD. In this study, we aimed to detect the transformational patterns of the intrinsic brain activity as the disease burden got heavy.

Method: In this study, we enrolled 44 SCD, 55 amnestic MCI (aMCI), 47 AD dementia (d-AD) patients and 57 normal controls (NC) in total. A machine learning classification was utilized to detect identification accuracies between groups by using ALFF, fALFF, and fusing ALFF with fALFF features. Then, we measured the amplitude of the low-frequency fluctuation (ALFF) and fractional ALFF (fALFF) levels in three frequency bands (classic: 0.01–0.1 Hz; slow-5: 0.01–0.027 Hz; and slow-4: 0.027–0.073 Hz) and compared alterations in patients with NC.

Results: In the machine learning verification, the identification accuracy of SCD, aMCI, d-AD from NC was higher when fused ALFF and fALFF features (76.44, 81.94, and 91.83%, respectively) than only using ALFF or fALFF features. Several brain regions showed significant differences in ALFF/fALFF within these bands among four groups: brain regions presented decreasing trend of values, including the Cingulum_Mid_R (aal), bilateral inferior cerebellum lobe, bilateral precuneus, and the Cingulum_Ant_R (aal); increasing trend of values were detected in the Hippocampus_L (aal), Frontal_Mid_Orb_R (aal), Frontal_Sup_R (aal) and Paracentral_Lobule_R (aal) as disease progressed. The normalized ALFF/fALFF values of these features were significantly correlated with the neuropsychological test scores.

Conclusion: This study revealed gradual disturbances in intrinsic brain activity as the disease progressed: the normal objective performance in SCD may be dependent on compensation; as disease advanced, the cognitive function gradually impaired and decompensated in aMCI, severer in d-AD. Our results indicated that the ALFF and fALFF may help detect the underlying pathological mechanism in AD continuum.

Clinical Trial Registration: ClinicalTrials.gov, identifier NCT02353884 and NCT02225964.

Keywords: Alzheimer's disease, subjective cognitive decline, amnestic mild cognitive impairment, dementia, resting-state functional MRI, ALFF, fALFF, classifier

INTRODUCTION

Alzheimer's disease (AD) is the most common progressive neurodegenerative disease of the elderly without a definite pathogenesis or effective treatment being found to decelerate the progression of this disorder, leading to poor outcomes and severe burdens to both the family and society (Scheltens et al., 2016). Explanations for the failure of drug clinical trials may be summarized by interventions during a stage of disease that is too late (McDade and Bateman, 2017). Thus, early detection of AD seems to be advantageous for the application of preventive means and may therefore help delay the progression. Clinical studies suggest the occurrence of very subtle cognitive alterations that are detectable years before meeting the criteria for MCI, predicting the progression to d-AD (Sperling et al., 2011). SCD refers to those elderly people who self-report a persistent decline in cognition but perform normally on the standard assessment with a higher conversion risk to MCI or d-AD, which is the transitional stage 2 of Alzheimer's continuum in the presence of AD pathology and seems to be the best target to research the underlying mechanism of AD (Sperling et al., 2011; Jessen et al., 2014; Mitchell et al., 2014; Jack et al., 2018; Jessen and Rodriguez Nee Then, 2018).

Neuroimaging techniques could help detect structural and functional brain abnormalities at an early stage before objective deficits are detectable. The rs-fMRI is a promising non-invasive functional imaging technique to measure spontaneous brain activities *in vivo* and helps detect the intrinsic brain functional architecture under normal and pathological conditions such as AD without performance confounders (Zhang and Raichle, 2010). It has been widely used to explore the neurophysiological mechanism and neural process of human cognition and to identify the functional integrity of brain networks supporting memory and other cognitive domains in AD (Sperling, 2011; Binnewijzend et al., 2012). The ALFF was introduced as a measure for the magnitude of LFOs of rs-fMRI. It is defined as the total power within the frequency range between 0.01 and 0.1 Hz and considered as an effective approach to detect the regional intensity of spontaneous fluctuations and to reflect spontaneous brain activity of the brain in the BOLD signal of the rs-fMRI (Fox and Raichle, 2007; Tomasi et al., 2013). Studies have indicated that this index may be used as a marker for disease states of the brain (Han et al., 2011; Chen et al., 2015; Wang et al., 2016). However, it can be impaired and influenced by non-neural physiological fluctuations such as respiration, cardiac action, and motion. The fALFF is the ALFF of a given frequency band as a fraction of the sum amplitudes across the whole frequency range. It is a normalized and modified index of ALFF that can improve the sensitivity and specificity for the detection of spontaneous brain activities by surpassing the physiological noise, especially in perivascular, periventricular and periaqueductal regions (Zou et al., 2008). However, it is less reliable than ALFF as a proportional measure (Zuo et al., 2010). These two indexes reflect different aspects of the LFOs amplitude: ALFF represents the strength of intensity of LFOs, while fALFF indexes the relative contribution of a specific LFOs to the entire frequency range (Zuo et al., 2010). They are both useful to characterize the physiology of AD, reveal intrinsic network disruption and are sensitive indexes to detect AD-related neurodegeneration (Han et al., 2011, 2012).

Rs-fMRI signals in the cortical and cistern areas may have different characteristics in the field of their power distribution in different frequency ranges (Zou et al., 2008). The independent frequency bands are generated by distinct oscillators with particular properties and physiological functions, and the pattern of intrinsic brain activity is sensitive to particular frequency bands (Buzsaki and Draguhn, 2004). Several studies have demonstrated that the pattern of disrupted LFOs in aMCI and d-AD is frequency-dependent (Han et al., 2011; Wang et al., 2011; Liu et al., 2014). ALFF/fALFF in the slow-5 band seem to be more sensitive to changes in the DMN than the slow-4 band in aMCI (Han et al., 2011). There seems to be different patterns of disruption in the slow-5 band compared with the slow-4 band (Liu et al., 2014). Therefore, it is necessary to differentiate the frequency bands to further examine the specific alterations in

---

Abbreviations: AD, Alzheimer's disease; ADL, Activity of Daily Living; ALFF, amplitude of the low-frequency fluctuation; aMCI, amnestic MCI; ANCOVA, analysis of covariance; AUC, the area under the receiver operating characteristic curve; AVLT, auditory verbal learning test; AVLT-D, AVLT-delayed recall; AVLT-I, AVLT-immediate recall; AVLT-R, AVLT-recognition recall; BOLD, blood oxygenation level-dependent; CDR, Clinical Dementia Rating Scale; d-AD, AD dementia; DMN, default-mode networks; fALFF, fractional ALFF; GM, gray matter; HAMD, Hamilton depression rating scale; HIS, Hachinski Ischemic Scale; LFOs, low-frequency oscillations; mALFF, normalized ALFF; MCI, mild cognitive impairment; MMSE, Mini–Mental State Examination; MoCA, Montreal Cognitive Assessment; MPFC, medial prefrontal cortex; NC, normal controls; PCC, posterior cingulate cortex; ROC, receiver operating characteristic; ROIs, regions of interest; rs-fMRI, resting-state functional magnetic resonance imaging; SCD, subjective cognitive decline; SVM, support vector machines; WM, white matter.

distinct brain regions. In this study, we divided the frequency bands into three signals (classic frequency band: 0.01–0.1 Hz; slow-5: 0.01–0.027 Hz; and slow-4: 0.027–0.073 Hz) to detect diverse and comprehensive oscillation properties of the brain (Buzsaki and Draguhn, 2004; Zuo et al., 2010).

A gradual neurodegenerative processing seems to occur in AD. From the perspective of structural transformation, the WM degradation and GM atrophy in SCD was similar to aMCI and d-AD with slight extents (Meiberth et al., 2015; Cantero et al., 2016). With respect to functional alterations, previous studies have detected several brain regions with higher ALFF in SCD related to those exhibiting functional disruptions in MCI and d-AD, which may indicate a possible compensation mechanism in the early stage of AD (Sperling et al., 2009; Sun et al., 2016). Studies in aMCI and d-AD have identified both regions with decreased and increased ALFF/fALFF compared with the NC (Wang et al., 2011; Liu et al., 2014; Cai et al., 2017; Lin et al., 2017), suggesting an impairment and compensation concurrently exist in aMCI and d-AD (Qi et al., 2010; Liu et al., 2014). Thus, we wondered whether a special pattern of functional alterations is present throughout the course of AD.

Amplitude of low-frequency fluctuations and fALFF both have strengths and weaknesses, and they cannot substitute for each other in the detection of intrinsic brain activity. In the current study, we extracted mALFF and normalized fALFF (mfALFF) values of rs-fMRI in three frequency bands, and further utilized machine learning algorithms to construct a classifier to detect the clinical classification efficacy of ALFF, fALFF features, and the combination of them; explored regional differences in intrinsic activities among NC, SCD, aMCI, and d-AD groups; then detected brain regions with alterations, attempting to generalize the alterations of intrinsic brain activity patterns in the resting-state of the AD continuum and explain their behavioral deficiency. We hypothesized that (1) the classifier constructed by ALFF and fALFF features would get a high identification accuracy; (2) the values of mALFF/mfALFF may get changed in patient groups; (3) as the disease progressed, the alterations in mALFF/mfALFF values turned to be obvious and closely correlated with their cognitive levels.

MATERIALS AND METHODS

Participants

A total of 220 right-hand, Han Chinese subjects were enrolled in this study from September 2009 to December 2015. Among them, 61 NC were recruited from the local community by advertisements. One hundred fifty-nine subjects with memory complaints were enlisted from the memory clinic of the Neurology Department of Xuanwu Hospital in Beijing, China, including 46 SCD, 60 aMCI, and 53 d-AD patients. The research was authorized by the Medical Research Ethics Committee and Institutional Review Board of Xuanwu Hospital (ClinicalTrials.gov identifier: NCT02353884 and NCT02225964). Each participant was provided with a written informed consent and signed it prior to any procedures. All subjects underwent a set of standardized clinical evaluations, including a medical history enquiry, neurological examination, and a suite of neuropsychological tests, which included the Chinese version of the MMSE, the Beijing version of MoCA (Lu et al., 2011), the AVLT (Guo et al., 2007), CDR (Morris, 1993), ADL, HIS, HAMD (Hamilton, 1960), and Center for Epidemiologic Studies depression scale (Dozeman et al., 2011). The diagnosis was made by experienced neurologists according to established guidelines. The NC must meet the following conditions: (a) no memory concerns; (b) MMSE (>19 for illiteracy, >22 for 1–6 educational years, >26 for more than 6 educational years) (Zhang et al., 1999) and MoCA scores (>13 for illiteracy, >19 for 1–6 educational years, >24 for more than 6 educational years) (Lu et al., 2011); and (c) CDR score of 0. SCD fulfilled the SCD research criteria proposed by the Subjective Cognitive Decline Initiative (SCD-I) (Jessen et al., 2014): (a) self-report persistent memory decline within the last 5 years compared with the previous normal status and confirmed by an informant; (b) normal range scores of MMSE and MoCA; and (c) CDR score of 0. The aMCI subjects were included based on the following items: (a) with or without self-perceived memory complaint and with informant complaints; (b) objectively impaired memory confirmed by MMSE (≤19 for illiteracy, ≤22 for 1–6 educational years, ≤26 for more than 6 educational years) and MoCA scores (≤13 for illiteracy, ≤19 for 1–6 educational years, ≤24 for more than 6 educational years); (c) clear-cut history of worsening cognition; (d) failure to meet the criteria for dementia according to the Diagnostic and Statistical Manual of Mental Disorders, Fourth Edition, revised (DSM-IV-R); and (e) CDR score of 0.5. The d-AD patients were diagnosed according to the National Institute of Aging-Alzheimer's (NIA-AA) criteria for clinically probable AD (McKhann et al., 2011): (a) meeting criteria for dementia; (b) insidious and gradual onset (not sudden) over more than 6 months; (c) clear-cut history of worsening cognition; (d) initial and most prominent cognitive deficits evident in performance of the amnestic presentation or non-amnestic presentations; (e) hippocampal atrophy confirmed by structural MRI; and (f) CDR score ≥1.

The exclusion criteria for all subjects included: (a) a history of stroke (HIS score >4); (b) severe depression (HAMD score >24 or center for Epidemiological Studies Depression Scale score >21); (c) other central nervous system diseases that may cause cognitive decline (e.g., epilepsy, brain tumors, Parkinson's disease, or encephalitis); (d) systemic diseases that could induce cognitive impairment (e.g., anthracemia, syphilis, thyroid dysfunction, or severe anemia, or HIV); (e) a history of psychosis or congenital mental growth retardation; (f) sever hypoplasia or dysacusis; (g) cognitive deficit caused by traumatic brain injury; (h) severe end-stage diseases or severe diseases in acute stages; or (i) those who could not complete neuropsychological tests or were contraindicated for MRI.

Image Data Acquisition

All participants were imaged with a 3.0 Tesla MR imager (Siemens Magnetom Trio Tim MRI system, Germany) using a standard head coil. Cushions and earplugs were used to reduce subject motion and scanner noise. Before imaging, subjects were asked to keep their eyes closed and relaxed, but not to fall asleep and to move as little as possible during the imaging. The echo plane imaging sequence was applied to collect functional images. The scanning parameters were as follows: repetition time (TR) = 2000 ms, echo time (TE) = 40 ms, flip angle (FA) = 90°, field of view (FOV) = 240 mm × 240 mm, number of layers = 28, layer thickness = 4 mm, matrix = 64 × 64, voxel size = 3.75 mm × 3.75 mm × 4 mm, layer interval = 1 mm, bandwidth = 2232 Hz per pixel. The sequence lasted for 478 s, so each scan of a subject included 239 phases. In addition, a T1-weighted image was acquired as an anatomical reference. T1-weighted MR images were obtained by a 3D magnetization-prepared rapid gradient echo (MPRAGE) with the following parameters: slices = 176, TR = 1900 ms, TE = 2 ms, inversion time (TI) = 900 ms, FA = 9°, FOV = 224 mm × 256 mm, acquisition matrix = 448 × 512, no gap, and thickness = 1.0 mm.

Image Data Preprocessing

Based on the MATLAB software platform, all images were processed using the static MR data processing toolkit *GRETNA v2.0.0*[1]. The image pre-processing steps consisted of the following. (1) The data for the first ten volumes were deleted to reduce the effect of magnetic field in homogeneity during the initial scan and to adapt subjects to the scanning environment. (2) Time correction was used to correct the difference in acquisition time between layers of a volume. (3) Head correction was performed by removing subjects who had large head movements. Each subject generated two types of figures: the translation diagram shows the translation of the head in the three directions, *X*, *Y*, and *Z*, and the rotation diagram shows the rotation angle of the three axes around *X*, *Y*, and *Z* in the experiment. Six-parameter motion regression estimates were used to calculate the framewise displacement (FD). In this study, subjects were deleted with maximum movements in translation > 3 mm or a rotation angle > 3°. (4) Space standardization: differences exist among human brains, both in shapes and volumes. To obtain the uniform coordinate system to describe the same anatomical location, we used spatial standardization so that the brains of different subjects were registered with the same standard space, Montreal Institute of Neurology, Standard Head Anatomical Template (MNI) space. In this study, structural images (T1 images) were used to register functional images to achieve spatial standardization of the subjects. A matrix was generated after registration and segmentation. The data of the matrix was applied to the functional images, which was used to realize the registration from the functional space of subjects to the standard space (MNI space). Finally, the functional images were then registered with the segmented structure images, and the resulting data were re-sampled to obtain functional data of 3 mm × 3 mm × 3 mm voxels. (5) Smoothing with a 4-mm full width at half maximum Gaussian kernel: smoothing can reduce the incomplete effects of registration so that the residuals are more consistent with the Gaussian distribution and improve the image signal-to-noise ratio. (6) Remove linear drift. (7) Regress out covariates including the global signal, WM signal, cerebrospinal fluid signal and Friston-24 parameters.

[1]https://www.nitrc.org/frs/downloadlink.php/10441/?i_agree=1&release_id=3694

For normalization, the ALFF of each voxel is divided by the average ALFF of all voxels in the whole brain to obtain the mALFF for each voxel, and mALFF should have a value of approximately 1 (Zang et al., 2007). In this study, ALFF and fALFF analysis was performed under the slow-5 (0.01–0.027 Hz), slow-4 (0.027–0.073 Hz) and classical frequency band (0.01–0.1 Hz) according to Zuo (Zuo et al., 2010). Then mALFF maps and mfALFF maps of each subject in the three bands were calculated using *REST V1.8*[2] software based on the MATLAB platform to prepare for the subsequent statistical analysis.

Classifiers

To assess the diagnostic efficacy of neuronal spontaneous activity, average mALFF values and mfALFF values of 116 brain regions divided based on AAL (Anatomical Automatic Labeling) template under three frequency bands were extracted as the whole brain features. A classifier analysis was performed to investigate the accuracy of ALFF, fALFF and the multimodal fusion of ALFF and fALFF with all features. We measured the separate accuracy of each two groups (d-AD vs. NC, aMCI vs. NC, SCD vs. NC, d-AD vs. aMCI, d-AD vs. SCD, aMCI vs. SCD) with ALFF, fALFF and the multimodal fusion of ALFF and fALFF features, respectively.

A cross-validation was applied to divide the sample data set into two complementary subsets, one for training (classifiers) as a training set, and the other for verifying the validity of the analysis as a testing set. The classifier applied SVM with a linear kernel. The SVM yielded a maximal-margin hyperplane in the feature space, which separated the groups in a training data set. K-fold cross-validation was performed to reduce the variability of the cross-validation results. This cross-validation encompassed the feature selection as well as the classifier. We performed feature selection based on elastic net model (Huang et al., 2018). Elastic net is a linear regression model using L1 and L2 as feature selection parameters. Specially, a multimodal fusion based on SVM was applied to evaluate the classification effect by using a combination of ALFF and fALFF features. In each experiment, we employed inner iterations to determine the feature selection parameters, the model parameters and the modality weights β in the multi-kernel SVM. To further avoid possible biases during partitioning, we repeated the experiments 10 times.

A multimodal SVM adequately utilized the particular characteristics of each modality's data and provided more possibilities to choose a suitable weighted combination. The kernel function was defined as follows:

$$K(x_i, x_j) = \langle \Phi(x_i), \Phi(x_j) \rangle \tag{1}$$

The kernel function is K; x_i, x_j are the input vectors; and Φ is a map to transform the source data from the input space to feature space. The final kernel function combined with the multimodal data source with a weight coefficient has a form of

$$K(x_i, x_j) = \beta_1 K_1(x_i^1, x_j^1) + \beta_2 K_2(x_i^2, x_j^2) \tag{2}$$

where $\{\beta_n\}$ is the weight coefficient, and K_n is the kernel function of each modality's data x^n. M data samples and two modality

[2]http://www.restfmri.net/forum/REST_V1.8

kernels are used in the learning. The decision function in the classification with a best parameter set is defined as follows:

$$\hat{y}(x) = \sum_{m=1}^{M} \alpha_m y_m K(x, x_m) + b \quad (3)$$

where $\{\alpha_m\}$ is a weight series, y_m is the label of the sample x_m, K is the final kernel defined previously, and b is a constant coefficient. It can be noted that the K is different from that in equation (2) because it was used for prediction. The SVM algorithm in our study was based on the *LIBSVM* library toolbox[3] (Chang and Lin, 2011) within the MATLAB environment.

The accuracy (percentage of participants detected correctly), sensitivity (percentage of patients detected correctly), and specificity (percentage of controls detected correctly) for each classifier was calculated to quantify the classification performance. The classification accuracy reflected the predictive power of the algorithm and was of direct diagnostic relevance. In addition, the area under the ROC curve (AUC) was also drawn to evaluate the overall performance of the classification method. The larger the AUC value, the better was the classification performance of the classification method.

Statistical Analysis

Analysis of covariance (ANCOVA) was used to analyze differences in mALFF/mfALFF throughout the brain based on the voxel level among NC, SCD, aMCI, and d-AD groups. Age, gender, education, mean GM volumes and mean FD were taken as covariates. In the study, we used a GM mask to exclude activities originating from white mater for analyzing ALFF/fALFF differences. All the statistical maps were corrected for multiple comparisons by GRF correction combining the voxel *P*-value < 0.001 and cluster level < 0.05 in DPABI_V3.*0_171210*[4] based on the Gaussian Random Field Theory.

The clusters showing significant differences were saved as ROIs. We extracted mALFF values from the four groups of subjects for these ROIs using the *REST V1.8* toolkit. *Post hoc* comparisons were then conducted within these ROIs with *SPSS 23.0*, and the two groups with significant differences ($P < 0.05$, $P < 0.01$, $P < 0.001$) were marked. Correction for the *post hoc* comparisons was performed using Bonferroni correction. The fALFF analysis was performed similarly to the ALFF analysis.

[3]http://www.csie.ntu.edu.tw/~cjlin/libsvm

[4]http://rfmri.org/dpabi

Relationship With Neuropsychological Tests

To test the clinical significance of these ROIs above, we correlated mALFF or mfALFF in these ROIs with neuropsychological tests across all participants including NC, SCD, aMCI, and d-AD. Age, gender, education level, mean GM volumes, mean FD and diagnosis were included as covariates. Bonferroni correction was used to account for multiple comparisons in correlation analyses ($P < 0.05/5$).

RESULTS

Demographics and Neuropsychological Test Results

Fifty-seven NC, 44 SCD, 55 aMCI, and 47 d-AD subjects were finally enrolled in this study after excluding subjects with poor registration and restricting head motion to less than 3 mm or 3 degrees. **Table 1** summarizes the demographic characteristics and neuropsychological performance of the four groups. No significant group differences were found in gender and mean FD ($P > 0.05$). Age, education, mean GM volume and all cognitive variables showed significant differences between at least two groups (**Table 1** and **Supplementary Table S1**). The d-AD and aMCI performed significantly worse than NC and SCD in all tests. The best memory performance was observed in NC, with intermediate performance in SCD, worse performance in aMCI, and the worst performance in d-AD.

Classifiers

The classifier model performance and ROC curves were depicted in **Table 2** and **Figure 1**. As shown in **Table 2**, cross-validation

TABLE 1 | Demographics and clinical characteristics of the participants.

Demographic data	NC (n = 57)	SCD (n = 44)	aMCI (n = 55)	d-AD (n = 47)	P-value	*Post hoc*[d]
Gender (male/female)	22/35	19/25	27/28	15/32	0.345[a]	
Age (years)	63.77 ± 8.09	65.13 ± 8.57	67.51 ± 9.62	70.99 ± 10.07	0.001[b]	NC < d-AD, SCD < d-AD
Education (years)	11.05 ± 4.92	11.80 ± 4.65	10.13 ± 4.98	8.89 ± 5.75	0.039[b]	SCD > d-AD
Mean GM volume (L)	0.60 ± 0.07	0.59 ± 0.07	0.56 ± 0.07	0.49 ± 0.05	0.000[b]	NC > aMCI > d-AD,SCD > d-AD
AVLT-I	9.16 ± 1.91	8.27 ± 1.79	6.15 ± 1.71	3.59 ± 1.61	0.000[c]	NC > SCD > aMCI > d-AD
AVLT-D	10.19 ± 2.78	8.50 ± 2.72	4.06 ± 2.88	1.00 ± 1.64	0.000[c]	NC > SCD > aMCI > d-AD
AVLT-R	12.05 ± 2.55	10.96 ± 2.73	7.96 ± 3.74	3.73 ± 3.39	0.000[c]	NC,SCD > aMCI > d-AD
MMSE	28.14 ± 2.13	27.93 ± 1.86	24.66 ± 4.20	16.55 ± 6.21	0.000[c]	NC, SCD > aMCI > d-AD
MoCA	26.10 ± 3.12	25.17 ± 2.91	19.77 ± 4.30	12.55 ± 5.11	0.000[c]	NC > SCD > aMCI > d-AD
Framewise displacement (FD)	0.25 ± 0.12	0.21 ± 0.12	0.25 ± 0.15	0.27 ± 0.13	0.216[b]	

$P < 0.05$ means significance existed between the groups. [a]P-value for sex distribution obtained by the chi-square test; [b]P-values obtained by ANOVA. [c]All clinical/cognitive variables from ANCOVA with age, gender, education, mean GM volume, mean FD as covariates; [d]Post hoc testing of cognitive variables based on means adjusted for age, gender, education, mean GM volume and mean FD.

TABLE 2 | Accuracy of the ALFF and fALFF analyses.

Accuracy (AUC)	ALFF	fALFF	ALFF_fALFF
d-AD vs. NC	80.2000(0.8142)	89.0909(0.9276)	91.8273(0.9261)
aMCI vs. NC	75.3561(0.7278)	70.1439(0.6981)	81.9394(0.7933)
SCD vs. NC	71.3818(0.6706)	63.8091(0.5890)	76.4364(0.6871)
d-AD vs. aMCI	66.6727(0.6363)	78.2727(0.7944)	83.8364(0.8182)
d-AD vs. SCD	72.1111(0.7221)	85.9444(0.8720)	87.0778(0.8724)
aMCI vs. SCD	77.4111(0.7561)	70.0333(0.6658)	81.4111(0.7737)

NC, normal controls; SCD, subjective cognitive decline; aMCI, amnestic mild cognitive impairment; d-AD, dementia of Alzheimer's disease; AUC, area under the receiver operating characteristic curve.

of the classifier using ALFF features yielded an accuracy of 80.20% for d-AD vs. NC, followed by an accuracy of 75.36% for aMCI vs. NC and 71.38% for SCD vs. NC. The classifier using fALFF features achieved an accuracy of 89.09, 70.14, and 63.81% for d-AD, aMCI and SCD from NC, respectively. A higher classification effect emerged after fusing ALFF and fALFF features based on multimodal fusion. The separate classifying accuracy of d-AD vs. NC, aMCI vs. NC, and SCD vs. NC was 91.83, 81.94, and 76.44%, respectively.

The AUC scores were 0.81, 0.73, and 0.67, respectively, for the classification of d-AD vs. NC, aMCI vs. NC, and SCD vs. NC with ALFF features. AUC scores were acquired for the distinction of d-AD, aMCI, and SCD from NC (0.93, 0.70, and 0.59, respectively) by using fALFF features. When combined ALFF and fALFF features via the multimodal fusion, better AUC scores were achieved (AUC = 0.93, 0.79, and 0.69 for d-AD, aMCI and SCD from NC, respectively).

To verify that the identified features are capable of separating patients in different stages, we also constructed the classifier between patient groups (d-AD vs. aMCI, d-AD vs. SCD, aMCI vs. SCD). We found ALFF and fALFF showed different classification results in each of these classifications. ALFF showed higher accuracy in classifications between these groups including aMCI vs. NC, SCD vs. NC, and aMCI vs. SCD, while fALFF showed higher accuracy in other classifications (d-AD vs. NC, d-AD vs. aMCI, and d-AD vs. SCD). However, the multimodal fusion of ALFF and fALFF showed higher accuracy in all classifications than just using ALFF or fALFF separately (**Table 2** and **Figure 1**). Thereby, ALFF and fALFF can't replace each other, and we investigated both of ALFF and fALFF index among the four groups.

ALFF/fALFF Analyses Under Different Frequency Bands

We selected clusters with significant differences and labeled their corresponding anatomical location, MNI coordinates, intensity of the significance, Brodmann and AAL partition (**Table 3**). These clusters were divided into several brain regions according to Andrews-Hanna et al. (2014). The results were shown in **Figure 2**.

During the analysis of ALFF, significant group differences were identified including the Hippocampus_L (aal), Frontal_Mid_Orb_R (aal), Precuneus_R (aal) extend to Posterior Cingulate, and Cerebelum_8_R (aal) in the full

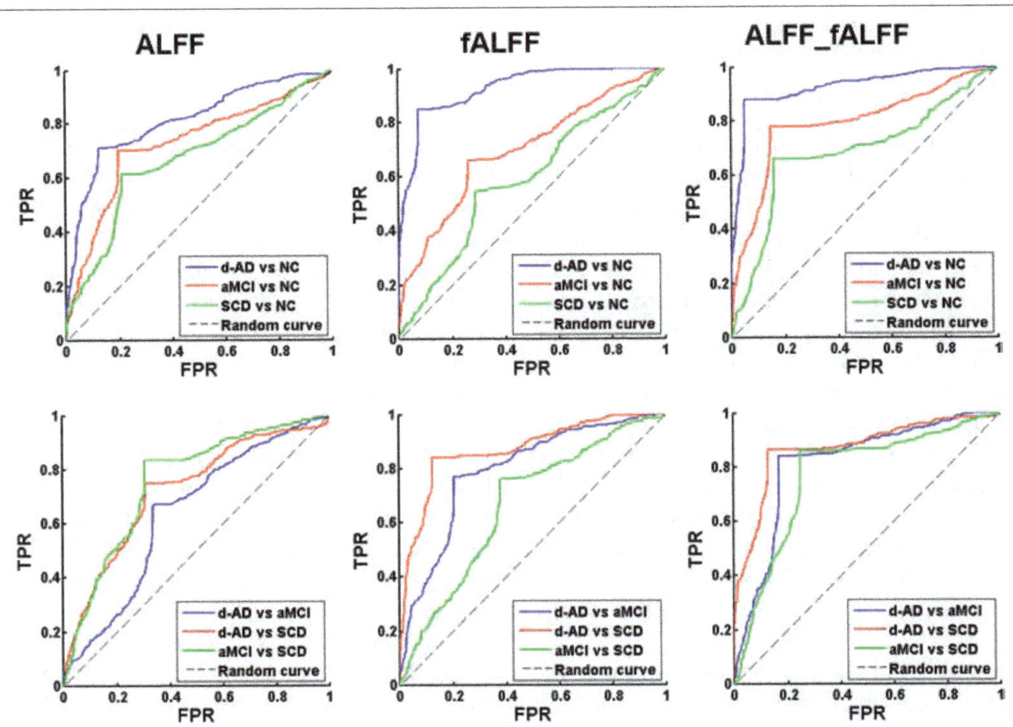

FIGURE 1 | Receiver operating characteristic (ROC) curve of ALFF, fALFF, and ALFF combined with fALFF. TPR, true positive rate; FPR, false positive rate; NC, normal controls; SCD, subjective cognitive decline; aMCI, amnestic mild cognitive impairment; d-AD, dementia of Alzheimer's disease.

TABLE 3 | ANCOVA results with age, gender, education, mean GM volume and mean FD as covariates across the four groups under three frequency bands.

Frequency bands		Anatomical area	BA	AAL	Peak MNI	Cluster Size	Peak intensity
ALFF	Full	**Medial Temporal Lobe**					
		Hippocampus_L (aal)	20	37	−36,−9,−21	16	7.697
		Lateral frontal cortex					
		Frontal_Mid_Orb_R (aal)	11	10	24,66,−9	17	8.0164
		Posterior cingulate cortex/precuneus					
		Precuneus_R (aal) extend to Posterior Cingulate	23	68	3,−57,24	11	7.6223
		Cerebellum regions					
		Cerebelum_8_R (aal)	0	104	18,−51,−60	145	9.5659
	Slow-4	**Posterior cingulate cortex**					
		Cingulum_Mid_R (aal)	23	34	3,−27,30	15	10.6692
		Cerebellum regions					
		Cerebelum_8_L (aal)	0	103	−36,−63,−57	140	9.5891
	Slow-5	**Posterior cingulate cortex/precuneus**					
		Precuneus_L (aal) extend to Posterior Cingulate	30	67	−3,−51,15	11	7.8118
		Cerebellum regions					
		Cerebelum_8_L (aal)	0	103	−33,−69,−57	67	10.7576
fALFF	Full	**Anterior cingulate cortex**					
		Cingulum_Ant_R (aal)	24	32	6,27,30	8	8.9079
		Lateral frontal cortex					
		Frontal_Sup_R (aal)	8	4	18,24,60	12	11.4105
	Slow-4	**Anterior cingulate cortex**					
		Cingulum_Ant_R (aal)	24	32	6,27,30	12	10.2268
		Medial frontal cortex					
		Paracentral_Lobule_R extend to Medial Frontal Gyrus	4	70	12,−30,60	9	11.2975
	Slow-5	**Precuneus**					
		Precuneus_L (aal)	7	67	−9,−75,48	10	8.1812

Full frequency band (0.01–0.1 Hz); slow-4 band (0.027–0.073 Hz); slow-5 band (0.01–0.027 Hz); BA, Brodmann area; AAL, anatomical automatic labeling; MNI, Montreal Institute of Neurology, Standard Head Anatomical Template; Hippocampus_L (aal): left hippocampus; Frontal_Mid_Orb_R (aal): right orbital part of middle frontal gyrus; Precuneus_R (aal): right precuneus; Cerebelum_8_R (aal): a part of right posterior cerebellum; Cingulum_Mid_R (aal): right median cingulate and paracingulate gyri; Cingulum_Ant_R (aal): right anterior cingulate and paracingulate gyri; Frontal_Sup_R (aal): right dorsolateral superior frontal gyrus; Paracentral_Lobule_R: right paracentral lobule; L., left; R., right.

band (0.01–0.1 Hz). In the slow-4 band (0.027–0.073 Hz), the Cingulum_Mid_R (aal) and Cerebelum_8_L (aal) were identified. In the slow-5 band (0.01–0.027 Hz), significant group differences were observed in the Precuneus_L (aal) extend to Posterior Cingulate and the Cerebelum_8_L (aal) (**Figures 3, 4**).

In the fALFF analysis, significant group differences were observed primarily in the Cingulum_Ant_R (aal) and Frontal_Sup_R (aal) in the full band. In the slow-4 band, the Cingulum_Ant_R (aal) and Paracentral_Lobule_R extend to Medial Frontal Gyrus showed significant group differences. In the slow-5 band, only the Precuneus_L (aal) manifested significant differences after GRF correction (**Figures 3, 4**).

Several brain regions presented a decreasing trend of mALFF/mfALFF values in the four groups, including the Cingulum_Mid_R (aal), bilateral inferior Cerebellum lobe, bilateral precuneus and the Cingulum_Ant_R (aal) as disease progressed (**Figure 3**).

Compared with NC, SCD showed significantly decreased ALFF levels in the Precuneus_R (aal) and Cerebelum_8_R (aal) in the full band; the Cerebelum_8_L (aal) in the slow-4 band; and decreased mALFF values in the Precuneus_L (aal) and Cerebelum_8_L (aal) in the slow-5 band. SCD also presented significantly decreasing mfALFF values in the Precuneus_L (aal) in the slow-5 band compared to NC. Compared to NC, aMCI performed similar to SCD in regions with significantly decreased mALFF values, with additional Cingulum_Mid_R (aal) in the slow-4 band. The aMCI also presented significantly decreasing mfALFF values in the Frontal_Sup_R (aal) in the full band; Cingulum_Ant_R (aal) in the slow-4 band; and the Precuneus_L (aal) in the slow-5 band compared to NC. Compared to NC, d-AD performed similarly to the aMCI in brain regions with significantly decreasing mALFF values. The d-AD also presented significantly decreasing mfALFF values in the Cingulum_Ant_R (aal) in the full band; Cingulum_Ant_R (aal) in the slow-4 band; and the Precuneus_L (aal) in the slow-5 band. Compared with SCD, LFOs decreased significantly in aMCI in several ROIs including the Frontal_Sup_R (aal) and Cingulum_Mid_R (aal); in Cingulum_Mid_R (aal) and Cingulum_Ant_R (aal) in d-AD. Compared with aMCI, d-AD was observed significantly decreased mfALFF values in the Cingulum_Ant_R (aal) (**Figures 3, 4**).

After *post hoc* comparisons, we found an increasing trend of mALFF/mfALFF values in the Hippocampus_L

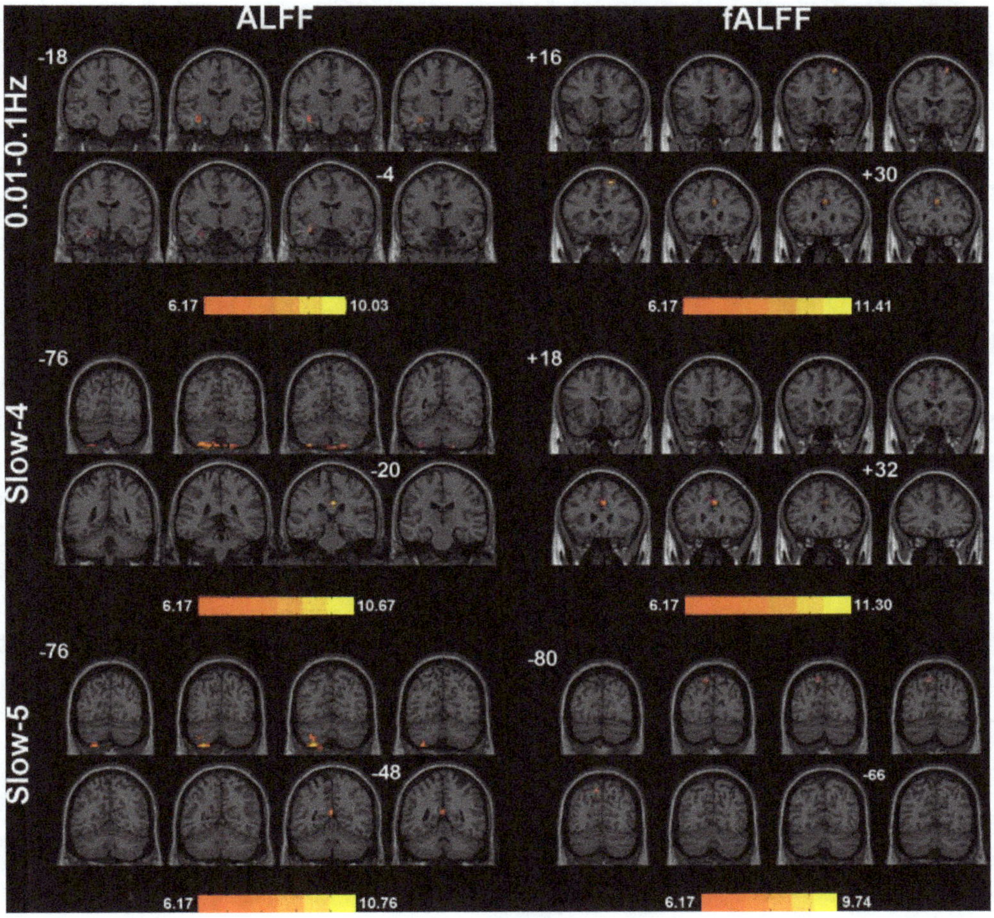

FIGURE 2 | Significant differences of ALFF/fALFF among NC, SCD, aMCI, and d-AD under different frequency bands. The results were obtained by ANCOVA analysis adjusted with mean age, gender, education, mean GM volume and mean FD (P < 0.001, cluster level < 0.05, GRF correction) by *DPABI_V3.0_171210*.

(aal), Frontal_Mid_Orb_R (aal), Frontal_Sup_R (aal) and Paracentral_Lobule_R (aal) as disease progressed (**Figure 4**).

Specifically, aMCI showed significantly higher LFOs in the Frontal_Mid_Orb_R (aal) and the Paracentral_Lobule_R (aal) than NC. The Hippocampus_L (aal) and Paracentral_Lobule_R (aal) presented significantly higher LFOs in d-AD than NC. Compared to SCD, aMCI and d-AD showed significantly increased LFOs in the Hippocampus_L (aal), and the Frontal_Mid_Orb_R (aal). The Hippocampus_L (aal), Frontal_Sup_R (aal) and Paracentral_Lobule_R showed significantly higher LFOs in d-AD, compared with aMCI (**Figure 4**).

Correlation With Neuropsychological Tests

We correlated mALFF/mfALFF values of ROIs in **Table 2** with behavioral scales controlling for age, gender, education, group, mean GM volumes, mean FD and diagnosis as covariates, and various correlations were detected (**Supplementary Table S1**). Seven brain regions showed significances. Two regions of fALFF features failed to undergo the Bonferroni correlation analysis (**Supplementary Table S1**). Here, we tried to analyze degenerative changes in AD by combining existing 5 features (Bonferroni, P < 0.05/5) with severity degree and alterations of LFOs.

The mALFF values of the Hippocampus_L (aal) and Cerebelum_8_R (aal) in the full band were significantly negative correlated with recognition of AVLT (AVLT-R) scores (Bonferroni, P < 0.05/5). And mALFF values of the Cingulum_Mid_R (aal) in the slow-4 band were significantly positive correlated with delayed recall of AVLT (AVLT-D) and MMSE scores (Bonferroni, P < 0.05/5). The mALFF values of the Cerebelum_8_L (aal) were significantly negative correlated with AVLT-R scores in slow-4 band; with AVLT-D and AVLT-R scores in slow-5 band (Bonferroni, P < 0.05/5).

In the Hippocampus_L (aal) in full band, aMCI showed significantly higher mALFF values than SCD, and d-AD showed significantly higher ALFF levels than NC, SCD, and aMCI. In the Cerebelum_8_R (aal) in full band, SCD, aMCI and d-AD all showed significantly decreased mALFF values than NC (**Figure 5**).

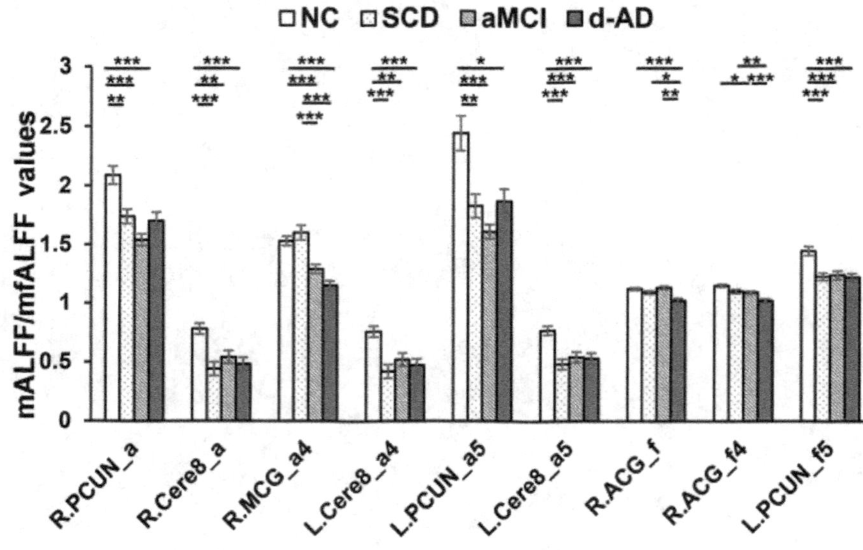

FIGURE 3 | Decreased ALFF and fALFF patterns tendency in patient groups. * represents significant level $P < 0.05$, ** means significant level $P < 0.01$, and *** means significant level $P < 0.001$. L., left; R., right; R.PCUN, Precuneus_R (aal); R.Cere8, Cerebelum_8_R (aal); R.MCG, Cingulum_Mid_R (aal); L.PCUN, Precuneus_L (aal); R.ACG, Cingulum_Ant_R (aal). ALFF analysis in full band (0.01–0.1 Hz); a4, ALFF analysis in slow-4 band (0.027–0.073 Hz); a5, ALFF analysis in slow-5 band (0.01–0.027 Hz); f, fALFF analysis in full band; f4, fALFF analysis in slow-4 band; f5, fALFF analysis in slow-5 band.

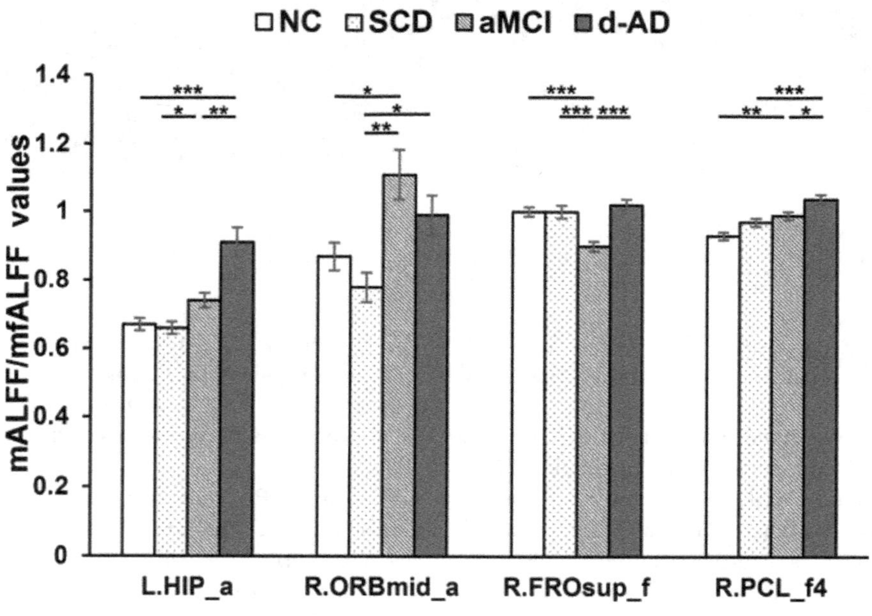

FIGURE 4 | Increased ALFF and fALFF patterns tendency in patient groups. * represents significant level $P < 0.05$, ** means significant level $P < 0.01$, and *** means significant level $P < 0.001$. L., left; R., right; L.HIP, Hippocampus_L (aal); R.ORBmid, Frontal_Mid_Orb_R (aal); R.FROsup, Frontal_Sup_R (aal); R.PCL, Paracentral_Lobule_R. a, ALFF analysis in full band (0.01–0.1 Hz); a4, ALFF analysis in slow-4 band (0.027–0.073 Hz); a5, ALFF analysis in slow-5 band (0.01–0.027 Hz); f, fALFF analysis in full band; f4, fALFF analysis in slow-4 band; f5, fALFF analysis in slow-5 band.

In the Cingulum_Mid_R (aal) in slow-4 band, both NC and SCD showed significantly higher mALFF values compared with aMCI and d-AD (**Figure 6**).

In the Cerebelum_8_L (aal) in slow-4 and slow-5 bands, patient groups all presented significantly lower mALFF values than NC (**Figure 7**).

DISCUSSION

In this study, the classifier model based on the fusion of ALFF and fALFF features performed better in the distinction of patients and NC, providing a higher classification accuracy and larger AUC than only using the ALFF or fALFF indexes. Wecalculated

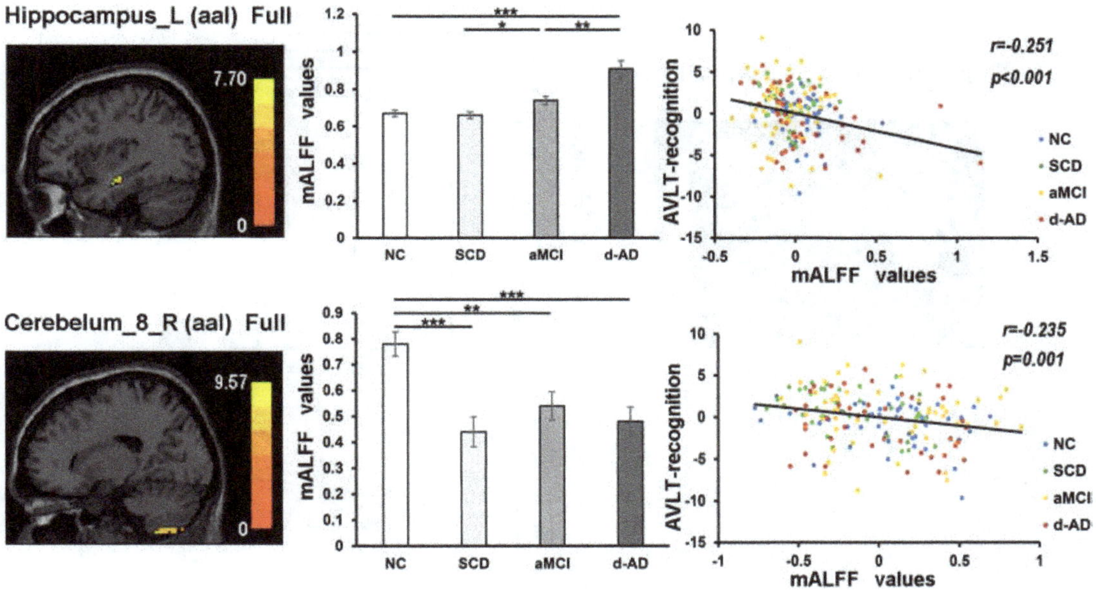

FIGURE 5 | The correlation between mALFF values of the Hippocampus_L (aal) and Cerebelum_8_R (aal) in full band and recognition of AVLT scores. The column 1 showed corresponding anatomic location of the left hippocampus and Cerebelum_8_R (aal) in the brain. The column 2 displayed significant differences of mALFF values of these two regions in full band among four groups obtained by *post hoc* test (Bonferroni correction, $P < 0.05$). * represents significant level $P < 0.05$; ** means significant level $P < 0.01$; *** means significant level $P < 0.001$. The column 3 were scatter plots demonstrating the negative correlation between the Hippocampus_L (aal) and Cerebelum_8_R (aal) and recognition of AVLT scores (Bonferroni correction, $P < 0.05/5$). Corresponding correlation coefficient "*r*" and significant level "*p*" were marked. NC, normal controls; SCD, subjective cognitive decline; aMCI, amnestic mild cognitive impairment; d-AD, dementia of Alzheimer's disease; mALFF, the normalized amplitude of the low-frequency fluctuation; AVLT, the auditory verbal learning test.

mALFF/mfALFF values in NC, SCD, aMCI, and d-AD at three frequency bands, examined alterations in patient groups compared with NC, and further conducted behavioral correlation analysis with neuropsychological tests. There were widespread differences of mALFF/mfALFF values among these bands in several brain regions in patient groups compared with NC. Some regions with changes of mALFF/mfALFF values presented a similar pattern in patient groups as an increasing or decreasing tendency. Furthermore, there seems to be a gradual pattern in AD spectrum: as the disease progressed, the number of altered brain regions with significantly increased/decreased mALFF/mfALFF values was increasing, and the extent of disruption was enhanced. Several regions with altered mALFF/mfALFF values were significantly correlated with the neuropsychological tests.

Classifier

The high identification accuracies demonstrated that both ALFF and fALFF could depict spontaneous functional alterations of brain regions in AD spectrum. This procedure was efficient and robust, enabling us to distinguish patients at various stages of AD with high accuracy and AUC values, and indicating that ALFF/fALFF could be a potential index to monitor disease progression. The classification framework composed of the integration of ALFF and fALFF achieved the best performance than only choosing any one of them or simply combined them in the AD staging. The ALFF directly reflect the intensity of regional spontaneous neural activity and potentially more sensitive for discerning differences between groups (Zang et al., 2007). The fALFF was developed after the original ALFF index to detect intrinsic spontaneous brain activity with higher sensitivity and specificity. It can provide a more specific measure of low oscillatory phenomena (Zou et al., 2008, 2010). Overall sensitivity to discriminate brain alterations was stronger for fALFF than ALFF; but the reliability to GM signals was lower for fALFF vs. ALFF (Meda et al., 2015). These two different parameters showed similarities in the main results and differences in the certain brain regions, which may demonstrate an inherent differences in specificity and sensitivity between these two indexes (Zhou et al., 2017). So they were usually applied to the same sample group simultaneously to maximize reliability across subjects and provide sufficient specificity to capture inter-individual differences (Zuo et al., 2010; Zhou et al., 2017). They captured both unique and shared effects across four groups.

Decreased Tendency of mALFF/mfALFF Values in Patient Groups

As disease progressed, mALFF/mfALFF values presented with decreasing tendency in several brain regions, including the right median cingulate and paracingulate gyri, bilateral inferior cerebellum lobe (belongs to posterior cerebellum), bilateral precuneus, and the right anterior cingulate and paracingulate gyri (**Figure 3**). These changes may directly imply weakening of the activities of neurons in these regions, potentially due to neurophysiological processes and indicating the presence of a functional deficiency or downregulation of excitability.

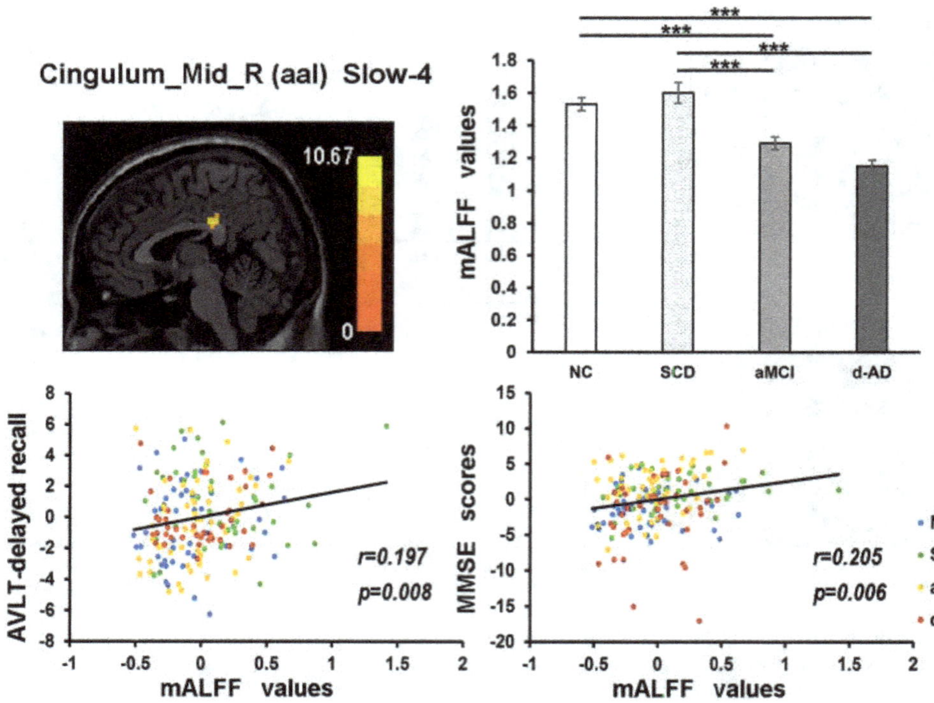

FIGURE 6 | The correlation between mALFF values of the Cingulum_Mid_R (aal) in slow-4 band and delayed recall of AVLT/MMSE scores. The row 1, column 1 showed the corresponding anatomic location of the right median cingulate and paracingulate gyri in the brain. The row 1, column 2 displayed significant differences of mALFF values of this region in slow-4 band among four groups obtained by *post hoc* test (Bonferroni correction, $P < 0.05$). *** means significant level $P < 0.001$. The row 2 were scatter plots demonstrating the positive correlation between the right median cingulate and paracingulate gyri and delayed recall of AVLT/MMSE scores (Bonferroni correction, $P < 0.05/5$). Corresponding correlation coefficient "*r*" and significant level "*p*" were marked. NC, normal controls; SCD, subjective cognitive decline; aMCI, amnestic mild cognitive impairment; d-AD, dementia of Alzheimer's disease; AVLT, the auditory verbal learning test; MMSE, the Mini-Mental State Examination.

These regions all belong to the DMN, which is involved in episodic memory processing, significantly correlated with hippocampal formation and has been consistently associated with the successful recollection of previously studied items (Buckner et al., 2008; Raichle, 2015). Progressive deficits in the DMN were observed in aMCI during a longitudinal follow-up (Bai et al., 2011). Converging evidence indicates that the functional connectivity within the DMN, especially the posterior part, is disrupted in relation to memory impairment in MCI and d-AD patients (Jacobs et al., 2013). Since the precuneus is the putative pivotal region of the DMN and functions as a cortical hub that is highly metabolically active and highly interconnected in the network architecture, it has a particular susceptibility to Alzheimer's-type neurodegeneration (Drzezga et al., 2011; Tomasi and Volkow, 2011). Previous studies have also detected a specific regional decrease in LFOs of the precuneus in MCI, early d-AD, and d-AD (Zhao et al., 2012; Liu et al., 2014; Huang et al., 2015), and a decline in metabolism in the precuneus at the pre-clinical stage of AD in PET studies (Minoshima et al., 1997). The precuneus was significantly thinner in amyloid-positive MCI than healthy amyloid-negative controls (Rane et al., 2018). SCD has presented significantly decreased mALFF values in the bilateral precuneus and descending mfALFF values in the left precuneus compared with NC, which may represent the existence of abnormity in SCD. Lower path length values were detected in precuneus in SCD, which was associated with a steeper decline in global cognition (Verfaillie et al., 2018). SCD also displayed lower functional connectivity of the precuneus compared with controls without memory complaints (Viviano et al., 2018).

Increased Tendency of mALFF/mfALFF Values in Patient Groups

In addition, mALFF/mfALFF values presented with incremental tendency were also observed in patient groups in the following brain regions, including the left hippocampus, right orbital part of middle frontal gyrus, right dorsolateral superior frontal gyrus and right paracentral lobule (**Figure 4**). It may be inferred that with the development of disease, neural damage strengthened the activity in an inverse manner.

The paradoxical increase in mALFF/mfALFF levels may be the result of the amyloid-induced hyper-excitability of neurons and impending neuronal network breakdown as a result of the increasing local and global neurodegenerative pathology (Ewers et al., 2011). The higher mALFF values may be caused by the greater neural activity involved in transmitting information to other regions and lead to greater connectivity among these regions (Di et al., 2013). This phenomenon may represent the most likely compensatory and neuroplasticity mechanism in

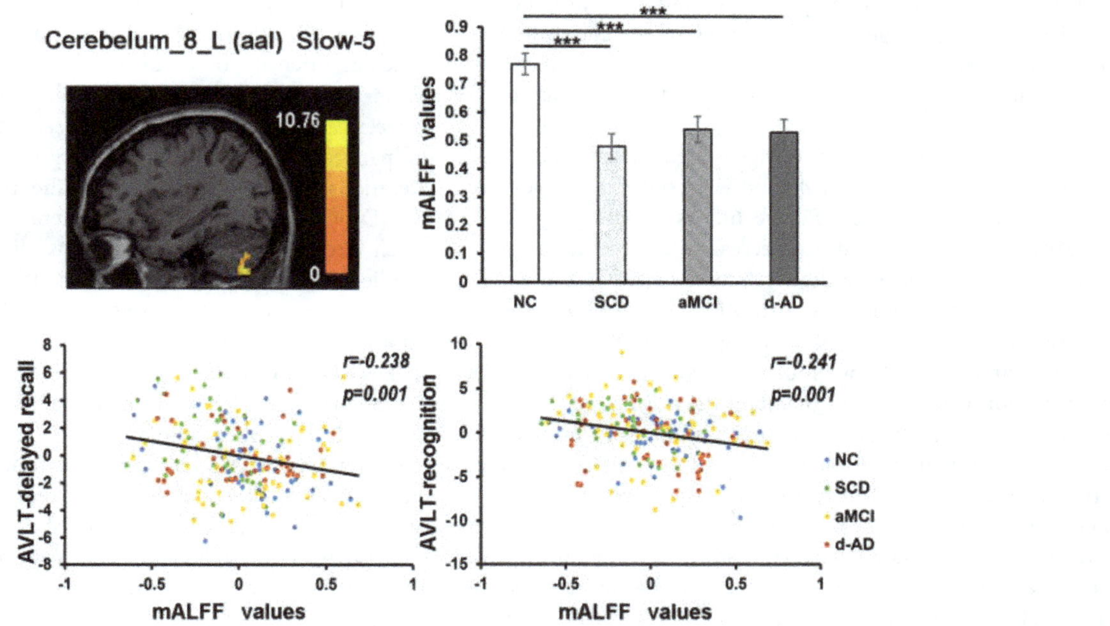

FIGURE 7 | The correlation between mALFF values of the Cerebelum_8_L (aal) in slow-5 band and delayed recall/recognition of AVLT scores. The row 1, column 1 showed the corresponding anatomic location of Cerebelum_8_L (aal) in the brain. The row 1, column 2 described corresponding group comparison obtained by *post hoc* test (Bonferroni correction, $P < 0.05$). *** means significant level $P < 0.001$. The row 2 showed negative correlation between this region and delayed recall/recognition of AVLT scores (Bonferroni correction, $P < 0.05/5$). Corresponding correlation coefficient "*r*" and significant level "*p*" were marked. NC, normal controls; SCD, subjective cognitive decline; aMCI, amnestic mild cognitive impairment; d-AD, dementia of Alzheimer's disease; AVLT, the auditory verbal learning test.

response to the accumulation of amyloid plaques, in which a greater number of resources is deployed to maintain the normal performance as much as possible as a reaction to the memory loss during the late course of AD (Huijbers et al., 2015). As disease progresses, cognitive processes gradually rely on an increased number of residual healthy synapses and neurons, as well as alternative brain networks (Stern, 2002). Brain areas with increasing activity are recruited as network resources to maintain cognitive functions following the reduced activity in some areas during the course of AD, which may reflect an increase in episodic memory consolidation or retrieval. The enhancement or inhibition of neuronal activities in these brain regions helps to maintain the physiological homeostasis of the whole brain. However, with further disease progression toward d-AD and an augmented pathology, these brain regions become more disturbed, with greater effects on the associated cognitive functions. Thus, patients with increased activation performed worse, reflecting the maladaptation and impairment. This hyperactivity may also be a harbinger of the impending loss of hippocampal function and subsequent rapid clinical decline, which may be present in the early stage of AD (O'Brien et al., 2010; Sperling et al., 2010).

Correlations Between Neuropsychological Test Scores and mALFF/mfALFF Values

In the correlation analysis, mALFF values of the left hippocampus in full band were significantly negative correlated with AVLT-R scores (**Figure 5**). The higher mALFF values were related to poor performance in aMCI and d-AD groups, which may also indicate their impairment and maladaptation in different ways (Shinoura et al., 2011). The neuronal spontaneous activity in this region was abnormally strengthened to maintain cognitive performance along with the disease progression. However, it was unable to maintain this function because the compensatory mechanism collapsed, suggesting that the increased spontaneous activity in this region might represent a decompensation related to the increased negative cognitive bias in aMCI and d-AD patients (Lau et al., 2016). The values were lower in SCD compared with NC (without significance), which may be a compensation strategy.

The mALFF values of the right posterior cerebellum lobe in the full band, as well as the left posterior cerebellum lobe in the slow-4 and slow-5 bands were significantly negative correlated with the AVLT-R scores (**Figures 5, 7**). The mALFF values of the bilateral posterior cerebellum lobe was lower in three patient groups compared to NC and exhibited descending tendency as disease burden got heavy, which indicated compensation in SCD (normal performance) and gradual decompensation in aMCI and d-AD (damaged performance). The cerebellum is involved in cognitive associative learning (Timmann et al., 2010; Buckner, 2013; Keren-Happuch et al., 2014). The posterior cerebellum contributes to complex cognitive operations (Schoch et al., 2006; Tavano et al., 2007; Stoodley and Schmahmann, 2009). The cerebellar alterations were hypothesized to correlate with different forms of cognitive impairment including MCI and d-AD (Thomann et al., 2008). Atrophy of the posterior cerebellum was related to impaired cognitive performance in AD, demonstrating degenerative changes of the cerebellum in AD (Castellazzi et al., 2014). Moreover, alterations of functional connectivity were also reported in MCI and d-AD (Castellazzi et al., 2014).

The mALFF values of the right median cingulate and paracingulate gyri in the slow-4 band were significantly positive correlated with test scores (**Figure 6**). As disease progressed, the mALFF values tended to decrease. Lower the intrinsic brain activities, lower were the test scores in aMCI and d-AD. This phenomenon implied the disruptions in aMCI and d-AD. Whereas, the ALFF value of this region was incremental in SCD compared with NC (without significance), which may be a compensation mechanism to maintain the normal performance (Sun et al., 2016). The neural compensation were initiated to maintain the impaired neural reserve and then alternate neural networks were recruited to further improve cognitive function (Steffener and Stern, 2012). The cingulum bundle is the main median associative fasciculus, consisting of long associative fibers that connect cortical brain areas and short associative fibers that band cingulate areas. It is one of the principal WM structures transferring anterior–posterior information, which affects its microstructure in AD (Catheline et al., 2010). A strong and specific correlation has been reported between atrophy of the hippocampal formation and the cingulum bundle, indicating that disruption of the cingulum bundle is related to perturbation of the hippocampal formation (Villain et al., 2008).

Three patient groups all exhibited different extents of altered spontaneous activity. And these graded disruptions of the intrinsic brain activity reflected by mALFF/mfALFF levels were detected in SCD, aMCI, and d-AD. These alterations indicate a gradual aggravating physiological pattern of alterations during a limited period of AD-related pathology along the normal aging-SCD-MCI-AD continuum. Mildly altered spontaneous activities presented in SCD might explain their self-perceived cognitive decline and associated subjective complaints prior to noticeable cognitive deficits. From the perspective of correlation analysis, we intended to speculate about the dynamic alterations of spontaneous activity occur in brain regions throughout the course of AD.

Our results indicated that AD should be considered as a disease in which large-scale distributed neural networks are disturbed. This disruption does not focus on changes in a single brain region but on large-scale network alterations or changes in components of these networks (Jacobs et al., 2013). The brain attempts to maintain normal performance via spontaneous regulatory mechanisms, such as the recruitment of additional neurons, as reflected by increasing ALFF/fALFF levels, or a reduction of activity to acclimatize the metabolic demand of other regions in the early stage before pathological invasion get heavy. As the disease burden increases, some regions are invaded by the pathology and fail to perceive the normal intensity of fluctuations, and the increasing/decreasing activation of additional regions can no longer induce a sufficient intensity of brain activity. With advancing disease, greater disturbances in the brain lead to a greater imbalance between activation and performance. The specific change in the pattern of intrinsic brain activity reflected by ALFF/fALFF alterations provides insights into the biological mechanisms of AD. Our results were consistent with the scenario in which progressive changes arise as disease propagated and supplied brain areas that are potentially involved in such degenerative processes (Rasero et al., 2017). Liang et al has found a general linear pattern of d-AD < late MCI < early MCI < NC or d-AD > late MCI > early MCI > NC in several brain regions with increased/decreased ALFF (Liang et al., 2014). Other studies have also detected progressive alterations in the AD continuum, as reflected by GM volume and cortical thickness decline indicators, atrophy degree and rate differences following the order of d-AD > MCI > NC (Ma et al., 2016). Longitudinal research with follow-up information concerning conversion to d-AD is needed to confirm this hypothesis.

Limitations

Our study has limitations. First, the samples were obtained using a cross-sectional design. Future longitudinal MRI data will be acquired to validate the disruption patterns with disease progression and further probe the classification accuracy of invert and stable patients. The high identification accuracy of patients groups does not mean the high conversion rate to d-AD. Second, we only analyzed rs-fMRI data. In advanced studies, the combination of multimodal neuroimaging and biological information could yield a comprehensive understanding of the progression patterns in AD. Finally, more extensive neuropsychological tests will be utilized to examine more cognitive aspects of patients to further explore the underlying mechanism in the brain.

CONCLUSION

In the present study, we observed comprehensive ALFF and fALFF alterations along with a deterioration of memory function in the AD spectrum. Our results indicated that ALFF/fALFF measurements of spontaneous or intrinsic brain activity may be useful to characterize the early and gradient of physiological alterations in AD. The nature and extent of large-scale brain region alterations varies and is aggravated with disease progression in AD. Our findings may help to better understand the relationship between the deterioration in brain spontaneous functional activity and the clinical characteristics of patients in the AD continuum.

AUTHOR CONTRIBUTIONS

LY, YY, TY, and YH drafted the manuscript, study concept or design, and Statistical analysis. LY, YY, YW, XH, JL, PC, TY, and YH revised the manuscript for content and analysis or interpretation of data. LY and YH acquisition of data. YH study supervision or coordination. All authors read and approved the final manuscript.

FUNDING

This article was supported by the National Key Research and Development Program of China (2016YFC1306300 and 2016YFC0103000); the National Natural Science Foundation of China (Grants 61633018, 81430037, 81471731, 31371007, 81671776, 61727807, and 81522021); Beijing Municipal Natural Science Foundation (7132147); the Beijing Municipal Commission of Health and Family Planning (PXM2018_026283_000002); and the Beijing Nova Program (Grant No. Z171100001117057).

ACKNOWLEDGMENTS

We thank our team for the collection of data. They were: Yu Sun, Xuanyu Li, Xiaoni Wang, Guanqun Chen, Jiachen Li, Wenying Du, Xiaoqi Wang, Weina Zhao, Ying Chen, Ziqi Wang, Li Lin, and Qin Yang.

REFERENCES

Andrews-Hanna, J. R., Smallwood, J., and Spreng, R. N. (2014). The default network and self-generated thought: component processes, dynamic control, and clinical relevance. *Ann. N. Y. Acad. Sci.* 1316, 29–52. doi: 10.1111/nyas.12360

Bai, F., Watson, D. R., Shi, Y., Wang, Y., Yue, C., Yuhuan, T., et al. (2011). Specifically progressive deficits of brain functional marker in amnestic type mild cognitive impairment. *PLoS One* 6:e24271. doi: 10.1371/journal.pone.0024271

Binnewijzend, M. A., Schoonheim, M. M., Sanz-Arigita, E., Wink, A. M., van der Flier, W. M., Tolboom, N., et al. (2012). Resting-state fMRI changes in Alzheimer's disease and mild cognitive impairment. *Neurobiol. Aging* 33, 2018–2028. doi: 10.1016/j.neurobiolaging.2011.07.003

Buckner, R. L. (2013). The cerebellum and cognitive function: 25 years of insight from anatomy and neuroimaging. *Neuron* 80, 807–815. doi: 10.1016/j.neuron.2013.10.044

Buckner, R. L., Andrews-Hanna, J. R., and Schacter, D. L. (2008). The brain's default network: anatomy, function, and relevance to disease. *Ann. N. Y. Acad. Sci.* 1124, 1–38. doi: 10.1196/annals.1440.011

Buzsaki, G., and Draguhn, A. (2004). Neuronal oscillations in cortical networks. *Science* 304, 1926–1929. doi: 10.1126/science.1099745

Cai, S., Chong, T., Peng, Y., Shen, W., Li, J., von Deneen, K. M., et al. (2017). Altered functional brain networks in amnestic mild cognitive impairment: a resting-state fMRI study. *Brain Imaging Behav.* 11, 619–631. doi: 10.1007/s11682-016-9539-0

Cantero, J. L., Iglesias, J. E., Van Leemput, K., and Atienza, M. (2016). Regional Hippocampal atrophy and higher levels of plasma Amyloid-Beta are associated with subjective memory complaints in nondemented elderly subjects. *J. Gerontol. A Biol. Sci. Med. Sci.* 71, 1210–1215. doi: 10.1093/gerona/glw022

Castellazzi, G., Palesi, F., Casali, S., Vitali, P., Sinforiani, E., Wheeler-Kingshott, C. A., et al. (2014). A comprehensive assessment of resting state networks: bidirectional modification of functional integrity in cerebro-cerebellar networks in dementia. *Front. Neurosci.* 8:223. doi: 10.3389/fnins.2014.00223

Catheline, G., Periot, O., Amirault, M., Braun, M., Dartigues, J. F., Auriacombe, S., et al. (2010). Distinctive alterations of the cingulum bundle during aging and Alzheimer's disease. *Neurobiol. Aging* 31, 1582–1592. doi: 10.1016/j.neurobiolaging.2008.08.012

Chang, C. C., and Lin, C. J. (2011). *LIBSVM: A Library for Support Vector Machines.* New York, NY: ACM.

Chen, Y.-C., Xia, W., Luo, B., Muthaiah, V. P. K., Xiong, Z., Zhang, J., et al. (2015). Frequency-specific alternations in the amplitude of low-frequency fluctuations in chronic tinnitus. *Front. Neural Circuits* 9:67. doi: 10.3389/fncir.2015.00067

Di, X., Kim, E. H., Huang, C. C., Tsai, S. J., Lin, C. P., and Biswal, B. B. (2013). The influence of the amplitude of low-frequency fluctuations on resting-state functional connectivity. *Front. Hum. Neurosci.* 7:118. doi: 10.3389/fnhum.2013.00118

Dozeman, E., van Schaik, D. J., van Marwijk, H. W., Stek, M. L., van der Horst, H. E., and Beekman, A. T. (2011). The center for epidemiological studies depression scale (CES-D) is an adequate screening instrument for depressive and anxiety disorders in a very old population living in residential homes. *Int. J. Geriatr. Psychiatry* 26, 239–246. doi: 10.1002/gps.2519

Drzezga, A., Becker, J. A., Van Dijk, K. R. A., Sreenivasan, A., Talukdar, T., Sullivan, C., et al. (2011). Neuronal dysfunction and disconnection of cortical hubs in non-demented subjects with elevated amyloid burden. *Brain* 134, 1635–1646. doi: 10.1093/brain/awr066

Ewers, M., Sperling, R. A., Klunk, W. E., Weiner, M. W., and Hampel, H. (2011). Neuroimaging markers for the prediction and early diagnosis of Alzheimer's disease dementia. *Trends Neurosci.* 34, 430–442. doi: 10.1016/j.tins.2011.05.005

Fox, M. D., and Raichle, M. E. (2007). Spontaneous fluctuations in brain activity observed with functional magnetic resonance imaging. *Nat. Rev. Neurosci.* 8, 700–711. doi: 10.1038/nrn2201

Guo, Q. H., Sun, Y. T., Yu, P. M., Hong, Z., and Lv, C. Z. (2007). Norm of auditory verbal learning test in the normal aged in Chinese community. *Chin. J. Clin. Psychol.* 15, 132–135.

Hamilton, M. (1960). A rating scale for depression. *J. Neurol. Neurosurg. Psychiatry* 23, 56–62. doi: 10.1136/jnnp.23.1.56

Han, Y., Lui, S., Kuang, W., Lang, Q., Zou, L., and Jia, J. (2012). Anatomical and functional deficits in patients with amnestic mild cognitive impairment. *PLoS One* 7:e28664. doi: 10.1371/journal.pone.0028664

Han, Y., Wang, J., Zhao, Z., Min, B., Lu, J., Li, K., et al. (2011). Frequency-dependent changes in the amplitude of low-frequency fluctuations in amnestic mild cognitive impairment: a resting-state fMRI study. *Neuroimage* 55, 287–295. doi: 10.1016/j.neuroimage.2010.11.059

Huang, J., Bai, F., Yang, X., Chen, C., Bao, X., and Zhang, Y. (2015). Identifying brain functional alterations in postmenopausal women with cognitive impairment. *Maturitas* 81, 371–376. doi: 10.1016/j.maturitas.2015.04.006

Huang, S., Hu, C. C., Bell, M. L., Billheimer, D., Guerra, S., Roe, D., et al. (2018). Regularized continuous-time Markov model via elastic net. *Biometrics* 74, 1045–1054. doi: 10.1111/biom.12868

Huijbers, W., Mormino, E. C., Schultz, A. P., Wigman, S., Ward, A. M., Larvie, M., et al. (2015). Amyloid-beta deposition in mild cognitive impairment is associated with increased hippocampal activity, atrophy and clinical progression. *Brain* 138(Pt 4), 1023–1035. doi: 10.1093/brain/awv007

Jack, C. R. Jr., Bennett, D. A., Blennow, K., Carrillo, M. C., Dunn, B., Haeberlein, S. B., et al. (2018). NIA-AA research framework: toward a biological definition of Alzheimer's disease. *Alzheimers Dement.* 14, 535–562. doi: 10.1016/j.jalz.2018.02.018

Jacobs, H. I., Radua, J., Luckmann, H. C., and Sack, A. T. (2013). Meta-analysis of functional network alterations in Alzheimer's disease: toward a network biomarker. *Neurosci. Biobehav. Rev.* 37, 753–765. doi: 10.1016/j.neubiorev.2013.03.009

Jessen, F., Amariglio, R. E., van Boxtel, M., Breteler, M., Ceccaldi, M., Chetelat, G., et al. (2014). A conceptual framework for research on subjective cognitive decline in preclinical Alzheimer's disease. *Alzheimers Dement.* 10, 844–852. doi: 10.1016/j.jalz.2014.01.001

Jessen, F., and Rodriguez Nee Then, F. S. (2018). Not all, but specific types of cognitive complaints predict decline to MCI. *Neurology* 91, 153–154. doi: 10.1212/WNL.0000000000005872

Keren-Happuch, E., Chen, S. H., Ho, M. H., and Desmond, J. E. (2014). A meta-analysis of cerebellar contributions to higher cognition from PET and fMRI studies. *Hum. Brain Mapp.* 35, 593–615. doi: 10.1002/hbm.22194

Lau, W. K., Leung, M. K., Lee, T. M., and Law, A. C. (2016). Resting-state abnormalities in amnestic mild cognitive impairment: a meta-analysis. *Transl Psychiatry* 6:e790. doi: 10.1038/tp.2016.55

Liang, P., Xiang, J., Liang, H., Qi, Z., Li, K., and Alzheimer's Disease Neuroimaging Initiative. (2014). Altered amplitude of low-frequency fluctuations in early and late mild cognitive impairment and Alzheimer's disease. *Curr. Alzheimer Res.* 11, 389–398. doi: 10.2174/1567205011666140331225335

Lin, F., Ren, P., Lo, R. Y., Chapman, B. P., Jacobs, A., Baran, T. M., et al. (2017). Insula and inferior frontal Gyrus' activities protect memory performance against Alzheimer's disease pathology in old age. *J. Alzheimers Dis.* 55, 669–678. doi: 10.3233/jad-160715

Liu, X., Wang, S., Zhang, X., Wang, Z., Tian, X., and He, Y. (2014). Abnormal amplitude of low-frequency fluctuations of intrinsic brain activity in Alzheimer's disease. *J. Alzheimers Dis.* 40, 387–397. doi: 10.3233/jad-131322

Lu, J., Li, D., Li, F., Zhou, A., Wang, F., Zuo, X., et al. (2011). Montreal cognitive assessment in detecting cognitive impairment in Chinese elderly individuals: a population-based study. *J. Geriatr. Psychiatry Neurol.* 24, 184–190. doi: 10.1177/0891988711422528

Ma, X., Li, Z., Jing, B., Liu, H., Li, D., Li, H., et al. (2016). Identify the atrophy of Alzheimer's disease, mild cognitive impairment and normal aging using morphometric MRI analysis. *Front. Aging Neurosci.* 8:243. doi: 10.3389/fnagi.2016.00243

McDade, E., and Bateman, R. J. (2017). Stop Alzheimer's before it starts. *Nature* 547, 153–155. doi: 10.1038/547153a

McKhann, G. M., Knopman, D. S., Chertkow, H., Hyman, B. T., Jack, C. R. Jr., Kawas, C. H., et al. (2011). The diagnosis of dementia due to Alzheimer's disease: recommendations from the National Institute on Aging-Alzheimer's Association workgroups on diagnostic guidelines for Alzheimer's disease. *Alzheimers Dement.* 7, 263–269. doi: 10.1016/j.jalz.2011.03.005

Meda, S. A., Wang, Z., Ivleva, E. I., Poudyal, G., Keshavan, M. S., Tamminga, C. A., et al. (2015). Frequency-specific neural signatures of spontaneous low-frequency resting state fluctuations in psychosis: evidence from Bipolar-Schizophrenia Network on Intermediate Phenotypes (B-SNIP) consortium. *Schizophr. Bull.* 41, 1336–1348. doi: 10.1093/schbul/sbv064

Meiberth, D., Scheef, L., Wolfsgruber, S., Boecker, H., Block, W., Traber, F., et al. (2015). Cortical thinning in individuals with subjective memory impairment. *J. Alzheimer. Dis.* 45, 139–146. doi: 10.3233/jad-142322

Minoshima, S., Giordani, B., Berent, S., Frey, K. A., Foster, N. L., and Kuhl, D. E. (1997). Metabolic reduction in the posterior cingulate cortex in very early Alzheimer's disease. *Ann. Neurol.* 42, 85–94. doi: 10.1002/ana.410420114

Mitchell, A. J., Beaumont, H., Ferguson, D., Yadegarfar, M., and Stubbs, B. (2014). Risk of dementia and mild cognitive impairment in older people with subjective memory complaints: meta-analysis. *Acta Psychiatr. Scand.* 130, 439–451. doi: 10.1111/a.12336

Morris, J. C. (1993). The Clinical Dementia Rating (CDR): current version and scoring rules. *Neurology* 43, 2412–2414. doi: 10.1212/WNL.43.11.2412-a

O'Brien, J. L., O'Keefe, K. M., LaViolette, P. S., DeLuca, A. N., Blacker, D., Dickerson, B. C., et al. (2010). Longitudinal fMRI in elderly reveals loss of hippocampal activation with clinical decline. *Neurology* 74, 1969–1976. doi: 10.1212/WNL.0b013e3181e3966e

Qi, Z., Wu, X., Wang, Z., Zhang, N., Dong, H., Yao, L., et al. (2010). Impairment and compensation coexist in amnestic MCI default mode network. *Neuroimage* 50, 48–55. doi: 10.1016/j.neuroimage.2009.12.025

Raichle, M. E. (2015). The brain's default mode network. *Annu. Rev. Neurosci.* 38, 433–447. doi: 10.1146/annurev-neuro-071013-014030

Rane, S., Donahue, M. J., and Claassen, D. O. (2018). Amnestic mild cognitive impairment individuals with dissimilar pathologic origins show common regional vulnerability in the default mode network. *Alzheimers Dement.* 10, 717–725. doi: 10.1016/j.dadm.2018.08.004

Rasero, J., Alonso-Montes, C., Diez, I., Olabarrieta-Landa, L., Remaki, L., Escudero, I., et al. (2017). Group-level progressive alterations in brain connectivity patterns revealed by diffusion-tensor brain networks across severity stages in Alzheimer's disease. *Front. Aging Neurosci.* 9:215. doi: 10.3389/fnagi.2017.00215

Scheltens, P., Blennow, K., Breteler, M. M., de Strooper, B., Frisoni, G. B., Salloway, S., et al. (2016). Alzheimer's disease. *Lancet* 388, 505–517. doi: 10.1016/S0140-6736(15)01124-1

Schoch, B., Dimitrova, A., Gizewski, E. R., and Timmann, D. (2006). Functional localization in the human cerebellum based on voxelwise statistical analysis: a study of 90 patients. *Neuroimage* 30, 36–51. doi: 10.1016/j.neuroimage.2005.09.018

Shinoura, N., Midorikawa, A., Kurokawa, K., Onodera, T., Tsukada, M., Yamada, R., et al. (2011). Right temporal lobe plays a role in verbal memory. *Neurol. Res.* 33, 734–738. doi: 10.1179/1743132811y.0000000005

Sperling, R. (2011). Potential of functional MRI as a biomarker in early Alzheimer's disease. *Neurobiol. Aging* 32(Suppl. 1), S37–S43. doi: 10.1016/j.neurobiolaging.2011.09.009

Sperling, R. A., Aisen, P. S., Beckett, L. A., Bennett, D. A., Craft, S., Fagan, A. M., et al. (2011). Toward defining the preclinical stages of Alzheimer's disease: recommendations from the National Institute on Aging-Alzheimer's association workgroups on diagnostic guidelines for Alzheimer's disease. *Alzheimers Dement.* 7, 280–292. doi: 10.1016/j.jalz.2011.03.003

Sperling, R. A., Dickerson, B. C., Pihlajamaki, M., Vannini, P., LaViolette, P. S., Vitolo, O. V., et al. (2010). Functional alterations in memory networks in early Alzheimer's disease. *Neuromol. Med.* 12, 27–43. doi: 10.1007/s12017-009-81097

Sperling, R. A., Laviolette, P. S., O'Keefe, K., O'Brien, J., Rentz, D. M., Pihlajamaki, M., et al. (2009). Amyloid deposition is associated with impaired default network function in older persons without dementia. *Neuron* 63, 178–188. doi: 10.1016/j.neuron.2009.07.003

Steffener, J., and Stern, Y. (2012). Exploring the neural basis of cognitive reserve in aging. *Biochim. Biophys. Acta* 1822, 467–473. doi: 10.1016/j.bbadis.2011.09.012

Stern, Y. (2002). What is cognitive reserve? Theory and research application of the reserve concept. *J. Int. Neuropsychol. Soc.* 8, 448–460. doi: 10.1017/S1355617702813248

Stoodley, C. J., and Schmahmann, J. D. (2009). Functional topography in the human cerebellum: a meta-analysis of neuroimaging studies. *Neuroimage* 44, 489–501. doi: 10.1016/j.neuroimage.2008.08.039

Sun, Y., Dai, Z., Li, Y., Sheng, C., Li, H., Wang, X., et al. (2016). Subjective cognitive decline: mapping functional and structural brain changes-A combined resting-state functional and structural MR imaging study. *Radiology* 281, 185–192. doi: 10.1148/radiol.2016151771

Tavano, A., Grasso, R., Gagliardi, C., Triulzi, F., Bresolin, N., Fabbro, F., et al. (2007). Disorders of cognitive and affective development in cerebellar malformations. *Brain* 130(Pt 10), 2646–2660. doi: 10.1093/brain/awm201

Thomann, P. A., Schlafer, C., Seidl, U., Santos, V. D., Essig, M., and Schroder, J. (2008). The cerebellum in mild cognitive impairment and Alzheimer's disease - a structural MRI study. *J. Psychiatr. Res.* 42, 1198–1202. doi: 10.1016/j.jpsychires.2007.12.002

Timmann, D., Drepper, J., Frings, M., Maschke, M., Richter, S., Gerwig, M., et al. (2010). The human cerebellum contributes to motor, emotional and cognitive associative learning. *Rev. Cortex* 46, 845–857. doi: 10.1016/j.cortex.2009.06.009

Tomasi, D., and Volkow, N. D. (2011). Association between Functional Connectivity Hubs and Brain Networks. *Cereb. Cortex* 21, 2003–2013. doi: 10.1093/cercor/bhq268

Tomasi, D., Wang, G. J., and Volkow, N. D. (2013). Energetic cost of brain functional connectivity. *Proc. Natl. Acad. Sci. U.S.A.* 110, 13642–13647. doi: 10.1073/pnas.1303346110

Verfaillie, S. C. J., Slot, R. E. R., Dicks, E., Prins, N. D., Overbeek, J. M., Teunissen, C. E., et al. (2018). A more randomly organized grey matter network is associated with deteriorating language and global cognition in individuals with subjective cognitive decline. *Hum. Brain Mapp.* 39, 3143–3151. doi: 10.1002/hbm.24065

Villain, N., Desgranges, B., Viader, F., de la Sayette, V., Mezenge, F., Landeau, B., et al. (2008). Relationships between hippocampal atrophy, white matter disruption, and gray matter hypometabolism in Alzheimer's disease. *J. Neurosci.* 28, 6174–6181. doi: 10.1523/jneurosci.1392-08. 2008

Viviano, R. P., Hayes, J. M., Pruitt, P. J., Fernandez, Z. J., van Rooden, S., van der Grond, J., et al. (2018). Aberrant memory system connectivity and working memory performance in subjective cognitive decline. *Neuroimage* doi: 10.1016/j.neuroimage.2018.10.015 [Epub ahead of print]. doi: 10.1016/j.neuroimage.2018.10.015

Wang, L., Kong, Q., Li, K., Su, Y., Zeng, Y., Zhang, Q., et al. (2016). Frequency-dependent changes in amplitude of low-frequency oscillations in depression: a resting-state fMRI study. *Neurosci. Lett.* 614, 105–111. doi: 10.1016/j.neulet.2016.01.012

Wang, Z., Yan, C., Zhao, C., Qi, Z., Zhou, W., Lu, J., et al. (2011). Spatial patterns of intrinsic brain activity in mild cognitive impairment and Alzheimer's disease: a resting-state functional MRI study. *Hum. Brain Mapp.* 32, 1720–1740. doi: 10.1002/hbm.21140

Zang, Y. F., He, Y., Zhu, C. Z., Cao, Q. J., Sui, M. Q., Liang, M., et al. (2007). Altered baseline brain activity in children with ADHD revealed by resting-state functional MRI. *Brain Dev.* 29, 83–91. doi: 10.1016/j.braindev.2006.07.002

Zhang, D. Y., and Raichle, M. E. (2010). Disease and the brain's dark energy. *Nat. Rev. Neurol.* 6, 15–28. doi: 10.1038/nrneurol.2009.198

Zhang, Z., Hong, X., and Hui, L. I. (1999). The minimental state examination in the Chinese residents population aged 55 years and over in the urban and rural areas of Beijing. *Chin. J. Neurol.* 32, 149–153. doi: 10.3760/j.issn:1006-7876.1999.03.006

Zhao, B., Shang, X.-L., He, Z.-Y., Fan, G.-G., and Liu, H. (2012). Amplitude of low-frequency fluctuation in patients with alzheimer's disease based on resting-state functional MRI. *J. China Med. Univ.* 41, 329–332.

Zhou, M., Hu, X., Lu, L., Zhang, L., Chen, L., Gong, Q., et al. (2017). Intrinsic cerebral activity at resting state in adults with major depressive disorder: a meta-analysis. *Prog. Neuropsychopharmacol. Biol. Psychiatry* 75, 157–164. doi: 10.1016/j.pnpbp.2017.02.001

Zou, Q. H., Zhu, C. Z., Yang, Y., Zuo, X. N., Long, X. Y., Cao, Q. J., et al. (2008). An improved approach to detection of amplitude of low-frequency fluctuation (ALFF) for resting-state fMRI: fractional ALFF. *J. Neurosci. Methods* 172, 137–141. doi: 10.1016/j.jneumeth.2008.04.012

Zuo, X. N., Di Martino, A., Kelly, C., Shehzad, Z. E., Gee, D. G., Klein, D. F., et al. (2010). The oscillating brain: complex and reliable. *Neuroimage* 49, 1432–1445. doi: 10.1016/j.neuroimage.2009.09.037

7

Brain Functional Networks in Type 2 Diabetes Mellitus Patients: A Resting-State Functional MRI Study

Jian Xu[1,2], Fuqin Chen[1], Taiyuan Liu[3], Ting Wang[4], Junran Zhang[1], Huijuan Yuan[5]* and Meiyun Wang[3]**

[1] *Department of Medical Information Engineering, School of Electrical Engineering and Information, Sichuan University, Chengdu, China,* [2] *School of Information Engineering, Hubei University for Nationalities, Enshi, China,* [3] *Department of Medical Imaging, Henan Provincial People's Hospital, Zhengzhou, China,* [4] *Department of Computer Science, Chengdu University of Information Technology, Chengdu, China,* [5] *Department of Endocrinology, Henan Provincial People's Hospital, Zhengzhou, China*

***Correspondence:**
Junran Zhang
zhangjunran@gmail.com
Huijuan Yuan
lmls3712@163.com
Meiyun Wang
mywang@ha.edu.cn

Background: Previous diabetes mellitus studies of cognitive impairments in the early stages have focused on changes in brain structure and function, and more recently the focus has shifted to the relationships between encephalic regions and diversification of network topology. However, studies examining network topology in diabetic brain function are still limited.

Methods: The study included 102 subjects; 55 type 2 diabetes mellitus (T2DM) patients plus 47 healthy controls. All subjects were examined by resting-state functional magnetic resonance imaging (rs-fMRI) scan. According to Automated Anatomical Labeling, the brain was divided into 90 anatomical regions, and every region corresponds to a brain network analysis node. The whole brain functional network was constructed by thresholding the correlation matrices of the 90 brain regions, and the topological properties of the network were computed based on graph theory. Then, the topological properties of the network were compared between different groups by using a non-parametric test. Finally, the associations between differences in topological properties and the clinical indicators were analyzed.

Results: The brain functional networks of both T2DM patients and healthy controls were found to possess small-world characteristics, i.e., normalized clustering coefficient (γ) > 1, and normalized characteristic path length (λ) close to 1. No significant differences were found in the small-world characteristics (σ). Second, the T2DM patient group displayed significant differences in node properties in certain brain regions. Correlative analytic results showed that the node degree of the right inferior temporal gyrus (ITG) and the node efficiencies of the right ITG and superior temporal gyrus of T2DM patients were positively correlated with body mass index.

Conclusion: The brain network of T2DM patients has the same small-world characteristics as normal people, but the normalized clustering coefficient is higher and the normalized characteristic path length is lower than that of the normal control group, indicating that the brain function network of the T2DM patients has changed. The changes of node properties were mostly concentrated in frontal lobe, temporal lobe and posterior cingulate gyrus. The abnormal changes in these indices in T2DM patients might be explained as a compensatory behavior to reduce cognitive impairments, which is achieved by mobilizing additional neural resources, such as the excessive activation of the network and the efficient networking of multiple brain regions.

Keywords: type 2 diabetes mellitus, resting-state functional magnetic resonance imaging, graph theory, functional network, small-world, topological properties

INTRODUCTION

Diabetes is a metabolic disease characterized by long-term hyperglycemia, which may cause various complications such as microvascular disease, retinopathy, kidney disease and peripheral neuropathy. In severe cases, diabetes can be fatal. Statistics produced by the International Diabetes Federation in 2015 indicated that the number of diabetes patients was about 415 million, and predicted that it would reach up to 642 million by 2040 (Ogurtsova et al., 2017). In China, the rate of diabetes cases has approximately doubled in the last 10 years. The incidence of diabetes in China is 11.6% and the number of diabetics is more than 100 million, both of which are the highest in the world. Type 2 diabetes mellitus (T2DM) patients account for around 90% of cases of diabetes mellitus (Holman et al., 2015), the morbidity of which has been increasing over the years. Consequently, diabetes has become one of the most critical health issues in China (Ning, 2018).

Previous studies have shown that T2DM can result in various cognitive deficits in the early stages of the disease, including lapses in concentration, hypomnesis, visual impairment, and declines in information processing speed and executive capacity (McCrimmon et al., 2012). In extreme cases, these cognitive deficits can develop into dementia. At present, the rapidly rising incidence of diabetes and its associated cognitive impairments has become a major issue. Although some progress has been made with regard to determining the cognitive impairments caused by T2DM, the underlying neuronal mechanisms of the disorder are still not well understood.

Recently, resting-state functional magnetic resonance imaging (rs-fMRI) has been used to study the underlying pathogenesis of many kinds of central nervous system diseases, including those which affect brain metabolism (Zhang L.J. et al., 2014; Zhou X.Q. et al., 2014). As an emerging non-invasive diagnostic tool, rs-fMRI can be applied to explore and distinguish impaired and normal cognitive function in patients with diabetes mellitus.

The brain network analysis method based on graph theory is mainly used to explore the potential mechanism of normal human brain and various brain diseases, and it is found that the brain function networks of normal people and brain diseases patients have small-world characteristics (Supekar et al., 2009; Zhang et al., 2011; Lei et al., 2015). He et al. (2007) successfully built the first human brain structure network in 2007 and found that it has small-world characteristics. They found that the brain network topology of AD patients has changed (He et al., 2008). They also confirmed the existence of stable small-world characteristics by studying the brain structure network of multiple sclerosis patients (He et al., 2009). Since then, this method has been adopted in many researches (Zhang et al., 2011; Suo et al., 2015; Xiao et al., 2015).

The graph theory-based network analysis has only been used in patients with T2DM to investigate brain structure. Zhang L.J. et al. (2014) discovered that the white matter network topology (including the efficient of global properties and central sulcus on right side cover) of T2DM patients is changed, and this kind of abnormal network structure is associated with the impairment of executive function observed in these patients. By taking advantage of fiber tracer diffusion magnetic resonance imaging and the method of graph theory, Reijmer et al. (2013) and others found that both local and global network properties of T2DM patients are changed. The abnormal network structure was associated with the information processing speed of patients and was independent of age, sex, education, white matter hyperintensities, lacunar infarct and other factors. There have not been any reports of the changes of brain gray matter functional network topology properties in T2DM patients. Cui et al. (2015) analyzed the differences in default mode network (DMN) of T2DM patients, finding out that T2DM patients were associated with impaired DMN function. With independent component analysis (ICA) methods, Chen et al. (2015) found abnormal functional connections between DMN, left frontal network and sensorimotor network in T2DM patients, but found no abnormal functional connections in other resting-state networks. With the same methods, Xia et al. (2015) investigated whether the attention network had changed in T2DM patients, and explored the relationship between abnormal functional connection of attention network and cognitive behavior.

The rs-fMRI brain network analysis method based on graph theory has become one of the hotspots in the study of normal human brain and neuropsychiatric diseases. It can explore the functional connections between the whole brain and the local brain regions, but it has not been widely used in the study of diabetes. Understanding the abnormal patterns of the brain's functional network can help to find a new way to treat and evaluate the diagnosis of diabetes.

In the present research, we compared the diversity of entire brain functional network topology properties between T2DM patients and healthy controls by adopting graph theory-based brain network analysis together with rs-fMRI. We also explored the relationship between the changes in brain functional network topology properties and clinical variables and the neurocognitive scale, and discussed the influence of relative cognitive obstacles and possible mechanism that it may have on patients. The results of the present study will provide a theoretical basis for diabetic pathophysiology and clinical presentation, and evidence for the need for early treatment and prognostic evaluations.

MATERIALS AND METHODS

Subjects

The study subjects were selected from a total of 154 potential participants: 91 patients with T2DM at Henan Provincial People's Hospital, and 63 healthy volunteers from the physical examination center. Fifty two subjects were excluded from the study, including 36 patients with T2DM (5 patients with incomplete clinical data, 6 patients with excessive head movement during fMRI scan and 25 patients who did not meet the inclusion criteria), and 16 healthy controls (1 individual with excessive head movement (translational movement > 1.5 mm or rotation > 1.5) during fMRI scan and 15 subjects that failed to meet the inclusion criteria). The remaining 102 subjects were included in the study: 55 patients in the T2DM group and 47 in the healthy control group. All subjects were right-handed, and were informed of the specific content of the study and voluntarily signed informed consent.

The inclusion criteria are as follows: (1) after oral glucose tolerance test (OGTT) T2DM was diagnosed in accordance with the diagnostic criteria published by the World Health Organization in 1999 (American Diabetes Association, 2014); (2) age 40–75, course of T2DM > 1 year. The exclusion criteria were as follows: (1) functional insufficiency of heart, lung, liver and kidney; (2) hyperthyroidism, hypothyroidism and other systemic diseases; (3) infection, ketoacidosis, hyperosmolarity, severe hypoglycemic coma or other urgent complication; (4) anxiety, depression or other neuropsychiatric disease that affects cognitive function; (5) cerebral hemorrhage, cerebral infarction, cerebral trauma, vascular dementia or other disease or medical history that incurs central nervous system injury; (6) recently taken medication that is likely to affect cognitive function; (7) drug taking or alcohol dependence; (8) failing to complete required test items because of intolerance or other factors; (9) MRI contraindication.

The inclusion criteria of healthy controls (Healthy Controls Corresponding to Type 2 Diabetes Mellitus, T2HC) were as follows: (1) age, gender, highest level of education and handedness are matched to those of the T2DM patients; (2) the OGTT result does not conform to the diagnostic criteria of T2DM published by the World Health Organization in 1999; (3) Montreal Cognitive Assessment Scale (MoCA) grade is normal. The exclusion criteria are the same as described above.

Clinical and Cognitive Scale Test

Before fMRI scanning, the following clinical characteristics were recorded: gender, age at diagnosis, diabetic course, MoCA, height, weight, glycosylated hemoglobin (HbAlc), fasting blood glucose, total cholesterol (TCHOL), glycerin trilaurate (TG), high density lipoprotein (HDL), and low density lipoprotein (LDL). The course of T2DM was defined as the time elapsed from when the patient was diagnosed with T2DM to the time of fMRI scanning. Height and weight were used to calculate body mass index (BMI) of subjects: BMI = weight (kg)/height (m^2). BMI < 18.5 is defined as slim, BMI = 18.5–23.9 is normal, BMI $\geq$ 24 is overweight, BMI = 24–26.9 is fat, BMI = 27–29.9 is corpulent, BMI $\geq$ 30 is severely obese, BMI $\geq$ 40 is extremely obese.

The MoCA was used to evaluate the integral cognitive function of all subjects, and the test was performed according to standard procedures. The test was carried out in a quiet environment. At the same time, subjects were expected to be relaxed, conscious and non-contradictory. The test assessed 8 cognitive domains: visual space and executive function, attention, memory, naming, abstract thinking, language, delayed recall and orientation. The MoCA is commonly used to screen for Mild Cognitive Impairment (MCI), for which it displays high sensitivity (Hobson, 2015). The MoCA test result has a total score of 30 points, with a final score $\geq$ 26 being considered normal.

Rs-fMRI Data Acquisition

Subjects were scanned under resting conditions using a 3.0T superconducting magnetic resonance imaging system and a Siemens 8-channel head coil. During scanning, subjects were instructed to take the supine position, close their eyes but do not sleep, and try to keep their body motionless. Head movement was limited with a foam pad, and the subject's hearing was protected with foam earplugs or earphones. First, regular MRI scanning was conducted to detect brain abnormalities, then echo planar imaging (EPI) was used to collect resting-state brain function. The scan parameters were as follows: TR = 2000 ms, TE = 30 ms, seam thickness = 5 mm, FOV = 240 $\times$ 240 mm^2, matrix = 64 $\times$ 64, voxel size = 3.75 $\times$ 3.75 $\times$ 5 mm^3, FA = 90°, acquisition 210 time points, the total scan time is 420 s. Subjects were asked to close their eyes, relax and keep their head motionless, and try to keep a clear head without much thinking before the functional scanning. After the scan was complete, the respondents were asked to cooperate, and those who did not cooperate well were excluded from the study.

Data Preprocessing

Data preprocessing analysis was conducted in the MATLAB 2017a software environment by using the GRETNA graph-based network analysis toolkit. First, data from the first 10 time points were removed to exclude the problem of magnetic field uniformity, then time layer correction of rs-fMRI data was performed, and moving 3 mm horizontally or rotating in the direction of x, y, and z axis as standard strip head dynamic data. The fMRI images were normalized after head-movement correction by using the MNI-152 standard template of brain anatomy of the Neurological Research Institute, Montreal, Canada, by matching the structure and function images of the subjects and resampling data (voxel size was 3 mm $\times$ 3 mm $\times$ 3 mm). Next, linear drift and low frequency filter (frequency 0.01–0.08 Hz) were taken to correct the influence of linear frequency drift and high-frequency physical noise; doing Gaussian smoothing to normalized graph, it was treated with 4 mm height and a half full width, smooth kernel size is 4 × 4 × 4. Finally, removal covariate included the impact of 6 head parameters (3 translation parameters and 3 rotation parameters), the whole mean signal, white matter, cerebrospinal fluid signal, age and gender.

Network Construction

Node Definition

A network is composed of many nodes and the edges of the connection between these nodes. In brain networks, nodes represent brain regions and edges represent the degree of statistical dependence of blood oxygenation level dependent (BOLD) imaging between different brain regions. In the article, brain is divided into 90 cortices and cortical interest areas.

Edge Definition

For every subject, we chose average time list of 90 brain regions, then, calculated the correlation coefficient between the mean time series value of the two brain regions (spread all brain regions, such as the i-th brain area and the j-th brain area), which as the functional connection metric between them. Last, obtained was a 90 × 90 correlation matrix, which is called a weighed functional connection matrix. According to the predefined threshold (see threshold selection below), we converted the weighed functional connection matrix to a binary adjacency matrix. If the absolute value of the correlation coefficient between any two brain regions was less than the given threshold, it was recorded as 0, otherwise it was recorded as 1.

Network Analysis

Threshold Selection

The number of sides of each brain network is different. To correct for this difference, we applied the sparse threshold (S) range to the relative matrix to ensure the brain network of every subject contained the same number of sides. For every subject, S is defined as the ratio between the actual number of edges and the highest possible number of edges. Because there has not any exact means to define the choice of single threshold at present, previous brain network analysis study used the range of S to thresholding every relative matrix repeatedly. The selection criteria should meet the following two conditions: (1) the minimum of S should meet average node degree in every thresholding network that id 2log(N), and N is node number; (2) the maximum of node should be satisfied with small-world characteristics scalar σ and that is bigger than 1.1. After above process, it would produce a range of S, that is pitch is 0.01 and S between 0.1 and 0.34. Network of this threshold range produced can guarantee small-world characteristics estimation with sparse attribute and minimal pseudo-side. The subsequent brain network analysis will calculate the global network properties and node properties in the order of each sparsity level.

Network Parameters

Global properties include: (1) small-world parameters, which includes cluster coefficient, characteristic path length, normalized cluster coefficient, normalized characteristic path length, and small-world characteristics; (2) network efficiency, which includes global efficiency, and component efficiency. Node properties include: (1) node degree; (2) node efficiency; and (3) the betweenness of node.

Statistical Analysis

Demographic and Clinical Data Statistical Analysis

Statistical analysis of the clinical data of the subjects included in the study was performed by using the SPSS 22.0 software package. The chi-squared test was used to compare the gender differences between groups. The measurements of other variables (age, BMI, course of disease, glycosylated hemoglobin, fasting blood glucose, total cholesterol, triglyceride, high density lipoprotein, low density lipoprotein and MoCA analog scale) were analyzed by using two-sample *t*-tests. $p < 0.05$ was deemed to be statistically significant.

Statistical Test of Network Properties Between Groups

Because area under the curve (AUC) describes the topology properties of brain network generally, and it can select single threshold calculation independently, moreover, it is highly sensitive about topology structure of brain disease abnormally. As a result, AUC of every topology attribute was selected as statistical sample (Suo et al., 2015). The AUC for a general metric Y can be defined as the AUC for calculating the sparsity range from S1 to Sn (the interval is ΔS) (**Figure 1**), and it's formula can be described as Lei et al. (2015):

$$Y^{\text{AUC}} = \frac{1}{2}\sum_{k=1}^{N-1}\left[Y(S_k) + Y(S_{k-1})\right] \bullet \Delta S$$

To determine whether there are inter-group differences in network properties, the non-parametric permutation test is used to test the AUC of each network attribute in the two sets of samples. It is divided into the following steps:

(1) Building the null hypothesis. It is assumed that there is no difference between the means of the two statistical samples.
(2) Determining inspection level α, which is designated as 0.05.

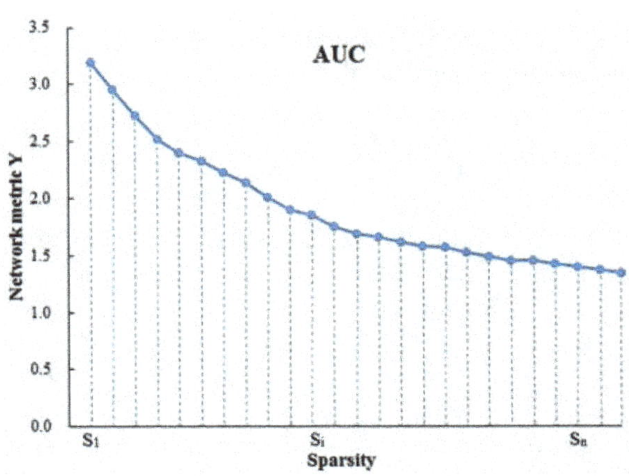

FIGURE 1 | The calculation of area under the curve (AUC). $S_1 = 0.10$, $S_n = 0.34$, $\Delta S = 0.01$.

(3) Calculating test statistic of previous two groups' samples.
(4) To determine whether the differences between groups of network properties could occur accidentally, a sample is selected at random without replacement from sample observation (two samples get together) so as to regroup, then replacement statistical tests of two samples, AUC after stochastic grouping were computed.
(5) Setting the number of random packets, for example 10,000 times, repeat step 4 1,000 times, then get a empirical exampling distribution of replacement statistical tests.
(6) Adopting 95% of every empirical exampling distribution as critical value of null tail test of the null hypothesis. This kind of mistakes is kept within 0.05, and calculating odds is p.
(7) With regard to the inspection level (significance level) given by step 2, and according to the principle of small probability, conclusion is drawn.

It is worthwhile to note that before taking statistical test, the effects of age, sex and other parameters need to be removed by multiple linear regression to ensure the differences between groups of every network properties are caused by diseases. To solve multiple comparative problems, use calibration methods of false discovery rate (FDR) proposed by Benjamini-Hochberg, which is to correct the p-value after difference between each network attribute group.

Correlation Analysis Between Network Properties and Clinical Parameters

After determining the differences in network properties between the groups, we examined the relationship between these differences and the clinical parameters of T2DM, with the age and gender as cointegration variables. Clinical parameters include BMI, course of disease, glycated hemoglobin, fasting blood-glucose, total cholesterol, triglyceride, high-density lipoprotein, low-density lipoprotein, and MoCA score.

TABLE 1 | Demographic data and clinical Features of type 2 diabetes mellitus patients and the corresponding control group.

Characteristics	Mean ± *SD*		*P*-value
	Type 2 diabetes mellitus (*n* = 55)	Control group (*n* = 47)	
Gender (male/female)	35/20	21/26	0.073
Age	53.31 (± 9.05)	53.34 (± 7.68)	0.919
Course of disease (years)	8.87 (± 6.42)	–	0.112
BMI	25.37 (± 2.85)	25.20 (± 2.80)	0.761
HbA1c	8.15 (± 1.78)	–	**0.001**
GLU	9.59 (± 3.04)	–	0.842
CHOL	4.42 (± 1.10)	4.81 (± 0.87)	0.054
TG	2.05 (± 2.41)	1.55 (± 0.82)	0.152
HDL	0.98 (± 0.24)	1.21 (± 0.33)	**0.001**
LDL	2.51 (± 0.90)	2.77 (± 0.64)	0.100
MoCA	25.36 (± 1.74)	27.79 (± 1.90)	**0.001**

All calculations were carried out in SPSS 22.0. Double-tailed chi-squared test was used for gender variables. Other measurement variables were tested with two-sample t-test. For all tests, $p < 0.05$ was considered statistically significant. Values in bold indicate statistically significant differences. BMI, body mass index; HbA1c, glycated hemoglobin; GLU, fasting blood glucose; CHOL, cholesterol; TG, triglyceride; HDL, high-density lipoprotein; LDL, low-density lipoprotein; MoCA, Montreal Cognitive Assessment score.

RESULTS

Demographic Data, Clinical Data, and Cognitive Scale

The results of demographic data, clinical features and cognitive scales of all subjects are shown in **Table 1**. The MoCA grade of the T2DM group is greater than 26, which is seen as cognitive dysfunction. There were no significant differences between the T2DM and T2HC groups in gender, age, BMI, TCHOL, TG, or LDL, but there were differences between the groups in HDL and MoCA scores.

Small-World Brain Functional Network

In the given threshold range, compared with the random network, the brain function networks of the two groups have small-world characteristics, i.e., the normalized cluster coefficient is >1, and the normalized feature path length is close to 1 (**Figure 2**). These results are consistent with previous studies of small-world networks.

Comparison of Network Topology Properties Between T2DM Patients Group and Healthy Controls

There was at least one brain region with significant difference in the comparison between record node properties groups (after correlation of FDR, $p < 0.05$). Compared with T2HC, T2DM patients displayed higher global properties (E_{glob}), local attribute (E_{loc}) and cluster coefficient (C_p), and lower characteristic path length L_p (**Figure 3**). There was no significant difference between the groups in normalized cluster coefficient (γ), normalized characteristic path length (λ) or small-world characteristics (σ) ($p > 0.05$).

Compared with those of the T2HC control group, the T2DM group displayed increased node degree in the following brain regions: bilateral lenticular putamen and right inferior temporal gyrus (ITG). The T2DM group displayed increased node efficiency in the following brain regions: left central sulcus, left insula, bilateral lenticular putamen and right ITG. The T2DM group displayed increased betweenness of node in the following brain region: right ITG (**Table 2**).

Correlation Analysis Between Abnormal Network Topology Properties and Clinical Parameters

The node degree, node efficiencies and the betweenness of node of the right ITG of the T2DM group were positively correlated with BMI ($r = 0.3115$, $p = 0.0206$; $r = 0.3060$, $p = 0.0231$; $r = 0.3175$, $p = 0.0182$, **Figure 4**). There was no significant

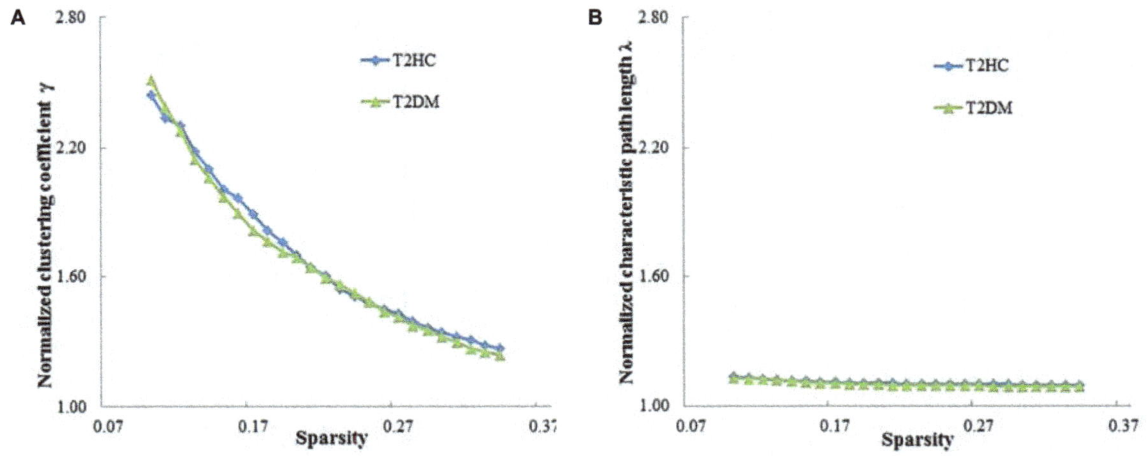

FIGURE 2 | Relationship between the small-world characteristics parameters of brain networks (normalized cluster coefficient and normalized characteristic path length) and sparsity of the brain function network. **(A)** Normalized cluster coefficient (γ) is > 1, and **(B)** normalized characteristic path length is close to 1, which shows that the brain functional networks in both groups have small-world characteristics. T2DM, type 2 diabetes mellitus patients; T2HC, matched healthy controls.

correlation between all global and other node properties and all clinical indicators ($p > 0.05$).

DISCUSSION

This study examined the topological differences in brain function networks of T2DM patients, based on graph theoretical analysis of rs-fMRI data. The main results were as follows: (1) Global properties: the brain function network of T2DM has small-world characteristics as healthy controls. (2) Node properties: compared with healthy controls, the T2DM group have notable changes in insula, lenticular putamen, central sulcus, ITG and other brain regions. (3) Related analysis: the node degree of the right ITG, and the node efficiency of the right inferior and superior temporal gyrus of the T2DM group are all positively correlated with BMI. The excessive activation indices of the T2DM group may be explained as a compensatory behavior, which may reduce cognitive impairment by mobilizing additional neural resources. These findings provide a new perspective of how changes in brain functional topology properties may be related to cognitive function.

Change of Global Properties

The human brain is a complex network in multiple space and time scales with many important topology, which include small-world characteristics, modular and highly connected networks of the core brain areas (Sporns, 2011). Complex network usually contains regular, small-world and stochastic networks, and these networks are judged by cluster coefficient and characteristic path length. The rule network has higher cluster coefficient and longer characteristic path length, and the random network has shorter characteristic path length and lower cluster coefficient. However, the small-world lies between the rule and random networks, which not only has rule network similar to highly clustering coefficient, but also short feature path length similar to a random network (Liang et al., 2010). The small-world network is the best balance between global integration of brain function activities and global specialization, which supports the two most basic organizational principles of the human brain (functional integration and separation of functions) (Rubinov and Sporns, 2010). Small-world characteristics can keep the network efficient, specific modular information and fast global information transmission (He and Evans, 2010). Previous studies showed that small-world characteristics exist in brain structures and functional networks, and changes in topology properties may lead to a variety of neuropsychiatric disorders, such as Alzheimer's disease (Supekar et al., 2008), depression (Zhang et al., 2011), epilepsy (Liao et al., 2010), and post-traumatic stress disorder (Lei et al., 2015). Although the topology properties of these diseases display various changes, as a general rule, the more the network topology properties deviate from small-world, the more disordered the brain function is.

Cluster coefficient and characteristic path length can all indicate that the process of transferring networks from small-world networks to rule network or random networks. Zhang found that the overall efficiency of the white matter network is reduced in T2DM, and characteristic path length is increased, and that the global properties and node efficiency of the central sulcus are positively correlated with executive function (Zhang et al., 2016); Reijmer found that global efficiency and cluster coefficient are reduced, and characteristic path length is increased. The abnormality of these structural networks is related to the slow speed of information processing observed in patients (Reijmer et al., 2013). These findings are essentially in agreement with the results observed in the diabetic brain network by Wang et al. (2016) by using the fMRI technique. In contrast to the results of the aforementioned study, in the present study we found that T2DM patients have higher normalized cluster coefficient and lower characteristic path length, which are typical features of a small-world network. Similar changes have been observed in MCI. For example, Wang et al. (2014) found there was a

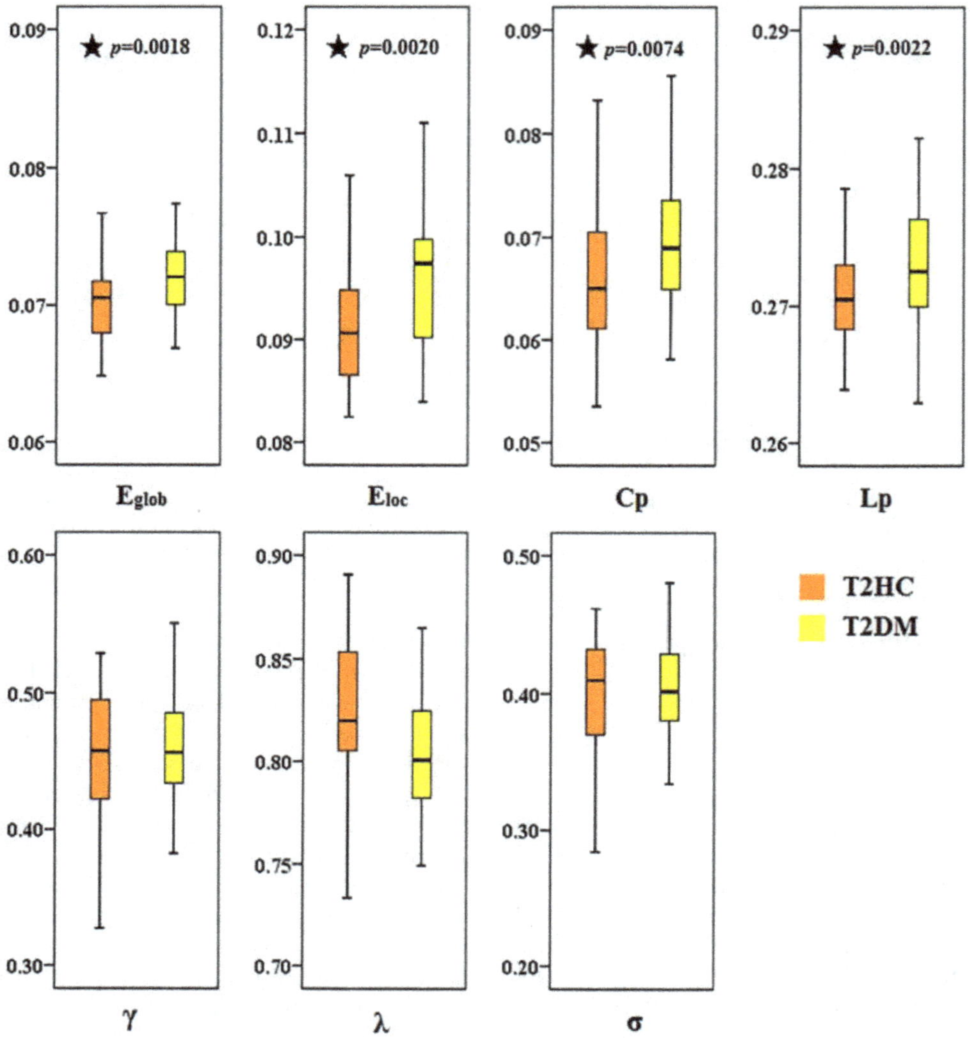

FIGURE 3 | Topological differences in brain function networks between type 2 diabetes mellitus (T2DM) and matched healthy control (T2HC) groups. Compared with the T2HC group, the global properties (E_{glob}), local attribute (E_{loc}), and cluster coefficient (C_p) of the T2DM group were higher, and the characteristic path length (L_p) was lower. There were no significant differences between groups in normalized cluster coefficient (γ), normalized characteristic path length (λ), or small-world characteristics (σ). The ordinate is the area under the curve (AUC) value for each attribute. Black asterisks indicate a significant difference between the two groups.

higher normalized cluster coefficient when sparsity threshold was in the range 0.10–0.18, but normalized characteristic path length was lower over the entire range of threshold. This means that the cognitive impairments of the diabetics that participated in the study were mild, and that they do not show the same small-world characteristics as healthy controls. The increasing of the cluster coefficient indicates that the local brain network is enhanced in patients with diabetes mellitus. However, the decrease of the characteristic pathway length indicates that the ability for information transfer between remote regions of the brain in patients with diabetes is enhanced. It is speculated that the brain function of patients with diabetes mellitus may be impaired in the early stages of cognitive impairment. Under compensatory mechanisms, its ability for local information and remote information processing is enhanced, showing the information processing mechanism consistent with MCI; but with the further development of diabetes (Wang et al., 2014). The impairment in brain function is more severe than in T2DM patients. Having lost the ability to compensate, its long-distance information transmission ability drops.

This study also found that patients with diabetes mellitus have higher global and local efficiency, which may mean that the functional integration ability of the whole brain network and the information processing ability of the local sub-networks are enhanced, which is in accordance with the small-world characteristics results. The changes of these network parameters were much ascribe to metabolic disturbance of diabetics, needing the whole brain network to compensation for the increase of the overall integration efficiency. However, inconsistent results were found in previous studies of diabetic brain network structure (Reijmer et al., 2013; Zhang et al., 2016), and this difference may stem from differences in subjects and modes. Although the trends

TABLE 2 | Brain areas with significant differences in node centricity between the Type 2 diabetes mellitus (T2DM) and matched healthy control (T2HC) groups.

Brain region	*P*-value		
	Node betweenness	Node degree	Node efficiency
T2HC < T2DM			
Left rolandic operculum	0.3123	0.0110	**0.0026**
Left insula	0.3203	0.0072	**0.0022**
Left putamen	0.4287	**0.0014**	**0.0004**
Right putamen	0.3673	**0.0002**	**0.0002**
Right inferior temporal gyrus	**0.0020**	**0.0016**	**0.0008**

Values in bold indicate statistically significant differences (correlation of FDR, expected threshold level α = 0.05). T2DM, type 2 diabetes mellitus; T2HC, matched healthy controls.

of the changes in these network parameters are inconsistent, they all illustrate the abnormality of the brain network efficiency in patients with diabetes mellitus.

The changes in the global topological properties of these brain networks indicate the abnormality of neural network structure in diabetes mellitus. Given that the small-world characteristics are not affected, the brain network is thus compensated with the high efficiency by global integration and local separation after cognitive function of diabetics is impaired, which makes this characteristic more obvious than the normal person.

Change of Node Properties

Consistent with the increased network efficiency, we also found the brain areas of the nodes in the patients with diabetes, the brain regions involved in the patients included the superior frontal gyrus, olfactory cortex, posterior cingulate gyrus, occipital gyrus and superior temporal gyrus. In functional studies of diabetes, the superior frontal gyrus was associated with cognitive impairment, and T2DM patients showed worse executive and memory skills in high working load memory tasks (Chen et al., 2014; Zhang et al., 2015). In addition, a reduction in the brain surface area of patients was also found in a previous study (Peng et al., 2015). Findings in the temporal gyrus and ITG in patients with diabetes mellitus are as follows: the cortex of cortical white matter decreased and was related to memory defects (Yau et al., 2009); the relationship between white matter damage and memory loss is closely related (Zhang J. et al., 2014); the decrease of functional activity is closely related to memory decline, and occurs earlier than atrophy (Zhou X. et al., 2014); these findings are consistent with the region of the advanced cognitive function. The node properties of the right temporal gyrus and ITG were positively correlated with BMI of T2DM patients, but obesity is a crucial factor affecting many metabolic disorders in patients with diabetes mellitus (Zhou and Xue, 2006). The results confirm that the changes of brain network topology in patients with diabetes have a relationship with obesity.

Previous studies have shown that the temporal and frontal lobes are the main brain areas involved in the cognitive impairment of diabetes. Evidence of structural and functional abnormalities of the frontal-temporal brain region in patients with diabetes mellitus is as follows: using diffusion tensor imaging (DTI) technology, Yau et al. (2009, 2014) found that the gray matter and white matter microscopic abnormalities of T2DM patients were mainly located in the frontal and temporal lobes, and participated in language memory disorders. Last et al. (2007) used continuous arterial spin label imaging to reveal temporal and frontal blood flow in T2DM patients. Using structural MRI and PET techniques, García-Casares observed a reduction in gray matter density and glucose metabolism in the fronto-temporal brain regions in T2DM patients after controlling for other vascular risk factors (Garcíacasares et al., 2014). Zhou et al. used rs-fMRI technology to detect diffuse amplitude of low frequency fluctuation (ALFF) changes in MCI patients with diabetes, including in the temporal lobe and frontal lobe (Zhou X. et al., 2014). These findings indicate that the fronto-temporal brain region is associated with impairments in cognitive functions such as information processing speed, memory and emotion (Yau et al., 2009, 2014; Hsu et al., 2012). The posterior

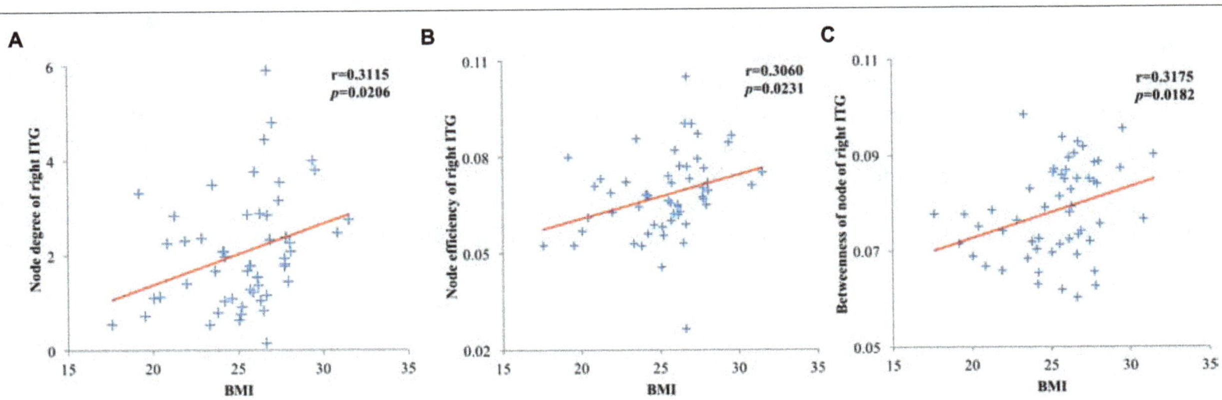

FIGURE 4 | Scatter plots of brain region and clinical index node properties with statistically significant correlations. **(A)** Node degree of the right inferior temporal gyrus of the type 2 diabetes mellitus (T2DM) group was positively correlated with body mass index (BMI); **(B)** Node efficiency of the right inferior temporal gyrus of the T2DM group was positively correlated with BMI; **(C)** The betweenness of node of the right inferior temporal gyrus of the T2DM group was positively correlated with BMI.

cingulate gyrus, as the core node of the DMN, plays a key role in the cognitive process, and it is used to predict the biological markers of MCI converting to early Alzheimer's disease. Recent studies have shown a reduction in the value of the posterior cingulate gyrus ALFF that is highly correlated to the MoCA scale, besides, its dysfunction of the functional connection with multiple brain is more indicative of the specific impairment of memory function (Qin et al., 2016). Studies conducted by Cui and others have also confirmed that the decrease of functional connectivity in the posterior cingulate cortex in the DMN is related to cognitive behavior (Cui et al., 2015). Therefore, it is speculated that the node properties abnormality in the posterior cingulate cortex is related to cognitive impairments in T2DM patients, such as information processing speed, emotion, memory and executive ability.

CONCLUSION

This study examined the brain network topology of T2DM patients by using graph theory-based analysis of rs-fMRI, and found that both global and node properties were changed. Compared with healthy controls, the normalized cluster coefficient and characteristic path length showed stronger small-world characteristics, indicating that the impairment in cognitive function is slight, and multiple brain regions make up an efficient sub-network that compensates for the small-world characteristic of the normal human brain. The changes of node properties were most prominent in the temporal and frontal lobes, and posterior cingulate gyrus, and the abnormality of node properties in these brain areas is related to the changes of brain cognitive function, which is a similar finding to those in previous studies. Consequently, inferring the efficient integration of functional networks of T2DM patients, sub-networks composed of multiple brain regions compensate for their impairment of cognitive function. Thus, the global properties and node properties results are activated excessively. The main limitations of the present study include: (1) This study used the AAL template to divide the cerebrum into 90 brain regions (nodes), and omits the epencephal. In previous brain network research, there is no gold standard template for the division of brain regions. (70 brain regions of automatic matching and non-linear imaging anatomical marker mapping, 116 brain regions including epencephal, 90 brain regions adopted by this study). To avoid the influence of the varying node definitions of the different brain atlas templates, future studies should establish and use a unified standard template. (2) This study only examined the MRI data of diabetic patients in the resting state, and did not investigate the structural image data at the same time. The brain is a complex network system with both anatomical and functional connections. If a combination of brain function and structure of patients can be analyzed, more powerful evidence for the changes of the topological properties of the diabetic brain network will be obtained. Future studies should combine multi-modal imaging data to establish these relationships, and these will provide more accurate interpretation of the neural mechanisms of patients with diabetes mellitus. In short, the combination of fMRI and graph theory for investigation of brain function in diabetes has just begun. Future research will focus more on the complex function and connection network properties of the patient's brain in the resting state, and will have potential significance for the early treatment, control and management of the disease and prevention of its complications. (3) Three diagnostic criteria for T2DM patients were published by WHO in 1999. One of them (OGTT) was used in this study, which may cause bias in the research results. In future studies, the other two criteria should be considered to improve the reliability of the results. (4) In this study, age and gender were used as covariates when performing correlation analysis between network properties and clinical parameters, but the diagnosis was not used as covariates. In future studies, clinical diagnostic parameters (such as BMI, etc.) should be used as covariates, which may improve the reliability of the results.

AUTHOR CONTRIBUTIONS

JZ contributed to the conception of the study. JX and FC contributed significantly to analysis and manuscript preparation. JX, MW, and TL performed the data analyses and wrote the manuscript. JZ, TW, and HY contributed to the interpretation and discussion of the results of the analysis.

FUNDING

This study was supported by National Natural Science Foundation of China (Grant Nos. 81371536 and 81500959), Sichuan Province Science and Technology Plan Project (Grant No. 2015HH036), Chengdu University of Information Engineering Research Fund (Grant No. KYTZ201719), the Project of Sichuan Provincial Education Hall (Grant No. 18ZA0089), and Chengdu Science and Technology Project of Benefiting People (Grant No. 2015-HM01-00561-SF).

REFERENCES

American Diabetes Association (2014). Diagnosis and classification of diabetes mellitus. *Diabetes Care* 37(Suppl. 1), S81–S90. doi: 10.2337/dc14-S081

Chen, Y., Liu, Z., Zhang, J., Tian, G., Li, L., Zhang, S., et al. (2015). Selectively disrupted functional connectivity networks in type 2 diabetes mellitus. *Front. Aging Neurosci.* 7:233. doi: 10.3389/fnagi.2015.00233

Chen, Y., Liu, Z., Zhang, J., Xu, K., Zhang, S., Wei, D., et al. (2014). Altered brain activation patterns under different working memory loads in patients with type 2 diabetes. *Diabetes Care* 37:3157. doi: 10.2337/dc14-1683

Cui, Y., Jiao, Y., Chen, H. J., Ding, J., Luo, B., Peng, C. Y., et al. (2015). Aberrant functional connectivity of default-mode network in type 2 diabetes patients. *Eur. Radiol.* 25, 3238–3246. doi: 10.1007/s00330-015-3746-8

Garcíacasares, N., Berthier, M. L., Jorge, R. E., Gonzalezalegre, P., Gutiérrez, C. A., Rioja, V. J., et al. (2014). Structural and functional brain changes in middle-aged type 2 diabetic patients: a cross-sectional study. *J. Alzheimers Dis.* 40, 375–386. doi: 10.3233/JAD-131736

He, Y., Chen, Z., and Evans, A. (2008). Structural insights into aberrant topological patterns of large-scale cortical networks in alzheimer's disease. *J. Neurosci.* 28, 4756–4766. doi: 10.1523/JNEUROSCI.0141-08.2008

He, Y., Chen, Z. J., and Evans, A. C. (2007). Small-world anatomical networks in the human brain revealed by cortical thickness from MRI. *Cereb. Cortex* 17, 2407–2419. doi: 10.1093/cercor/bhl149

He, Y., Dagher, A., Chen, Z., Charil, A., Zijdenbos, A., Worsley, K., et al. (2009). Impaired small-world efficiency in structural cortical networks in multiple sclerosis associated with white matter lesion load. *Brain* 132, 3366–3379. doi: 10.1093/brain/awp089

He, Y., and Evans, A. (2010). Graph theoretical modeling of brain connectivity. *Curr. Opin. Neurol.* 23, 341–350. doi: 10.1097/WCO.0b013e32833aa567

Hobson, J. (2015). The montreal cognitive assessment (MoCA). *Occup. Med. Oxford* 65, 764–765. doi: 10.1093/occmed/kqv078

Holman, N., Young, B., and Gadsby, R. (2015). Current prevalence of type 1 and type 2 diabetes in adults and children in the UK. *Diabetic Med.* 32, 1119–1120. doi: 10.1111/dme.12791

Hsu, J. L., Chen, Y. L., Leu, J. G., Jaw, F. S., Lee, C. H., Tsai, Y. F., et al. (2012). Microstructural white matter abnormalities in type 2 diabetes mellitus: a diffusion tensor imaging study. *Neuroimage* 59, 1098–1105. doi: 10.1016/j.neuroimage.2011.09.041

Last, D., Bazelaire, C. D., Alsop, D. C., Hu, K., Abduljalil, A. M., Cavallerano, J., et al. (2007). Global and regional effects of type 2 diabetes on brain tissue volumes and cerebral vasoreactivity. *Diabetes Care* 30:1193. doi: 10.2337/dc06-2052

Lei, D., Li, K. M., Li, L. J., Chen, F. Q., Huang, X. Q., Lui, S., et al. (2015). Disrupted functional brain connectome in patients with posttraumatic stress disorder. *Radiology* 276, 818–827. doi: 10.1148/radiol.15141700

Liang, X., Wang, J. H., and He, Y. (2010). Human connectome: structural and functional brain networks. *Chin. Sci. Bull.* 16:18. doi: 10.1360/972009-2150

Liao, W., Zhang, Z., Pan, Z., Mantini, D., Ding, J., Duan, X., et al. (2010). Altered functional connectivity and small-world in mesial temporal lobe epilepsy. *Brain Res.* 5, 152–160. doi: 10.1371/journal.pone.0008525

McCrimmon, R. J., Ryan, C. M., and Frier, B. M. (2012). Diabetes and cognitive dysfunction. *Lancet* 379, 2291–2299. doi: 10.1016/S0140-6736(12)60360-2

Ning, G. (2018). Status quo and prospect of prevention and control of diabetes in china. *Sci. Sin. Vitae* 48, 810–811.

Ogurtsova, K., Fernandes, J. D. D. R., Huang, Y., Linnenkamp, U., Guariguata, L., Cho, N. H., et al. (2017). IDF diabetes atlas: global estimates for the prevalence of diabetes for 2015 and 2040. *Diabetes Res. Clin. Pract.* 128, 40–50. doi: 10.1016/j.diabres.2017.03.024

Peng, B., Chen, Z., Ma, L., and Dai, Y. (2015). Cerebral alterations of type 2 diabetes mellitus on MRI: a pilot study. *Neurosci. Lett.* 606, 100–105. doi: 10.1016/j.neulet.2015.08.030

Qin, D. X., Zhang, Q., and Lin, L. (2016). Rs-fMRI changes of posterior cingulate cortex in type 2 diabetes mellitus patients with cognitive im-pairment. *Chin. J. Behav. Med. Brain Sci.* 25:5.

Reijmer, Y. D., Leemans, A., Brundel, M., Kappelle, L. J., and Biessels, G. J. (2013). Disruption of the cerebral white matter network is related to slowing of information processing speed in patients with type 2 diabetes. *Diabetes* 62:2112. doi: 10.2337/db12-1644

Rubinov, M., and Sporns, O. (2010). Complex network measures of brain connectivity: uses and interpretations. *Neuroimage* 52:1059. doi: 10.1016/j.neuroimage.2009.10.003

Sporns, O. (2011). The human connectome: a complex network. *Ann. N. Y. Acad. Sci.* 1224, 109–125. doi: 10.1111/j.1749-6632.2010.05888.x

Suo, X., Lei, D., Li, K., Chen, F., Li, F., Li, L., et al. (2015). Disrupted brain network topology in pediatric posttraumatic stress disorder: a resting-state fMRI study. *Hum. Brain Mapp.* 36, 3677–3686. doi: 10.1002/hbm.22871

Supekar, K., Menon, V., Rubin, D., Musen, M., and Greicius, M. D. (2008). Network analysis of intrinsic functional brain connectivity in alzheimer's disease. *PLoS Compu. Biol.* 4:e1000100. doi: 10.1371/journal.pcbi.1000100

Supekar, K., Musen, M., and Menon, V. (2009). Development of large-scale functional brain networks in children. *PLoS Biol.* 7:e1000157. doi: 10.1371/journal.pbio.1000157

Wang, X. B., Zhao, X. H., and Jiang, H. (2014). Small-worldness of brain fMRI network in patients with mild cognitive impairment. *Chin. J. Med. Imag. Technol.* 30:4.

Wang, X. Y., Wang, P. C., and Hou, L. X. (2016). Small-world features of brain functional MRI network in patients with type 2 diabetic encephalopathy. *Chin. J. Med. Imag. Technol.* 33:4.

Xia, W., Wang, S., Rao, H., Spaeth, A. M., Wang, P., Yang, Y., et al. (2015). Disrupted resting-state attentional networks in T2DM patients. *Sci. Rep.* 5:11148. doi: 10.1038/srep11148

Xiao, F., Lei, D., An, D., Li, L., Chen, S., Chen, F., et al. (2015). Functional brain connectome and sensorimotor networks in rolandic epilepsy. *Epil. Res.* 113, 113–125. doi: 10.1016/j.eplepsyres.2015.03.015

Yau, P. L., Javier, D., Tsui, W., Sweat, V., Bruehl, H., Borod, J. C., et al. (2009). Emotional and neutral declarative memory impairments and associated white matter microstructural abnormalities in adults with type 2 diabetes. *Psychiatry Res.* 174, 223–230. doi: 10.1016/j.pscychresns.2009.04.016

Yau, P. L., Kluger, A., Borod, J. C., and Convit, A. (2014). Neural substrates of verbal memory impairments in adults with type 2 diabetes mellitus. *J. Clin. Exp. Neuropsychol.* 36, 74–87. doi: 10.1080/13803395.2013.869310

Zhang, H. M., Li, W., and Zhang, Y. (2015). Inefficient activity in working memory related brain regions in patients with type 2 diabetes mellitus. *J. China Clin. Med. Imag.* 26:4.

Zhang, J., Liu, Z., Li, Z., Wang, Y., Chen, Y., Li, X., et al. (2016). Disrupted white matter network and cognitive decline in type 2 diabetes patients. *J. Alzheimers Dis.* 53, 185–195. doi: 10.3233/JAD-160111

Zhang, J., Wang, J., Wu, Q., Kuang, W., Huang, X., He, Y., et al. (2011). Disrupted brain connectivity networks in drug-naive, first-episode major depressive disorder. *Biol. Psychiatry* 70, 334–342. doi: 10.1016/j.biopsych.2011.05.018

Zhang, J., Wang, Y., Wang, J., Zhou, X., Shu, N., Wang, Y., et al. (2014). White matter integrity disruptions associated with cognitive impairments in type 2 diabetic patients. *Diabetes* 63, 3596–3605. doi: 10.2337/db14-0342

Zhang, L. J., Zheng, G., Zhang, L. P., Zhong, J. H., Li, Q., Zhao, T. Z., et al. (2014). Disrupted small world networks in patients without overt hepatic encephalopathy: a resting state fMRI study. *Eur. J. Radiol.* 83, 1890–1899. doi: 10.1016/j.ejrad.2014.06.019

Zhou, L., and Xue, Y. M. (2006). Metabolic status analysis of type 2 diabetes obese patients. *Chin. J. Prim. Med. Pharm.* 13:2.

Zhou, X., Zhang, J., Chen, Y., Ma, T., Wang, Y., Wang, J., et al. (2014). Aggravated cognitive and brain functional impairment in mild cognitive impairment patients with type 2 diabetes: a resting-state functional MRI study. *J. Alzheimers Dis.* 41:925. doi: 10.3233/JAD-132354

Zhou, X. Q., Zhang, J. Y., Chen, Y. J., Ma, T., Wang, Y. X., Wang, J., et al. (2014). Aggravated cognitive and brain functional impairment in mild cognitive impairment patients with type 2 diabetes: a resting-state functional MRI study. *J. Alzheimers Dis.* 41, 925–935. doi: 10.3233/Jad-132354

8

Integrating the Local Property and Topological Structure in the Minimum Spanning Tree Brain Functional Network for Classification of Early Mild Cognitive Impairment

Xiaohong Cui [1], Jie Xiang [1], Bin Wang [1], Jihai Xiao [2], Yan Niu [1] and Junjie Chen [1]*

[1] College of Information and Computer, Taiyuan University of Technology, Taiyuan, China, [2] Center of Information Management and Development, Taiyuan University of Technology, Taiyuan, China

Correspondence:
Junjie Chen
chenjj@tyut.edu.cn

Abnormalities in the brain connectivity in patients with neurodegenerative diseases, such as early mild cognitive impairment (EMCI), have been widely reported. Current research shows that the combination of multiple features of the threshold connectivity network can improve the classification accuracy of diseases. However, in the construction of the threshold connectivity network, the selection of the threshold is very important, and an unreasonable setting can seriously affect the final classification results. Recent neuroscience research suggests that the minimum spanning tree (MST) brain functional network is helpful, as it avoids the methodological biases while comparing networks. In this paper, by employing the multikernel method, we propose a framework to integrate the multiple properties of the MST brain functional network for improving the classification performance. Initially, the Kruskal algorithm was used to construct an unbiased MST brain functional network. Subsequently, the vector kernel and graph kernel were used to quantify the two different complementary properties of the network, such as the local connectivity property and the topological property. Finally, the multikernel support vector machine (SVM) was adopted to combine the two different kernels for EMCI classification. We tested the performance of our proposed method for Alzheimer's Disease Neuroimaging Initiative (ANDI) datasets. The results showed that our method achieved a significant performance improvement, with the classification accuracy of 85%. The abnormal brain regions included the right hippocampus, left parahippocampal gyrus, left posterior cingulate gyrus, middle temporal gyrus, and other regions that are known to be important in the EMCI. Our results suggested that, combining the multiple features of the MST brain functional connectivity offered a better classification performance in the EMCI.

Keywords: minimum spanning tree, local property, topological structure, the multikernel SVM, early mild cognitive impairment, classification

INTRODUCTION

Alzheimer's disease (AD) is a common progressive neurodegenerative disease that affects the nervous system. In 2018, the number of AD patients in the United States will reach 5.7 million and the cost of treatments will reach 277 billion, causing great economic losses to the families and the society (Alzheimer's Association, 2018). Therefore, in the early stage, such as early mild cognitive impairment (EMCI), it is important to find the symptoms of the disease and develop strategies to treat it. However, the subtle differences in the cognitive function between the EMCI and normal control (NC) make it difficult to diagnose the EMCI. Therefore, it is very important to propose a framework to identify the individuals with EMCI from NC.

At present, the brain functional magnetic resonance imaging (fMRI) data is represented as a brain network composed of nodes and edges (Lópezsanz et al., 2017). Through the analysis and study of the brain network, the brain functional network of the mild cognitive impairment (MCI) patients exhibit abnormal local properties and topological structures (Supekar et al., 2008; Sanz-Arigita et al., 2010; Petrella et al., 2011; Liu et al., 2012; Wang et al., 2017; Yan et al., 2018). Jie et al. (2014b) constructed an undirected functional brain network of NC and MCI, and extracted the topological features to classify the two groups of subjects, where abnormal regions were found in the brain network including those in the hippocampus, amygdala, and the inferior temporal gyrus. Khazaee et al. (2016) also constructed an undirected brain network of NC, MCI, and AD groups by using 264 putative functional areas. Network topology attributes were extracted as classification features to be used in the classification of three groups of subjects. The result showed that this method was able to accurately classify three groups (i.e., NC, MCI, and AD) with an accuracy of 88.4%, and it was found that the left posterior central gyrus, the right inferior temporal gyrus, the left lingual gyrus, the right middle frontal gyrus, and the right thalamus were significantly different from the normal elderly. Wee et al. (2016) designed a disease identification framework based on the estimated temporal networks, and analyzed the group differences in the level network property. Yu et al. (2016) studied the directed functional connectivity using the Granger causality analysis (GCA), and found that the posterior cingulate cortex (PCC) in the Default Mode Network (DMN) showed directional disorders in receiving and transmitting information.

A common problem in the above studies was the use of a single type of network property for the MCI, and NC classification, such as the local connectivity or global topological properties. In order to improve the accuracy in the MCI diagnosis, Jie et al. (2014a) extracted local connectivity and global topological properties from five different threshold brain networks and combined these properties in the classification of MCI and NC. However, this may affect the final classification performance to some extent, since we need to set a threshold for the original weighted network in the construction of the threshold brain network. In 2015, Tewarie et al. proposed the minimum spanning tree (MST) as an unbiased approach in the construction and the analysis of the brain networks (Tewarie et al., 2015). MST method preserves the core framework of the networks while voiding the influences of the threshold. It does not only reduce the computational cost, but also guarantees the network's neurological interpretability. In 2006, Lee et al. applied the MST to brain network for the first time, and MST was widely applied in the research and development of many kinds of neuropsychiatric disorders (Lee et al., 2006; Boersma et al., 2012; Demuru et al., 2013; Stam et al., 2014).

Accordingly, in this paper, based on an unbiased MST brain network, a classification framework combining the local properties and topological structures is proposed. **Figure 1** illustrates the framework of our proposed method. Initially, the MST brain functional network was constructed, then the local property and topological structure property of the MST brain functional network were extracted, and the two features were combined to identify the EMCI from the NC. Experiments showed that the classification framework not only realized the complementation of local and topological structure properties, but also improved the classification performance.

MATERIALS AND METHODS

Data Acquisition and Preprocessing

The data used in this study was from the Alzheimer's Disease Neuroimaging Initiative (ADNI) database at website http://adni.loni.usc.edu/. A total of 60 subjects were selected from ADNI-2 database, including 32 EMCI patients and 28 NC. **Table 1** shows the demographics of all participants. A 3.0 T scanner (Philips Medical Systems) was used to acquire resting-state BOLD fMRI scans of all subjects. The scanning parameters were set as follows: repetition time (TR) = 3,000 ms; echo time (TE) = 30 ms; slice thickness = 3.3 mm; flip angle = 80°; slice number = 48 and 140 time points. During scanning, all the subjects were instructed to keep their eyes closed.

Many preprocessing steps of the fMRI images were performed using Data Processing Assistant for Resting-State fMRI (DPARSF; Yan and Zang, 2010), Statistical Parametric Mapping (SPM12; http://www.fil.ion.ucl.ac.uk/spm), and the Resting-State fMRI Data Analysis Toolkit (REST 1.8) packages (Song et al., 2011). Specifically, the first 10 time points of each subject were removed; slice-timing correction and image realignment were carried out on the remaining 130-time points. Because the brain size, shape, orientation, and gyral anatomy of each subject is different, the fMRI data of each subject was usually normalized into the Montreal Neurological Institute (MNI) space (resampled into $3 \times 3 \times 3$ mm^3 voxels) by using a unified segmentation on the T1 image. Then, the linear trends of the time courses were removed, and the effect of nuisance covariates was removed by signal regression using the global signal, the six motion parameters, the cerebrospinal fluid (CSF) and white matter (WM) signals. Temporal filtering (0.01 Hz $< f <$ 0.08 Hz) was applied. Lastly, since we used only gray matter (GM) tissue to construct the functional connectivity network, the gray matter mask was used to mask the corresponding fMRI images to eliminate the possible effects from CSF and WM.

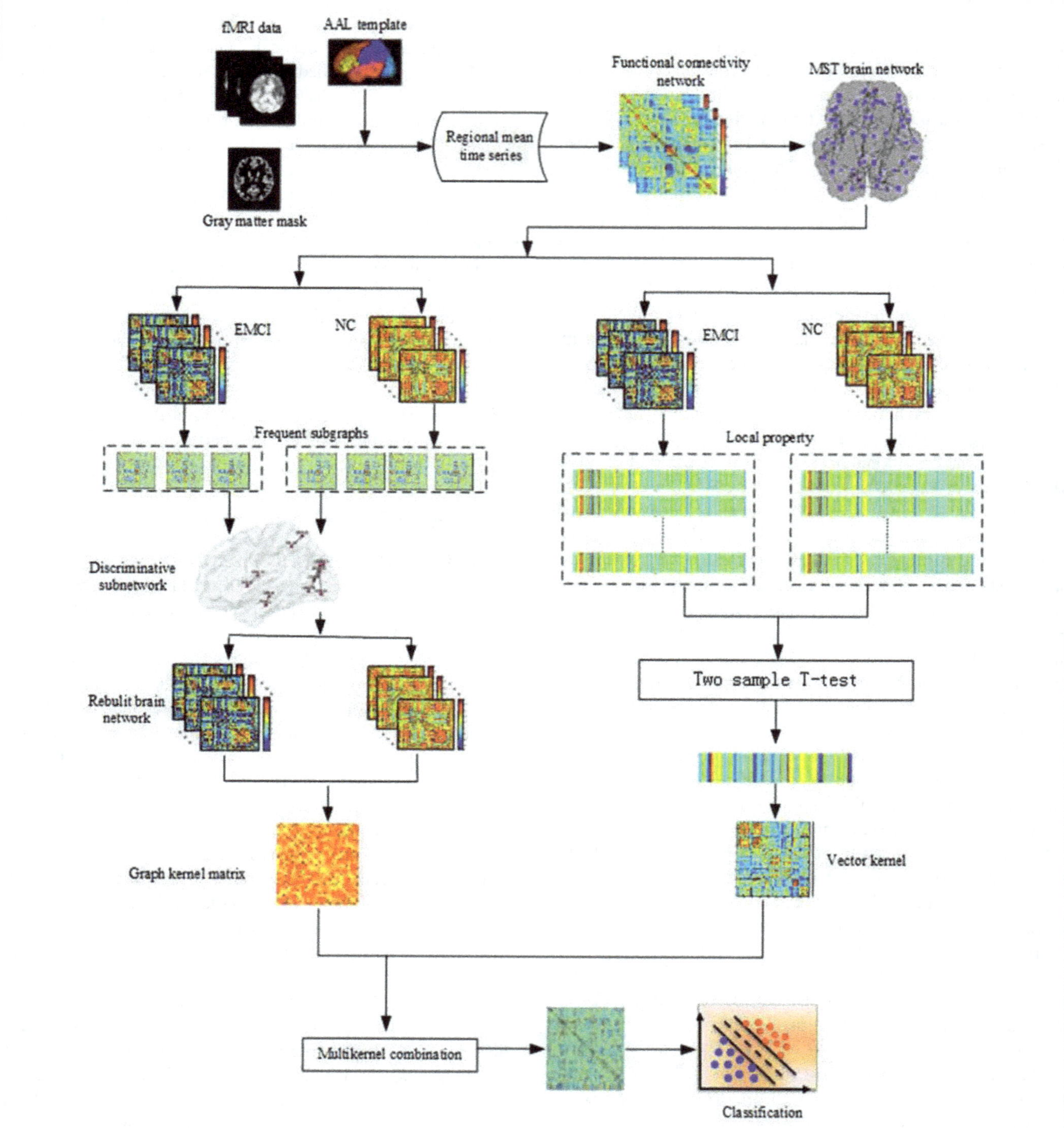

FIGURE 1 | Framework of proposed method. Firstly, data preprocessing of fMRI; Then the MST brain functional network is constructed, the local property and topological structure property of the MST brain functional network are extracted, Finally, the two features are combined to classify by using Multi-kernel SVM.

Methods

The key technologies in this paper included: Kruskal algorithm (Kruskal, 1956), graph-based Substructure pattern mining (gSpan; Yan and Han, 2002), the local feature selection, the discriminative subgraph algorithm selection and the multikernel learning technique (Zhang D. et al., 2011). Firstly, the unbiased brain functional network was constructed using the Kruskal algorithm, and betweenness was extracted as the local property. Then, frequent subgraphs were mined from the brain network using the gSpan algorithm, and the discriminative subgraphs of

TABLE 1 | The demographics of all participants.

Group	EMCI	NC
No. of subjects (M/F)	17/15	11/17
Age (mean ± SD)	72.1 ± 6.0	74.3 ± 6.2
MMSE (mean ± SD)	27.7 ± 1.9	28.9 ± 1.3
CDR (mean ± SD)	0.48 ± 0.1	0 ± 0

EMCI, Early Mild Cognitive Impairment; NC, Normal Control; MMSE, Mini-Mental State Examination; CDR, Clinical Dementia Rating; M, Male; F, Female.

brain networks were extracted as the topological property. Lastly the local property and topological property were combined to classify the EMCI.

Construction of the Unbiased MST Brain Functional Network

The brain network can be abstracted into a graph. The construction of the brain network involved the determination of the nodes and edges in the graph. In this study, construction steps of MST brain functional network included:

(1) Definition of node: We parcellated the gray-matter masked voxels into 90 regions of interest (ROIs) by the Automated Anatomical Labeling (AAL) template (Tzourio-Mazoyer et al., 2002). A ROI is a node of the brain network. Therefore, the brain network consisted of 90 nodes.
(2) Definition of edge: The average value of the fMRI time series of all voxels in each ROI is considered as the average time series of the node, and the Pearson correlation coefficient between the pair of nodes is taken as the weight of the connected edges. So, a functional full connected network is constructed for each subject. Moreover, in order to extract the meaningful network measures, we removed all negative correlations from the obtained connectivity networks.
(3) Construction of unbiased brain functional network: In order to construct an unbiased brain network, we used the Kruskal algorithm to construct the MST brain network. MST is a weighted graph that connects the nodes together, without any cycles, and with the minimum weight. Since we were only interested in the strongest connections in the brain network, the Kruskal algorithm was used to construct a weighted graph that connects all the nodes together, without any cycles and with the maximum weight. The algorithm sorted initially, all the correlation coefficients into descending order, and then connected the edges with the largest correlation coefficients that were added successively until all nodes were connected in an acyclic subnetwork. In this process, if the addition of a link formed a loop, this link was ignored.

Local Property of the MST Brain Functional Network

Local property

Betweenness is an important local property in the MST, and it was also recognized as the most relevant feature in the classification between the MCI and the NC (Ebadi et al., 2017). So betweenness was extracted as a feature. Betweenness of node was defined as the number of all the shortest paths through this node.

The betweenness bc_i of the node i was defined as (Tewarie et al., 2015):

$$bc_i = \frac{1}{(n-1)(n-2)} \sum_{\substack{h,j \in V \\ h \neq j, h \neq i}} \frac{\rho_{hj}^{i}}{\rho_{hj}} \tag{1}$$

Where ρ_{hj} represents the number of the shortest paths between the node h and j; ρ_{hj}^{i} represents the number of the shortest paths between the node h and j through the node i; V represents the set of nodes; and n represents the number of nodes.

Discriminative brain regions selection

We calculated the betweenness of each node in the MST functional network. To select the most discriminative brain region, two sample t-test was used. The brain regions with $p < 0.05$ were selected as the discriminative brain regions.

Linear kernel

The betweenness of the discriminative brain regions composed a feature vector representing the local property of a brain network. We measured the similarity of two functional connectivity networks in term of local property by using linear kernel as follows:

$$k_v(x, y) = x^T y \tag{2}$$

Where x and y represent the feature vectors from two subjects, respectively.

Topological Property of Brain Network

Frequent subgraph mining

In order to capture the differences in the topological structure of the brain networks, this study uses the gSpan algorithm to extract the frequent subgraphs from the brain network, and the most discriminative subgraphs were selected.

Definition 1 (Undirected labeled network): For an undirected labeled network G = (V, E, L), V represents the set of nodes; $E \subseteq V \times V$, the set of edges; L, the set of labels.

Definition 2 (Subnetwork): Given two undirected labeled networks G = (V, E, L) and $G_s = (V_s, E_s, L_s)$, if $V_s \subseteq V$, $L_s \subseteq L$ and $E_s \subseteq E$, G_s is a subnetwork of G.

Definition 3 (Subnetwork frequency): For a given network set $\mathbb{G}$, $\mathbb{G} = \{G_1, G_2, \cdots G_n\}$, n is the number of networks. The frequency f_q of a subnetwork g_s is defined in Equation (3):

$$f_q(g_s|\mathbb{G}) = \frac{|g_s \text{ is subgraph of G and } G \in \mathbb{G}|}{|\mathbb{G}|} \tag{3}$$

where $|\mathbb{G}|$ presents the number of networks.

Definition 4 (Frequent subnetwork mining): For a given undirected labeled network set $\mathbb{G}$ and frequency thresholding value s where $0 \leq s \leq 1$, the process of finding all subnetworks of $\mathbb{G}$ with the frequency of at least s is called frequent subnetwork mining.

Discriminative subgraphs selection

In fact, there exist a large number of frequent subgraphs in a network, but only a small portion of the frequent subgraphs have the discriminability. Therefore, the most discriminative subgraphs were selected by using the further feature selection method based on their respective frequency difference (Wang et al., 2015).

The frequency difference $D(g_s)$ of subgraph g_s is defined in Equation (4):

$$D(g_s) = \left|f_q(g_s|G_p) - f_q(g_s|G_n)\right| \tag{4}$$

Where G_p denotes the set of frequent subgraphs for positive samples, and G_n denotes the set of frequent subgraphs for negative samples.

The greater the frequency difference, the stronger is the discriminability. The frequency difference of frequent subgraphs were calculated and then the frequency difference threshold T was set. The subgraphs with a frequency differences greater than T were considered to be the most discriminative subgraphs.

Then, the brain network was reconstructed using the most discriminative subgraphs. Specifically, for a network, we only needed to delete the edges that did not appear in any discriminative subgraphs. In this way, the topology of the brain network and the discriminative subgraphs was preserved.

Graph kernel

The brain network is a complex structural dataset. The traditional feature extraction methods cannot deal with the complex topological features of the brain network. Graph kernel can map data from the original graph space to the feature space, and the similarity between the two graphs is further measured by comparing the topological structure of the graph. Therefore, the graph kernel establishes a bridge between the graph data and many kernel-based learning algorithms, and has been successfully applied in the fields of computer vision (Camps-Valls et al., 2010) and bioinformatics (Zhang Y. et al., 2011).

Recent research has shown that the Weisfeiler-Lehman (WL) subtree kernel (Shervashidze et al., 2011) could be efficiently computed in time O(|E|), and was a suitable option for brain graph classification (Vega-Pons et al., 2014). In this paper, we have used the WL subtree-based kernel method to measure the topological similarity between the brain networks. For a pair of brain networks G and H, the basic processes of WL subtree-based kernels were as follows:

1) Initially, every vertex of a graph was labeled with a degree of that node.
2) At each iteration, the label of each node was augmented in the graph by a sorted set of node labels of neighboring nodes, and these augmented labels were compressed into a new short label.
3) This process proceeded iteratively until the node label sets of two graphs differed, or the number of iteration reached the maximum h.
4) The WL subtree-based kernel on two graphs G and H is defined in Equation (5):

$$k_g(G,H) = <\varphi(G), \varphi(H)> \tag{5}$$

Where

$$\varphi(G) = (\sigma_0(G, s_{01}), \cdots, \sigma_0(G, s_{0|L_0|}), \cdots, \sigma_h(G, s_{h1}), \cdots, \sigma_h(G, s_{h|L_h|}))$$

$$\varphi(H) = (\sigma_0(H, s_{01}), \cdots, \sigma_0(H, s_{0|L_0|}), \cdots, \sigma_h(H, s_{h1}), \cdots, \sigma_h(H, s_{h|L_h|}))$$

$\sigma_i(G, s_{i,j})$ and $\sigma_i(H, s_{i,j})$ is the numbers of occurrences of the label $s_{i,j}$ in G and H, respectively, $s_{i,j}$ denotes the label of i-th node in iteration j. $|L_i|$ is the number of labels in the iteration i, L_i denotes the label set of G, and H in iteration i, L_0 represents the initial labels set of G and H. K is the kernel matrix of $n \times n$, n is the number of brain networks.

The Multikernel SVM

Recent studies on multikernel SVM has proved that the multikernel integration not only improves the accuracy of classification, but also improves the interpretability of the results (Lanckriet et al., 2002). Neuroimaging studies have also shown that multikernel integration can systematically aggregate different kernels into a single mode (Wee et al., 2012).

In this paper, we consider two types of kernels, i.e., the linear kernel and the graph kernel. We assumed that these kernels could provide the complementary information for EMCI identification.

Firstly, as this research uses two different types of kernel, normalization was done individually. Then we used a multi-kernel SVM technique to linearly combine the two kernels, as shown in Equation (6):

$$K(G,H) = \beta k_v(x,y) + (1-\beta) k_g(G,H) \tag{6}$$

Where G and H are two MST functional networks, $k_g(G,H)$ is a graph kernel of G and H, x and y are their local feature vectors of G and H, $k_v(x,y)$ is a linear kernel, and β is a nonnegative weighting parameter.

Once β was determined, we used the traditional single-kernel SVM (Chang and Lin, 2011) for the classification.

Methodology

On the basis of pre-processing, Kruskal algorithm was used to construct an unbiased brain network. The betweenness of the node was extracted and the feature was selected from the training set by using two sample t-test. In addition, the linear kernel was adopted as the vector kernel. Then using gSpan algorithm (s is set to 0.7), the frequency subgraphs of brain network was mined and the most discriminative subgraphs (the frequency differences >0.13) were selected. Subsequently, we used the WL subtree kernel (h and n are set as 2 and 1, respectively) to extract the topological features of the reconstructed brain network, and, the optimal weighting parameter β was obtained from the training set via a grid search (the range from 0 to 1 at a step size of 0.1). Finally, the conventional SVM framework was used to identify the EMCI from NCs. All experiments are performed using 10-fold cross-validation. Specially, the subject

TABLE 2 | The abnormal brain region of local property.

Brain region	Statistical significance (P-value)
L.Middle frontal gyrus	0.037
R.Rolandic operculum	0.004
L.Supplementary motor area	0.048
L.Anterior cingulate and paracingulate gyri	0.043
L.Median cingulate and paracingulate gyri	0.024
L.Posterior cingulate gyrus	0.035
R.Thalamus	0.018
L.Middle temporal gyrus	0.039
R.Middle temporal gyrus	0.007
R.Inferior temporal gyrus	0.020

dataset was randomly divided into 10 parts, one of which was left as the testing set, while the remaining nine were used as training sets. The feature selection was carried out on the training set, and the selected discriminative features were used to build the classification model, then this model was used to classify on the testing set. Ten-fold cross-validation was preformed 50 times. Finally, we computed the arithmetic mean of the 50 repetitions as the final result.

RESULTS

Discriminative Brain Regions and Subgraphs

Betweenness of 90 nodes was calculated from the training sets and two sample t-test was performed to evaluate its discriminative power for identifying the EMCI from NC. Betweenness of 90 nodes and p-value of two sample t-test are shown in **Supplemental Text S1**. **Table 2** lists the 10 discriminative regions ($p < 0.05$) that were selected based on the betweenness. These discriminative regions were found to be consistent with the previous findings.

On the other hand, we also extracted the most discriminative subgraphs based on the global topological property of the training sets. The frequent subgraphs were mined using the gSpan from the MST functional connectivity network of EMCI and NC, with frequency thresholding value of $s = 0.7$. We obtained 20 frequent subgraphs for EMCI and 22 frequent subgraphs for NC. Then we computed the frequency difference of these subgraphs (Details refer to **Supplemental Text S2.**), and selected only those subgraphs that exhibited a frequency difference more than 0.13. Thus, we obtained 6 discriminative subgraphs that consisted of 12 abnormal regions. **Figure 2** shows the most discriminative subgraphs. **Table 3** shows the 12 abnormal brain regions from the subgraph feature.

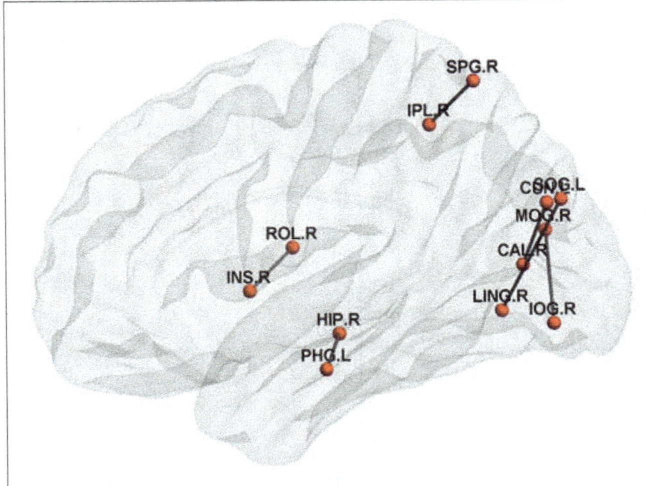

FIGURE 2 | The discriminative subgraphs of EMCI. ROL.R, R Rolandic operculum; INS.R, R Insula; HIP.R, R Hippocampus; PHG.L, L Parahippocampal gyrus; CAL.R, R Calcarine fissure and surrounding cortex; CUN.L, L Cuneus; LING.R, R Lingual gyrus; SOG.L, L Superior occipital gyrus; MOG.R, R Middle occipital gyrus; IOG.R, R Inferior occipital gyrus; SPG.R, R Superior parietal gyrus; IPL.R, R Inferior parietal, but supramarginal and angular gyri.

TABLE 3 | The abnormal brain regions of subgraph feature.

Brain region
R. Rolandic operculum
R. Insula
R. Calcarine fissure and surrounding cortex
L. Cuneus
R.Middle occipital gyrus
R.Inferior occipital gyrus
R. Superior parietal gyrus
R. Inferior parietal, but supramarginal and angular gyri
R. Lingual gyrus
L. Superior occipital gyrus
R. Hippocampus
L. Parahippocampal gyrus

TABLE 4 | The classification performances for different methods.

Feature	ACC (%)	SEN (%)	SPE (%)	AUC
LP	81.6	86.6	77.5	0.86
TP	61.7	73.3	54.5	0.59
Our method	85	90	79.2	0.88

ACC, classification accuracy; SEN, sensitivity; SPE, specificity; AUC, the area under the receiver operating characteristic curve; LP represents only use local property as feature to classify; TP represents only use topological property as feature to classify.

Classification Performance

In this experiment, the MST was constructed, and the local property and topological property were combined to identify the EMCI from NC. The classification performance was evaluated based on the accuracy, sensitivity, specificity, and area under receiver operating characteristic (ROC) curve (AUC), respectively.

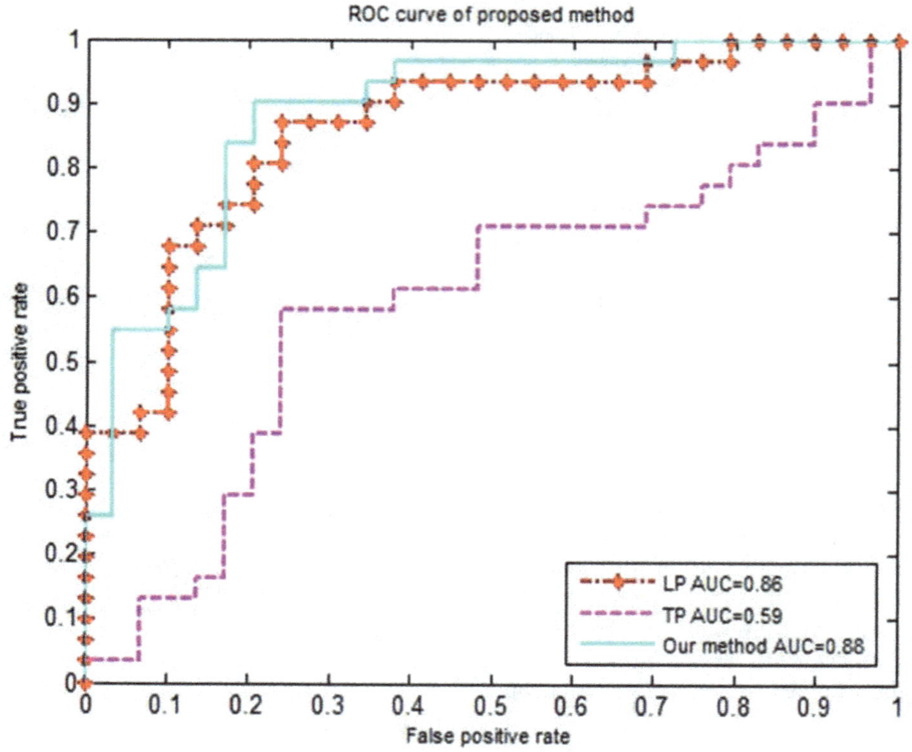

FIGURE 3 | The ROC curve of different methods. The ROC curve of different methods on EMCI vs. NC classification. LP represents the local property is used as classification feature; TP represents the topological property is used as classification feature.

We compared our proposed method using solely the single network property. Specifically, (1) For the local property, denoted as LP, we computed the vector kernel based on the local property. (2) For the topological property, denoted as TP, graph kernel was only computed from the rebuilt networks. All experiments were performed using a 10-fold cross-validation. The classification performances for different methods are summarized in **Table 4**. **Figure 3** shows the ROC curves for these methods.

TABLE 5 | The classification performance and the number of subgraphs under the different parameter T.

T	The number of subgraphs	ACC (%)	SEN (%)	SPE (%)
0.06	14	83.3	83	83.2
0.07	13	83.3	87.1	80.83
0.08	12	83.3	87.5	77.5
0.09	8	83.3	82.2	79.7
0.1/0.11/0.12	7	81.6	89.3	80.6
0.13	6	85	90	79

T represents the frequency differences threshold; ACC, classification accuracy; SEN, sensitivity; SPE, specificity.

DISCUSSION

Discriminative Brain Regions

Many studies have suggested that the brains of MCI differ from brains of NC in connectivity patterns, such as local properties (Guo et al., 2017), and the topological properties of brain network (Vega-Pons et al., 2014). We used two types of kernels to quantify these two different properties.

On the one hand, the betweenness of the node was calculated to quantize the local property. Then, two sample *t*-test was used to extract the relevant property for classification. From **Table 2**, we found that (1) compared with NC, the abnormal regions were mainly concentrated in the Default Mode Network (DMN), such as, L. Middle frontal gyrus, L. Anterior cingulate and paracingulate gyri, L. Posterior cingulate gyrus, Middle temporal gyrus, and R. Inferior temporal gyrus. This conclusion is consistent with the view accepted by most researchers that DMN was damaged in the early stages of AD (Garcés et al., 2014; Montembeault et al., 2014; Knh et al., 2017). Similarly, the low-frequency amplitudes of the AD patients were studied and the brain regions were found to be consistent with our study (Yetkin et al., 2006). For example, Liu et al. (2014) found that the low frequency amplitude of AD patients in the bilateral posterior cingulate gyrus, middle temporal gyrus and superior temporal gyrus decreased when compared with the NC. (2) The right Rolandic operculum, the left supplementary motor area and the right thalamus also showed differences, which was consistent with the related literature. Wang et al. (2011) found that the low-frequency amplitude between AD and NC located in the bilateral supplementary motor area and the left fusiform gyrus was different. Yetkin et al. (2006) confirmed that AD was more active in the right middle frontal gyrus, left inferior temporal gyrus, left thalamus, and right lenticular putamen nucleus than the NC. Fei et al. (2014) showed the difference of topological structures between the MCI, and NC were mainly in left rolandic operculum, insula, left supplementary motor area, left hippocampus, left parahippocampal gyrus, right parahippocampal gyrus, and so on.

On the other hand, a graph kernel was calculated to measure the similarity of the topological property. **Figure 2** shows that the brain connectivity network changed during EMCI, mainly in the right Rlandic operculum, the right Insula, the right hippocampus, the left parahippocampal gyrus, the right lingual gyrus, the left superior occipital gyrus, the right Calcarine fissure and surrounding cortex, the left cuneus, the right middle occipital gyrus, the right inferior occipital gyrus, the right superior parietal gyrus, and the right inferior parietal. This suggests that the hippocampus, parahippocampal gyrus, and the insula are the first to be damaged in the early stage of AD, which is associated with a decline in memory (Bai et al., 2009), attention, speech, and behavior in early AD patients. Specifically, the hippocampus plays an important role in the spatial memory and in the consolidation of information from short-term memory to long-term memory. The hippocampus demonstrated a significantly negative correlation to episodic memory performance (Bai et al., 2009). The Parahippocampal gyrus plays an important role in the encoding and recognition of environmental scenes (Machulda et al., 2008).

Finally, it can be seen from **Table 2** and **Figure 2** that the local property and topological property complement each other and provide biomarkers for early diagnosis of MCI from both the local and global aspects.

TABLE 6 | The classification performance and the running time under different parameter h.

h	ACC (%)	SEN (%)	SPE (%)	Runtime(s)
2	85	90	79.2	0.41
4	83.3	84.2	75.5	0.58
6	85	89.1	80	0.76
8	83.3	85.5	70.7	0.97
10	81.7	86.7	77.5	1.11

h, the number of iteration; ACC, classification accuracy; SEN, sensitivity; SPE, specificity; Runtime, the running time (second) of WL- subtree kernel.

Classification Performance

A large number of studies have proved that the different features (the local property, the topological property or multi-property) of the traditional threshold network have obtained better classification results. For example, Jie et al. (2014b) constructed multiple threshold connectivity networks of NC and MCI, and extracted the topological features from the multiple threshold connectivity networks. Finally, the multi-kernel SVM was used to classify the two groups of subjects. Fei et al. (2014) had constructed threshold connectivity networks of NC and MCI, and extracted frequent subgraphs, and subsequently selected a discriminative subgraph as a feature. Finally, SVM was used for the classification. These researches show that the subgraph features can better capture the topological information of brain network. Jie et al. (2014a) extracted the local connectivity and global topological properties from five different threshold brain networks and combined these properties by using multikernel SVM for the classification of the MCI and NC. It is shown that the local and topological properties of multi-threshold connected networks were complementary to each other, thus improving the classification performance.

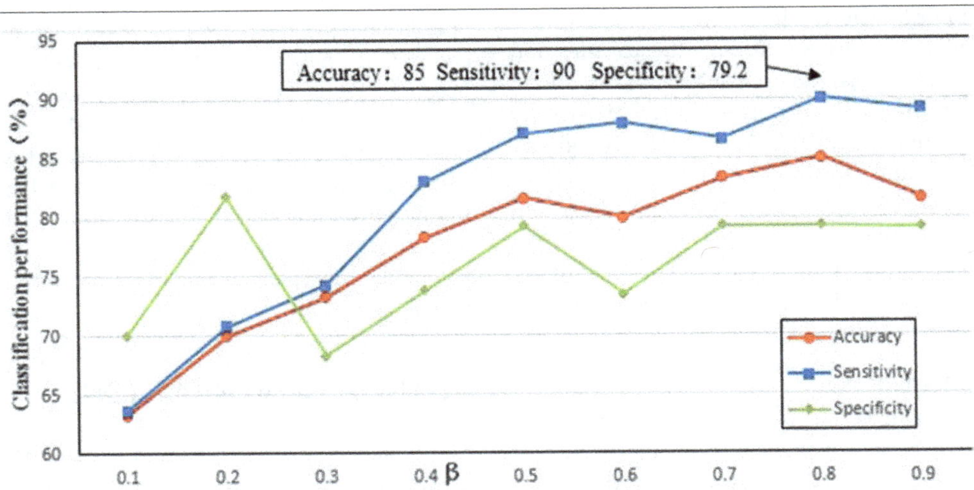

FIGURE 4 | The classification performance of different parameter β. The ordinate indicates accuracy, specificity and sensibility of this method, and the abscissa denotes different parameter β. As shown in the figure, when β = 0.8, better classification performance was obtained, including that accuracy is 85%, and specificity is 90%, and then sensibility is 79.2%.

The traditional threshold network construction method is influenced by the threshold, which makes the brain network to exhibit some deviation. In order to avoid these deviations, the MST method was used to construct an unbiased brain network, and this method exhibited a less computational cost, and at the same time, retained the neurological interpretability of the network.

In order to accurately compare the classification performance of different features, we used the same data set, constructed the MST brain network, and calculated the classification performance of the local property, topological property and multi-property feature respectively. **Table 4** and **Figure 3** showed that our method in combination with the local and topological properties based on MST brain functional network performed significantly better than the single network property. Specifically, for the classification of EMCI and NC, the proposed method achieved 85% accuracy, 90% sensitivity, 79.2% specificity, and 0.88 AUC in the classification. These results show that the proposed classification framework constructed an unbiased brain functional network, captured and combined the local and topological properties, and achieved better classification performance. Compared with the traditional threshold method, our method offered two advantages by avoiding the need to select an optimal threshold, and by making the full use of local and topological properties.

Effect of the Frequency Difference Threshold T

A large number of frequent subgraphs were obtained by using the gSpan module. In order to select the most discriminative subgraphs, we computed the frequency differences of each of the frequent subgraphs. Then frequent subgraphs with a frequency difference greater than T were considered to be the most discriminative subgraphs. In order to test the effect of the frequency difference threshold (T) on the classification performance, T (the range from 0.06 to 0.13 at a step size of 0.01) was tested separately in the experiment, and the results are shown in the **Table 5**. The results showed that when T is 0.13, the number of subgraphs was 6, and the classification performance was best. On analyzing six subgraphs, we found that two of them were frequent subgraphs of the EMCI group and the other four were frequent subgraphs of the NC group. Additionally, we also found that the discriminative subgraphs obtained by T = 0. 5 and T = 0. 13 were the same, and they could be the only frequent subgraphs of EMCI or NC. Thus, when T = 0.5, we can obtain the most discriminative subgraphs. In future research, 0.5 can be used as a reference value for T.

Effect of Parameter h

When performing a graph kernel calculation, the number of iterations (h) needs to be set. In the subtree, h represents the height of a subtree. The height of a subtree is the maximum distance between the root and any other node in the subtree. Different h values result in different values of graph kernels. In order to test the effect of parameter h on classification performance, h ($h \in \{2,4,6,8,10\}$) was tested separately in the experiment, and the results are shown in the **Table 6**. The results showed that when h = 2 or h = 6, the classification performance was the best. But from the point of view of running time, when h = 2, the running time was shorter.

Effect of Parameter β

We needed to find an optimal weighting parameter β in the MKL method. In order to test the effect of weighting parameter β on classification performance, β (the range from 0.1 to 0.9 at a step size of 0.1) was tested separately in the experiment, and the results are shown in **Figure 4**. It can be seen from **Figure 4** that when β is 0.8 the best classification performance is obtained, with 85% accuracy, 90% sensitivity, and 79.2% specificity. The results indicate that the local property (i.e., betweenness) is more important than the topological property of the MST brain functional network for the classification.

Limitations of the Study

This study is limited by the following factors. First, during the network construction, defining of the nodes is a critical step. Previous studies have demonstrated that network nodes can be defined using different brain atlases and image voxels, and the constructed network exhibited different network properties (Hayasaka and Laurienti, 2010). The impact of different brain parcellation atlases on the classification performance will be explored in the future. A second limitation is due to the small amount of data used in the experiment, the results of the classification lack a generality. This method will be applied to larger AD dataset in future work.

CONCLUSION

In this paper, we proposed a classification framework based on the MST brain functional connectivity network to identify the EMCI patients and NC. The proposed method mainly used the MST, vector kernel, graph kernel and the multikernel SVM. Specifically, MST was used to construct the brain functional connectivity network; vector kernel was used to extract local property, graph kernel was used to extract global topological property, and the multikernel SVM was adopted to fuse these heterogeneous kernels for classification. In experiments with the ADNI dataset, our proposed method not only significantly improved the classification performance in terms of accuracy, sensitivity, specificity, and AUC value, but also potentially detected the ROIs that are sensitive in the disease pathology.

AUTHOR CONTRIBUTIONS

XC designed the classification framework and wrote the manuscript. YN performed data analysis and statistical processing. JhX made experiment and gave the proof of results. JX and BW supervised the paper. JC was the head of the funds and supervised the paper. All authors approved the final version of the manuscript.

FUNDING

This study was supported by research grants from the National Natural Science Foundation of China (61472270, 61402318, 61672374), Natural Science Foundation of Shanxi Province (201601D021073), and Scientific and Technological Innovation Programs of Higher Education Institutions in Shanxi (2016139). The sponsors had no role in the design or execution of the study, the collection, management, analysis, and interpretation of the data, or preparation, review, and approval of the manuscript.

Data collection and sharing for this project was funded by the Alzheimer's Disease Neuroimaging Initiative (ADNI; National Institutes of Health Grant U01 AG024904) and DOD ADNI (Department of Defense award number W81XWH-12-2-0012). ADNI is funded by the National Institute on Aging and the National Institute of Biomedical Imaging and Bioengineering and through generous contributions from the following: AbbVie, Alzheimer's Association; Alzheimer's Drug Discovery Foundation; Araclon Biotech; BioClinica, Inc.;Biogen; Bristol-Myers Squibb Company; CereSpir, Inc.; Cogstate; Eisai Inc.; Elan Pharmaceuticals, Inc.; Eli Lilly and Company; EuroImmun; F. Hoffmann-La Roche Ltd and its affiliated company Genentech, Inc.; Fujirebio; GE Healthcare; IXICO Ltd.; Janssen Alzheimer Immunotherapy Research & Development, LLC.; Johnson & Johnson Pharmaceutical Research & Development LLC.; Lumosity; Lundbeck; Merck & Co., Inc.; Meso Scale Diagnostics, LLC.; NeuroRx Research; Neurotrack Technologies; Novartis Pharmaceuticals Corporation; Pfizer Inc.; Piramal Imaging; Servier; Takeda Pharmaceutical Company; and Transition Therapeutics. The Canadian Institutes of Health Research provides funds to support ADNI clinical sites in Canada. Private sector contributions are facilitated by the Foundation for the National Institutes of Health (www.fnih.org). The grantee organization is the Northern California Institute for Research and Education, and the study is coordinated by the Alzheimer's Therapeutic Research Institute at the University of Southern California. ADNI data are disseminated by the Laboratory for Neuro Imaging at the University of Southern California.

REFERENCES

Alzheimer's Association (2018). 2018 Alzheimer's disease facts and figures. *Alzheimers Dement.* 14, 367–429. doi: 10.1016/j.jalz.2018.02.001

Bai, F., Zhang, Z., Watson, D. R., Yu, H., Shi, Y., Yuan, Y., et al. (2009). Abnormal functional connectivity of hippocampus during episodic memory retrieval processing network in amnestic mild cognitive impairment. *Biol. Psychiatry* 65, 951–958. doi: 10.1016/j.biopsych.2008.10.017

Boersma, M., Smit, D., Boomsma, D., Geus, E., Delemarre-van de Waal, H., and Stam, C. (2012). Growing trees in child brains: graph theoretical analysis of EEG derived minimum spanning tree in 5 and 7 year old children reflects brain maturation. *Brain Connect.* 3, 50–60. doi: 10.1089/brain.2012.0106

Camps-Valls, G., Shervashidze, N., and Borgwardt, K. M. (2010). Spatio-spectral remote sensing image classification with graph Kernels. *IEEE Geosci. Remote Sens. Lett.* 7, 741–745. doi: 10.1109/LGRS.2010.2046618

Chang, C.-C., and Lin, C.-J. (2011). LIBSVM: a library for support vector machines. *ACM Trans. Intell. Syst. Technol.* 2:27. doi: 10.1145/1961189.1961199

Demuru, M., Fara, F., and Fraschini, M. (2013). Brain network analysis of EEG functional connectivity during imagery hand movements. *J. Integr. Neurosci.* 12, 441–447. doi: 10.1142/S021963521350026X

Ebadi, A., Dalboni da Rocha, J. L., Nagaraju, D. B., Tovar-Moll, F., Bramati, I., Coutinho, G., et al. (2017). Ensemble classification of Alzheimer's disease and mild cognitive impairment based on complex graph measures from diffusion tensor images. *Front. Neurosci.* 11:56. doi: 10.3389/fnins.2017.00056

Fei, F., Jie, B., and Zhang, D. (2014). Frequent and discriminative subnetwork mining for mild cognitive impairment classification. *Brain Connect.* 4, 347–360. doi: 10.1089/brain.2013.0214

Garcés, P., Angel, P.-P. J., Canuet, L., Aurtenetxe, S., López, M. E., Marcos, A., et al. (2014). The Default Mode Network is functionally and structurally disrupted in amnestic mild cognitive impairment—A bimodal MEG–DTI study. *Neuroimage Clin.* 6, 214–221. doi: 10.1016/j.nicl.2014.09.004

Guo, H., Liu, L., Chen, J., Xu, Y., and Jie, X. (2017). Alzheimer classification using a minimum spanning tree of high-order functional network on fMRI dataset. *Front. Neurosci.* 11:639. doi: 10.3389/fnins.2017.00639

Hayasaka, S., and Laurienti, P. J. (2010). Comparison of characteristics between region- and Voxel-based network analyses in resting-state fMRI data. *Neuroimage* 50, 499–508. doi: 10.1016/j.neuroimage.2009.12.051

Jie, B., Zhang, D., Gao, W., Wang, Q., Wee, C. Y., and Shen, D. (2014a). Integration of network topological and connectivity properties for neuroimaging classification. *IEEE Trans. Biomed. Eng.* 61, 576–589. doi: 10.1109/TBME.2013.2284195

Jie, B., Zhang, D., Wee, C. Y., and Shen, D. (2014b). Topological graph kernel on multiple thresholded functional connectivity networks for mild cognitive impairment classification. *Hum. Brain Mapp.* 35, 2876–2897. doi: 10.1002/hbm.22353

Khazaee, A., Ebrahimzadeh, A., and Babajani-Feremi, A. (2016). Application of advanced machine learning methods on resting-state fMRI network for identification of mild cognitive impairment and Alzheimer's disease. *Brain Imag. Behav.* 10, 799–817. doi: 10.1007/s11682-015-9448-7

Knh, D., Hil, J., Kukolja, J., Richter, N., Von, R. B., Onur, Ö. A., et al. (2017). Functional disintegration of the default mode network in prodromal Alzheimer's disease. *J. Alzheimers Dis.* 59, 169–187. doi: 10.3233/JAD-161120

Kruskal, J. B. (1956). On the shortest spanning subtree of a graph and the traveling salesman problem. *Proc. Am. Math. Soc.* 7, 48–50. doi: 10.1090/S0002-9939-1956-0078686-7

Lanckriet, G. R. G., Christianini, N., Bartlett, P. L., El Ghaoui, L., and Jordan, M. I. (2002). "Learning the kernel matrix with semi-definite programming," in *Proceedings of the Nineteenth International Conference on Machine Learning* (San Francisco, CA: Morgan Kaufmann Publishers Inc.), 323–330.

Lee, U., Kim, S., and Jung, K.-Y. (2006). Classification of epilepsy types through global network analysis of scalp electroencephalograms. *Phys. Rev. E* 73:041920. doi: 10.1103/PhysRevE.73.041920

Liu, X., Wang, S., Zhang, X., Wang, Z., Tian, X., and He, Y. (2014). Abnormal amplitude of low-frequency fluctuations of intrinsic brain activity in Alzheimer's disease. *J. Alzheimers Dis.* 40, 387–397. doi: 10.3233/JAD-131322

Liu, Z., Zhang, Y., Bai, L., Yan, H., Dai, R., Zhong, C., et al. (2012). Investigation of the effective connectivity of resting state networks in Alzheimer's disease: a functional MRI study combining independent components analysis and multivariate Granger causality analysis. *NMR Biomed.* 25, 1311–1320. doi: 10.1002/nbm.2803

Lópezsanz, D., Bruña, R., Garcés, P., Martínburo, M. C., Walter, S., Delgado, M. L., et al. (2017). Functional connectivity disruption in subjective cognitive decline and mild cognitive impairment: a common pattern of alterations. *Front. Aging Neurosci.* 9:109. doi: 10.3389/fnagi.2017.00109

Machulda, M. M., Senjem, M. L., Smith, G. E., Ivnik, R. J., Boeve, B. F., Knopman, D. S., et al. (2008). Functional magnetic resonance imaging activation patterns in cognitively normal elderly, amnestic, and non-amnestic mild cognitive impairment during a recognition memory task. *Alzheimers Dementia* 4, T23–T24. doi: 10.1016/j.jalz.2008.05.048

Montembeault, M., Rouleau, I., and Brambati, S. M. (2014). "Decreased structural association in regions of the default-mode network in the early stages of

Alzheimer's disease," in *International Conference on Frontotemporal Dementias* (Vancouver, BC), Vol. 3, 330.

Petrella, J. R., Sheldon, F. C., Prince, S. E., Calhoun, V. D., and Doraiswamy, P. M. (2011). Default mode network connectivity in stable vs progressive mild cognitive impairment. *Neurology* 76, 511–517. doi: 10.1212/WNL.0b013e31820af94e

Sanz-Arigita, E. J., Schoonheim, M. M., Damoiseaux, J. S., Rombouts, S. A. R. B., Maris, E., Barkhof, F., et al. (2010). Loss of 'small-world' networks in Alzheimer's disease: graph analysis of FMRI resting-state functional connectivity. *PLoS ONE* 5:e13788. doi: 10.1371/journal.pone.0013788

Shervashidze, N., Schweitzer, P., Leeuwen, E. J.,v., Mehlhorn, K., and Borgwardt, K. M. (2011). Weisfeiler-lehman graph kernels. *J. Mach. Learn. Res.* 12, 2539–2561. Available online at: http://www.jmlr.org/papers/volume12/shervashidze11a/shervashidze11a.pdf

Song, X. W., Dong, Z. Y., Long, X. Y., Li, S. F., Zuo, X. N., Zhu, C. Z., et al. (2011). REST: a toolkit for resting-state functional magnetic resonance imaging data processing[J]. *PLoS ONE* 6:e25031. doi: 10.1371/journal.pone.0025031

Stam, C. J., Tewarie, P., Van Dellen, E., van Straaten, E. C., Hillebrand, A., and Van Mieghem, P. (2014). The trees and the forest: characterization of complex brain networks with minimum spanning trees. *Int. J. Psychophysiol.* 92, 129–138. doi: 10.1016/j.ijpsycho.2014.04.001

Supekar, K., Menon, V., Rubin, D., Musen, M., and Greicius, M. D. (2008). Network analysis of intrinsic functional brain connectivity in Alzheimer's disease. *PLoS Comput. Biol.* 4:e1000100. doi: 10.1371/journal.pcbi.1000100

Tewarie, P., van Dellen, E., Hillebrand, A., and Stam, C. J. (2015). The minimum spanning tree: an unbiased method for brain network analysis. *Neuroimage* 104, 177–188. doi: 10.1016/j.neuroimage.2014.10.015

Tzourio-Mazoyer, N., Landeau, B., Papathanassiou, D., Crivello, F., Etard, O., Delcroix, N., et al. (2002). Automated anatomical labeling of activations in SPM using a macroscopic anatomical parcellation of the MNI MRI single-subject brain. *Neuroimage* 15, 273–289. doi: 10.1006/nimg.2001.0978

Vega-Pons, S, A. P., Andric, M., and Hasson, U. (2014). "Classification of inter-subject fMRI data based on graph kernels," in *International Workshop on Pattern Recognition in Neuroimaging* (Tubingen).

Wang, B., Niu, Y., Miao, L., Cao, R., Yan, P., Guo, H., et al. (2017).Decreased complexity in Alzheimer's disease: resting-state fMRI evidence of brain entropy mapping. *Front. Aging Neurosci.* 9:378. doi: 10.3389/fnagi.2017.00378

Wang, L., Fei, F., Jie, B., and Zhang, D. (2015). "Combining multiple network features for mild cognitive impairment classification," in *IEEE International Conference on Data Mining Workshop.Shenzhen* (Shenzhen), 996–1003.

Wang, Z., Yan, C., Zhao, C., Qi, Z., Zhou, W., Lu, J., et al. (2011). Spatial patterns of intrinsic brain activity in mild cognitive impairment and Alzheimer's disease: a resting-state functional MRI study. *Hum. Brain Mapp.* 32, 1720–1724. doi: 10.1002/hbm.21140

Wee, C. Y., Yang, S., Yap, P. T., and Shen, D. (2016). Sparse temporally dynamic resting-state functional connectivity networks for early MCI identification. *Brain Imag. Behav.* 10, 342–356. doi: 10.1007/s11682-015-9408-2

Wee, C. Y., Yap, P. T., Zhang, D., Denny, K., Browndyke, J. N., Potter, G. G., et al. (2012). Identification of MCI individuals using structural and functional connectivity networks. *Neuroimage* 59, 2045–2056. doi: 10.1016/j.neuroimage.2011.10.015

Yan, C., and Zang, Y. (2010). DPARSF: a MATLAB toolbox for "pipeline" data analysis of resting-state fMRI. *Front. Syst. Neurosci.* 4:13. doi: 10.3389/fnsys.2010.00013

Yan, T., Wang, W., Yang, L., Chen, K., Chen, R., and Han, Y. (2018).Rich club disturbances of the human connectome from subjective cognitive decline to Alzheimer's disease.*Theranostics* 8, 3237–3255. doi: 10.7150/thno.23772

Yan, X., and Han, J. (2002). "gspan: Graph-based substructure pattern mining," in *Proceedings IEEE International Conference on Data Mining* 2002 (Maebashi), 12.

Yetkin, F. Z., Rosenberg, R. N., Weiner, M. F., Purdy, P. D., and Cullum, C. M. (2006). FMRI of working memory in patients with mild cognitive impairment and probable Alzheimer's disease. *Eur. Radiol.* 16, 193–206. doi: 10.1007/s00330-005-2794-x

Yu, E., Liao, Z., Mao, D., Zhang, Q., Ji, G., Li, Y., et al. (2016). Directed functional connectivity of posterior cingulate cortex and whole brain in Alzheimer's disease and mild cognitive impairment. *Curr. Alzheimer Res.* 14,628–635. doi: 10.2174/1567205013666161201201000

Zhang, D., Wang, Y., Zhou, L., Yuan, H., Shen, D., and Alzheimer's Disease Neuroimaging Initiative. (2011). Multimodal classification of Alzheimer's disease and mild cognitive impairment. *Neuroimage* 55, 856–867.doi: 10.1016/j.neuroimage.2011.01.008.

Zhang, Y., Lin, H., Yang, Z., and Li, Y. (2011). Neighborhood hash graph kernel for protein-protein interaction extraction. *J. Biomed. Inform.* 44, 1086–1092. doi: 10.1016/j.jbi.2011.08.011

9

Structural and Functional Amygdala Abnormalities in Hemifacial Spasm

Hui Xu [1,2,3], Chenguang Guo [1], Haining Li [1], Lin Gao [2], Ming Zhang [1] and Yuan Wang [1*]*

[1] *Department of Medical Imaging, The First Affiliated Hospital of Xi'an Jiaotong University, Xi'an, China,* [2] *Key Laboratory of Biomedical Information Engineering of Education Ministry, Institute of Biomedical Engineering, Xi'an Jiaotong University, Xi'an, China,* [3] *Faculty of Dentistry, University of Toronto, Toronto, ON, Canada*

Correspondence:
Ming Zhang
zmmri@163.com
Yuan Wang
wangyuan8003@126.com

Background and Purpose: Hemifacial spasm (HFS) is a rare neuromuscular disorder characterized by unilateral, involuntary, and paroxysmal contractions of orofacial muscles. To elucidate the central neural mechanisms of HFS, we investigated brain gray matter and resting-state functional connectivity (rsFC) in HFS patients.

Methods: Thirty patients with HFS and 30 age- and sex-matched healthy participants consented to the study. T1-weighted structural magnetic resonance imaging (MRI) and resting-state BOLD images were collected in all participants. Cortical gray matter thickness was assessed, and subcortical volumetric analysis was performed. Seed-based rsFC analysis was performed on structurally abnormal regions in HFS patients. *Post hoc* correlations with HFS severity and measures of mood (i.e., depression and anxiety) were performed to characterize rsFC alterations.

Results: There were no significant differences in cortical thickness in HFS patients compared to healthy controls. Patients with HFS presented smaller right amygdala volume in contrast to healthy controls ($q < 0.05$, false-discovery rate corrected). We found that the right amygdala had increased rsFC with bilateral medial prefrontal cortex (mPFC), bilateral orbital frontal cortex (OFC), and left posterior insula (L postIns; voxel-wise $p < 0.05$, family-wise error corrected). Moreover, the connections of amygdala–postIns and amygdala–mPFC were positively related to HFS severity and anxiety, respectively.

Conclusions: This is the first study to show structural and functional brain abnormalities in HFS. The volumetric and rsFC amygdala abnormalities were potentially driven by HFS, providing novel insights into HFS pathophysiology.

Keywords: hemifacial spasm, subcortical volumetric analysis, functional connectivity, facial spasm score, affective disorders

INTRODUCTION

Hemifacial spasm (HFS) is a neuromuscular movement disorder characterized by unilateral, involuntary, and paroxysmal contractions of the muscles innervated by the facial nerve (1, 2). The spasm usually originates from the orbicularis oculi muscle of the eyelid, and as the disease progresses, spasms spread to the orbicularis oris and buccinator muscles (1, 3). Even though HFS is not a life-threatening condition, it inevitably causes various degrees of visual and verbal disabilities, which can be distressing and lead to social phobia (4).

It is widely considered that HFS is caused by vascular contact to the facial nerve in the cerebellopontine angle cistern (5, 6); however, to date, only two studies have evaluated gray matter abnormalities in HFS patients. The first study by Bao et al. (7) found that patients with HFS showed reduced gray matter volume (GMV) in the thalamus, putamen, pallidum, amygdala, and parahippocampal gyrus compared to healthy volunteers. The second study, however, found that HFS patients had decreased GMV in the right inferior parietal lobule and increased GMV in the cerebellar lobule compared to controls (8). It should be noted that both studies employed voxel-based morphometry (VBM) to investigate GMV abnormalities (9). Surface-based analyses (SBAs) can detect thickness differences in the cortical sheets between patients and healthy controls. This method accounts for interindividual anatomical variability of the cortical surface through gyral and sulcal geometry, which can directly measure cortical thickness and areas with subvoxel precision (10). This increases the sensitivity to gray matter abnormalities. To the best of our knowledge, no study has applied SBA to determine whether there are cortical thickness abnormalities in HFS patients. However, SBA is limited to cortical regions, and thus, subcortical structures must be evaluated through other volumetric means.

Resting-state functional connectivity (rsFC) is a functional magnetic resonance imaging (fMRI) method used to probe temporal correlations in spontaneous, low-frequency fluctuations across functionally related but structurally distinct brain regions without designated tasks (11). Furthermore, this technique is also suitable for revealing the functional reorganization in intrinsic brain networks in various pathological states (12, 13). To date, no studies have investigated rsFC in HFS. The only study to detect functional abnormalities in HFS investigated signal coherence [or regional homogeneity (ReHo)], a measure of time series similarity in a voxel and its neighbors. The authors found that patients with HFS showed decreased ReHo values in the middle frontal gyrus (MFG) and middle cingulate cortex (MCC), and increased ReHo in the precentral gyrus and brainstem (14). Nevertheless, they were unable to investigate the rsFC alterations in the brain associated with structural abnormalities in the patient group. Besides, it remains unknown whether alterations of gray matter or rsFC are related to disease characteristics and mood disorders, such as anxiety and depression in HFS. It is possible that the social phobia experienced by patients may be linked to brain abnormalities.

Therefore, the objectives of this study are to (1) identify cortical thickness and subcortical volume changes in HFS patients and (2) determine whether these structural abnormalities are related to rsFC abnormalities. Next, we will test whether these abnormalities are associated with the severity of disease and degree of mood disorders.

METHODS

Participants and Neuropsychological Assessment

Thirty primary HFS patients were recruited from the department of neurology at the First Affiliated Hospital of Xi'an Jiaotong University. Inclusion criteria were as follows: disease duration >6 months and typical hemifacial muscle spasms with involuntary and intermittent onset, as independently diagnosed by two experienced physicians. Exclusion criteria included secondary HFS caused by tumors and cysts, organic brain disorders, significant premorbid psychiatric or neurological history, no history of microvascular decompression surgery or botulinum neurotoxin injection, and contraindication to MRI scans (e.g., claustrophobia). Thirty age- and sex-matched healthy volunteers also enrolled in this study. Participants had no history of psychiatric or neurological illness, and no history of alcohol or drug abuse. Written informed consent was obtained from all subjects prior to participation in accordance with the Declaration of Helsinki.

All subjects underwent a structured clinical interview and completed a brief psychological assessment, including the Hamilton Depression Scale (HAM-D) and Hamilton Anxiety Scale (HAM-A). In addition, patients with HFS were also assessed by the Cohen evaluation scale to quantify severity of facial muscle spasms [0–4 scale: 0 = none; 1 = increased blinking caused by external stimuli; 2 = mild, noticeable fluttering, not incapacitating; 3 = moderate, very noticeable spasm, mildly incapacitating; 4 = severely incapacitating (unable to drive, read, etc.)] (15).

Structural and Functional Magnetic Resonance Imaging Data Acquisition

Neuroimaging data from patients with HFS and healthy controls were acquired using the GE Signa HDxt 3.0-T MRI system with an eight-channel head coil. Three-dimensional anatomical images were acquired using a magnetization-prepared rapid acquisition gradient echo (MPRAGE) sequence [time of repetition (TR) = 10.7 ms, time of echo (TE) = 4.9 ms, flip angle (FA) = 15°, in-plane resolution = 1 × 1 × 1 mm, matrix size = 256 × 256, field of view (FOV) = 256 × 256 mm, scan duration = 4 min and 51 s]. Next, a resting-state fMRI scan was collected for each subject using gradient echo–echo planar imaging (GRE-EPI; 150 volumes per slice, TR = 2,000 ms, TE = 35 ms, FA = 90°, in-plane resolution = 3.75 × 3.75 × 4 mm, matrix size = 64 × 64, FOV = 240 × 240 mm). Participants were asked to keep their eyes closed and to remain awake during resting-state fMRI. Finally, diffusion-tensor imaging was also collected after the T1-weighted and resting-state fMRI, but was not discussed in this study.

Measurements of Cortical Thickness and Subcortical Volumes

Each T1-weighted MRI was processed using FreeSurfer (version 5.3.0, http://surfer.nmr.mgh.harvard.edu) with its standard processing pipeline to generate cortical surface models and measure cortical thickness and subcortical volumes. Briefly, for each T1-weighted volume, gray and white matter tissues were segmented, followed by a three-dimensional reconstruction of the gray matter surface and the cortical mantle. The cortical sheet is now represented by vertices, rather than voxels, as it is represented by a surface. Then, cortical thickness at every vertex was determined by computing the distance between the boundary of white matter and the pial boundaries of the gray matter surface. Surface maps were generated following registration of all individuals' cortical reconstructions to a common average template. Finally, surface maps were smoothed with a 10-mm full width at half maximum (FWHM) Gaussian kernel.

Whole-brain vertex-wise analysis of cortical thickness was performed using the Qdec module implemented in FreeSurfer, with a general linear model (GLM) examining group differences. Maps showing significant group differences between patients and healthy controls were generated by thresholding the images of t statistics with false-discovery rate (FDR) correction of $p < 0.05$ at cluster level followed by a cluster-forming threshold of $p < 0.001$, marking the cortical regions with significant changes. In addition, a volumetric analysis of subcortical structures was performed based on the FreeSurfer subcortical segmentation pipeline. These volumes were compared using t tests and further corrected for multiple comparisons using FDR control with a $q < 0.05$.

Resting-State Functional Magnetic Resonance Imaging Connectivity

The resting-state fMRI data were analyzed using FSL (Version 5.0) and included removal of the first five volumes, slice timing and head motion correction, realignment, spatial normalization (to MNI space), spatial smoothing using an 8-mm isotropic Gaussian kernel, temporal band-pass filtering (0.01–0.1 Hz), and elimination of nuisance signals including head motion parameters from MCFLIRT (part of FSL), white matter signal, and cerebrospinal fluid signal by exacting their mean time series.

To examine rsFC changes related to the morphological abnormalities in HFS patients, regions with significant between-group differences of cortical thickness or subcortical volumes were extracted as seed regions. The subcortical seed region was defined by getting the 95% maximum intensity value of this region of the Harvard–Oxford Subcortical Structural Atlas in the standard MNI template space. Then, correlation coefficients between the mean time series of each seed and time series of every voxel throughout the rest of the brain were calculated as rsFC map, which was further converted to z values using Fisher's z transformation to improve normality. A permutation-based two-sample t test was run to generate group-level-difference maps of rsFC for each seed region and then corrected for multiple comparisons with a family-wise error (FWE) rate of $p < 0.05$.

Quality Control of Structural and Functional Magnetic Resonance Imaging

During the structural and functional MRI analysis, we inspected any artifact that could affect processing, including segmentation, normalization, etc. In addition, 7 subjects (5 patients and 2 controls) with head motion of any volume more than 1.5 mm or 1.5° were excluded in further MRI data analysis, leaving a total of 53 participants (25 patients and 28 controls, details seen in **Table 1**) in this study.

TABLE 1 | Summary of demographic characteristics and psychiatric tests between patients with HFS and healthy controls.

Characteristic	HFS ($n = 25$)	HC ($n = 28$)	p-value
Age (years)	48.32 ± 11.59	48.96 ± 12.27	>0.05
Sex			>0.05
Male	11	12	>0.05
Female	14	16	
Disease duration (years)	3.61 ± 3.55	N.A.	
Cohen scores	2.93 ± 0.77	N.A.	
Psychiatric tests			
HAM-A scores	5.21 ± 2.73	0.33 ± 0.91	0.000*
HAM-D scores	5.04 ± 2.85	0.28 ± 0.90	0.000*

HFS, hemifacial spasm; HC, healthy controls; Cohen scores, spasm severity rating via the Cohen evaluation scale; HAM-A, Hamilton Anxiety; HAM-D, Hamilton Depression; N.A., not assigned. Values given as mean ± standard deviation.
**Significant difference between groups.*

Association of Functional Connectivity to Clinical Indices in Patients With Hemifacial Spasm

Spearman correlation coefficients were calculated to evaluate the relationship between clinical variables (Cohen evaluation scale, HAMD score, and HAMA score) and functional connectivity values from group-level-difference clusters of rsFC analysis using SPSS software version 18.0. A p-value of <0.05 was considered statistically significant after correction for multiple comparisons with Bonferroni test.

RESULTS

Demographics and Neuropsychological Assessment

Patients with HFS and healthy controls were matched well for age (48.32 ± 11.59 years old for patients and 48.96 ± 12.27 years old for controls, $t_{51} = -0.195$, $p = 0.846$) and sex (56.0% female patients vs. 57.1% female controls, $\chi^2_1 = 0.007$, $p = 0.933$). In addition, patients with HFS reported significant levels of anxiety ($t_{51} = 8.924$, $p < 0.001$) and felt more depressed ($t_{51} = 8.110$, $p < 0.001$) than healthy controls, which were measured by HAM-A and HAM-D, respectively. Demographic and clinical data are all presented in **Table 1**.

Abnormal Cortical Thickness and Subcortical Volumes in Patients With Hemifacial Spasm

The unbiased whole-brain vertex-wise comparison showed no significant differences that survived multiple comparisons (FDR correction of $p < 0.05$ at a cluster level followed by a cluster-forming threshold of $p < 0.001$) in patients with HFS compared with healthy controls. Furthermore, the volumetric analysis of subcortical structures showed significantly reduced subcortical volume merely in the right amygdala in patients with HFS compared to healthy controls ($q < 0.05$, FDR corrected; **Figure 1**).

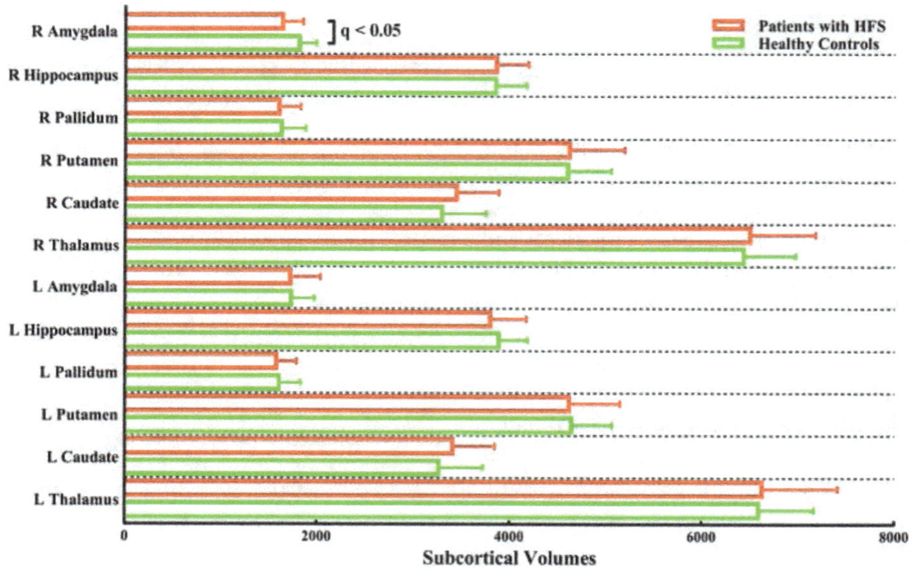

FIGURE 1 | Subcortical volumes in patients with HFS compared with healthy controls. Patients merely showed significantly reduced subcortical volume in the right amygdala compared to the control group [$q < 0.05$, false-discovery rate (FDR) corrected for multiple comparisons]. L, left; R, right.

Abnormal Right Amygdala-Based Functional Connectivity Following Patients With Hemifacial Spasm

Increased right amygdala-anchored rsFC to the bilateral medial prefrontal cortex (mPFC), bilateral orbital frontal cortex (OFC), and left posterior insula (L postIns) was observed in patients with HFS compared with healthy controls ($p < 0.05$, FWE corrected; **Figure 2**, **Table 2**).

Association of Functional Connectivity to Clinical Variables in Patients With Hemifacial Spasm

Correlations of FC values from group-level-difference clusters of rsFC were detected to the clinical indices of patients with HFS. We found that the mean FC value of right amygdala to L postIns positively correlated with spasm severity ($\rho = 0.588$, $p = 0.002$, **Figure 3A**). In addition, the mean FC value of the right amygdala to right mPFC also correlated with anxiety symptom ($\rho = 0.479$, $p = 0.015$, **Figure 3B**). No other significant correlation was found between FC values and other clinical parameters (i.e., disease duration and HAM-D score).

DISCUSSION

This study investigated structural and functional reorganization in the brain associated with HFS and how these changes are relevant to the severity of muscle contraction and concomitant affective disturbance. Patients with HFS had significantly reduced volume in the right amygdala. Furthermore, compared with healthy controls, the right amygdala displayed increased rsFC to the bilateral mPFC, bilateral OFC, and L postIns in patients with HFS. To date, there has been only one resting-state fMRI study related to HFS, which focused on evaluating synchronous brain activity of a given region to its nearest neighbors by ReHo analysis (14) without capturing the functional relationships to the distant brain areas. To our knowledge, this is the first study to show structural and functional amygdala abnormalities in HFS.

One of the major findings of this study presented as decreased volume of right amygdala in patients with HFS compared to healthy controls. The amygdala belongs to a key region with afferent and efferent neural connections that modulate complex stimuli such as pain, anxiety, fear, and reward (16). Corresponding to its functional diversity, the amygdaloid complex has been shown to consist of dozens of distinct but closely interconnected nuclei in nonhuman primates (17). In addition, cytoarchitectonic study of human postmortem brains suggested that amygdala includes three major sets of nuclei that are called laterobasal, centromedial, and superficial groups (18). For one, the centromedial nuclei of amygdala can produce hormones and induce autonomic responses according to the anatomical and physiological knowledge (19–22), which involves the process of unpleasant stimuli including anxious and depressive information (23, 24), and the spasm-anchored affective disorders in patients with HFS may partially contribute to the amygdala atrophy. For another, the morphological and functional alterations of amygdala may be linked to visual attentional deficit triggered by the spasm in patients with HFS. The lateral portion of amygdala was established to coordinate visual information, which was supported by a tract-tracing study (25) and single-cell recordings (26) in monkeys. Besides, bidirectional communication between amygdala and fusiform gyrus was further verified during facial information processing by fMRI experiment (27). Given that those enrolled in this study underwent chronic and severe facial spasm (mean Cohen score

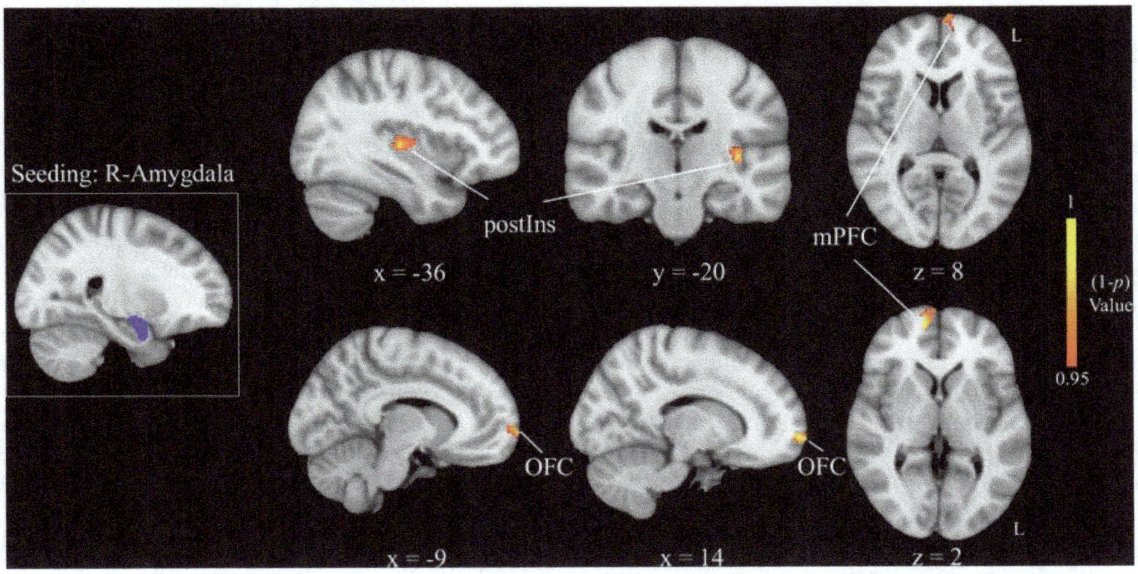

FIGURE 2 | Increased right amygdala-based functional connectivity following patients with hemifacial spasm (HFS) in contrast to healthy controls [$p < 0.05$, family-wise error (FWE) corrected]. postIns, posterior insula; mPFC, medial prefrontal cortex; OFC, orbital frontal cortex; L, left; R, right.

TABLE 2 | Clusters demonstrating differences in functional connectivity between HFS and HC participants.

ROI	Brain region	Hemisphere	Size of cluster (voxels)	Peak MNI coordinate			Peak voxel *t*-value
				x	y	z	
HFS > HC							
Right amygdala	Medial prefrontal cortex	L	137	−8	70	12	3.625
	Medial prefrontal cortex	R	370	12	56	2	3.434
	Orbital frontal cortex	L	52	−8	70	−2	3.298
	Orbital frontal cortex	R	62	14	68	−6	3.315
	Posterior insula	L	100	−36	−20	4	4.758
HFS < HC							
No between-group differences							

ROI, region of interest; MNI, Montreal Neurologic Institute; L, left; R, right.

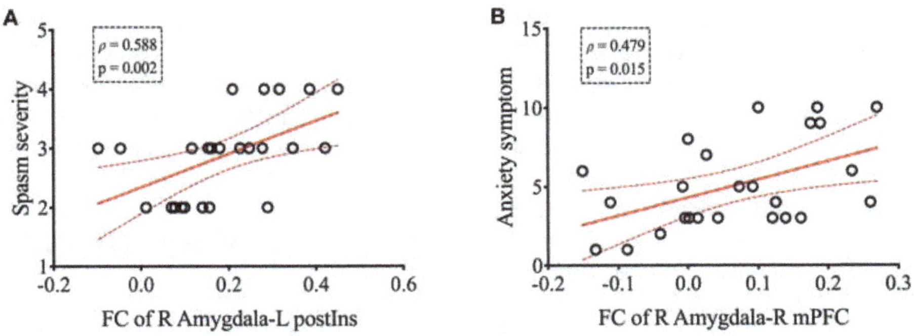

FIGURE 3 | The right amygdala-based functional connectivity was positively correlated with spasm severity **(A)** and anxiety symptom **(B)** in patients with HFS, respectively. Curved dashed lines indicate 95% confidence intervals. The spasm severity was measured by Cohen evaluation scale, and Hamilton Anxiety Scale was performed to assess patients' anxiety symptom. FC, functional connectivity; postIns, posterior insula; mPFC, medial prefrontal cortex; L, left; R, right.

was near 3), patients with HFS were difficult to concentrate on others' face in a short period of time during social contact, which probably lead to the structural alteration in the laterobasal nuclei of amygdala. Since anatomical tracing studies revealed that most of the nuclei in the amygdaloid complex had extensive intranuclear and internuclear connections (22), our imaging data on amygdala abnormality may be attributed to the interaction of emotional and visual deficiency in patients with HFS.

Another finding in our study was altered right amygdala-driven connections to several emotion-related brain areas, such as bilateral mPFC and bilateral OFC in patients with HFS compared to healthy controls, which was in accordance with previous fMRI results (28). Previous animal and human studies suggested a distinctive amygdala–frontal circuit on emotion generation and regulation (29–31). Anatomical tracing studies have detected reciprocal connections between the amygdala and the anterior cingulate cortex (ACC), OFC, and dorsal medical prefrontal cortex (DMPFC) (32, 33). Of note, the OFC was usually segmented into medial and lateral divisions, which initially derived from differential cognitive and affective deficits of medial OFC (mOFC) vs. lateral OFC (lOFC) in primates (34), and this parcellation was confirmed by differentiated connections with tracing studies; that is, the mOFC received inputs from limbic structures such as hippocampus, amygdala, and insular cortex (35), while lOFC showed anatomic connections with several visual processing regions including fusiform gyrus and lateral occipital cortex (36). Moreover, in a meta-analysis focusing on divergent patterns of rsFC between different OFC subregions, the lOFC showed notable coactivations with the amygdala and the fusiform gyrus, both of which are known to participate in visual processing (37). Accordingly, we assume that the strengthened rsFC of amygdala to lOFC may be helpful for patients with HFS to compensate for the deficit of focusing on objects for a long period of time.

Meanwhile, our study displayed increased right amygdala rsFC to bilateral mPFC in patients with HFS. The mPFC was involved in various categories of affective disorders detected by fMRI and PET, such as schizophrenia, bipolar disorder (38), major depression (39), and social anxiety (40). Electron microscopy (41) and retrograde tracing techniques (42, 43) confirmed that the mPFC directly received extensive input from amygdala, which was important for emotion regulation. Considering that the current findings demonstrated positive correlation of amygdala–mPFC connection to the degree of anxiety in patients with HFS, we proposed that the rsFC abnormality of the two regions in the patient group was caused in part by the spasm-induced negative emotion. In addition, it is well known that mPFC is a major hub of default mode network. Because mPFC activity has linked to maintain vigilance toward the surrounding environment (44), and the laterobasal nuclei group in amygdala was established to coordinate high-level sensory input including visual information preprocessing (17), the increased connectivity between mPFC and amygdala could also reflect exaggerated vigilance to the environment so as to compensate for the deficit of visual attention in patients with HFS.

Last but not the least, the patients with HFS exhibited increased amygdala–postIns connection compared to controls. It is well established that insula has structural and functional connections with almost all of the amygdaloid nuclei. Neurophysiological and histochemical experiments had confirmed projections of anterior insula to the anterior and medial amygdaloid area and projections of posterior insula to the dorsolateral part of amygdala in the rhesus monkey (45), where the corresponding nuclei are responsible for modulation of autonomic activity and high-level sensory information, respectively (17), and it was partially supported by a functional imaging study with positron emission tomography (46). Because the posterior insula and lateral part of amygdala share a functional similarity on visual stimuli coordination, increased rsFC of the two regions is likely to make up the visual defect of HFS with frequent facial contraction, which provides a basis for positive correlation of amygdala–insular connectivity to the degree of facial spasm.

Several limitations of this study bear acknowledgment here. First, the sample size of both groups is relatively small. The reliability of the results would be improved by recruiting more subjects. Second, the cross-sectional experiment design was not useful to observe dynamic changes in structural and functional dataset to assess the characteristics of HFS over time. A longitudinal study should be performed to monitor the volume and rsFC of right amygdala along with alterations of the facial spasm and emotional disturbance.

In summary, the current study revealed atrophic right amygdala in patients with HFS together with increased rsFC of this seed to bilateral OFC, bilateral mPFC, and left postIns. Moreover, the altered amygdala–postIns and amygdala–mPFC networks were correlated with spasm severity and anxiety symptom, which provide distinct aspects of clues of HFS-related disorders.

ETHICS STATEMENT

This study was carried out in accordance with the recommendations of the Medical Research Ethics Committee and Institutional Review Board of the first affiliated hospital of Xi'an Jiaotong University with written informed consent from all subjects. All subjects gave written informed consent in accordance with the Declaration of Helsinki. The protocol was approved by the Department of medical imaging, the first affiliated hospital of Xi'an Jiaotong University.

AUTHOR CONTRIBUTIONS

YW, MZ, and HX drafted the manuscript, study concept or design, and statistical analysis. HX, HL, and LG revised the manuscript for content and analysis or interpretation of data. CG and HL acquired the data. YW, MZ, and HX supervised or coordinated the experiment. All authors read and approved the final manuscript.

FUNDING

This work was supported in part by the Natural Science Foundation of Shaanxi Province (No. 2018JM7026), the Xi'an Science and Technology Project [No. 201805102YX10SF36 (3)], Fundamental Research Funds for the Central Universities in Xi'an Jiaotong University (No. xjj2018272), and the Clinical Research Award of the First Affiliated Hospital of Xi'an Jiaotong University, China (No. XJTU1AF-CRF-2015-028).

ACKNOWLEDGMENTS

We thank Dr. Faxiu Bao for her assistance with recruiting HFS patients, and thank Dr. Massieh Moayedi for his advice writing this article and language help.

REFERENCES

Rosenstengel C, Matthes M, Baldauf J, Fleck S, Schroeder H. Hemifacial spasm: conservative and surgical treatment options. *Dtsch Arztebl Int.* (2012) 109:667–73. doi: 10.3238/arztebl.2012.0667

Yaltho TC, Jankovic J. The many faces of hemifacial spasm: differential diagnosis of unilateral facial spasms. *Mov Disord.* (2011) 26:1582– 92. doi: 10.1002/mds.23692

Au WL, Tan LC, Tan AK. Hemifacial spasm in Singapore: clinical characteristics and patients' perceptions. *Ann Acad Med Singapore.* (2004) 33:324–8.

Tan E-K, Lum S-Y, Fook-Chong S, Chan L-L, Gabriel C, Lim L. Behind the facial twitch: depressive symptoms in hemifacial spasm. *Parkinsonism Relat Disord.* (2005) 11:241–5. doi: 10.1016/j.parkreldis.2004.12.003

Kawashima M, Yamada M, Sato S, Oka H, Fujii K, Matsushima T. Hemifacial spasm caused by vascular compression of the distal portion of the facial nerve associated with configuration variation of the facial and vestibulocochlear nerve complex. *Turk Neurosurg.* (2009) 19:269–75.

Campos-Benitez M, Kaufmann AM. Neurovascular compression findings in hemifacial spasm. *J Neurosurg.* (2008) 109:416– 20. doi: 10.3171/JNS/2008/109/9/0416

Bao F, Wang Y, Liu J, Mao C, Ma S, Guo C, et al. Structural changes in the CNS of patients with hemifacial spasm. *Neuroscience.* (2015) 289:56– 62. doi: 10.1016/j.neuroscience.2014.12.070

Tu Y, Yu T, Wei Y, Sun K, Zhao W, Yu B. Structural brain alterations in hemifacial spasm: a voxel-based morphometry and diffusion tensor imaging study. *Clin Neurophysiol.* (2016) 127:1470–4. doi: 10.1016/j.clinph.2015.07.036

Wang Y, Yang Q, Cao D, Seminowicz D, Remeniuk B, Gao L, et al. Correlation between nerve atrophy, brain grey matter volume and pain severity in patients with primary trigeminal neuralgia. *Cephalalgia.* (2018) 39:515–25. 333102418793643. doi: 10.1177/0333102418793643

Fischl B, Dale AM. Measuring the thickness of the human cerebral cortex from magnetic resonance images. *Proc Natl Acad Sci USA.* (2000) 97:11050–5. doi: 10.1073/pnas.200033797

Fox MD, Raichle ME. Spontaneous fluctuations in brain activity observed with functional magnetic resonance imaging. *Nat Rev Neurosci.* (2007) 8:700–11. doi: 10.1038/nrn2201

Greicius M. Resting-state functional connectivity in neuropsychiatric disorders. *Curr Opin Neurol.* (2008) 21:424– 30. doi: 10.1097/WCO.0b013e328306f2c5

Wang Y, Cao D, Remeniuk B, Krimmel S, Seminowicz DA, Zhang M. Altered brain structure and function associated with sensory and affective components of classic trigeminal neuralgia. *Pain.* (2017) 158:1561–70. doi: 10.1097/j.pain.0000000000000951

Tu Y, Wei Y, Sun K, Zhao W, Yu B. Altered spontaneous brain activity in patients with hemifacial spasm: a resting-state functional MRI study. *PLoS ONE.* (2015) 10:e0116849. doi: 10.1371/journal.pone.0116849

Cohen DA, Savino PJ, Stern MB, Hurtig HI. Botulinum injection therapy for blepharospasm: a review and report of 75 patients. *Clin Neuropharmacol.* (1986) 9:415–29.

Simons LE, Pielech M, Erpelding N, Linnman C, Moulton E, Sava S, et al. The responsive amygdala: treatment-induced alterations in functional connectivity in pediatric complex regional pain syndrome. *Pain.* (2014) 155:1727–42. doi: 10.1016/j.pain.2014.05.023

Danilo B, Laird AR, Karl Z, Fox PT, Eickhoff SB. An investigation of the structural, connectional, and functional subspecialization in the human amygdala. *Hum Brain Mapp.* (2013) 34:3247–66. doi: 10.1002/hbm.22138

Amunts K, Kedo O, Kindler M, Pieperhoff P, Mohlberg H, Shah NJ, et al. Cytoarchitectonic mapping of the human amygdala, hippocampal region and entorhinal cortex: intersubject variability and probability maps. *Anat Embryol.* (2005) 210:343–52. doi: 10.1007/s00429-005-0025-5 Davis M, Whalen PJ. The amygdala: vigilance and emotion. *Mol Psychiatry.* (2001) 6:13–34. doi: 10.1038/sj.mp.4000812

Moreno N, González A. Evolution of the amygdaloid complex in vertebrates, with special reference to the anamnio-amniotic transition. *J Anat.* (2007) 211:151–63. doi: 10.1111/j.1469-7580.2007.00780.x

Pessoa L. Emotion and cognition and the amygdala: from "what is it?" to "what's to be done?" *Neuropsychologia.* (2010) 48:3416–29. doi: 10.1016/j.neuropsychologia.2010.06.038

Sah P, Faber ESL, Armentia MLDe, Power J. The amygdaloid complex: anatomy and physiology. *Physiol Rev.* (2003) 83:803– 34. doi: 10.1152/physrev.00002.2003

Leppänen JM. Emotional information processing in mood disorders: a review of behavioral and neuroimaging findings. *Curr Opin Psychiatry.* (2006) 19:34–9. doi: 10.1097/01.yco.0000191500.46411.00

Monk CS, Telzer EH, Mogg K, Bradley BP, Mai X, Louro HM, et al. Amygdala and ventrolateral prefrontal cortex activation to masked angry faces in children and adolescents with generalized anxiety disorder. *Arch Gen Psychiatry.* (2008) 65:568–76. doi: 10.1001/archpsyc.65.5.568

Iwai E, Yukie M. Amygdalofugal and amygdalopetal connections with modality-specific visual cortical areas in macaques (*Macaca fuscata, M. mulatta,* and *M. fascicularis*). *J Comp Neurol.* (1987) 261:362–87.

Mosher CP, Zimmerman PE, Gothard KM. Response characteristics of basolateral and centromedial neurons in the primate amygdala. *J Neurosci.* (2010) 30:16197–207. doi: 10.1523/JNEUROSCI.3225-10.2010

Sato W, Kochiyama T, Uono S, Matsuda K, Usui K, Usui N, et al. Bidirectional electric communication between the inferior occipital gyrus and the amygdala during face processing. *Hum Brain Mapp.* (2017) 38:4511– 24. doi: 10.1002/hbm.23678

Banks SJ, Eddy KT, Angstadt M, Nathan PJ, Phan KL. Amygdala–frontal connectivity during emotion regulation. *Soc Cogn Affect Neurosci.* (2007) 2:303–12. doi: 10.1093/scan/nsm029

Davidson RJ, Putnam KM, Larson CL. Dysfunction in the neural circuitry of emotion regulation—a possible prelude to violence. *Science.* (2000) 289:591–4. doi: 10.1126/science.289.5479.591

K Luan P, Taylor SF, Welsh RC, Decker LR, Noll DC, Nichols TE, et al. Activation of the medial prefrontal cortex and extended amygdala by individual ratings of emotional arousal: a fMRI study. *Biol Psychiatry.* (2003) 53:211–5. doi: 10.1016/S0006-3223(02)01485-3

Quirk GJ, Beer JS. Prefrontal involvement in the regulation of emotion: convergence of rat and human studies. *Curr Opin Neurobiol.* (2006) 16:723–7. doi: 10.1016/j.conb.2006.07.004

Ghashghaei HT, Hilgetag CC, Barbas H. Sequence of information processing for emotions based on the anatomic dialogue between prefrontal cortex and amygdala. *Neuroimage.* (2007) 34:905–23. doi: 10.1016/j.neuroimage.2006.09.046

Ghashghaei HT, Barbas H. Pathways for emotion: interactions of prefrontal and anterior temporal pathways in the amygdala of the rhesus monkey. *Neuroscience.* (2002) 115:1261–79. doi: 10.1016/S0306-4522(02)00446-3

Zald DH, Kim SW. Anatomy and function of the orbital frontal cortex, I: anatomy, neurocircuitry; and obsessive-compulsive disorder. *J Neuropsychiatry Clin Neurosci.* (1996) 8:125–38.

Carmichael ST, Price JL. Limbic connections of the orbital and medial prefrontal cortex in macaque monkeys. *J Comp Neurol.* (1995) 363:615–41.

Carmichael ST, Price JL. Sensory and premotor connections of the orbital and medial prefrontal cortex of macaque monkeys. *J Comp Neurol.* (1995) 363:642–64.

Zald DH, McHugo M, Ray KL, Glahn DC, Eickhoff SB, Laird AR. Meta-analytic connectivity modeling reveals differential functional connectivity of the medial and lateral orbitofrontal cortex. *Cereb Cortex.* (2014) 24:232–48. doi: 10.1093/cercor/bhs308

Chai XJ, Whitfieldgabrieli S, Shinn AK, Gabrieli JDE, Castañón AN, Mccarthy JM, et al. Abnormal medial prefrontal cortex resting-state connectivity in bipolar disorder and schizophrenia. *Neuropsychopharmacology.* (2011) 36:2009–17. doi: 10.1038/npp.2011.88

Lemogne C, Delaveau P, Freton M, Guionnet S, Fossati P. Medial prefrontal cortex and the self in major depression. *J Affect Disord.* (2012) 136:e1–11. doi: 10.1016/j.jad.2010.11.034

Evans KC, Simon NM, Dougherty DD, Hoge EA, Worthington JJ, Chow C, et al. A PET study of tiagabine treatment implicates ventral medial prefrontal cortex in generalized social anxiety disorder. *Neuropsychopharmacol Off Publ Am Coll Neuropsychopharmacol.* (2009) 34:390–8. doi: 10.1038/npp.2008.69

Bacon SJ, Headlam AJ, Gabbott PL, Smith AD. Amygdala input to medial prefrontal cortex (mPFC) in the rat: a light and electron microscope study. *Brain Res.* (1996) 720:211–9.

Gabbott PLA, Warner TA, Jays PRL, Salway P, Busby SJ. Prefrontal cortex in the rat: projections to subcortical autonomic, motor, and limbic centers. *J Comp Neurol.* (2005) 492:145–77. doi: 10.1002/cne.20738

Hoover WB, Vertes RP. Anatomical analysis of afferent projections to the medial prefrontal cortex in the rat. *Brain Struct Funct.* (2007) 212:149–79. doi: 10.1007/s00429-007-0150-4

Tang Y-Y, Rothbart MK, Posner MI. Neural correlates of establishing, maintaining, and switching brain states. *Trends Cogn Sci.* (2012) 16:330–7. doi: 10.1016/j.tics.2012.05.001

Mufson EJ, Mesulam MM, Pandya DN. Insular interconnections with the amygdala in the rhesus monkey. *Neuroscience.* (1981) 6:1231–48.

Dupont S, Bouilleret V, Hasboun D, Semah F, Baulac M. Functional anatomy of the insula: new insights from imaging. *Surg Radiol Anat.* (2003) 25:113– 9. doi: 10.1007/s00276-003-0103-4

10

Imaging Genetics Towards a Refined Diagnosis of Schizophrenia

Wenhao Jiang[1], Tricia Z. King[1] and Jessica A. Turner[1,2]*

[1] Department of Psychology and the Neuroscience Institute, Georgia State University, Atlanta, GA, United States, [2] Mind Research Network, Albuquerque, NM, United States

***Correspondence:**
Wenhao Jiang
wjiang5@student.gsu.edu

Current diagnoses of schizophrenia and related psychiatric disorders are classified by phenomenological principles and clinical descriptions while ruling out other symptoms and conditions. Specific biomarkers are needed to assist the current diagnostic system. However, complicated gene and environment interactions induce great disease heterogeneity. This unclear etiology and heterogeneity raise difficulties in distinguishing schizophrenia-related effects. Simultaneously, the overlap in symptoms, genetic variations, and brain alterations in schizophrenia and related psychiatric disorders raises similar difficulties in determining disease-specific effects. Imaging genetics is a unique methodology to assess the impact of genetic factors on both brain structure and function. More importantly, imaging genetics builds a bridge to understand the behavioral and clinical implications of genetics and neuroimaging. By characterizing and quantifying the brain measures affected in psychiatric disorders, imaging genetics is contributing to identifying potential biomarkers for schizophrenia and related disorders. To date, candidate gene analysis, genome-wide association studies, polygenetic risk score analysis, and large-scale collaborative studies have made contributions to the understanding of schizophrenia with the potential to serve as biomarkers. Despite limitations, imaging genetics remains promising as more aggregative, clustering methods and imaging genetics-compatible clinical assessments are employed in future studies. We review imaging genetics' contribution to our understanding of the heterogeneity within schizophrenia and the commonalities across schizophrenia and other diagnostic borders, and we will discuss whether imaging genetics is ready to form its own diagnostic system.

Keywords: imaging genetics, diagnostic catalogues, heterogeneity, genetic overlap, brain alterations

INTRODUCTION

The current diagnosis of schizophrenia and psychiatric disorders is mainly based on phenomenological observation and clinical descriptions. Although these descriptions are reliable, they are not established on valid pathological bases (1). The heterogeneity of the symptoms, treatment response, and outcomes implies that there are different subtypes within schizophrenia, while phenomenological observation fails to generate precise subgroups revealing etiological and pathological differences (2). Additionally, similar psychotic symptoms aggregate in different disorders and in families. Behind this aggregation, shared biological mechanisms including genetics and neurophysiology are found (1). These findings suggest that the boundaries of psychiatric disorders are merging beyond the traditional categorical diagnostic system. The precise subgroups and disorder boundaries may optimize treatment and prognosis, and research-based biomarkers may help to fulfill this goal. Importantly, efforts have already been made as part of the *Diagnostic and Statistical Manual of Mental Disorders, Fifth Edition* (DSM-5).

Combining genetics and imaging to assess accumulating genetic variations on brain function and morphometry has become the integrated research method known as imaging genetics (3). Imaging genetics not only serves as a tool to understand the impact of genetic variations on both structural and functional brain, but it also enables researchers to capture the behavioral implication of those genes and associated brain alterations (4). Importantly, imaging genetics characterizes different pathways from genes, imaging, and behavior data. Its quantified findings make it possible to contribute to the currently unknown map of future diagnosis (5). The common technologies in imaging genetic include candidate gene analysis, genome-wide association study (GWAS) using imaging phenotypes, polygenic approaches (polygenic scores, pathway analysis, and multivariate methods), and developing novel approaches (6–8). We focus in this paper on the subset of imaging genetics that focuses on the relationships from gene to brain to behavior, which have generally focused on common variants in the single nucleotide polymorphisms (SNPs).

Various genetically related brain abnormalities have been revealed in SZ. SZ patients generally show smaller brain volume, overall reductions in gray matter in fronto-temporal, thalamo-cortical, and subcortical-limbic circuits and enlargement of ventricles (9). These brain alterations induced in partly by genetic variations (10) are bridging the gap between gene and the phenotype and even clinical symptoms of SZ (see **Figure 1**) (11). It is encouraging that some shared genetics, imaging, and imaging genetics findings have been recognized across SZ, bipolar disorder (BD), and disorders under other categories. At the same time, imaging and genetics are helping to form subtypes with different mechanisms in SZ.

In this paper, we review the major imaging genetics findings on SZ with closely related psychotic disorders with an eye toward the following questions: 1) to date, what contribution have genetics, neuroimaging, and imaging genetics made to our understanding of the heterogeneity of SZ and the boundaries among psychiatric disorders and 2) whether imaging genetics is ready to form its own diagnostic system.

TRADITIONAL AND CURRENT DIAGNOSES OF SZ

Feighner and colleagues published the criteria for highly reproducible diagnoses based on behavioral observation in 1972 (12). From this historical view, clinical description, laboratory studies, delineation from other disorders, follow-up studies with retreatment response, and family studies are considered as major theoretical bases for

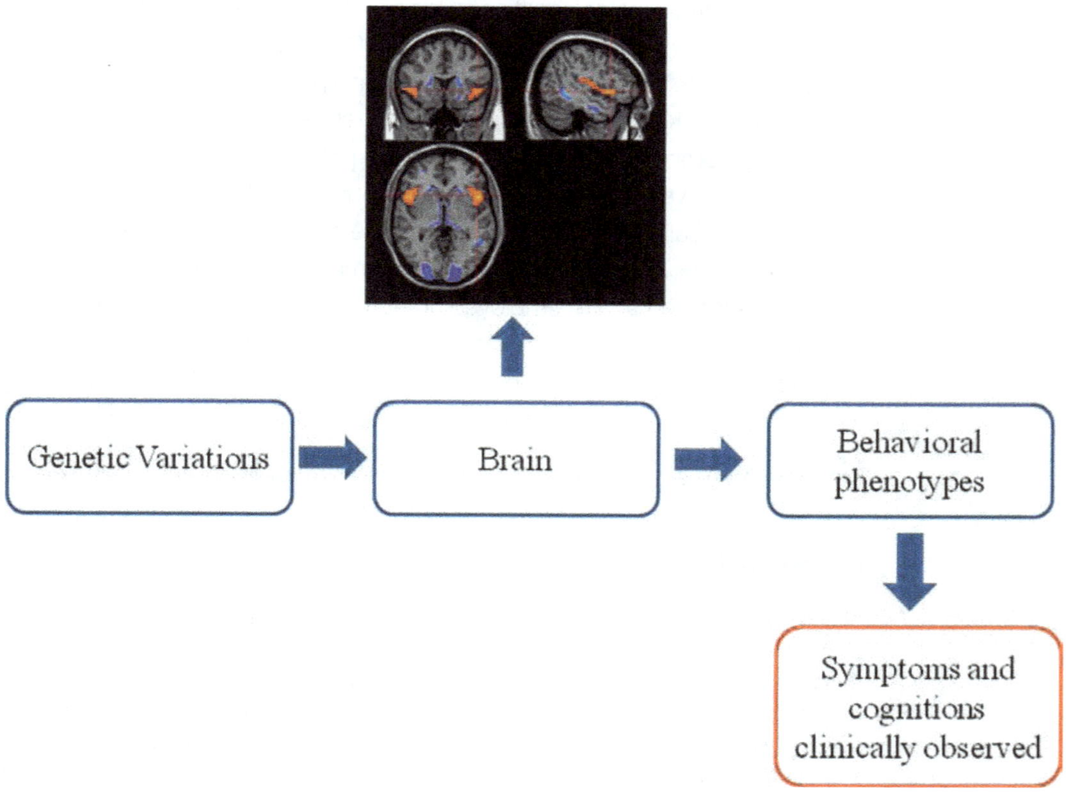

FIGURE 1 | The classic "bottom-up" model in imaging genetics. Genetic variations acclimate their influences on the brain. The brain alterations further develop into behavioral phenotype changes, which can be clinically observed as symptoms and cognitive impairments. This observed clinical profile established the base of current phenomenological diagnostic system of psychiatric disorders.

validating a diagnosis (13). However, the follow-up study and treatment response may be questioned for whether they could validate the diagnosis, *per se*. Antipsychotics are a major choice not only for SZ spectrum but also for depression and BD.

Accumulating new biological understanding does not always agree with the criteria and classification proposed at Feighner's time. It is now accepted that family coaggregation implies shared abnormal genetic markers and mechanism in the family line. For example, SZ, BD, and schizoaffective disorder (SAD) are in different diagnostic categories, but observations of diagnoses in families of patients showed significant overlap among them, which is still being studied to explore the genetic background (14). Thus, the traditional methods for determining the diagnostic category boundaries are not sufficient.

GENETICS AND ITS IMPACT ON THE DIAGNOSTIC PROBLEM

Genetic Overlap Among SZ and Other Psychiatric Disorders

Genes contribute greatly to the etiology of SZ, and meta-analysis in SZ twin study shows a heritability around 80% (15). Val158Met single polymorphism (SNP) of catechol-O-methyltransferase (COMT), the Val66Met SNP of brain-derived neurotrophic factor (BDNF), and the Ser704Cys SNP of disrupted-in-SZ 1 (DISC1) is the most well-known gene alteration examined by candidate gene analysis (7). The first few reports of GWAS, in contrast, demonstrated several loci associated with SZ including Zinc finger protein 804A (ZNF804A), neurogranin (NRGN), and the major histocompatibility complex (MHC) region. More recent GWAS studies with increased sample size discovered more SZ related loci (16), and some of these loci are shared by BD and other psychiatric disorders (17–25).

SZ and BD are often studied together to elucidate the genetic overlap and disorder boundaries. A genetic correlation around 0.6 is suggested by family, twin, and adoption study (26). However, applying a hierarchical or nonhierarchical diagnostic system has provided conflicting co-occurrence results at the same time (27). SAD is often included in the study of SZ and BD and that genetic relationship could also be potentially affected (28).

In addition to epidemiological evidence, the GWAS study has brought more insight into the actual genetic overlap. ZNF804A is the first discovered marker that may increase the risk for both SZ and BD, and meta-analysis has supported its role (29). The combined SZ and BD GWAS study from Psychiatric Genomics Consortium (PGC) has identified calcium voltage-gated channel subunit alpha1 C (CACNA1C), ankyrin-3(ANK3) and inter-alpha-trypsin inhibitor heavy chain 3-4 (ITIH3-ITIH4) as risk for both disorders (30, 31). Later by introducing pleiotropy-informed conditional false discovery rate, 14 loci were associated with both disorders, and CACNA1C and ITIH4 were identified again (32). PGC's diagnostic specificity of five disorders analyses has also shown 5′-nucleotidase, cytosolic II (NT5C2), and coiled-coil domain containing 68 (CCDC68) is associated with both disorders (33). The combined GWAS studies will continue to reveal more important loci, but the functional implications and roles of these distinct genes in SZ and BD will need further investigation.

Another idea is using a polygenetic method to combine and count the accumulating effects of a large number of loci, which may or may not reach the GWAS threshold for significance. Again in the PGC study, the cross-disorder group stated SZ and BD were affected by genetic correlation of 0.68 based on their common SNPs (33). Additional polygenic studies blur the distinction across categories and indicate a broad genetic mechanism for these psychiatric disorders (34–36).

However, there is also genetic evidence showing distinctions between SZ and BD (37). Large and rare copy number variations (CNV) have been identified in SZ and certain developmental disorders, but less consistently in BD. In addition, Sz pathogenic CNV carriers showed reduced subcortical regions including thalamus, putamen, pallidum, hippocampus, and accumbens, which were previously identified in Sz participants (38). This finding is consistent with the diagnosis hierarchy, by which BD is only diagnosed with the absence of SZ and developmental disorders.

Genetics Helps Reveal Heterogeneity and Future Subtypes of SZ

Many researchers have tried to provide genetic explanations for SZ's heterogeneities. Arnedo and colleagues made a promising attempt trying to uncover the hidden genetic architecture of different subtypes of SZ (39). The basic idea of their research was to measure the complexity of hidden architecture in genotype and phenotype. It was expected that the association between distinct sets of phenotypes and SNPs could be revealed in heterogeneous SZ, and it would represent subtypes of SZ with the respective genetic mechanism.

Arnedo et al. generated phenotypic sets using non-negative matrix factorization from the data of series questionnaire and structured interview results. The factorization divided the SZ patients into distinct subgroups with different disease severity, process, and symptom domain (positive, negative, and disorganized symptoms) regardless of their genetic background. SNP sets were generated by a generalized factorization method combined with non-negative matrix factorization. The overlap of patients and SNPs in these sets ensured to be disjoint, to reflect the heterogeneity of SZ. Finally, the association between phenotypic sets and SNP sets were tested in the molecular genetics of schizophrenia (MGS) study. It was also largely replicated by them in the National Institute of Mental Health Clinical Antipsychotic Trials of Intervention Effectiveness (CATIE) project and Portuguese Island family samples.

The results were encouraging: Arnedo et al. found 42 SNP sets had >70% risk for SZ, and these SNP sets were significantly associated with different phenotypic sets. For instance, a phenotypic set indicating a general process of severe deterioration (severe process, with positive and negative symptom; moderate severity of impairment; unable to function since onset) was highly correlated with certain SNP set including polypyrimidine tract binding protein 2 (PTBP2) and several other genes which might play a role in neuron differentiation. This severe deterioration SZ may be a potential clinical valid subtype, and following the track of PTBP2 and its SNP cluster may facilitate the examination of the mechanisms underlying severe deterioration.

Based on their findings, it was believed that SZ could be seen as "syndromes group" in which distinct clinical syndromes are associated with disjoint genotypic networks. The interaction map of disjoint genotype and distinct syndromes have shown a possible way of shaping SZ into biological markers or a networks-based subtype.

IMAGING AND ITS IMPACT ON THE DIAGNOSTIC ISSUE

Anatomical changes in fronto-temporal, thalamo-cortical, subcortical-limbic circuits, enlargement of ventricles, and widespread white matter fibers abnormalities have been found in many structural studies of schizophrenia (40–43). With the growing sample size and collaboration through different sites, many large-scale meta-analyses have provided new information. The Enhancing Neuroimaging Genetics through Meta-Analysis (ENIGMA) SZ working group's meta-analysis of subcortical regions across several thousand subjects reported the consistent findings of smaller hippocampus, amygdala, thalamus, accumbens, and intracranial volumes, but larger pallidum and lateral ventricle volumes (44). The putamen and caudate volume results were not reliable across different populations and studies even with this sample size, indicating the possibility of clinical heterogeneity affecting those regions (44). The development of these differences prior to, with, and after disease onset and diagnosis is also important for understanding the disease (45), and comparing the course of the morphometric reductions and increases across diagnoses will be informative. Functional imaging studies have also discovered various abnormal brain regions and connections in SZ. Partially overlapped with structural findings, functional alterations including the prefrontal cortex, superior temporal gyrus, thalamus, frontal lobe, and parietal lobe have been reported in either resting state or task fMRI (46).

Many of the above regions have been identified as structural or functional commonalities among DSM categories (1, 47, 48). Starting from the same point as genetics, there are also imaging research efforts trying to redraw the boundaries between psychotic disorders. One pioneer study is from the Bipolar-SZ Network on Intermediate Phenotypes (B-SNIP) Consortium, Clementz et al. applied neurobiological measures among SZ, BD, and SAD and tried to regroup them into different "biotypes" rather than DSM catalogs (49). A selection of psychotic biomarkers and functional brain activity were collected in this study. Not only patients with psychosis but also their first-degree relatives and healthy controls were included. Clementz et al. then identified three "biotypes," which were also believed to be more heritable than their original DSM diagnoses. Sensorimotor reactivity and cognitive control distinguish three biotypes: biotype 1 patients showed serious impairment across sensorimotor reactivity and cognitive control; biotype 2 patients show only deficits in cognitive control; and biotype 3 patients seem to be the mildest in cognitive symptoms. The B-SNIP group has also been trying to find the factors that contribute to its biotyping; one attempt is using the flow–frequency fluctuations (ALFF/fALFF) across the SZ, BD, and SAD from the large B-SNIP family study (50). More recently, gray matter density was checked in these three biotypes, and the density loss followed the same order as cognitive decline: biotype 1 showed whole brain gray matter density loss, while type 2 showed largely overlapping results with type 1, and the largest effects were found in fronto-temporal circuits, parietal cortex, and cerebellum. The findings were much more localized and of less magnitude for type 1. Type 3 only showed small reductions in frontal, cingulate, and temporal regions despite their similar DSM diagnoses (51).

IMAGING GENETICS TO REFINE THE DIAGNOSIS

Imaging Genetics Linking Genetics, Intermediate Imaging, and Cognitive Phenotypes

There are hundreds of papers using imaging genetics method to study SZ in the past 10 years, but here, we will focus on the findings with relatively clear functional implications. First, we selected the genes that have been highlighted in SZ and cognitive functions and if there is more than one report implicating those genes. The details of included genes can be found in **Tables 1** and **2** under "Risk SNPs/allele" column. We then searched PubMed database using the terms: ["gene symbols"] (genes we selected) AND ["schizophrenia"] AND ["symptom" OR "cognition" OR "cognitive function"] AND ["MRI"]. Abstracts and main texts were assessed with the following inclusion/exclusion criteria. The inclusion criteria were the following: 1) publications between January 2000 and January 2017, 2) diagnosis of any psychiatric disorders or risk gene, 3) brain structure with volume, concentration, thickness, and surface area, 4) brain function including resting state or task, and 5) including modalities of gene, imaging, and behavior simultaneously. Exclusion criteria were the following: 1) publications including letters, short reports, and brief communication; 2) MRI scanning sequences other than T1, T2, or BOLD; 3) in functional studies, the association between genes, images, and behavior were not directly assessed; and 4) in structural studies, symptoms, cognition, or behavior was not evaluated and collected at the same time window as images were acquired. After excluding 7 studies, 24 studies remained in **Table 1** for functional studies. **Table 1** lists the selected functional papers, and we highlight findings below by symptom/cognitive domains and possible intermediate imaging phenotype. However, most of these imaging genetic studies were done in healthy risk allele carriers.

Working memory deficit is fundamental and critical in SZ. The most well-studied possible intermediate imaging phenotype was the connection abnormalities between dorsolateral prefrontal cortex and hippocampus (DLPFC-HC). ZNF804A (52, 55, 56) and CACNA1C (58) were associated with DLPFC-HC connection alteration. In the healthy controls, risk allele of ZNF804A was associated with the increased DLPFC-HC connection. COMT (60), regulator of G protein signaling 4 (RGS4) (61), and

TABLE 1 | Clinical/cognitive domain specific imaging genetic evidence and potential intermediate functional imaging phenotypes.

Clinical/ cognitive domains	Risk SNPs/ allele	Study	Population	Scan modality	Scanner type	Intermediate imaging phenotype	Specific cognitive task	Risk allele associated functional imaging phenotypes
Working Memory	ZNF804A rs1344706 (A)	Esslinger et al. (52)	HC (115)	BOLD fMRI	Siemens 3T	R DLPFC functional connectivity	N-back task	Increased DLPFC coupling with L hippocampus but decreased coupling within DLPFCs
		Esslinger et al. (53)	HC (111)	BOLD fMRI	Siemens 3T	R DLPFC functional connectivity	N-back task	Increased DLPFC coupling with bilateral hippocampus but decreased coupling within DLPFCs in n-back task
		Linden et al. (54)	HC (43)	BOLD fMRI	Philips 1.5T	Rostral R DLPFC activation	Memory task with Ekman face images	Decreased activation
		Paulus et al. (55)	HC (94)	BOLD fMRI	Siemens 3T	DLPFC functional connectivity	–	Increased DLPFC coupling with hippocampus formation
		Rasetti and Weinberger (56)	SZ (78), US (171) and HC (153)	BOLD fMRI	GE 3T	DLPFC functional connectivity	N-back task	Risk allele carriers' DLPFC "inefficiency" in the SZ and US group greater than HC
	CACNA1C rs1006737 (A)	Bigos et al. (57)	HC (131/316 in respective tasks)	BOLD fMRI	GE 3T	PFC activation	Emotional face task and n-back task	Increased regional activation
		Paulus et al. (58)	HC (94)	BOLD fMRI	Siemens 3T	DLPFC activation and functional connectivity	N-back task	Decreased task related activation and increased coupling between DLPFC and hippocampus
	ANK3 rs9804190 (C)	Roussos et al. (59)	HC (52)	BOLD fMRI	GE 1.5T	L IFG, L MFG activation	N-back task	Increased regional activation in L IFG and L MFG
	COMT Val158Met	Tan et al. (60)	HC (46)	BOLD fMRI	GE 3T	DLPFC to striatal effective connectivity	Event-related working memory task	Increased DLPFC parietal 'excitatory' effective connectivity in Met-carriers
	RGS4 rs951436 (A)	Buckholtz et al. (61)	HC (94)	BOLD fMRI	Siemens 1.5T	R VLPFC connectivity	N-back task	Decreased right VLPFC connectivity to DLPFC and parietal cortex
	COMT X GRM3 epistasis	Tan et al. (62)	HC (29)	BOLD fMRI	GE 3T	DLPFC, VLPFC activation and functional connectivity	N-back task	Inefficient PFC engagement and altered PFC-parietal coupling with COMT Val/Val and GRM3 AA/G
	NRGN rs12807809 (T)	Rose et al. (63)	HC (52)	BOLD fMRI	Philips 3T	Activation in frontal lobe	Block design spatial working memory task	A load-independent decrease in left superior frontal gyrus during task
Episodic memory	CACNA1C rs1006737 (A)	Erk et al. (64)	HC (50)	BOLD fMRI	Siemens 3T	Activation in hippocampus and functional connectivity	3 consecutive memory tasks including coding, recall and face-profession pairs	Decreased activation in hippocampus and various brain regions, and decreased bilateral hippocampus connectivity
		Krug et al. (65)	HC (205)	BOLD fMRI	Siemens 3T	Hippocampus activation	Memory encoding and retrieval task	Decreased activation in hippocampus during task
		Erk et al. (66)	US (188)	BOLD fMRI	Siemens 3T	Activation in hippocampus, DLPFC and functional connectivity	Memory encoding and retrieval task	Replication to previous and decreased activation in DLPFC associated with genetic risk score
	NRGN rs12807809 (T)	Krug et al. (67)	HC (94)	BOLD fMRI	Siemens 3T	Activation in various regions	Memory encoding and retrieval task	Increased activation in L lingual gyrus, ACC and Inhibited deactivation in L precentral gyrus, and L insula during task

TABLE 1 | Continued

Clinical/ cognitive domains	Risk SNPs/ allele	Study	Population	Scan modality	Scanner type	Intermediate imaging phenotype	Specific cognitive task	Risk allele associated functional imaging phenotypes
Cognitive control/attention	ZNF804A rs1344706 (A)	Thurin et al. (68)	HC (208)	BOLD fMRI	GE 3T	DLPFC and ACC activation and effective connectivity	Modified Flanker task	Decreased PPI connection between DLPFC and ACC
	CACNA1C rs1006737 (A)	Thimm et al. (69)	HC (80)	BOLD fMRI	Siemens 3T	Activation in parietal and frontal lobes	Attention network test including: alerting, orienting and executive control	Decreased activation in R inferior parietal lobule and MFG
	NOS1 rs3782206 (T)	Zhang et al. (70)	HC (78)	BOLD fMRI	Siemens 3T	Activation in R IFG and coupling of DLPFC	N-back task and stroop task	Decreased activation in R IFG and reduced connectivity between IFG and DLPFC
Emotion	ZNF804A rs1344706 (A)	Esslinger et al. (52)	HC (115)	BOLD fMRI	Siemens 3T	Functional connectivity of R amygdala	N-back task	Increased functional connectivity between R amygdala and numerous brain regions
	CACNA1C rs1006737 (A)	Bigos et al. (57)	HC (116/131 in respective tasks)	BOLD fMRI	GE 3T	Activation in hippocampus	Emotional memory task, emotional face task	Increased activation in bilateral hippocampus during emotion memory task
	COMT Val158Met	Drabant et al. (71)	HC (101)	BOLD fMRI	GE 3T	Activation in hippocampus and VLPFC	Corticolimbic reactivity task	Increased hippocampus and VLPFC activation and in met/met there was increased limbic and prefrontal regions coupling during emotional face task
	DRD2 rs1076560 (G)	Blasi et al. (72)	HC (24)	BOLD fMRI	GE 3T	Activation and functional connectivity of amygdala and DLPFC	Facial expression task	Increased activation in both regions, and coupling of both of them associated with emotion control scores
	MIR137 rs1625579(T)	Mothersill et al. (73)	HC (98)	BOLD fMRI	Philips 3T	Fronto-amygdala functional connectivity	Face processing task	Increased amygdala connectivity with various regions in frontal lobe
Theory of mind	ZNF804A rs1344706 (A)	Walter et al. (74)	HC (109)	BOLD fMRI	Siemens 3T	Functional connectivity of DLPFC and activation	A theory of mind task judging picture to picture changes	Decreased activation in various brain regions and increased functional connectivity between DLPFC and R precentral gyrus, medial temporal gyrus and L lingual gyrus
		Mohnke et al. (75)	HC (188)	BOLD fMRI	Siemens 3T	Functional connectivity of left temporal parietal junction	Theory of mind task same as above	Increased functional connectivity between left temporal parietal junction and various brain regions

The phenotypic changes in last column corresponds to the risk allele. ACC, anterior cingulate cortex; BOLD fMRI, blood-oxygen-level dependent functional magnetic resonance imaging; DLPFC, dorsolateral prefrontal cortex; HC, healthy controls; IFG, inferior frontal gyrus; L, left; MFG, medial frontal gyrus; PFC, prefrontal cortex; R, right; SZ, schizophrenia; US, unaffected siblings; VLPFC, ventrolateral prefrontal cortex.

TABLE 2 | Potential structural imaging genetic phenotypes and possible function association.

Genetic factors	SNPs and risk allele	Study	Population	Scan modality	Scanner type	Imaging phenotype associated with risk allele	Function/symptom implication
ANK3	rs1938526 and rs10994336	Cassidy et al. (76)	First-episode psychosis patients (82)	T1	Siemens 1.5T	Widespread cortical thinning	General cognitive impairment
APOE	e4	Hata et al. (77)	SZ (21)	T1	GE 1.5T	Trend of reduce R hippocampal volume	Memory and cognitive function
BDNF	Val66Met(Met)	Ho et al. (78)	HC (80) and SZ (183)	T1, proton density and T2	GE 1.5T	Reduced hippocampal, temporal and occipital grey matter	Hallucinations. Impaired cognitive functions including working memory, episodic memory and etc.
		Pezawas et al. (79)	HC (214)	T1	GE 1.5T	Reduced hippocampal and prefrontal grey matter volume	Memory, learning, executive function and attention
		Bueller et al. (80)	HC (36)	T1	GE 1.5T	Reduced hippocampal grey matter volume	Emotional reactivity traits and episodic memory
		Aas et al. (81)	Schizophrenia spectrum disorders (48), BD (58), and MDD (3)	T1	Siemens 1.5T	Reduced hippocampal volume	Impaired cognitive functions including working memory and episodic memory
		Carballedo et al. (82)	MDD (62) and HC (71)	T1	Philips 3T	Reduced hippocampal volumes	Met carriers were in line with MDD patients (smaller hippocampal volume)
		Gatt et al. (83)	HC (89)	T1	Siemens 1.5T	Reduced hippocampal and prefrontal volumes	Impaired working memory, depression and anxiety traits
		Gerritsen et al. (84)	HC (275 for 1.5T and 293 for 3T)	T1	Siemens 1.5T and 3T	Reduced anterior cingulate volume	Sensitive to childhood adversity
		Nemoto et al. (85)	HC (109)	T1	Siemens 1.5T	Reduced DLPFC volume	DLPFC reduction related to age and gender
CACNA1C	rs1006737(A)	Wang et al. (86)	HC (55)	T1 and BOLD fMRI	Siemens 3T	Greater gray matter volume in cortico-limbic fronto-temporal region	Decrease functional connectivities from altered structural regions observed during emotion tasks
		Cerasa et al. (87)	HC (57)	T1	GE 1.5T	Increased hippocampal volumes	Executive cognition
COMT	Val158	Honea et al. (88)	HC (151)	T1	GE 1.5T	Reduced hippocampal and DLPFC gray matter volume	Nonlinear dependence of prefrontal neurons on extracellular dopamine
		Mechelli et al. (89)	HC (50)	T1 and BOLD fMRI	GE 3T	Reduced hippocampal volume and decreased activation of parahippocampal gyrus during facial expressions	Emotional processing
		Taylor et al. (90)	HC (31)	T1	GE 1.5T	Reduced temporal lobe and hippocampal volumes	Memory and emotional processing
		McIntosh et al. (91)	SZ (11), High risk subjects (67) and HC (15)	T1 and BOLD fMRI	Siemens 1T	Reduced ACC grey matter volume and increased activation in L PFC and PCC	Increasing sentence difficulty
		Ohnishi et al. (92)	SZ (47) and HC (76)	T1	Siemens 1.5T	Reduced L ACC and R MTG grey matter volume	Mental efforts, working memory, etc.
		Ho et al. (93)	SZ (159) and HC (84)	T1	GE 1.5T and PET	Negative in MRI, but higher frontal lobe activation in performing the one-back task	Working memory and executive function
DISC1	Ser704Cys (Cys)	Gruber et al. (94)	SZ (30) and non-affected family members (52)	T1	Siemens 1.5T	Reduced hippocampal volume	Grey matter reduction shared in family structure

TABLE 2 | Continued

Genetic factors	SNPs and risk allele	Study	Population	Scan modality	Scanner type	Imaging phenotype associated with risk allele	Function/symptom implication
NRG1	HAP_{ICE}	Tosato et al. (95)	SZ (27)	T1	Siemens 1.5T	Reduced superior temporal gyrus volume	Implications of the language disturbances
		Addington et al. (96)	Childhood onset SZ (78) and HC (165)	T1	GE 1.5T	Risk allele carriers have greater total grey matter and white matter volume in childhood and a steeper rate of subsequent decline in volume into adolescence.	Genetic effects in various cognitive and social function development
ZNF804A	rs1344706 (A)	Lencz et al. (97)	HC (39)	T1	GE 1.5T	Larger total white matter volumes and reduced grey matter volumes in angular gyrus, parahippocampal gyrus, posterior cingulate, and medial orbitofrontal gyrus	Risk allele carrier showed worse visuomotor performance task
		Donohoe et al. (98)	SZ (70) and HC (38)	T1	Siemens 1.5T	Larger hippocampal volumes in patients Larger white matter volume in total, frontal and parietal lobe.	No genetic effects were found in the measures of positive, negative or general symptom severity
		Wassink et al. (99)	Schizophrenia spectrum disorders (306) and HC (198)	T1	GE 1.5T	Reduced L superior temporal gyrus volume with higher PRS for SZ	Risk allele carriers also showed severer psychotic symptoms including hallucination and delusion
Polygenic Risk		Ohi et al. (100)	SZ (160) and HC (378)	T1	GE 1.5T		Contributing SNPs located in genes involved in developmental delay and cognitive impairment
		Terwisscha et al. (101)	SZ (152) and HC (142)	T1	Philips 1.5T	Reduced whole brain white matter volume with higher PRS for SZ	SNPs located in neuronal functions are associated with white matter reduction
		Harrisberger et al. (102)	At-risk mental state (43) and first episode psychosis (36)	T1	Siemens 3T	Reduced hippocampal volumes with higher PRS for SZ	First episode psychosis patients have higher genetic risk than the at-risk mental state participants

The phenotypic changes in last column corresponds to the risk allele. ACC, anterior cingulate cortex; BOLD fMRI, blood-oxygen-level-dependent functional magnetic resonance imaging; DLPFC, dorsolateral prefrontal cortex; HC, healthy controls; L, left; MFG, medial frontal gyrus; MTG, middle temporal gyrus; PET, positron emission tomography; PFC, prefrontal cortex; PRS, polygenic risk score; R, right; SNP, single nucleotide polymorphism; SZ, schizophrenia.

COMT X glutamate metabotropic receptor 3 (GRM3) epistasis were connected to prefrontal cortex-parietal coupling.

Episodic memory or long-term memory was also often disturbed in SZ. Possible intermediate imaging phenotypes included decreased coupling of the hippocampus–parietal cortex, hippocampus and ventrolateral prefrontal cortex (VLPFC), and bilateral hippocampus. However, the genetic association within this thread is elusive (46). In healthy controls, CACNA1C risk allele carriers showed the decreased activation during recall in decreased coupling between bilateral hippocampus (64). The NRGN rs12807809 was found with increased activation in the left lingual gyrus and decreased deactivation in the left precentral gyrus, cingulate, and left insula during the different stages of memory retrieval (67).

SZ patients often show attention or cognitive control deficits. Disturbances in PFC and DLPFC and connection alterations were the most important issue regarding this deficit. NOS1 risk allele carriers showed reduced inferior frontal gyrus and DLPFC connection associated with attention performance (103). For other risk genes, CACNA1C risk allele carriers showed decreased activation in the right inferior parietal lobule and medial frontal gyrus during an attention task (69). Again, ZNF804A showed association with the anterior cingulate cortex (ACC) and DLPFC coupling during attention and cognitive control (68). During emotional memory, SZ CACNA1C risk allele carriers showed increased activation in the bilateral hippocampus, which was in line with finding in BD (57).

Emotion processing is another important disruption common in SZ. ZNF804A (52) and DRD2 (72) have shown correlation with the amygdala and ACC/medial prefrontal cortex (mPFC) within emotion processing. Increased connectivity between amygdala and VLPFC, which was considered as another intermediate imaging phenotype for emotion processing, has been found in healthy risk allele carriers of the COMT (71) and MIR137 (73).

As part of social cognition that is often impaired in SZ, the theory of mind capabilities tends to help people understand mental states of themselves and others. ZNF804A risk alleles correlated with the PFC and various cortical regions in social information processes (74). Decreased activation in bilateral dorsal medial PFC, the left temporoparietal cortex, left inferior parietal cortex, posterior cingulate, and the left lateral PFC was found while investigating ZNF804A (74). There was also a trend for increased functional connectivity of the left temporal parietal junction with several regions (75).

Rather than a localized abnormality, most findings are notably in line with a "disconnection disorder" (104). Additionally, as noted above, these genes are not specific to risk for schizophrenia but show risk as well for other psychiatric disorders; the common functional impairments showing the genetic relationship in SZ and BD tend to be closely associated with connection disturbances and involve multiple brain regions (46, 105, 106).

Structural Brain Imaging Genetics Findings in SZ

It is more difficult for researchers to relate risk gene factors, brain structural alteration, and symptoms or cognitive impairments; large numbers of these structural brain imaging genetic studies have conflicting results (10). We reviewed structural brain imaging studies with the relatively clear and consistent symptom or cognitive implications following the criteria we described above. Note that only research involving genetics, structural brain, symptoms, or cognitions and the analysis between them were included. After excluding 8 studies, 27 structural studies remained (see **Table 2**).

Some genes like BDNF are engaged in many cognitive domains that are commonly impaired in SZ, although their associations with SZ *per se* may not be strong. BDNF is essential in nervous system development and prevention of cell loss in various brain regions including the hippocampus, striatum, and more. The Val66Met has been found to be related with reduced hippocampal (107), temporal (78), and frontal volume (80), which may affect various cognitive functions including working memory, episodic memory, executive function, and hallucinations. Its interaction with early life abuse may also result in reduced hippocampal volume in SZ, BD, and MDD (81, 82). As the disease progresses, BDNF is found to be connected with reduced frontal volume and impaired executive function (85, 108).

Other genes may have a closer relationship with SZ, but their imaging genetic findings with brain regions and clinical phenotypes are less consistent. COMT may be involved not only in reduced hippocampal volume but also in reduced cingulate and DLPFC volume, which may potentially affect memory, attention, and executive function (87, 91). Risk allele carriers with rs1006737(A) in CACNA1C show greater gray matter volume in a cortico-limbic and fronto-temporal region but generally in BD (86). The neuregulin 1 gene (NRG1) and its risk haplotype may also contribute to the hippocampal and temporal volume (95, 109). Other critical genes including ANK3 (76), Apoe (77), DISC 1 (110), and ZNF804A (97–99) and more have been found connected to reduced brain volume in hippocampus, cingulate, frontal, temporal, and various brain region volume, suggesting their role in SZ-related cognitive impairment and symptoms.

Polygenic risk score studies also provide imaging genetic evidence for SZ imaging genetic. Temporal volume (100), whole brain white matter volume (101), and hippocampal volume abnormality (102) have been suggested through these approaches.

Overall, the genetic influence on brain structure are widely spread, and their functional or clinical implications are complex. At the moment, the gene to the brain and behavior/symptom links are extensive, affecting many cognitive domains when tested in nonaffected individuals. The specificity of genetic effects on SZ need to be carefully examined, and uncovering better methods to form a link from imaging genetics to clinical phenotypes is important to contribute to the diagnostic issue.

LIMITATIONS AND FUTURE DIRECTIONS

Imaging genetics has contributed greatly to our understanding of the biological mechanism behind psychiatric disorders by revealing the potential association between genetics and imaging phenotypes. The merging boundaries between disorders and subtypes within SZ revealed by imaging genetics will continue to shape the future diagnostic approach of psychiatric disorders. However, it also has inevitable limitations, and the pathways linking genetics, neuroimaging intermediate phenotypes, and clinically assessable phenotypes remain far from clear. A diagnostic system built on imaging genetics requires further research efforts.

Limitations

Typically, the effect size of candidate gene analyses is rather small and explains limited brain structural or functional variations (111). Alternatively, large sample imaging genetics research often report encouraging findings supporting vast common variations influence on the human brain (112).

However, these findings and even the logic behind imaging genetics has been questioned. Franke et al. mega-analyzed the largest GWAS data for SZ to date from PGC (33,636 cases and 43,008 controls) and eight structural MRI brain measures from ENIGMA (11,840 individuals) to evaluate the relationship between the common variations and SZ-associated subcortical brain regions (113). For instance, the hippocampal volume deficit was thought fundamental in SZ (114). The hippocampus deficits in SZ are one of the most reliable findings of volumetric deficits (44). The ENIGMA analysis identified common genetic variations related to hippocampal volume without regard to disorder (112); the PGC identified common genetic variations highlighted by 108 loci from GWAS, which were thought to play important roles in the etiology of SZ without regard to hippocampal volume (16). Franke et al. did several analyses to investigate the correlation between these genetic and imaging findings. They used linkage disequilibrium score regression to estimate the SNP-based heritability of volumetric measures, computed and compared genetic predisposition scores to volumes, and quantified rank–rank hypergeometric overlap test and listed genetic variants influencing the brain volume. Unfortunately, all these analyses reported no significant results. They also analyzed the 128 index SNPs from PGC and their association with brain volume including the hippocampus, meta-analyses, conjunction analysis and compare the genetic effect sizes for SZ and volumes. Again, these analyses resulted in nonsignificant findings.

Although Franke et al. emphasized that there were several limitations that may result in this null finding, it strongly reminded us to think carefully about the logic of imaging genetics. Brain measures or structural brain deficits believed to be important pathological alterations of SZ may not be induced by those primary genetic causes of SZ as a diagnostic category. They may be reflecting prenatal and later development environmental effects that correlate with but are not specific to SZ, or the diagnostic category of SZ may not be uniformly organized so the large-scale studies of disease risk may have introduced too many heterogeneities.

Instead, the field must consider whether brain volume is a good bridge to look into the genetic influence on disorders. The idea of "intermediate phenotype" succeeded the idea of endophenotype, which was first used by Gottesman and Shields (115). Either structural or functional imaging was believed to be good intermediate phenotypes, as they provide a large amount of data that can show the effect of genes. Although many imaging genetics studies used the concept of intermediate phenotypes to conduct the hypothesis and research flow, they did not fully meet the criteria of intermediate phenotype. To fulfill the criteria, the phenotype must have the following: good psychometric properties, disorder and symptoms related in general population, stable over time, increased expression in unaffected relatives, cosegregation in families, and common genetic influences shown in the disorder. We have to verify whether a chosen brain measure meets each of these criteria.

Hippocampal volumes, in particular, did seem to fulfill these criteria, in that the volumes were more similar in unaffected siblings (116, 117), seemed to decrease with younger disease onset (118), and the smaller volumes were a strong effect in comparing SZ and controls (119). The other brain regions especially caudate and putamen, which showed a small effect size in ENIGMA, would also need to pass these criteria if they are to be used as intermediate phenotypes. However, these brain volume alterations may not be specific to SZ. As for hippocampal volume among psychiatric disorders, it is also affected in MDD (120, 121), obsessive–compulsive disorder (122), and attention deficit hyperactivity disorder (123). Other than psychiatric disorders, cardiovascular disease, diabetes, hypertension, obesity, physical activity, and various somatic factors may also play a role in modifying hippocampal volume to different extents (124, 125). The hippocampus is vulnerable to various environmental factors from the prenatal stage throughout the lifetime, which makes the hippocampal structure sensitive to neurodisruption but not necessarily specific to SZ (126). The specificity of these altered brain volume will need careful examination before being considered as part of SZ's pathology in complicated clinical situations.

Another approach is to reconsider other imaging intermediate phenotypes bridging genetics and SZ. For example, there are various anatomic measures other than volumes that should be assessed for genetic effects (127, 128). Gray/white matter density, cortical thickness, cortical folding, cortical surface area, and white matter integrity are potential useful intermediate phenotypes from which to choose. However, although it may also be difficult to fully grasp, the functional implication of these brain measures and their compatibility with genetics will need further investigation (129). As for these other brain volumes and functional measurements, their stability, situation in unaffected relatives, families, and general population will need to be further investigated to answer the criteria question as well as their specificity to the diagnosis or clinical subgrouping.

It may be helpful to expand the genetic modality of imaging genetic study. More heritability could be captured by involving rare variance and chromosome structural variations like CNVs (38). Both options will need better imaging genetic analysis methods and models.

Future Directions

The current review summarized genetics, imaging, and imaging genetics in schizophrenia to date. Imaging genetics may continue to shape the future conceptualization of SZ and psychotic disorders in both clinical and research field.

One future direction is collecting a large number of genetic effects. The method applied by Arnedo et al. is promising in coupling both genetic and phenotypic clusters, but it may need to establish its association with imaging data or physiological measures. The clustering method shows great complexity, while its compatibility with neuroimaging is unknown. The other polygenic method like polygenic risk score is also promising. However, it will call for more common variations and the combination with other data (e.g., the B-SNIP biotype study).

Parallel independent component analysis (pICA) may be another useful tool in this field. This method allows independent components from two modalities to be identified simultaneously, and the association between these two modalities is optimized. pICA is designed to be totally theoretically blind and data-driven, but pICA with reference allows *a priori* knowledge as the reference to improve robustness. For instance, a set of genes from the same pathway can be used as a reference to highlight their effect on certain brain components as well as behavioral data (130). Chen et al. used pICA and reported that the gray matter density of frontal, precuneus, and cingulate regions might potentially be affected by various genes participating in synaptic plasticity, axon guidance, and molecular signal transduction (131).

Another possible direction is refining the clinical assessment tools to better complement imaging genetics. As raised in the B-SNIP study, a series of symptom rating scales including the Global Assessment of Functioning scale, the Positive and Negative Syndrome Scale, the Young Mania Rating Scale, the Montgomery–Åsberg Depression Rating Scale, the Schizo-Bipolar Scale, and the Birchwood Social Functioning Scale were obtained from the participants. These measures were not able to distinguish SZ, BD, and SAD significantly or contribute much in the building of biotypes (132). Imaging genetic compatible comprehensive symptom scales are needed. These scales are not aiming at distinguishing traditional diagnostic groups or a certain diagnostic group usage. However, they would provide comprehensive clinical profiles "scanning" the symptom domains (2). Some scales like the Symptom Checklist-90 (SCL-90) and its revised version (133) might be worth trying (134). More detailed multidimensional symptoms reflecting scale need to be developed to fit the need of imaging genetics and clarify the path linking genotypic variation, intermediate brain imaging, and clinical phenotypes.

Finally, future research will need to be enhanced by improving power and replicability. Studies with small number of subjects (below 100 participants) will be able to show moderate power with effect size of 0.5. However, it is critical to replicate them independently with same genetic variants, imaging, and behavioral measurements, and direction of the effects by Carter et al. (135). It is also argued, in such studies, null results or conflicting associations with failed replication should still be considered for publications as potentially informative or innovative studies (6, 136). In this case, meta-analytic studies addressing the conflicted results and the issues of publication bias will help to avoid the misleading information potentially generated from small sample research results (6, 137).

AUTHOR CONTRIBUTIONS

All authors listed have made substantial, direct, and intellectual contribution to the work and approved it for publication.

FUNDING

WJ and JT were supported in this work by a grant from the National Institute of Mental Health (R01 MH094524).

REFERENCES

Lawrie SM, O'Donovan MC, Saks E, Burns T, Lieberman JA. Towards diagnostic markers for the psychoses. *Lancet Psychiatry* (2016) 3(4):375–85. doi: 10.1016/S2215-0366(16)00021-3

Bhati MT. Defining psychosis: the evolution of DSM-5 schizophrenia spectrum disorders. *Curr Psychiatry Rep* (2013) 15(11):409. doi: 10.1007/ s11920-013-0409-9

Turner JA, Smyth P, Macciardi F, Fallon JH, Kennedy JL, Potkin SG. Imaging phenotypes and genotypes in schizophrenia. *Neuroinformatics* (2006) 4(1):21–49. doi: 10.1385/NI:4:1:21

Bigos KL, Weinberger DR. Imaging genetics—days of future past. *NeuroImage* (2010) 53(3):804–9. doi: 10.1016/j.neuroimage.2010.01.035

Lawrie SM, O'Donovan MC, Saks E, Burns T, Lieberman JA. Improving classification of psychoses. *Lancet Psychiatry* (2016) 3(4):367–74. doi: 10.1016/S2215-0366(15)00577-5

Bogdan R, Salmeron BJ, Carey CE, Agrawal A, Calhoun VD, Garavan H, et al. Imaging genetics and genomics in psychiatry: a critical review of progress and potential. *Biol Psychiatry* (2017) 82(3):165–75. doi: 10.1016/j. biopsych.2016.12.030

Hashimoto R, Ohi K, Yamamori H, Yasuda Y, Fujimoto M, Umeda-Yano S, et al. Imaging genetics and psychiatric disorders. *Curr Mol Med* (2015) 15(2):168–75. doi: 10.2174/1566524015666150303104159

Fan CC, Smeland OB, Schork AJ, Chen CH, Holland D, Lo MT, et al. Beyond heritability: improving discoverability in imaging genetics. *Hum Mol Genet* (2018) 27(R1):R22–R28. doi: 10.1093/hmg/ddy082

Palaniyappan L, Maayan N, Bergman H, Davenport C, Adams CE, Soares-Weiser K. Voxel-based morphometry for separation of schizophrenia from other types of psychosis in first episode psychosis. *Cochrane Database Syst Rev* (2015) (8), CD011021. doi: 10.1002/14651858.CD011021. pub2

van Haren NE, Bakker SC, Kahn RS. Genes and structural brain imaging in schizophrenia. *Curr Opin Psychiatry* (2008) 21(2):161–7. doi: 10.1097/ YCO.0b013e3282f4f25b

Nenadic I, Gaser C, Sauer H. Heterogeneity of brain structural variation and the structural imaging endophenotypes in schizophrenia. *Neuropsychobiology* (2012) 66(1):44–9. doi: 10.1159/000338547

Feighner JP, Robins E, Guze SB, Woodruff RA, Jr., Winokur G, Munoz R. Diagnostic criteria for use in psychiatric research. *Arch Gen Psychiatry* (1972) 26(1):57–63. doi: 10.1001/archpsyc.1972.01750190059011

Gershon ES, Grennan KS. Genetic and genomic analyses as a basis for new diagnostic nosologies. *Dialog Clin Neurosci* (2015) 17(1):69–78.

Cross-Disorder Group of the Psychiatric Genomics C, Lee SH, Ripke S, Neale BM, Faraone SV, Purcell SM, et al. Genetic relationship between five psychiatric disorders estimated from genome-wide SNPs. *Nat Genet* (2013) 45(9):984–94. doi: 10.1038/ng.2711

Sullivan PF, Kendler KS, Neale MC. Schizophrenia as a complex trait: evidence from a meta-analysis of twin studies. *Arch Gen Psychiatry* (2003) 60(12):1187–92. doi: 10.1001/archpsyc.60.12.1187

Schizophrenia Working Group of the Psychiatric Genomics C. Biological insights from 108 schizophrenia-associated genetic loci. *Nature* (2014) 511(7510):421–7. doi: 10.1038/nature13595

Schwab SG, Wildenauer DB. Genetics of psychiatric disorders in the GWAS era: an update on schizophrenia. *Eur Arch Psychiatry Clin Neurosci* (2013) 263 Suppl 2:S147–154. doi: 10.1007/s00406-013-0450-z

O'Donovan MC, Craddock N, Norton N, Williams H, Peirce T, Moskvina V, et al. Identification of loci associated with schizophrenia by genome-wide association and follow-up. *Nat Genet* (2008) 40(9):1053–5.

Guan J, Cai JJ, Ji G, Sham PC. Commonality in dysregulated expression of gene sets in cortical brains of individuals with autism, schizophrenia, and bipolar disorder. *Transl Psychiatry* (2019) 9(1):152. doi: 10.1038/ s41398-019-0488-4

Musliner KL, Mortensen PB, McGrath JJ, Suppli NP, Hougaard DM, Bybjerg-Grauholm J, et al. Association of polygenic liabilities for major depression, bipolar disorder, and schizophrenia with risk for depression in the danish population. *JAMA Psychiatry* (2019) 76(5):516–25. doi: 10.1001/ jamapsychiatry.2018.4166

Smeland OB, Bahrami S, Frei O, et al. Genome-wide analysis reveals extensive genetic overlap between schizophrenia, bipolar disorder, and intelligence. *Mol Psychiatry* (2019) . doi: 10.1038/s41380-018-0332-x

Markota M, Coombes BJ, Larrabee BR, McElroy SL, Bond DJ, Veldic M, et al. Association of schizophrenia polygenic risk score with manic and depressive psychosis in bipolar disorder. *Transl Psychiatry* (2018) 8(1):188. doi: 10.1038/ s41398-018-0242-3

Gandal MJ, Haney JR, Parikshak NN, Leppa V, Ramaswami G, Hartl C, et al. Shared molecular neuropathology across major psychiatric disorders parallels polygenic overlap. *Science* (2018) 359(6376):693–7. doi: 10.1126/ science.aad6469

Khanzada NS, Butler MG, Manzardo AM. GeneAnalytics pathway analysis and genetic overlap among autism spectrum disorder, bipolar disorder and schizophrenia. *Int J Mol Sci* (2017) 18(3):527. doi: 10.3390/ijms18030527

Forstner AJ, Hecker J, Hofmann A, Maaser A, Reinbold CS, Muhleisen TW, et al. Identification of shared risk loci and pathways for bipolar disorder and schizophrenia. *PloS one* (2017) 12(2):e0171595.

Lichtenstein P, Yip BH, Björk C, Pawitan Y, Cannon TD, Sullivan PF, et al. Common genetic determinants of schizophrenia and bipolar disorder in Swedish families: a population-based study. *Lancet* (2009) 373(9659):234–9. doi: 10.1016/S0140-6736(09)60072-6

Cardno AG, Owen MJ. Genetic relationships between schizophrenia, bipolar disorder, and schizoaffective disorder. *Schizophr Bull* (2014) 40(3):504–15. doi: 10.1093/schbul/sbu016

Kotov R, Leong SH, Mojtabai R, Erlanger AC, Fochtmann LJ, Constantino E, et al. Boundaries of schizoaffective disorder: revisiting Kraepelin. *JAMA Psychiatry* (2013) 70(12):1276–86. doi: 10.1001/jamapsychiatry.2013.2350

Williams HJ, Norton N, Dwyer S, Moskvina V, Nikolov I, Carroll L, et al. Fine mapping of ZNF804A and genome-wide significant evidence for its involvement in schizophrenia and bipolar disorder. *Mol Psychiatry* (2011) 16(4):429–41. doi: 10.1038/mp.2011.21

Schizophrenia Psychiatric Genome-Wide Association Study C. Genome- wide association study identifies five new schizophrenia loci. *Nat Genet* (2011) 43(10):969–76. doi: 10.1038/ng.940

Sullivan PF, Daly MJ, O'Donovan M. Genetic architectures of psychiatric disorders: the emerging picture and its implications. *Nat Rev Genet* (2012) 13(8):537–51. doi: 10.1038/nrg3240

Andreassen OA, Thompson WK, Schork AJ, Ripke S, Mattingsdal M, Kelsoe JR, et al. Improved detection of common variants associated with schizophrenia and bipolar disorder using pleiotropy-informed conditional false discovery rate. *PLoS Genet* (2013) 9(4):e1003455.

Cross-Disorder Group of the Psychiatric Genomics C. Identification of risk loci with shared effects on five major psychiatric disorders: a genome-wide analysis. *Lancet* (2013) 381(9875):1371–9. doi: 10.1016/ S0140-6736(12)62129-1

Duncan LE, Ratanatharathorn A, Aiello AE, Almli LM, Amstadter AB, Ashley-Koch AE, et al. Largest GWAS of PTSD (N = 20 070) yields genetic overlap with schizophrenia and sex differences in heritability. *Mol Psychiatry* (2018) 23(3):666–73.

St Pourcain B, Robinson EB, Anttila V, Sullivan BB, Maller J, Golding J, et al. ASD and schizophrenia show distinct developmental profiles in common genetic overlap with population-based social communication difficulties. *Mol Psychiatry* (2018) 23(2):263–70. doi: 10.1038/mp.2016.198

Maier R, Moser G, Chen GB, Ripke S, Cross-Disorder Working Group of the Psychiatric Genomics C, Coryell W, et al. Joint analysis of psychiatric disorders increases accuracy of risk prediction for schizophrenia, bipolar disorder, and major depressive disorder. *Am J Human Genet* (2015) 96(2):283–94.

Lee KW, Woon PS, Teo YY, Sim K. Genome wide association studies (GWAS) and copy number variation (CNV) studies of the major psychoses: what have we learnt? *Neurosci Biobehav Rev* (2012) 36(1):556–71. doi: 10.1016/j. neubiorev.2011.09.001

Warland A, Kendall KM, Rees E, Kirov G, Caseras X. Schizophrenia- associated genomic copy number variants and subcortical brain volumes in the UK Biobank. *Mol Psychiatry* (2019). doi: 10.1038/s41380-019-0355-y

Arnedo J, Svrakic DM, Del Val C, Romero-Zaliz R, Hernandez-Cuervo H, Molecular Genetics of Schizophrenia C, et al. Uncovering the hidden risk architecture of the schizophrenias: confirmation in three independent genome-wide association studies. *Am J Psychiatry* (2015) 172(2):139–53. doi: 10.1176/appi.ajp.2014.14040435

Karlsgodt KH, Sun D, Cannon TD. Structural and functional brain abnormalities in schizophrenia. *Curr Dir Psychol Sci* (2010) 19(4):226–31. doi: 10.1177/0963721410377601

Dazzan P, Arango C, Fleischacker W, Galderisi S, Glenthoj B, Leucht S, et al. Magnetic resonance imaging and the prediction of outcome in first- episode schizophrenia: a review of current evidence and directions for future research. *Schizophr Bull* (2015) 41(3):574–83. doi: 10.1093/schbul/sbv024

Pearlson GD, Marsh L. Structural brain imaging in schizophrenia: a selective review. *Biol Psychiatry* (1999) 46(5):627–49. doi: 10.1016/ S0006-3223(99)00071-2

Dietsche B, Kircher T, Falkenberg I. Structural brain changes in schizophrenia at different stages of the illness: a selective review of longitudinal magnetic resonance imaging studies. *Aust N Z J Psychiatry* (2017) 51(5):500–8. doi: 10.1177/0004867417699473

van Erp TG, Hibar DP, Rasmussen JM, Glahn DC, Pearlson GD, Andreassen OA, et al. Subcortical brain volume abnormalities in 2028 individuals with schizophrenia and 2540 healthy controls *via the* ENIGMA consortium. *Mol Psychiatry* (2016) 21(4):547–53. doi: 10.1038/mp.2015.63

Shenton ME, Dickey CC, Frumin M, McCarley RW. A review of MRI findings in schizophrenia. *Schizophr Res* (2001) 49(1–2):1–52. doi: 10.1016/ S0920-9964(01)00163-3

Cao H, Dixson L, Meyer-Lindenberg A, Tost H. Functional connectivity measures as schizophrenia intermediate phenotypes: advances, limitations, and future directions. *Curr Opin Neurobiol* (2016) 36:7–14. doi: 10.1016/j. conb.2015.07.008

Isobe M, Miyata J, Hazama M, Fukuyama H, Murai T, Takahashi H. Multimodal neuroimaging as a window into the pathological physiology of schizophrenia: current trends and issues. *Neurosci Res* (2016) 102:29–38. doi: 10.1016/j.neures.2015.07.009

Schwarz E, Tost H, Meyer-Lindenberg A. Working memory genetics in schizophrenia and related disorders: an RDoC perspective. *Am J Med GenetPart B Neuropsychiatr Genet* (2016) 171B(1):121–31. doi: 10.1002/ ajmg.b.32353

Clementz BA, Sweeney JA, Hamm JP, Ivleva EI, Ethridge LE, Pearlson GD, et al. Identifi ation of distinct psychosis biotypes using brain-based biomarkers. *Am J Psychiatry* (2016) 173(4):373–84. doi: 10.1176/appi.ajp.2015.14091200

Meda SA, Wang Z, Ivleva EI, Poudyal G, Keshavan MS, Tamminga CA, et al. Frequency-specific neural signatures of spontaneous low-frequency resting state fluctuations in psychosis: evidence from Bipolar-Schizophrenia Network on Intermediate Phenotypes (B-SNIP) Consortium. *Schizophr Bull* (2015) 41(6):1336–48. doi: 10.1093/schbul/sbv064

Ivleva EI, Clementz BA, Dutcher AM, Arnold SJM, Jeon-Slaughter H, Aslan S, et al. Brain structure biomarkers in the psychosis biotypes: findings from the bipolar-schizophrenia network for intermediate phenotypes. *Biol Psychiatry* (2017) 82(1):26–39.

Rasetti R, Sambataro F, Chen Q, Callicott JH, Mattay VS, Weinberger DR. Neural mechanisms of a genome-wide supported psychosis variant. *Science* (2009) 324(5927):605. doi: 10.1126/science.1167768

Esslinger C, Kirsch P, Haddad L, Mier D, Sauer C, Erk S, et al. Cognitive state and connectivity effects of the genome-wide significant psychosis variant in ZNF804A. *NeuroImage* (2011) 54(3):2514–23.

Linden DE, Lancaster TM, Wolf C, Baird A, Jackson MC, Johnston SJ, et al. ZNF804A genotype modulates neural activity during working memory for faces. *Neuropsychobiology* (2013) 67(2):84–92.

Esslinger C, Walter H, Kirsch P, Erk S, Schnell K, Arnold C, et al. Partial support for ZNF804A genotype-dependent alterations in prefrontal connectivity. *Hum Brain Mapp* (2013) 34(2):304–13. doi: 10.1002/hbm.21434

Rasetti R, Sambataro F, Chen Q, Callicott JH, Mattay VS, Weinberger DR. Altered cortical network dynamics: a potential intermediate phenotype for schizophrenia and association with ZNF804A. *Arch Gen Psychiatry* (2011) 68(12):1207–17. doi: 10.1001/archgenpsychiatry.2011.103

Bigos KL, Mattay VS, Callicott JH, Straub RE, Vakkalanka R, Kolachana B, et al. Genetic variation in CACNA1C affects brain circuitries related to mental illness. *Arch Gen Psychiatry* (2010) 67(9):939–45. doi: 10.1001/archgenpsychiatry.2010.96

Paulus FM, Bedenbender J, Krach S, Pyka M, Krug A, Sommer J, et al. Association of rs1006737 in CACNA1C with alterations in prefrontal activation and fronto-hippocampal connectivity. *Hum Brain Mapp* (2014) 35(4):1190–200. doi: 10.1002/hbm.22244

Roussos P, Katsel P, Davis KL, Bitsios P, Giakoumaki SG, Jogia J, et al. Molecular and genetic evidence for abnormalities in the nodes of Ranvier in schizophrenia. *Arch Gen Psychiatry* (2012) 69(1):7–15.

Tan HY, Chen AG, Kolachana B, Apud JA, Mattay VS, Callicott JH, et al. Effective connectivity of AKT1-mediated dopaminergic working memory networks and pharmacogenetics of anti-dopaminergic treatment. *Brain: J Neurol* (2012) 135(Pt 5):1436–45. doi: 10.1093/brain/aws068

Buckholtz JW, Meyer-Lindenberg A, Honea RA, Straub RE, Pezawas L, Egan MF, et al. Allelic variation in RGS4 impacts functional and structural connectivity in the human brain. *J Neurosci* (2007) 27(7):1584–93. doi: 10.1523/JNEUROSCI.5112-06.2007

Tan HY, Chen Q, Sust S, Buckholtz JW, Meyers JD, Egan MF, et al. Epistasis between catechol-O-methyltransferase and type II metabotropic glutamate receptor 3 genes on working memory brain function. *Proc Natl Acad Sci U S A* (2007) 104(30):12536–41.

Rose EJ, Morris DW, Fahey C, Robertson IH, Greene C, O'Doherty J, et al. The effect of the neurogranin schizophrenia risk variant rs12807809 on brain structure and function. *Twin Res Hum Genet* (2012) 15(3):296–303.

Erk S, Meyer-Lindenberg A, Schnell K, Opitz von Boberfeld C, Esslinger C, Kirsch P, et al. Brain function in carriers of a genome-wide supported bipolar disorder variant. *Arch Gen Psychiatry* (2010) 67(8):803–11. doi: 10.1001/ archgenpsychiatry.2010.94

Krug A, Witt SH, Backes H, Dietsche B, Nieratschker V, Shah NJ, et al. A genome-wide supported variant in CACNA1C influences hippocampal activation during episodic memory encoding and retrieval. *Eur Arch Psychiatry Clin Neurosci* (2014) 264(2):103–10.

Erk S, Meyer-Lindenberg A, Schmierer P, Mohnke S, Grimm O, Garbusow M, et al. Hippocampal and frontolimbic function as intermediate phenotype for psychosis: evidence from healthy relatives and a common risk variant in CACNA1C. *Biol Psychiatry* (2014) 76(6):466–75.

Krug A, Krach S, Jansen A, Nieratschker V, Witt SH, Shah NJ, et al. The effect of neurogranin on neural correlates of episodic memory encoding and retrieval. *Schizophr Bull* (2013) 39(1):141–50. doi: 10.1093/schbul/ sbr076

Thurin K, Rasetti R, Sambataro F, Safrin M, Chen Q, Callicott JH, et al. Effects of ZNF804A on neurophysiologic measures of cognitive control. *Mol Psychiatry* (2013) 18(8):852–4. doi: 10.1038/mp.2012.134

Thimm M, Kircher T, Kellermann T, Markov V, Krach S, Jansen A, et al. Effects of a CACNA1C genotype on attention networks in healthy individuals. *Psychol Med* (2011) 41(7):1551–61. doi: 10.1017/S0033291710002217

Zhang Z, Chen X, Yu P, Zhang Q, Sun X, Gu H, et al. Evidence for the contribution of NOS1 gene polymorphism (rs3782206) to prefrontal function in schizophrenia patients and healthy controls. *Neuropsychopharmacology* (2015) 40(6):1383–94.

Drabant EM, Hariri AR, Meyer-Lindenberg A, Munoz KE, Mattay VS, Kolachana BS, et al. Catechol O-methyltransferase val158met genotype and neural mechanisms related to affective arousal and regulation. *Arch Gen Psychiatry* (2006) 63(12):1396–406. doi: 10.1001/archpsyc.63.12.1396

Blasi G, Lo Bianco L, Taurisano P, Gelao B, Romano R, Fazio L, et al. Functional variation of the dopamine D2 receptor gene is associated with emotional control as well as brain activity and connectivity during emotion processing in humans. *J Neurosci* (2009) 29(47):14812–9. doi: 10.1523/JNEUROSCI.3609-09.2009

Mothersill O, Morris DW, Kelly S, Rose EJ, Fahey C, O'Brien C, et al. Effects of MIR137 on fronto-amygdala functional connectivity. *NeuroImage* (2014) 90:189–95. doi: 10.1016/j.neuroimage.2013.12.019

Walter H, Schnell K, Erk S, Arnold C, Kirsch P, Esslinger C, et al. Effects of a genome-wide supported psychosis risk variant on neural activation during a theory-of-mind task. *Mol Psychiatry* (2011) 16(4):462–70. doi: 10.1038/mp.2010.18

Mohnke S, Erk S, Schnell K, Schutz C, Romanczuk-Seiferth N, Grimm O, et al. Further evidence for the impact of a genome-wide-supported psychosis risk variant in ZNF804A on the Theory of Mind Network. *Neuropsychopharmacology* (2014) 39(5):1196–205. doi: 10.1038/npp.2013.321

Cassidy C, Buchy L, Bodnar M, Dell'elce J, Choudhry Z, Fathalli F, et al. Association of a risk allele of ANK3 with cognitive performance and cortical thickness in patients with first-episode psychosis. *J Psychiatry Neurosci* (2014) 39(1):31–9. doi: 10.1503/jpn.120242

Hata T, Kunugi H, Nanko S, Fukuda R, Kaminaga T. Possible effect of the APOE epsilon 4 allele on the hippocampal volume and asymmetry in schizophrenia. *Am J Med Genet* (2002) 114(6):641–2. doi: 10.1002/ajmg.10556

Ho BC, Milev P, O'Leary DS, Librant A, Andreasen NC, Wassink TH. Cognitive and magnetic resonance imaging brain morphometric correlates of brain-derived neurotrophic factor Val66Met gene polymorphism in patients with schizophrenia and healthy volunteers. *Arch Gen Psychiatry* (2006) 63(7):731–40. doi: 10.1001/archpsyc.63.7.731

Pezawas L, Verchinski BA, Mattay VS, Callicott JH, Kolachana BS, Straub RE, et al. The brain-derived neurotrophic factor val66met polymorphism and variation in human cortical morphology. *J Neurosci* (2004) 24(45):10099–102.

Bueller JA, Aftab M, Sen S, Gomez-Hassan D, Burmeister M, Zubieta JK. BDNF Val66Met allele is associated with reduced hippocampal volume in healthy subjects. *Biol Psychiatry* (2006) 59(9):812–5. doi: 10.1016/j.biopsych.2005.09.022

Aas M, Haukvik UK, Djurovic S, Bergmann O, Athanasiu L, Tesli MS, et al. BDNF val66met modulates the association between childhood trauma, cognitive and brain abnormalities in psychoses. *Prog Neuro-psychopharmacol Biol Psychiatry* (2013) 46:181–8. doi: 10.1016/j.pnpbp.2013.07.008

Carballedo A, Morris D, Zill P, Fahey C, Reinhold E, Meisenzahl E, et al. Brain-derived neurotrophic factor Val66Met polymorphism and early life adversity affect hippocampal volume. *Am J Med GenetPart B Neuropsychiatr Genet* (2013) 162B(2):183–90. doi: 10.1002/ajmg.b.32130

Gatt JM, Nemeroff CB, Dobson-Stone C, Paul RH, Bryant RA, Schofield PR, et al. Interactions between BDNF Val66Met polymorphism and early life stress predict brain and arousal pathways to syndromal depression and anxiety. *Mol Psychiatry* (2009) 14(7):681–95.

Gerritsen L, Tendolkar I, Franke B, Vasquez AA, Kooijman S, Buitelaar J, et al. BDNF Val66Met genotype modulates the effect of childhood adversity on subgenual anterior cingulate cortex volume in healthy subjects. *Mol Psychiatry* (2012) 17(6):597–603.

Nemoto K, Ohnishi T, Mori T, Moriguchi Y, Hashimoto R, Asada T, et al. The Val66Met polymorphism of the brain-derived neurotrophic factor gene affects age-related brain morphology. *Neurosci Lett* (2006) 397(1-2):25–9. doi: 10.1016/j.neulet.2005.11.067

Wang F, McIntosh AM, He Y, Gelernter J, Blumberg HP. The association of genetic variation in CACNA1C with structure and function of a frontotemporal system. *Bipolar Disord* (2011) 13(7-8):696–700. doi: 10.1111/j.1399-5618.2011.00963.x

Cerasa A, Gioia MC, Labate A, Liguori M, Lanza P, Quattrone A. Impact of catechol-O-methyltransferase Val(108/158) Met genotype on hippocampal and prefrontal gray matter volume. *Neuroreport* (2008) 19(4):405–8. doi: 10.1097/WNR.0b013e3282f5f784

Honea R, Verchinski BA, Pezawas L, Kolachana BS, Callicott JH, Mattay VS, et al. Impact of interacting functional variants in COMT on regional gray matter volume in human brain. *NeuroImage* (2009) 45(1):44–51.

Mechelli A, Tognin S, McGuire PK, Prata D, Sartori G, Fusar-Poli P, et al. Genetic vulnerability to affective psychopathology in childhood: a combined voxel-based morphometry and functional magnetic resonance imaging study. *Biol Psychiatry* (2009) 66(3):231–7.

Taylor WD, Zuchner S, Payne ME, Messer DF, Doty TJ, MacFall JR, et al. The COMT Val158Met polymorphism and temporal lobe morphometry in healthy adults. *Psychiatry Res* (2007) 155(2):173–7.

McIntosh AM, Baig BJ, Hall J, Job D, Whalley HC, Lymer GK, et al. Relationship of catechol-O-methyltransferase variants to brain structure and function in a population at high risk of psychosis. *Biol Psychiatry* (2007) 61(10):1127–34. doi: 10.1016/j.biopsych.2006.05.020

Ohnishi T, Hashimoto R, Mori T, Nemoto K, Moriguchi Y, Iida H, et al. The association between the Val158Met polymorphism of the catechol-O-methyl transferase gene and morphological abnormalities of the brain in chronic schizophrenia. *Brain* (2006) 129(Pt 2):399–410.

Ho BC, Wassink TH, O'Leary DS, Sheffield VC, Andreasen NC. Catechol-O-methyl transferase Val158Met gene polymorphism in schizophrenia: working memory, frontal lobe MRI morphology and frontal cerebral blood flow. *Mol Psychiatry* (2005) 10(3):229, 287-298.

Gruber O, Falkai P, Schneider-Axmann T, Schwab SG, Wagner M, Maier W. Neuregulin-1 haplotype HAP(ICE) is associated with lower hippocampal volumes in schizophrenic patients and in non-affected family members. *J Psychiatr Res* (2008) 43(1):1–6.

Tosato S, Bellani M, Bonetto C, Ruggeri M, Perlini C, Lasalvia A, et al. Is neuregulin 1 involved in determining cerebral volumes in schizophrenia? Preliminary results showing a decrease in superior temporal gyrus volume. *Neuropsychobiology* (2012) 65(3):119–25. doi: 10.1159/000330584

Addington AM, Gornick MC, Shaw P, Seal J, Gogtay N, Greenstein D, et al. Neuregulin 1 (8p12) and childhood-onset schizophrenia: susceptibility haplotypes for diagnosis and brain developmental trajectories. *Mol Psychiatry* (2007) 12(2):195–205.

Lencz T, Szeszko PR, DeRosse P, Burdick KE, Bromet EJ, Bilder RM, et al. A schizophrenia risk gene, ZNF804A, influences neuroanatomical and neurocognitive phenotypes. *Neuropsychopharmacology* (2010) 35(11):2284–91. doi: 10.1038/npp.2010.102

Donohoe G, Rose E, Frodl T, Morris D, Spoletini I, Adriano F, et al. ZNF804A risk allele is associated with relatively intact gray matter volume in patients with schizophrenia. *NeuroImage* (2011) 54(3):2132–7. doi: 10.1016/j.neuroimage. 2010.09.089

Wassink TH, Epping EA, Rudd D, Axelsen M, Ziebell S, Fleming FW, et al. Influence of ZNF804a on brain structure volumes and symptom severity in individuals with schizophrenia. *Arch Gen Psychiatry* (2012) 69(9):885–92. doi: 10.1001/archgenpsychiatry.2011.2116

Ohi K, Hashimoto R, Ikeda M, Yamashita F, Fukunaga M, Nemoto K, et al. Genetic risk variants of schizophrenia associated with left superior temporal gyrus volume. *Cortex* (2014) 58:23–6. doi: 10.1016/j.cortex.2014.05.011

Terwisscha van Scheltinga AF, Bakker SC, van Haren NE, Derks EM, Buizer-Voskamp JE, Boos HB, et al. Genetic schizophrenia risk variants jointly modulate total brain and white matter volume. *Biol Psychiatry* (2013) 73(6):525–31. doi: 10.1016/j.biopsych.2012.08.017

Harrisberger F, Smieskova R, Vogler C, Egli T, Schmidt A, Lenz C, et al. Impact of polygenic schizophrenia-related risk and hippocampal volumes on the onset of psychosis. *Transl Psychiatry* (2016) 6(8):e868. doi: 10.1038/tp.2016.143

Zhang Z, Chen X, Yu P, Zhang Q, Sun X, Gu H, et al. Evidence for the contribution of NOS1 gene polymorphism (rs3782206) to prefrontal function in schizophrenia patients and healthy controls. *Neuropsychopharmacology* (2015) 40(6):1383–94. doi: 10.1038/npp.2014.323

Friston KJ, Frith CD. Schizophrenia: a disconnection syndrome? *Clin Neurosci* (1995) 3(2):89–97.

Tost H, Bilek E, Meyer-Lindenberg A. Brain connectivity in psychiatric imaging genetics. *NeuroImage* (2012) 62(4):2250–60. doi: 10.1016/j.neuroimage. 2011.11.007

Wheeler AL. Voineskos AN. A review of structural neuroimaging in schizophrenia: from connectivity to connectomics. *Front Hum Neurosci* (2014) 8:653. doi: 10.3389/fnhum.2014.00653

Molendijk ML, Bus BA, Spinhoven P, Kaimatzoglou A, Oude Voshaar RC, Penninx BW, et al. A systematic review and meta-analysis on the association between BDNF val(66)met and hippocampal volume—a genuine effect or a winners curse? *Am J Med GenetPart B Neuropsychiatr Genet* (2012) 159B(6):731–40. doi: 10.1002/ajmg.b.32078

Ho BC, Andreasen NC, Dawson JD, Wassink TH. Association between brain-derived neurotrophic factor Val66Met gene polymorphism and progressive brain volume changes in schizophrenia. *Am J Psychiatry* (2007) 164(12):1890–9. doi: 10.1176/appi.ajp.2007.05111903

Munafo MR, Thiselton DL, Clark TG, Flint J. Association of the NRG1 gene and schizophrenia: a meta-analysis. *Mol Psychiatry* (2006) 11(6):539–46. doi: 10.1038/sj.mp.4001817

Duff BJ, Macritchie KA, Moorhead TW, Lawrie SM, Blackwood DH. Human brain imaging studies of DISC1 in schizophrenia, bipolar disorder and depression: a systematic review. *Schizophr Res* (2013) 147(1):1–13. doi: 10.1016/j.schres.2013.03.015

Hibar DP, Stein JL, Renteria ME, Arias-Vasquez A, Desrivieres S, Jahanshad N, et al. Common genetic variants influence human subcortical brain structures. *Nature* (2015) 520(7546):224–9.

Thompson PM, Stein JL, Medland SE, Hibar DP, Vasquez AA, Renteria ME, et al. The ENIGMA Consortium: large-scale collaborative analyses of neuroimaging and genetic data. *Brain Imaging Behav* (2014) 8(2):153–82.

Franke B, Stein JL, Ripke S, Anttila V, Hibar DP, van Hulzen KJ, et al. Genetic influences on schizophrenia and subcortical brain volumes: large-scale proof of concept. *Nat Neurosci* (2016) 19(3):420–31. doi: 10.1038/nn.4228

Haijma SV, Van Haren N, Cahn W, Koolschijn PC, Hulshoff Pol HE, Kahn RS. Brain volumes in schizophrenia: a meta-analysis in over 18 000 subjects. *Schizophr Bull* (2013) 39(5):1129–38. doi: 10.1093/schbul/sbs118

Gottesman II, Shields J. A polygenic theory of schizophrenia. *Proc Nat Acad Sci U S A* (1967) 58(1):199–205. doi: 10.1073/pnas.58.1.199

Hu M, Li J, Eyler L, Guo X, Wei Q, Tang J, et al. Decreased left middle temporal gyrus volume in antipsychotic drug-naive, fi st-episode schizophrenia patients and their healthy unaffected siblings. *Schizophr Res* (2013) 144(1–3):37–42. doi: 10.1016/j.schres.2012.12.018

Ordonez AE, Luscher ZI, Gogtay N. Neuroimaging findings from childhood onset schizophrenia patients and their non-psychotic siblings. *Schizophr Res* (2016) 173(3):124–31. doi: 10.1016/j.schres.2015.03.003

Meyer-Lindenberg A, Tost H. Neuroimaging and plasticity in schizophrenia. *Restor Neurol Neurosci* (2014) 32(1):119–27.

Adriano F, Caltagirone C, Spalletta G. Hippocampal volume reduction in first-episode and chronic schizophrenia: a review and meta-analysis. *Neuroscientist* (2012) 18(2):180–200. doi: 10.1177/1073858410395147

Schmaal L, Veltman DJ, van Erp TG, Samann PG, Frodl T, Jahanshad N, et al. Subcortical brain alterations in major depressive disorder: findings from the ENIGMA Major Depressive Disorder working group. *Mol Psychiatry* (2016) 21(6):806–12.

Frodl T, Janowitz D, Schmaal L, Tozzi L, Dobrowolny H, Stein DJ, et al. Childhood adversity impacts on brain subcortical structures relevant to depression. *J Psychiatr Res* (2017) 86:58–65. doi: 10.1016/j.jpsychires.2016. 11.010

Boedhoe PS, Schmaal L, Abe Y, Ameis SH, Arnold PD, Batistuzzo MC, et al. Distinct Subcortical volume alterations in pediatric and adult OCD: a worldwide meta- and mega-analysis. *Am J Psychiatry* (2017) 174(1):60–9.

Hoogman M, Bralten J, Hibar DP, Mennes M, Zwiers MP, Schweren LS, et al. Subcortical brain volume differences in participants with attention deficit hyperactivity disorder in children and adults: a cross-sectional mega-analysis. *Lancet Psychiatry* (2017) 4(4):310–9. doi: 10.1016/S2215-0366(17)30160-8

Fotuhi M, Do D, Jack C. Modifiable factors that alter the size of the hippocampus with ageing. *Nat Rev Neurol* (2012) 8(4):189–202. doi: 10.1038/ nrneurol.2012.27

Jochem C, Baumeister SE, Wittfeld K, Leitzmann MF, Bahls M, Schminke U, et al. Domains of physical activity and brain volumes: A population-based study. *NeuroImage* (2017) 156:101–8. doi: 10.1016/j.neuroimage.2017.05.020

Schmitt A, Malchow B, Hasan A, Falkai P. The impact of environmental factors in severe psychiatric disorders. *Front Neurosci* (2014) 8:19. doi: 10.3389/fnins.2014.00019

Bois C, Ronan L, Levita L, Whalley HC, Giles S, McIntosh AM, et al. Cortical surface area differentiates familial high risk individuals who go on to develop schizophrenia. *Biol Psychiatry* (2015) 78(6):413–20. doi: 10.1016/j. biopsych.2014.12.030

Brandt CL, Doan NT, Tonnesen S, Agartz I, Hugdahl K, Melle I, et al. Assessing brain structural associations with working-memory related brain patterns in schizophrenia and healthy controls using linked independent component analysis. *NeuroImage Clin* (2015) 9:253–63. doi: 10.1016/j. nicl.2015.08.010

Gurung R, Prata DP. What is the impact of genome-wide supported risk variants for schizophrenia and bipolar disorder on brain structure and function? A systematic review. *Psychol Med* (2015) 45(12):2461–80. doi: 10.1017/S0033291715000537

Chen J, Calhoun VD, Pearlson GD, Perrone-Bizzozero N, Sui J, Turner JA, et al. Guided exploration of genomic risk for gray matter abnormalities in schizophrenia using parallel independent component analysis with reference. *NeuroImage* (2013) 83:384–96. doi: 10.1016/j.neuroimage.2013.05.073

Chen J, Calhoun VD, Arias-Vasquez A, Zwiers MP, van Hulzen K, Fernandez G, et al. G-protein genomic association with normal variation in gray matter density. *Hum Brain Mapp* (2015) 36(11):4272–86. doi: 10.1002/hbm.22916

Pearlson GD, Clementz BA, Sweeney JA, Keshavan MS, Tamminga CA. Does biology transcend the symptom-based boundaries of psychosis? *Psychiatr Clin North Am* (2016) 39(2):165–74. doi: 10.1016/j.psc.2016.01.001

Derogatis LR, Cleary PA. Factorial invariance across gender for the primary symptom dimensions of the SCL-90. *Br J Soc Clin Psychol* (1977) 16(4):347–56. doi: 10.1111/j.2044-8260.1977.tb00241.x

Schmitz N, Hartkamp N, Kiuse J, Franke GH, Reister G, Tress W. The Symptom Check-List-90-R (SCL-90-R): a German validation study. *Qual Life Res* (2000) 9(2):185–93. doi: 10.1023/A:1008931926181

Carter CS, Bearden CE, Bullmore ET, Geschwind DH, Glahn DC, Gur RE, et al. Enhancing the informativeness and replicability of imaging genomics studies. *Biol Psychiatry* (2017) 82(3):157–64. doi: 10.1016/j.biopsych.2016.08.019

Ioannidis JP. Why most published research findings are false. *PLoS Med* (2005) 2(8):e124. doi: 10.1371/journal.pmed.0020124

de Vries YA, Roest AM, Franzen M, Munafo MR, Bastiaansen JA. Citation bias and selective focus on positive findings in the literature on the serotonin transporter gene (5-HTTLPR), life stress and depression. *Psychol Med* (2016) 46(14):2971–9. doi: 10.1017/S0033291716000805

11

A Novel Biomarker of Compensatory Recruitment of Face Emotional Imagery Networks in Autism Spectrum Disorder

*Marco Simões[1,2,3], Raquel Monteiro[1,2], João Andrade[2], Susana Mouga[1,2,4], Felipe França[5], Guiomar Oliveira[1,2,4,6,7], Paulo Carvalho[3] and Miguel Castelo-Branco[1,2]**

[1] Coimbra Institute for Biomedical Imaging and Translational Research, Instituto de Ciências Nucleares Aplicadas à Saúde, University of Coimbra, Coimbra, Portugal, [2] Faculty of Medicine, University of Coimbra, Coimbra, Portugal, [3] Center for Informatics and Systems, University of Coimbra, Coimbra, Portugal, [4] Neurodevelopmental and Autism Unit from Child Developmental Center, Hospital Pediátrico, Centro Hospitalar e Universitário de Coimbra, Coimbra, Portugal, [5] PESC-COPPE, Universidade Federal do Rio de Janeiro, Rio de Janeiro, Brazil, [6] University Clinic of Pediatrics, Faculty of Medicine of the University of Coimbra, Coimbra, Portugal, [7] Centro de Investigação e Formação Clínica, Hospital Pediátrico, Centro Hospitalar e Universitário de Coimbra, Coimbra, Portugal

***Correspondence:**
Miguel Castelo-Branco
mcbranco@fmed.uc.pt

Imagery of facial expressions in Autism Spectrum Disorder (ASD) is likely impaired but has been very difficult to capture at a neurophysiological level. We developed an approach that allowed to directly link observation of emotional expressions and imagery in ASD, and to derive biomarkers that are able to classify abnormal imagery in ASD. To provide a handle between perception and action imagery cycles it is important to use visual stimuli exploring the dynamical nature of emotion representation. We conducted a case-control study providing a link between both visualization and mental imagery of dynamic facial expressions and investigated source responses to pure face-expression contrasts. We were able to replicate the same highly group discriminative neural signatures during action observation (dynamical face expressions) and imagery, in the precuneus. Larger activation in regions involved in imagery for the ASD group suggests that this effect is compensatory. We conducted a machine learning procedure to automatically identify these group differences, based on the EEG activity during mental imagery of facial expressions. We compared two classifiers and achieved an accuracy of 81% using 15 features (both linear and non-linear) of the signal from theta, high-beta and gamma bands extracted from right-parietal locations (matching the precuneus region), further confirming the findings regarding standard statistical analysis. This robust classification of signals resulting from imagery of dynamical expressions in ASD is surprising because it far and significantly exceeds the good classification already achieved with observation of neutral face expressions (74%). This novel neural correlate of emotional imagery in autism could potentially serve as a clinical interventional target for studies designed to improve facial expression recognition, or at least as an intervention biomarker.

Keywords: emotional facial expression, mental imagery, EEG biomarker, machine learning, autism spectrum disorder, dynamic expressions

INTRODUCTION

Faces represent a critical source of visual information for social perception, conveying relevant information about identity and emotional states of others (Kanwisher and Yovel, 2006). Since the first months of life, children are capable of understanding and processing facial cues, like FEs (Field et al., 1982). The ability to interpret these social signs represents an essential skill in child development and, therefore, a basic condition for the development of the ability to engage in successful social interactions early in life (Bayless et al., 2011).

ASD is a neurodevelopmental disorder characterized by deficits in the social domain which represent hallmark early characteristics (Sperdin et al., 2018). Even for simple visualization of FE, the literature is somewhat inconsistent: while some studies show group differences both in behavioral performance and neural responses, other studies show no identifiable deficits at all (for a compreensive review, see Monteiro et al., 2017).

Importantly, no previous study has considered the role of MI in the FE processing domain, possibly because of the challenges in identifying imagery signatures that mimic neural responses during simple observation. The perceptual strength and spatial frequency of the FE stimuli seem to be relevant to yield ASD group differences during simple visual presentation (Vlamings et al., 2010; Luckhardt et al., 2017), but the large majority of visual perception studies use static frame stimuli, lacking the dynamic characteristics of naturalistic FE (Monteiro et al., 2017). Those dynamics have been shown to play a crucial role on the perception of the respective FE and its emotional valence (Krumhuber et al., 2013) possibly because they allow to generate perception and action imagery cycles.

Another limiting aspect is the notion that specific processing experimental contrasts are needed to isolate effects of interest. For example, the use of blank screen baselines, before the presentation of faces, generates a non-specific contrast of face with expression against a baseline without any stimulus. Therefore, those responses comprise both the processing of low-level core aspects of the face and the specific processing of the FE. In this EEG study we used dynamic FE morphing in a virtual avatar and used its neutral expression as baseline, to ensure a FE specific contrast. This way, the neutral FE is already present in the baseline. We believe this stringent contrast provides a response specific to the processing of the FE aspects, isolating it from the simple response to the face static itself. A systematic review of EEG studies regarding FE processing in ASD conducted by Monteiro et al. (2017) has already identified the need for experimental paradigms targeting the dynamic characteristics of FEs. All the studies identified by that review applied non-specific experimental contrasts, using blank screens as baseline of their experimental conditions. To the best of our knowledge, our study is the first one to combine a task-specific contrast for dynamic FE stimuli.

MI is defined as the simulation or re-creation of perceptual experience (Kosslyn et al., 2001; Pearson et al., 2013). Most of these mental representations are extracted from memory and allow one to mentally revisit the original stimuli or their combination (Pearson et al., 2015). Disturbed MI has been postulated to be present in several psychiatric disorders, from post-traumatic stress disorder (Lanius et al., 2002) to socio-emotional disorders like social phobia or depression (Hirsch et al., 2006). In the specific case of ASD, MI is likely to be impaired, since one of the key deficits included in the ASD diagnosis, in the form of absence or impairment of 'pretend play' (Baron-Cohen et al., 2001; American Psychiatric Association [APA], 2013), which requires preserved action-perception imagery cycles. This deficit is particularly interesting since it spans into the social, imitation and repetitive behavior dimensions (Crespi et al., 2016). Therefore, the study of the neural correlates of MI in ASD gains relevance since it might lead to the understanding of the neural correlates of its core neurodevelopmental limitation and further help into the development of successful therapies.

Here, by providing a critical link between visual observation and subsequent replay imagery, we bound MI to the FE of an avatar, in a task where the participant mentally replays the previously observed dynamic image of the avatar performing a happy or a sad FE. We believe this link between visual observation and MI of FE in others addresses both the deficits of FE processing, emotion identification and theory of mind, due to the lack of thinking from the perspective of the other present in ASD. Therefore, the concept of visually imagining others smiling recruits the faculties of expression processing and pretend play, and our experimental design allowed to study such imagery process in ASD, and to use two distinct classification approaches, based on linear and non-linear features describing brain signals, to differentiate between the disease state and normal cognition. Non-linear features consist of quantitative measures that represent in a relatively simple way complex dynamic characteristics of the EEG signals, which the traditional linear methods (amplitude and frequency, for example) are not able to capture. They have been adopted more and more frequently in EEG analysis in general and ASD biomarker research in particular (Bosl et al., 2011, 2017).

MATERIALS AND METHODS

Participants

Seventeen male teenagers with the diagnosis of idiopathic ASD were recruited from the Unit of Neurodevelopment and Autism from the Pediatrics Unit from the University Hospital of Coimbra and from Portuguese ASD patient associations (Coimbra and Viseu). Since ASD is a disorder far more prevalent in male individuals, with a ratio of four males to every female, and there is accumulated evidence for sex differences in brain connectivity (Alaerts et al., 2016; Irimia et al., 2017; Fu et al., 2018), only male participants were included in the study. The diagnosis of

Abbreviations: ASD, autism spectrum disorder; ERP, event-related potential; FE, facial expression; fMRI, functional magnetic resonance imaging; IQ, intelligence quotient; MI, mental imagery; sLORETA, standardized low resolution brain electromagnetic tomography; SnPM, statistical non-parametric mapping; SVM, support vector machine; TD, typically developed; VEP, visual evoked potential; WiSARD, wilkes, stonham and aleksander recognition device; WNN, weightless neural network

ASD was performed based on the Autism Diagnostic Observation Schedule, the Autism Diagnostic Interview - Revisited and the Diagnostic and Statistical Manual of Mental Disorders - 5th edition criteria, confirmed by an expert multidisciplinary team. Seventeen healthy TD male controls were recruited from our local database of volunteers. Participants from both groups had their IQ assessed by the Wechsler Adult Intelligence Scale for participants older than 16 years old, and by the Wechsler Intelligence Scale for Children for younger participants. Groups were matched by chronological age (ASD mean age and standard error (SE): 16.4 ± 0.6 years; TD mean age and SE: 15.5 ± 0.6 years) and performance IQ (ASD mean score and SE: 99.8 ± 3.0; TD mean score and SE: 106.2 ± 4.2). Additional group characterization can be found in **Table 1**.

Written informed consent was obtained from the parents of the participants or, when appropriate, the participants themselves. The study was approved by the ethics committee from Faculty of Medicine from the University of Coimbra and was conducted in accordance with the declaration of Helsinki.

Experimental Tasks

The experiment is divided in two tasks: one of visual stimulation and one of MI requiring "mental replay" of previously observed FE, with the goal to identify similar neural signatures. The visual stimulation task and overall experiment were developed in *WorldViz Vizard 5 VR Toolkit* (development edition) using the *male002* virtual avatar from the *Complete Characters HD pack* and its FE poses. The total duration of the experiment is about 50 min, including 15 min for scalp cleaning and placement of the EEG cap, 30 min for the experimental tasks and 5 min to clean up at the end of the session.

Visual Stimulation Task

This task consists in observing a virtual avatar performing either sad or happy FEs (see **Figure 1A**), which represent two antagonistic expressions from the six core expressions (Ekman and Friesen, 1971). The FEs were verified in accordance with the action units defined in the Facial Action Coding System (FACS) (Ekman and Friesen, 1978). The happy expression comprises action units 6 (cheek raiser), 12 (lip corner puller) and 25 (lip part), while the sad FE uses action units 1 (inner brow raiser), 2 (outer brow raiser), 4 (brow depressor), 15 (lip corner depressor), and 17 (chin raiser).

Each trial is composed by a morphing period of 250 ms where the expression of the avatar gradually changes from neutral to the target expression, followed by a static period where the virtual avatar is displaying the target FE for 1000 ms and a final period where the avatar morphs back to the neutral expression, with the duration of 250 ms (see **Figure 1B**). Thus, each stimulus has a duration of 1.5 s and the inter-trial interval consisted in 1s plus a jitter of 500 ms. The neutral face of the avatar is always present during the baseline/inter-trial interval, which creates a stringent contrast with the FE since the stimuli does not come from no stimulus/blank screen, but from the neutral face, as naturally happens in real life.

This part of the experiment is composed by two blocks of 120 randomized trials (60 of each FE), for a total of 240 trials. The participants were asked to fixate the face of the avatar in the middle of the eyes and observe the expressions. A rest period was included between blocks to ensure focus and reduce fatigue throughout the experiment. A total of 120 trials per condition were recorded.

TABLE 1 | Group characterization: mean and standard error of the mean (between brackets) of age, full scale IQ (FSIQ), verbal IQ (VIQ) and performance IQ (PIQ) (*$p > 0.05$).

	ASD	TD	
N	17	17	
Age	16.4 (0.6)	15.5 (0.6)	*
FSIQ	92.2 (3.1)	109.2 (4.5)	
VIQ	88.1 (4.2)	110.3 (4.2)	
PIQ	99.8 (3.0)	106.2 (4.2)	*

Mental Imagery Task

The second part of the experiment consists of a MI paradigm. In this task, the participant is asked to mentally imagine the avatar performing the same types of FEs used in the stimulation part (used to facilitate mental replay). The computer screen shows the neutral face of the avatar during the whole period, except for the instruction, when it performs the FE the participant is asked to imagine. Then, after a cue, the participant imagines the avatar performing the FE, in a period of 4 s, returning to no imagery after that period. The (c) section of **Figure 1** details the structure of the trials. This task is composed by two blocks of 40 randomized trials (20 for each expression), achieving a total of 80 trials for the task.

Experimental Setup and Data Recording

The experiment was conducted in a 22-inch LCD Monitor (frame rate of 60 Hz, 1680 × 1050 pixel resolution). The participants sat about 60 cm away from the screen (distance measured from the eyes to the center of the screen) and were asked to keep their eyes open and fixed on the face of the avatar. EEG data were recorded using a 64 channel actiCHamp system from Brain Products.

The scalp of the participants was first cleaned using abrasive gel and then the 64 channel actiCAP cap was placed on their head. Data were recorded from 64 Ag/AgCl active electrodes (Brain Products), placed across the head according to the international 10–10 standard system. The ground electrode was placed at AFz position and the reference electrode at the right ear. The impedance of the electrodes was kept under 10 kΩ during the recordings. The electrodes were connected directly to the Brain Products actiCHamp amplifier and sampled at 1000 Hz. EEG data were recorded using the Brain Products Recorder software. For each paradigm, the individuals were informed about the respective task. The total duration of the experimental procedure (preparation + 2 tasks) was around 50 min.

EEG Preprocessing

We used MathWorks Matlab, 2017b and the EEGLAB toolbox v14.1.1 (Delorme and Makeig, 2004) for EEG signal preprocessing and analysis. EEG data were filtered with a finite

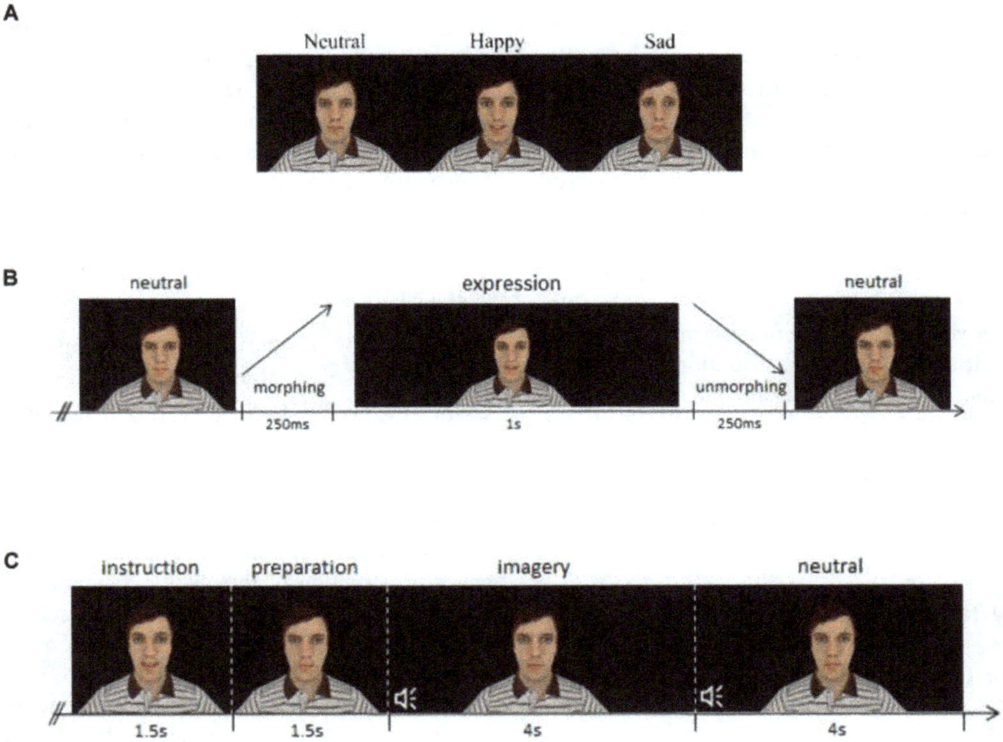

FIGURE 1 | Description of the tasks, both regarding structure, and stimuli used. **(A)** Base stimuli used for each expression at their expression endpoint, comprising the neutral, happy, and sad facial expressions. **(B)** Structure of the visual stimulation paradigm: each expression lasted 1.5 s, divided by facial expression morphing (250 ms), static facial expression (1 s) and facial expression unmorphing (250 ms). **(C)** Structure of the mental imagery paradigm: the instruction is composed by the avatar performing the expression to be imagined, as presented in the visual stimulation task, and to facilitate mental replay. After that, an interval of 1.5 s is left for preparation, and an auditory stimulus (beep) cues the start of the mental imagery process, for 4 s, whereas another beep indicates the end of the mental imagery of the expression, and the start of the neutral period.

impulse response bandpass filter of frequencies 1 and 100 Hz and notch filtered with an infinite impulse response filter between 47.5 and 52.5 Hz, as implemented in the EEGLAB toolbox. Bad channels were removed and data were re-referenced for the average reference. Epochs were created locked to the stimulus onsets (please refer to the task-specific analysis for details about the epoch lengths). Bad epochs were removed based on the EEGLAB semi-automatic procedures for extreme values and improbable signal segments. Independent Components Analysis (ICA) was then run on the data using EEGLAB implementation of *infomax* algorithm (Bell and Sejnowski, 1995). Components were used in order to extract noisy components, such as blinks, muscular activity or electrical interference. Components presenting such artifacts were removed and the weights were projected back to the data (Makeig et al., 2004). Bad channels previously removed were then interpolated. Further analysis of EEG data was conducted over these preprocessed signals.

Experimental Design and Statistical Analysis

The analysis focused on identifying group differences for both visualization and MI of the FEs. We specify the different analyses performed for each task separately.

Visual Stimulation Task Analysis

The visual stimulation epochs comprise 1 s, starting 100 ms prior to the stimuli onset (baseline) and go to 900 ms after the start of the expression morphing (during the first 250 ms of the epoch, the face of the avatar is continuously morphing the FE). ERPs were computed by subtracting each epoch by the mean of its baseline (from 100 ms pre-stimulus to 0) and then averaging all epochs corresponding to the same stimulus condition.

Source analysis were conducted using the sLORETA toolbox (Pascual-Marqui, 2002). The procedure included exporting from EEGLAB the preprocessed single-trial epochs, importing them into sLORETA software, averaging them (per subject and expression) and converting to the source space. Each participant electrode locations were co-registered with the realistic anatomical MR model using landmarks and standard electrode positions. The source space representation consists of a current source density (CSD) map computed with the sLORETA algorithm, a standardized discrete three-dimensional (3D) distributed linear weighted minimum norm inverse solution that takes several neurophysiologic and anatomical constraints into account and has been shown to yield depth-compensated zero localization error inverse solutions (Pascual-Marqui, 1999; Pascual-Marqui et al., 2002). sLORETA employs the current density estimate given by the minimum norm solution, and localization inference is based on standardized values of the current density estimates (Pascual-Marqui, 2002) and has been shown to outperform its competitor algorithms in terms of localization error and ghost sources (Grech et al., 2008).

For each expression and each group, we identified the peaks of the first and second ERP component for each electrode, and extracted the latencies for both peaks across the scalp. We performed the source localization of the mean activity of around those two ERP components (±125 ms, see **Supplementary Figure S1**).

We conducted a voxel-by-voxel between-group comparison of the mean current source density distribution in those time windows around the ERP peaks, using the sLORETA software implementation of SnPM, employing a log-*F*-ratio statistic for independent groups (for a similar procedure see, for example, Velikova et al., 2011). The SnPM method corrects for multiple comparisons without requiring Gaussian assumptions (Nichols and Holmes, 2001).

Mental Imagery Task Analysis

For the MI task, we also performed ERP analysis locked to the sound trigger. For the longer imagery blocks, we performed a spectral source analysis at more distant time windows and investigated the statistical classification of putative neural biomarkers.

Mental imagery ERP source analysis

For the imagery epochs, we investigated the ERP sources originated by the happy and sad imagery triggers. The participant receives the instruction beforehand of which expression to imagine. We segmented the trials from 100 ms prior to the cue beep and up to 900 ms after it, and subtracted them by the mean of their baseline (−100 ms to 0).

Similarly to the visual stimulation ERPs, for the source analysis we looked for the mean global field power in the window of 0–250 ms. The pipeline was analogous to the VEP, as well as the statistical framework.

Mental imagery spectral source analysis

For the MI periods, we investigated frequency bands of the signal during the time window of 500–3500 ms, avoiding the contribution of the beep ERP and covering the main period of MI, because MI processes are best captured using time-frequency analysis (Horki et al., 2014). The frequency bands of interest were θ, α, β, and δ, as defined in the sLORETA toolbox. This analysis of frequency bands of induced activity comprised the following steps: we export the single trials from EEGLAB and imported them to the sLORETA toolbox. Then we compute the cross-spectrum of each trial and average them per subject and condition. The average cross-spectrum is used to compute the source current density maps used in the second-level analysis.

For both ERP and frequency analysis we conducted voxel-by-voxel between-group comparisons of the current density distribution for each expression, in a way analogous to the VEP procedure.

Mental imagery biomarkers to classify groups

To explore the MI processes through the EEG data, we defined several features from the time, frequency, and non-linear domain. We then performed a ranking analysis and selected the best features to train a classifier to discriminate participants between groups. Features were extracted for each channel and trial by trial and averaged across all imagery trials and electrode clusters.

Feature extraction. We follow the procedure of Simoes et al. (2015) for extracting features representative of different EEG characteristics.

Time/frequency domain. For the time and frequency domain, we selected the signal envelope (env), Teager energy operator (teag) and instantaneous power (pow) as features. A detailed description of these features is present in **Supplementary Table S1**.

Non-linear domain. To extract signal complexity measures, the EEG signal was transformed to its phase-space. The phase-space is a reconstruction of the chaotic dynamics of the system and, as was proven by Takens (1981), it keeps some of the relevant properties of the state space representation of the system, such as the topographic properties, Lyaponov exponents and the Kolmogorov-Sinai Entropy. Every possible state of the system can be represented by a point in the multidimensional phase space and time evolution of the system creates a trajectory in the phase space (Kliková and Raidl, 2011). We used the time delay method to reconstruct the phase-space of the signal. Given a time series of a scalar variable it is possible to construct a vector $X(t_i),\ i=1, \ldots, N$ in phase-space in time t_i as follows:

$$X(t_i) = [x(t_i),\ x(t_i + \tau), \ldots,\ x(t_i + (m-1)\tau)], \quad i = 1, \ldots, N - (m-1)\tau \qquad (1)$$

where τ is time delay, m is the dimension of reconstructed space and $M = N - (m-1)\tau$ is the number of points (states) in the phase space.

We reconstructed a 2 and 3-dimensional phase-space associated to the EEG data, and the time delay was considered to be the mean of the first local minimum from the signal's autocorrelation (hereafter defined as lag).

From the non-linear domain we extracted the spatial filling index (SFI), largest Lyapunov exponent (Lyap), correlation dimension (CorrDim), approximate entropy (ApEn) and sample entropy (SpEn) as features. We provide a detailed description of these features in the **Supplementary Table S2**.

The features were extracted from 3 time windows in each trial: baseline [−500 ms to 0 ms pre instruction], emotion imagery [500–3500 ms after imagery trigger] and neutral [500–3500 ms after neutral trigger]. For the emotion and neutral time windows, we used the absolute value for the non-linear features and the normalized values (subtracted by the same feature extracted from the baseline) for the time/frequency domain.

Frequency bands. All features were extracted from signals filtered at different frequency bands. Band-pass Infinite Impulse Response (IIR) filters were used as implemented in EEGLAB toolbox, for the frequency bands: θ [4–8] Hz, α [8–12] Hz, low β [12–21] Hz, high β [21–30] Hz and γ [30–40] Hz.

Feature selection. In order to reduce the dimensionality of the feature set, we averaged the features extracted from each electrode in spatial clusters, as defined in **Supplementary Figure S2.** The clusters were defined by electrode spatial proximity in a way that covers the full scalp, keeps symmetry and lobule divisions (frontal, parietal – subdivided in central and posterior region, occipital and temporal). We then used the *a priori* information provided by the source localization and selected only the clusters closer to the right precuneus region, namely C1, C2, C4, and C5.

We ended up with 8 different features × 5 frequency bands × 4 clusters, for a total of 160 different features. We then computed the statistical discriminative value of each feature between groups with two sample *t*-tests, using only the samples from the training set, and the features were ordered by absolute T value, from the most important to the least.

Classification. We trained a SVM with a linear kernel, for being one of the most used classifiers applied to EEG signals (Lotte et al., 2007) and also a WNN. The WNNs are underused in the literature but present characteristics that generalize well for noisy domains, like the EEG (Simões et al., 2018a). We implemented a variation of the WiSARD combined with a bleaching technique (França et al., 2014) which has been shown to perform at the same level as the SVM in distinct fields and presents fast learning curves, achieving good results even with small datasets of data (Cardoso et al., 2016).

We trained the classifiers to discriminate the group of the participant, based on the feature vector extracted from his EEG data. We divided the participants into train and test sets: 80% of the cases were randomly chosen for training and the remaining 20% for testing. We repeated the procedure more than 30 times, to avoid overfitting, following the guidelines provided by Varoquaux et al. (2017) regarding the use of machine learning on brain imaging data. Feature selection was performed every time using only training-set data.

To explore the relation between accuracy and the number of features used, the procedure was conducted starting with 5 features and adding 5 more features up to the total of features.

We repeated the full classification procedure using the EEG signal from the neutral part of the MI task, in order to check if the results were specifically improved during over emotion expression imagery.

RESULTS

Visual Stimulation Task

This section presents the results of the analysis performed on the ERP responses to the visual stimulation task (observation of happy and sad FEs), which was used to identify neural signatures relevant to validate the imagery task.

ERP Source Analysis Results

The ERPs obtained from the visual stimulation task present two clear independent components, the first one peaking around 300 ms and the second around 600 ms (**Figure 2**). Since the morphing occurs during the first 250 ms, we expect a delay on the first component, as reported by Graewe et al. (2012). The topography of the first component matches the well-known topography of the N170 component, with a negativity around the right and left parietal-occipital regions, but it appears delayed in time, as expected by the morphing animation. The second component has a strong parietal positivity, slightly right lateralized, especially for the ASD group.

For the source analysis of the visual stimulation task ERPs we defined time-windows of 250 ms around the two component peaks of activity in the ERPs. We show the results for the first and the second ERP component, separately. The mean peak latencies used for each expression and each group is detailed in **Supplementary Table S3.**

The mean current source density of activity in the intervals around the component peaks showed group differences for both expressions in the first component, using voxel-by-voxel independent tests between groups, corrected for multiple comparisons at the 5% level using the SnPM method (two-tailed). Both expressions show the group differences right-lateralized and located at the superior parietal region, in the precuneus area (**Figure 3**). As for the second component, only the sad expression presented statistically significant differences, exactly in the same superior parietal region, which showed also enhanced recruitment for the ASD group, in the right hemisphere.

Mental Imagery Task

This section presents the results for the MI task. We analyzed the ERP for the initial imagery period and the longer MI blocks through source analysis of the power spectrum and the analysis of several characteristics of the signal using machine learning techniques.

Mental Imagery ERP Source Analysis Results

After the sound trigger, an initial ERP can be found corresponding to processing the beep and starting the imagery procedure (**Figure 4**). We defined a time window to target at the source level, between 0 and 250ms, in order to investigate specific responses at the source level. The mean current source density in that interval presented group differences for both expressions with $p < 0.01$, using voxel-by-voxel independent tests between groups, corrected for multiple comparisons using the SnPM method. Importantly, the same region identified group differences for both expressions. This was also the same region that was identified during visual stimulation. Accordingly, the ASD group presented higher activation in the superior parietal region (precuneus area – **Figure 5**).

Mental Imagery Spectral Source Analysis Results

For the longer periods of imagery (500–3500 ms), we conducted a source analysis of the defined frequency bands of the signal. A statistical significant result was found for in the imagery of sad expressions, for the theta band (**Figure 6**). The ASD group shows

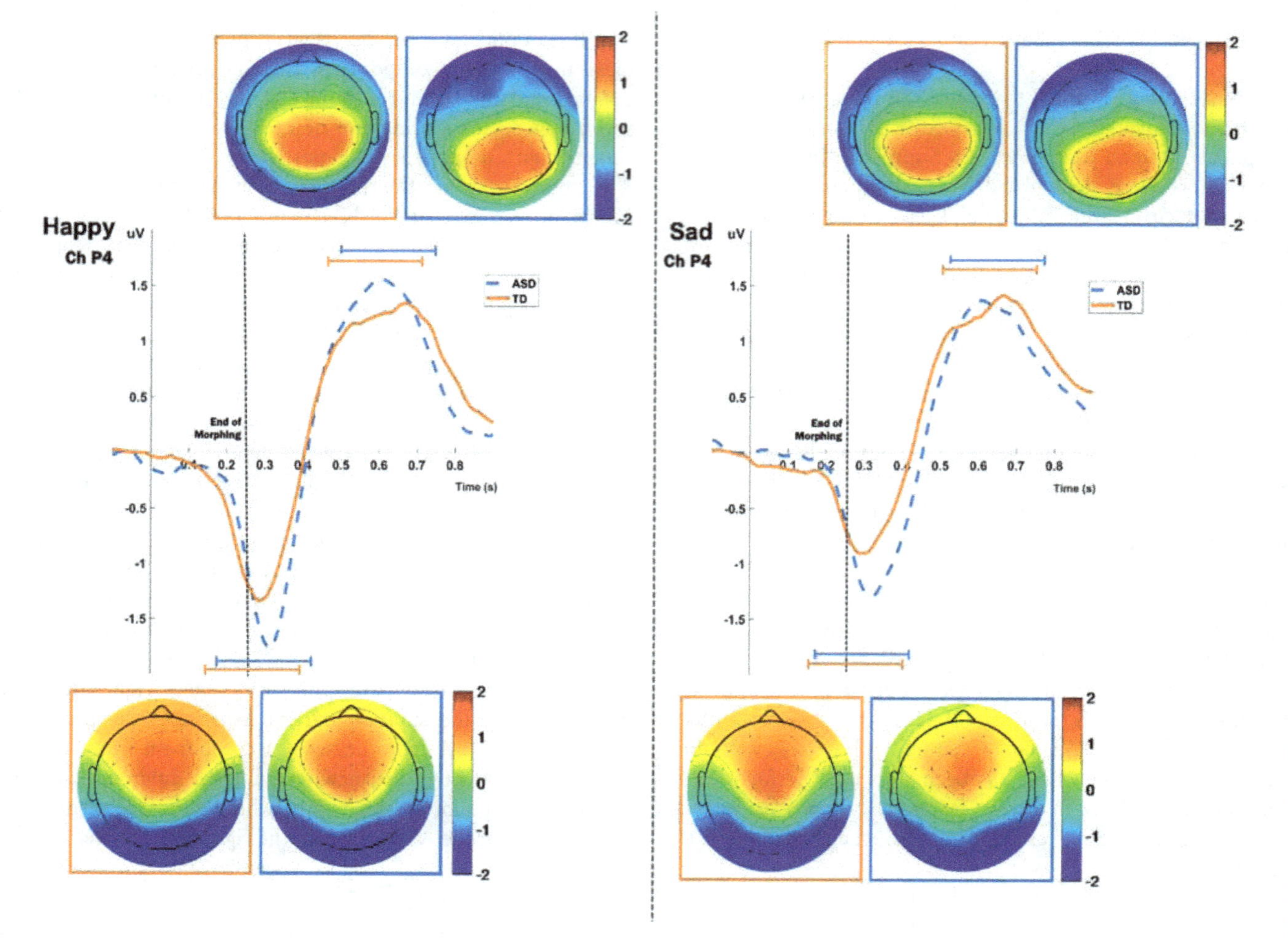

FIGURE 2 | ERPs for both groups and expressions, extracted from the P4 electrode. Topographic maps for each component are present near the ERP plots. Orange marks represent the TD group and blue marks the ASD. Topographic maps show the scalp distribution of the ERP amplitudes extracted from 250 ms windows, centered at the peaks of the components of each expression (refer to **Supplementary Table S3** for detailed peak latencies).

again higher recruitment of the very same right precuneus area at this frequency.

Statistical Classification of Mental Imagery Periods – Evidence for a Potential Biomarker in ASD

We then tested whether the identified neural signatures of imagery of FEs could be identified in a data driven manner using statistical classifiers. The linear SVM and the WiSARD classifier were able to achieve high test set accuracies (~77% and ~81% of accuracy, respectively), with the WiSARD yielding the best accuracy of 81% with just 15 features (**Figure 7**). Test set classification accuracy of the neutral face expression segments of the signal were far worse, with ~68% for the SVM and ~74% for the WiSARD, suggesting that important group differences are captured by the features are emotion expression-dependent (for statistical details see **Figure 7**). We present also a detailed exploration of the performance metrics using the top 15 features. We computed accuracy, specificity, sensitivity/recall, precision and the F1 score for both classifiers using the MI segments and the neutral segments.

We checked the correlation value between the extracted features and the IQ measurements (full-scale, verbal and performance IQ), and no feature was significantly correlated with any of the covariates.

We then focused on the top 15 features that generated the 81% of accuracy. We investigated the most selected frequency bands and clusters of these top features. **Figure 8** shows the top 15 feature distribution by clusters and frequency bands, showing the specific contribution of theta, high beta and gamma bands for group discrimination. Detailed feature information (**Table 2**) clarifies that the most discriminative features originate from the time-frequency domain, at the high-beta/gamma bands, and that the non-linear features are mainly from the theta-band.

DISCUSSION

Here we addressed for the first time FE imagery in ASD and identified a common neural correlate of observation and MI of dynamic FEs in this condition, in the precuneus. Robust

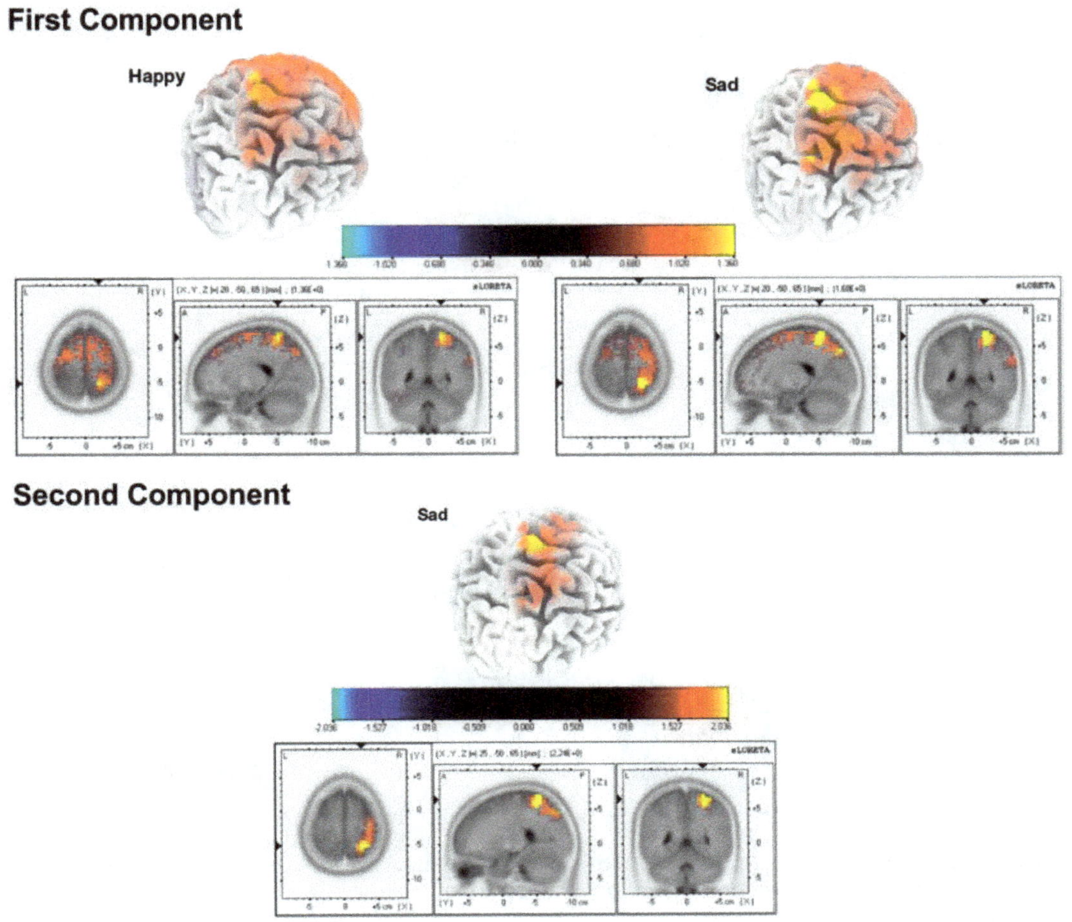

FIGURE 3 | Source group differences for the first and second ERP components, for happy and sad expressions. We found higher activation for the ASD group in the right precuneus using a two tailed alpha level of 5%, corrected with the SnPM method. Regarding the second component, this result was statistically significant specifically for the sad expression.

statistical classification of brain activity patterns using linear and non-linear features could also be achieved, and the identified biomarker of abnormal imagery in ASD can potentially be used as an outcome measure to evaluate clinical interventions addressing cognitive and behavioral improvement in this condition.

We focused on MI of FEs in ASD as a major research target in this study. This is a very important cognitive process in the context of this disease, because mental rehearsal is very important for action perception cycles, in particular in the context emotional face recognition. MI is the process of creating a mental representation and corresponding sensory experience of an episode or stimulus without a direct external source (Pearson et al., 2015). In the case of FEs, it also involves MI of motor patterns (FEs) which requires the involvement of the mirror neuron system. There are indeed several types of MI, namely visual, auditory and motor (for a review, see Kosslyn et al., 2001). Some studies showed the effect of MI on boosting performance in detection tasks (Tartaglia et al., 2009) and on decision making bias (Pearson et al., 2009). In our study, participants were asked to perform visual MI of an avatar performing a FE (mentally replaying previously observed patterns). This task combines MI, perspective taking and theory of mind, since the participant is asked to recreate an expression of another.

A critical aspect that renders the study of imagery difficult in ASD is that it is important to ascertain that imagery really reflects the expected visual content. We could achieve this by showing that similar neural signatures (source localization) can be found by both observation and imagery of FEs. The ERP elicited by the imagery cue did indeed reveal that source differences were very similar as compared to the ERP of the FE stimuli, with the precuneus showing higher activation for the ASD group. The right precuneus belongs to task-active networks (Yang et al., 2015) that are also active during imagery [for a review of the relation with the precuneus with visuo-spatial imagery and visuomotor transformations, please refer to (Cavanna and Trimble, 2006)].

One of the common aspects of visualization and MI of the others FEs is the need to incorporate the perspective of the other. Because we use a stringent contrast in the visual stimulation task, we expected the core processing of the face to have less weight than the perspective taking aspects task. The precuneus is one of the core regions present in the perspective taking

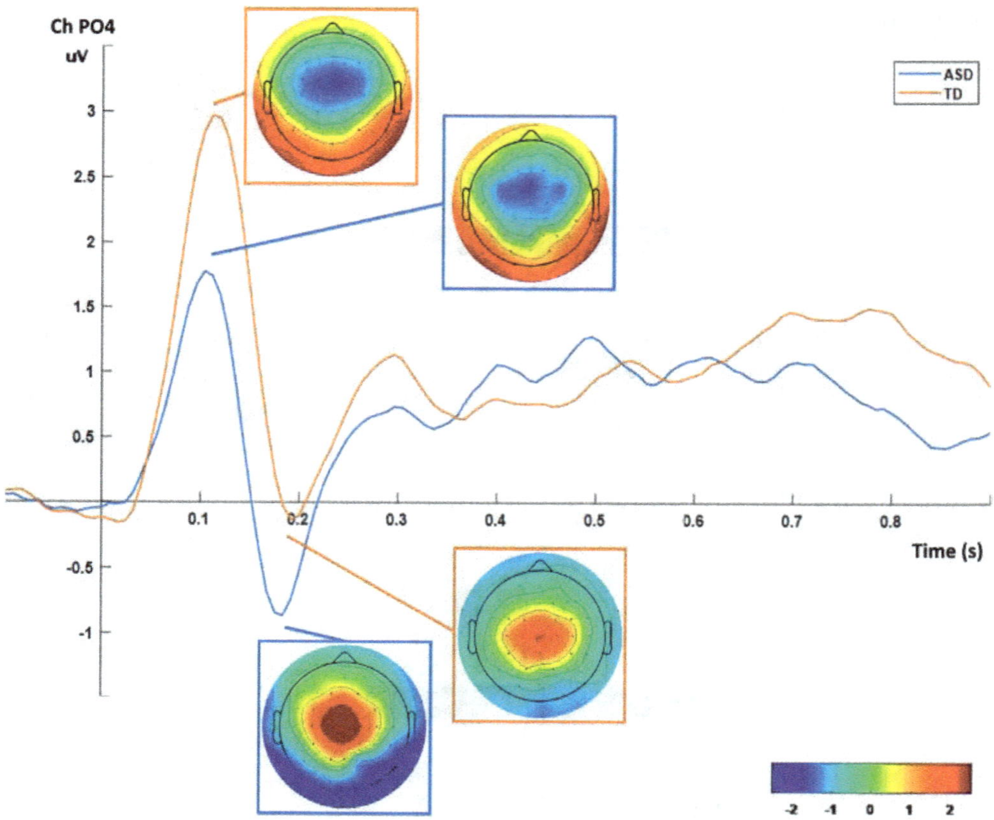

FIGURE 4 | ERP and topographic plots for the mental imagery task (PO4 channel). An initial ERP is visible peaking positively at 100 ms and negatively at 200 ms, with the tonic spectral characteristics overtaking the remaining time period (from 0.5 s onward).

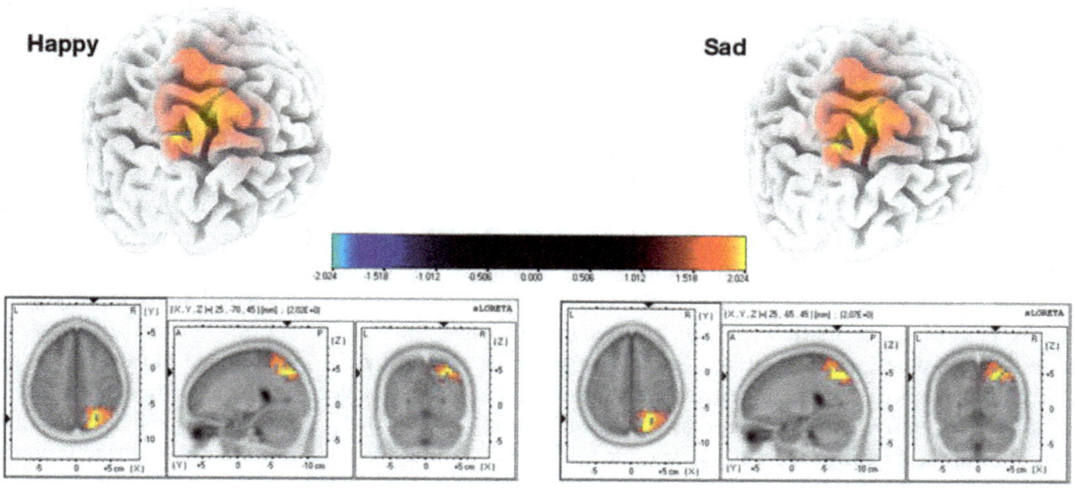

FIGURE 5 | Group differences for the source analysis of the ERPs of mental imagery. Statistical differences (two-tailed $p < 0.01$, SnPM corrected) were found in the region of precuneus, with higher activation for the ASD group.

network, as showed by Healey and Grossman (2018). The authors reviewed the literature and found the precuneus as a key region in both cognitive and affective perspective taking networks (Abu-Akel and Shamay-Tsoory, 2011). Those fMRI studies validate the source we identified in our study.

The link between the precuneus and its role in FEs processing has already been demonstrated by some studies (Saarimäki et al., 2016; An et al., 2018), but our study is the first one, to the best of our knowledge, to identify the over-recruitment of this region in the ASD population in a social cognition task. Since visual

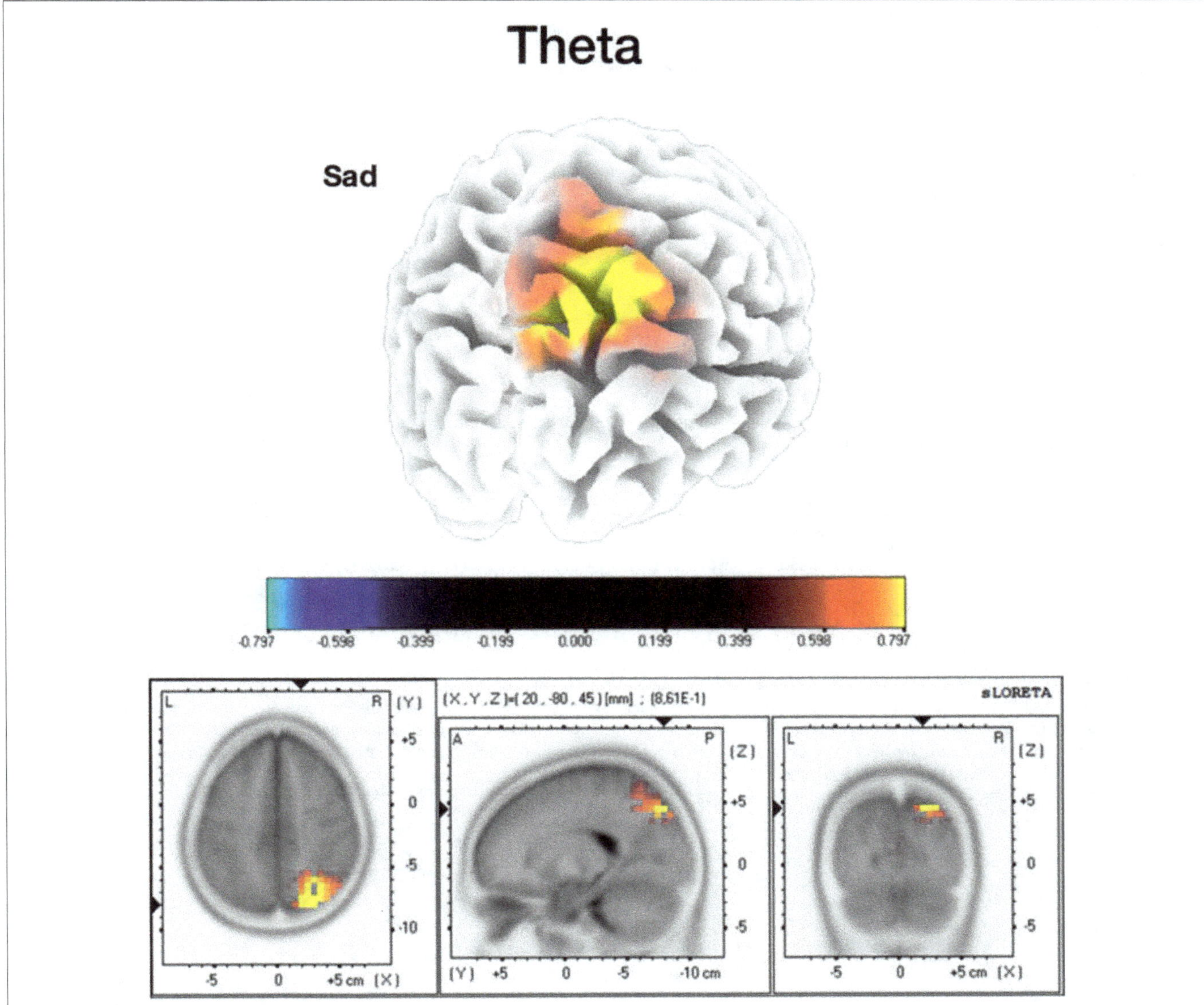

FIGURE 6 | Source analysis for the mental imagery segments, in the theta band. Higher activation for the ASD group in the precuneus area (two tailed $p < 0.05$, SnPM corrected).

perspective taking and theory of mind skills are impaired in ASD (Hamilton et al., 2009; David et al., 2010), we believe that ASD participants needed higher recruitment of the right precuneus as a compensatory mechanism for the MI of the other's FE.

Frequency band decomposition of the MI signals showed that theta and high-beta/gamma bands explained the main group differences. The source analysis of the theta band further revealed again a higher activation of the right precuneus for the ASD group (specifically for the sad FE). It was already known that FEs elicited higher theta responses than neutral expressions in healthy participants (for a review, please refer to Güntekin and Başar, 2014). Although theta band activity patterning has been linked to the medial frontal cortex and its role in cognitive control (Cavanagh and Frank, 2014) its source in our study seems to be different. In agreement with our own source, Wang et al. (2016) demonstrated a relationship between the theta band and activity patterns in the posterior cingulate cortex/precuneus, in a simultaneous EEG-fMRI study. Furthermore, the study from Knyazev et al. (2009) identified the same right parietal source from theta responses to FEs. Therefore, we believe the parietal theta band relation with the precuneus to be a core neural correlate of emotional MI processing. Despite using different types of signals (phasic or tonic in relation to the type of mental process) to perform the source localization (ERP and time-frequency decomposition), due to the characteristics of the tasks, it is very interesting to observe the same region involved in both visualization and MI processes.

The precuneus is recruited in several types of imagery, including motor imagery, mental navigation, memory-related

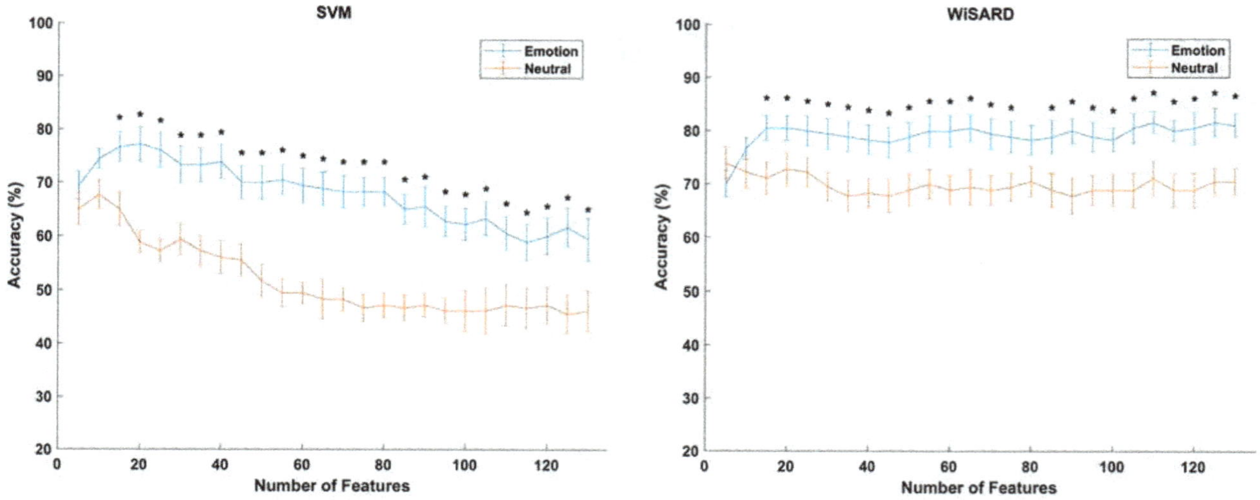

Type	Classifier	Accuracy	Specificity	Sensitivity	Precision	F1 Score
Emotion	SVM	76.7% (2.8)	**92.2% (3.1)**	61.1% (5.3)	90.6% (4.1)	71.1% (4.1)
	WiSARD	**80.6% (2.4)**	91.1% (3.2)	**70.0% (4.6)**	**92.5% (2.7)**	**76.2% (3.3)**
Neutral	SVM	65.0% (3.2)	68.9% (5.5)	61.1% (6.2)	70.5% (3.9)	69.5% (3.1)
	WiSARD	**71.1% (3.0)**	**72.2% (3.9)**	**70.0% (4.3)**	**73.2% (3.6)**	**69.7% (3.4)**

FIGURE 7 | Accuracy of the classifiers SVM (left) and WiSARD (right) as function of the considered number of features. Mean accuracies are represented with the lines and the error bars show the standard error of the mean. Classification results with the mental imagery part of the EEG signals are represented in blue and the neutral signals in orange. Statistically different accuracies between Emotion and Neutral are marked by * (one-sample *t*-tests with alpha level of 5% and false discovery rate correction for multiple comparisons). At the bottom we present the performance metrics for both classifiers using the top 25 features. Each cell presents the mean values followed by the standard error of the mean of the respective metric.

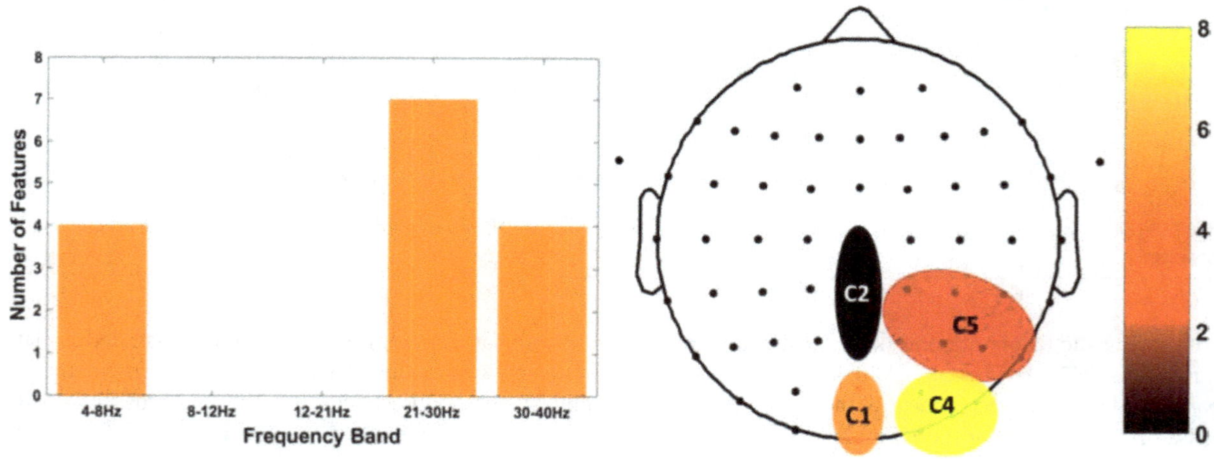

FIGURE 8 | Top 15 features distribution by frequency band (left) and clusters (right). The histogram on the left depicts the exploitability of theta and high-beta/gamma frequency features. The histogram of the right shows the scalp distribution of features within the right parietal-occipital region, showing a preference for the posterior clusters of the region.

imagery, episodic source memory retrieval and emotional state attribution (Cavanna and Trimble, 2006). Specifically regarding attributing emotions to others, several studies identified the role of the precuneus in Theory of Mind scenarios (Vogeley et al., 2001; Takahashi et al., 2015). Moreover, a connectivity analysis study of resting state fMRI data showed decreased connectivity of the precuneus region with the middle temporal gyrus and the ventromedial frontal cortex in the ASD population, in both hemispheres (Cheng et al., 2015). All these observations pinpoint the precuneus as playing a pivotal role in FE MI. Furthermore, the group difference in the right hemisphere, which is also known to dominate in attention and imagery, suggests that the

ASD group processes the FEs of the other in a more effortful, attention-based mechanism than the TD group. This view has been suggested by Harms et al. (2010). Our study is the first one, to our knowledge, to show that the same neural pattern that is observed during FE recognition is replicated for MI of the FEs, in ASD.

Based on the observed group differences, we investigated whether we could extract features that would function as biomarkers (not necessarily as diagnostic, but as intervention targets) of ASD, based on the MI process. The need for diagnostic, prognostic and intervention biomarkers in ASD is well recognized. While ASD biomarkers range from genetics to clinical (for a review, please refer to Ruggeri et al., 2014), the inter-subject variability observed in this disorder justifies the use of machine learning techniques combining multiple features to generate potential biomarkers (Huys et al., 2016). Therefore, we developed two classifiers – a SVM and a WNN to classify each subject (represented by a feature vector extracted from his EEG data) into ASD or TD group. Our purpose is to show that the features used by the classifiers provide exploitable group differences, that can also be used to characterize neural mechanisms underlying ASD (in this case, FE processing) and therefore be used to monitor, for example, rehabilitation efficacy (outcome measure) or aid at subgroup stratification in the ASD population (Castelhano et al., 2018), albeit not for early detection.

We verified that the WNN method achieved around 81% of accuracy using 15 features. When compared to the same classifiers trained with features extracted from EEG of the neutral periods, the accuracy was significantly lower (around 73%).

TABLE 2 | List of the top 15 features used in the classifiers, showing their frequency band, cluster, and statistical value.

FEATURE	FREQ. BAND	CLUSTER	RANK	T	P
ENV	[21–30] Hz	4	2.57 (0.41)	4.23	0.0002
TEAG	[21–30] Hz	1	4.30 (0.53)	3.84	0.0005
POW	[21–30] Hz	1	6.87 (0.77)	3.61	0.0010
ENV	[30–40] Hz	4	7.67 (0.83)	3.67	0.0009
TEAG	[21–30] Hz	4	8.73 (0.87)	3.56	0.0012
SPEN	[4–8] Hz	4	8.80 (1.16)	3.43	0.0017
LYAP	[4–8] Hz	4	9.83 (1.27)	−3.36	0.0020
ENV	[30–40] Hz	5	10.03 (0.99)	3.53	0.0013
POW	[21–30] Hz	4	11.37 (1.11)	3.41	0.0018
ENV	[21–30] Hz	1	12.03 (1.23)	3.22	0.0029
ENV	[30–40] Hz	1	13.37 (1.65)	3.24	0.0028
SPI	[4–8] Hz	4	13.43 (1.33)	3.25	0.0027
ENV	[21–30] Hz	5	13.83 (1.30)	3.37	0.0020
APEN	[4–8] Hz	4	14.37 (1.77)	3.15	0.0036
POW	[30–40] Hz	1	14.97 (1.14)	3.08	0.0042

Non-linear features are presented with gray background and time/frequency features with white background. Rank values correspond to the mean order of the feature across training sets, with the respective standard error of the mean. T and P values for each feature are presented, resulting from an independent t-test between the groups. All the 15 features are statistically significant (corrected for multiple comparisons using the false discovery rate algorithm).

We then performed a further analysis of the top 15 features selected for classification. The most representative frequency band, when using non-linear features, was the theta band, while the most discriminative features were from the time/frequency domain and high-beta/gamma frequency bands. Those bands and their relation with the precuneus have been explored in the literature by Fomina et al. (2016), which attempted to train the self-regulation of gamma and theta bands in the precuneus in amyotrophic lateral sclerosis patients. This is consistent with our results, showing that the precuneus activity at the theta and high-beta/gamma bands represent important MI information that can be used for clinical purposes, for instance in BCI based neurofeedback.

The overall use of dynamic FE morphing enabled a more realistic and ecologic approach, because the stimuli featured more realistically the daily life characteristics of social interactions than the commonly used static stimuli. Moreover, we used a specific face expression contrast (emotional expressions vs. neutral expression). As stated by Krumhuber et al. (2013), the dynamic characteristics of FEs are possibly also understudied which is a limitation for the validity of neurocognitive approaches.

Our approach to morph the expression into a virtual avatar makes a potential bridge between dynamic FEs and rehabilitation possibilities using, for instance, virtual reality. Understanding how the FEs are processed in virtual environments opens the door for intervention solutions, where the environment is completely controlled (Miller and Bugnariu, 2016; Simões et al., 2018b). This is important because the neural markers identified in this study could potentially be used as intervention target measures.

A common characteristic of most studies in the literature using EEG and observation of FEs is the use of a blank-screen as baseline for the visual stimulus (Monteiro et al., 2017), thus eliciting ERPs that mix the processing of the FE with face and other non-specific visual features. We argue that the use of a more specific contrast (expressionless/neutral face as baseline) elicits an ERP specific to the dynamic expression characteristics of the face, not the face itself. Moreover, Monteiro et al. (2017) demonstrate disparate findings in the literature when evaluating EEG responses to FEs in ASD. Several studies found expression effects accompanied by group effects. Using a very specific contrast, we were able to identify, even for FE observation, group differences in the right precuneus, with the ASD group showing higher activation in this region. The functional role of precuneus in attentional deployment and imagery is well recognized (Cavanna and Trimble, 2006), with some studies also suggesting a relation to perspective taking (Vogeley et al., 2001; Kircher et al., 2002; Schurz et al., 2015), face familiarity (specifically for the left precuneus) (Lee et al., 2013) and emotional state recognition and attribution (Ochsner et al., 2004; Spies et al., 2017). Our right precuneus group effect for both happy and sad expressions is consistent with several studies using fMRI that reported the same effect for ASD in the right precuneus (see the meta-analysis of Aoki et al., 2015, which found hyperactivation of bilaterate thalamus, caudade and right precuneus for the ASD group). Especially in tasks requiring taking the others perspective, the recruitment of the precuneus is key in both cognitive and affective perspective taking networks (Healey and Grossman, 2018). We hypothesize that the ASD group performs a higher recruitment of the precuneus region to compensate for emotional processing and perspective taking behavioral deficits.

Our study focused only on male subjects to avoid an effect of gender in the analysis. There is evidence for sex differences in brain connectivity in ASD which might influence the EEG analysis we conducted (Alaerts et al., 2016; Irimia et al., 2017; Fu et al., 2018). The replicability of these results in female ASD cohorts lacks further validation. Moreover, in spite of the limitations of our sample size, it paves the way for future replication studies in larger groups.

In conclusion, we found for the first time, a neural correlate of emotion expression imagery in ASD, which was validated as a replication of the neural signatures evoked by visual observation of specific FEs. We developed an innovative approach to study FE processing in ASD, combining visualization of dynamic FEs (with a very selective contrast, isolating pure FEs from the mere presence of a face) and MI of FEs in others. Our results emphasize the important role of the precuneus in the ASD facial processing circuit and suggest that its increased recruitment may serve as a compensatory strategy to overcome the natural deficits in their emotional processing. Furthermore, we extracted a set of features and trained a classifier that was able to discriminate between groups with high accuracy. The features were then observed to match topographically and spectrally the group effects, and can therefore be potentially used as intervention targets.

AUTHOR CONTRIBUTIONS

MS, RM, JA, SM, GO, PC, and MC-B conceived and designed the study. MS, RM, and JA performed the experiments with the participants. SM performed the screening and psychological evaluation. MS, RM, and JA analyzed the data. MS, RM, JA, PC, FF, and MC-B discussed the results and iterative approaches. MS, RM, and MC-B wrote the paper. All authors read, contributed and approved the final manuscript.

FUNDING

This work was supported by FCT – Portuguese national funding agency for science, research and technology [Grants PAC MEDPERSYST, POCI-01-0145-FEDER-016428, BIGDATIMAGE, CENTRO-01-0145-FEDER-000016 financed by Centro 2020 FEDER, COMPETE, FCT-UID/4539/2013 – COMPETE, POCI-01-0145-FEDER-007440, POCI-01-0145-FEDER-30852, Fellowships SFRH/BD/77044/2011 and SFRH/BD/102779/2014, and the BRAINTRAIN Project – Taking imaging into the therapeutic domain: Self-regulation of brain systems for mental disorders - FP7 HEALTH 2013 INNOVATION 1 602186 20, 2013, FLAD Life Sciences 2016.

ACKNOWLEDGMENTS

The authors acknowledge the contribution of the autism patient associations (APPDA) of Coimbra and Viseu for their collaboration in the recruitment of participants and logistics, for their participation in the study, as well as all the parents. They thank as well all the control participants who voluntarily participated in this study.

REFERENCES

Abu-Akel, A., and Shamay-Tsoory, S. (2011). Neuroanatomical and neurochemical bases of theory of mind. *Neuropsychologia* 49, 2971–2984. doi: 10.1016/j.neuropsychologia.2011.07.012

Alaerts, K., Swinnen, S. P., and Wenderoth, N. (2016). Sex differences in autism: a resting-state fMRI investigation of functional brain connectivity in males and females. *Soc. Cogn. Affect. Neurosci.* 11, 1002–1016. doi: 10.1093/scan/nsw027

American Psychiatric Association [APA] (2013). *Diagnostic and Statistical Manual of Mental Disorders.* Washington, DC: American Psychiatric Association.

An, S., Han, X., Wu, B., Shi, Z., Marks, M., Wang, S., et al. (2018). Neural activation in response to the two sides of emotion. *Neurosci. Lett.* 684, 140–144. doi: 10.1016/j.neulet.2018.07.011

Aoki, Y., Cortese, S., and Tansella, M. (2015). Neural bases of atypical emotional face processing in autism: a meta-analysis of fMRI studies. *World J. Biol. Psychiatry* 16, 291–300. doi: 10.3109/15622975.2014.957719

Baron-Cohen, S., Wheelwright, S., Skinner, R., Martin, J., and Clubley, E. (2001). The autism spectrum quotient: evidence from Asperger syndrome/high functioning autism, males and females, scientists and mathematicians. *J. Autism Dev. Disord.* 31, 5–17. doi: 10.1023/A:1005653411471

Bayless, S. J., Glover, M., Taylor, M. J., and Itier, R. J. (2011). Is it in the eyes? Dissociating the role of emotion and perceptual features of emotionally expressive faces in modulating orienting to eye gaze. *Vis. Cogn.* 19, 483–510. doi: 10.1080/13506285.2011.552895

Bell, A. J., and Sejnowski, T. J. (1995). An information-maximization approach to blind separation and blind deconvolution. *Neural Comput.* 7, 1129–1159. doi: 10.1162/neco.1995.7.6.1129

Bosl, W., Tierney, A., Tager-Flusberg, H., and Nelson, C. (2011). EEG complexity as a biomarker for autism spectrum disorder risk. *BMC Med.* 9:18. doi: 10.1186/1741-7015-9-18

Bosl, W. J., Loddenkemper, T., and Nelson, C. A. (2017). Nonlinear EEG biomarker profiles for autism and absence epilepsy. *Neuropsychiatr. Electrophysiol.* 3:1. doi: 10.1186/s40810-017-0023-x

Cardoso, D. O., Carvalho, D. S., Alves, D. S. F., Souza, D. F. P., Carneiro, H. C. C., Pedreira, C. E., et al. (2016). Financial credit analysis via a clustering weightless neural classifier. *Neurocomputing* 183, 70–78. doi: 10.1016/j.neucom.2015.06.105

Castelhano, J., Tavares, P., Mouga, S., Oliveira, G., and Castelo-Branco, M. (2018). Stimulus dependent neural oscillatory patterns show reliable statistical identification of autism spectrum disorder in a face perceptual decision task. *Clin. Neurophysiol.* 129, 981–989. doi: 10.1016/j.clinph.2018.01.072

Cavanagh, J. F., and Frank, M. J. (2014). Frontal theta as a mechanism for cognitive control. *Trends Cogn. Sci.* 18, 414–421. doi: 10.1016/j.tics.2014.04.012

Cavanna, A. E., and Trimble, M. R. (2006). The precuneus: a review of its functional anatomy and behavioural correlates. *Brain* 129, 564–583. doi: 10.1093/brain/awl004

Cheng, W., Rolls, E. T., Gu, H., Zhang, J., and Feng, J. (2015). Autism: reduced connectivity between cortical areas involved in face expression, theory of mind, and the sense of self. *Brain* 138(Pt 5), 1382–1393. doi: 10.1093/brain/awv051

Crespi, B., Leach, E., Dinsdale, N., Mokkonen, M., and Hurd, P. (2016). Imagination in human social cognition, autism, and psychotic-affective conditions. *Cognition* 150, 181–199. doi: 10.1016/j.cognition.2016.02.001

David, N., Aumann, C., Bewernick, B. H., Santos, N. S., Lehnhardt, F. G., and Vogeley, K. (2010). Investigation of mentalizing and visuospatial perspective taking for self and other in asperger syndrome. *J. Autism Dev. Disord.* 40, 290–299. doi: 10.1007/s10803-009-0867-4

Delorme, A., and Makeig, S. (2004). EEGLAB: an open sorce toolbox for analysis of single-trail EEG dynamics including independent component anlaysis. *J. Neurosci. Methods* 134, 9–21. doi: 10.1016/j.jneumeth.2003.10.009

Ekman, P., and Friesen, W. V. (1971). Constants across cultures in the face and emotion. *J. Pers. Soc. Psychol.* 17, 124–129. doi: 10.1037/h0030377

Ekman, P., and Friesen, W. V. (1978). *Facial Action Coding System: A Technique for the Measurement of Facial Movement.* Palo Alto, CA: Consulting Psychologists Press.

Field, T., Woodson, R., Greenberg, R., and Cohen, D. (1982). Discrimination and imitation of facial expression by neonates. *Science* 218, 179–181. doi: 10.1126/science.7123230

Fomina, T., Lohmann, G., Erb, M., Ethofer, T., Schölkopf, B., and Grosse-Wentrup, M. (2016). Self-regulation of brain rhythms in the precuneus: a novel BCI paradigm for patients with ALS. *J. Neural Eng.* 13:066021. doi: 10.1088/1741-2560/13/6/066021

França, F. M. G., de Gregorio, M., Lima, P. M. V., and de Oliveira, W. R. (2014). "Advances in weightless neural systems," in *Proceedings of the 22th European Symposium on the Artificial Neural Networks, Computational Intelligence and Machine Learning*, (Bruges).

Fu, Z., Tu, Y., Di, X., Du, Y., Sui, J., Biswal, B. B., et al. (2018). Transient increased thalamic-sensory connectivity and decreased whole-brain dynamism in autism. *Neuroimage* doi: 10.1016/j.neuroimage.2018.06.003 [Epub ahead of print].

Graewe, B., de Weerd, P., Farivar, R., and Castelo-Branco, M. (2012). Stimulus dependency of object-evoked responses in human visual cortex: an inverse problem for category specificity. *PLoS One* 7:e30727. doi: 10.1371/journal.pone.0030727

Grech, R., Cassar, T., Muscat, J., Camilleri, K. P., Fabri, S. G., Zervakis, M., et al. (2008). Review on solving the inverse problem in EEG source analysis. *J. Neuroeng. Rehabil.* 5:25. doi: 10.1186/1743-0003-5-25

Güntekin, B., and Başar, E. (2014). A review of brain oscillations in perception of faces and emotional pictures. *Neuropsychologia* 58, 33–51. doi: 10.1016/j.neuropsychologia.2014.03.014

Hamilton, A. F., Brindley, R., and Frith, U. (2009). Visual perspective taking impairment in children with autistic spectrum disorder. *Cognition* 113, 37–44. doi: 10.1016/j.cognition.2009.07.007

Harms, M. B., Martin, A., and Wallace, G. L. (2010). Facial emotion recognition in autism spectrum disorders: a review of behavioral and neuroimaging studies. *Neuropsychol. Rev.* 20, 290–322. doi: 10.1007/s11065-010-9138-6

Healey, M. L., and Grossman, M. (2018). Cognitive and affective perspective-taking: evidence for shared and dissociable anatomical substrates. *Front. Neurol.* 9:491. doi: 10.3389/fneur.2018.00491

Hirsch, C. R., Clark, D. M., and Mathews, A. (2006). Imagery and Interpretations in social phobia: support for the combined cognitive biases hypothesis. *Behav. Ther.* 37, 223–236. doi: 10.1016/j.beth.2006.02.001

Horki, P., Bauernfeind, G., Klobassa, D. S., Pokorny, C., Pichler, G., Schippinger, W., et al. (2014). Detection of mental imagery and attempted movements in patients with disorders of consciousness using EEG. *Front. Hum. Neurosci.* 8:1009. doi: 10.3389/fnhum.2014.01009

Huys, Q. J. M., Maia, T. V., and Frank, M. J. (2016). Computational psychiatry as a bridge from neuroscience to clinical applications. *Nat. Neurosci.* 19, 404–413. doi: 10.1038/nn.4238

Irimia, A., Torgerson, C. M., Jacokes, Z. J., and Van Horn, J. D. (2017). The connectomes of males and females with autism spectrum disorder have significantly different white matter connectivity densities. *Sci. Rep.* 7, 1–10. doi: 10.1038/srep46401

Kanwisher, N., and Yovel, G. (2006). The fusiform face area: a cortical region specialized for the perception of faces. *Philos. Trans. R. Soc. B Biol. Sci.* 361, 2109–2128. doi: 10.1098/rstb.2006.1934

Kircher, T. T. J., Brammer, M., Bullmore, E., Simmons, A., Bartels, M., and David, A. S. (2002). The neural correlates of intentional and incidental self processing. *Neuropsychologia* 40, 683–692. doi: 10.1016/S0028-3932(01)00138-5

Kliková, B., and Raidl, A. (2011). "Reconstruction of phase space of dynamical systems using method of time delay," in *Proceedings of the 20th Annual Conference WDS 2011*, Prague.

Knyazev, G. G., Slobodskoj-Plusnin, J. Y., and Bocharov, A. V. (2009). Event-related delta and theta synchronization during explicit and implicit emotion processing. *Neuroscience* 164, 1588–1600. doi: 10.1016/j.neuroscience.2009.09.057

Kosslyn, S. M., Ganis, G., and Thompson, W. L. (2001). Neural foundations of imagery. *Nat. Rev. Neurosci.* 2, 635–642. doi: 10.1038/35090055

Krumhuber, E. G., Kappas, A., and Manstead, A. S. R. (2013). Effects of dynamic aspects of facial expressions: a review. *Emot. Rev.* 5, 41–46. doi: 10.1177/1754073912451349

Lanius, R. A., Williamson, P. C., Boksman, K., Densmore, M., Gupta, M., Neufeld, R. W. J., et al. (2002). Brain activation during script-driven imagery induced dissociative responses in PTSD: a functional magnetic resonance imaging investigation. *Biol. Psychiatry* 52, 305–311. doi: 10.1016/S0006-3223(02)01367-7

Lee, T. M. C., Leung, M. K., Lee, T. M. Y., Raine, A., and Chan, C. C. H. (2013). I want to lie about not knowing you, but my precuneus refuses to cooperate. *Sci. Rep.* 3, 1–5. doi: 10.1038/srep01636

Lotte, F., Congedo, M., Lécuyer, A., Lamarche, F., and Arnaldi, B. (2007). A review of classification algorithms for EEG-based brain-computer interfaces. *J. Neural Eng.* 4, R1–R13.

Luckhardt, C., Kröger, A., Cholemkery, H., Bender, S., and Freitag, C. M. (2017). Neural correlates of explicit versus implicit facial emotion processing in ASD. *J. Autism Dev. Disord.* 47, 1944–1955. doi: 10.1007/s10803-017-3141-1

Makeig, S., Debener, S., Onton, J., and Delorme, A. (2004). Mining event-related brain dynamics. *Trends Cogn. Sci.* 8, 204–210. doi: 10.1016/j.tics.2004.03.008

Miller, H. L., and Bugnariu, N. L. (2016). Level of immersion in virtual environments impacts the ability to assess and teach social skills in autism spectrum disorder. *Cyberpsychol. Behav. Soc. Netw.* 19, 246–256. doi: 10.1089/cyber.2014.0682

Monteiro, R., Simões, M., Andrade, J., and Castelo Branco, M. (2017). Processing of facial expressions in autism: a systematic review of EEG/ERP evidence. *Rev. J. Autism Dev. Disord.* 4, 255–276. doi: 10.1007/s40489-017-0112-6

Nichols, T. E., and Holmes, A. P. (2001). Nonparametric permutation tests for {PET} functional neuroimaging experiments: a primer with examples. *Hum. Brain Mapp.* 15, 1–25. doi: 10.1002/hbm.1058

Ochsner, K. N., Knierim, K., Ludlow, D. H., Hanelin, J., Ramachandran, T., Glover, G., et al. (2004). Reflecting upon feelings: an fMRI study of neural systems supporting the attribution of emotion to self and other. *J. Cogn. Neurosci.* 16, 1746–1772. doi: 10.1162/0898929042947829

Pascual-Marqui, R. (1999). Review of methods for solving the EEG inverse problem. *Int. J. Bioelectromagn.* 1, 75–86.

Pascual-Marqui, R. D. (2002). Standardized low-resolution brain electromagnetic tomography (sLORETA): technical details. *Methods Find. Exp. Clin. Pharmacol.* 24(Suppl. D), 5–12.

Pascual-Marqui, R. D., Esslen, M., Kochi, K., and Lehmann, D. (2002). Functional imaging with low-resolution brain electromagnetic tomography (LORETA): a review. *Methods Find. Exp. Clin. Pharmacol.* 24(Suppl. C), 91–95.

Pearson, D. G., Deeprose, C., Wallace-Hadrill, S. M. A., Heyes, S. B., and Holmes, E. A. (2013). Assessing mental imagery in clinical psychology: a review of imagery measures and a guiding framework. *Clin. Psychol. Rev.* 33, 1–23. doi: 10.1016/j.cpr.2012.09.001

Pearson, J., Clifford, C., and Tong, F. (2009). The functional impact of mental imagery on conscious perception. *Curr. Biol.* 18, 982–986. doi: 10.1016/j.cub.2008.05.048

Pearson, J., Naselaris, T., Holmes, E. A., and Kosslyn, S. M. (2015). Mental imagery: functional mechanisms and clinical applications. *Trends Cogn. Sci.* 19, 590–602. doi: 10.1016/j.tics.2015.08.003

Ruggeri, B., Sarkans, U., Schumann, G., and Persico, A. M. (2014). Biomarkers in autism spectrum disorder: the old and the new. *Psychopharmacology* 231, 1201–1216. doi: 10.1007/s00213-013-3290-7

Saarimäki, H., Gotsopoulos, A., Jääskeläinen, I. P., Lampinen, J., Vuilleumier, P., Hari, R., et al. (2016). Discrete neural signatures of basic emotions. *Cereb. Cortex* 26, 2563–2573. doi: 10.1093/cercor/bhv086

Schurz, M., Kronbichler, M., Weissengruber, S., Surtees, A., Samson, D., and Perner, J. (2015). Clarifying the role of theory of mind areas during visual perspective taking: issues of spontaneity and domain-specificity. *Neuroimage* 117, 386–396. doi: 10.1016/j.neuroimage.2015.04.031

Simões, M., Amaral, C., França, F., Carvalho, P., and Castelo-Branco, M. (2018a). "Applying weightless neural networks to a P300-based brain-computer interface," in *Proceedings of the World Congress on Medical Physics and Biomedical Engineering 2018*, eds L. Lhotska, L. Sukupova, I. Lacković, and G. S. Ibbott (Singapore: Springer), 113–117.

Simões, M., Bernardes, M., Barros, F., and Castelo-Branco, M. (2018b). Virtual travel training for autism spectrum disorder: proof-of-concept interventional study. *JMIR Serious Games* 6:e5. doi: 10.2196/games.8428

Simoes, M., Lima, J., Direito, B., Castelhano, J., Ferreira, C., Carvalho, P., et al. (2015). "Feature analysis for correlation studies of simultaneous EEG-fMRI data: a proof of concept for neurofeedback approaches," in *Proceedings of the 37th Annual International Conference of the IEEE Engineering in Medicine and Biology Society (EMBC)*, Milan.

Sperdin, H. F., Coito, A., Kojovic, N., Rihs, T. A., Jan, R. K., Franchini, M., et al. (2018). Early alterations of social brain networks in young children with autism. *eLife* 7, 1–18. doi: 10.7554/eLife.31670

Spies, M., Kraus, C., Geissberger, N., Auer, B., Klöbl, M., Tik, M., et al. (2017). Default mode network deactivation during emotion processing predicts early antidepressant response. *Trans. Psychiatry* 7, e1008–e1009. doi: 10.1038/tp.2016.265

Takahashi, H. K., Kitada, R., Sasaki, A. T., Kawamichi, H., Okazaki, S., Kochiyama, T., et al. (2015). Brain networks of affective mentalizing revealed by the tear effect: the integrative role of the medial prefrontal cortex and precuneus. *Neurosci. Res.* 101, 32–43. doi: 10.1016/j.neures.2015.07.005

Takens, F. (1981). "Detecting strange attractors in turbulence," in *Dynamical Systems and Turbulence Lecture Notes in Mathematics*, eds D. A. Rand and L. S. Young (New York, NY: Springer), 366–381.

Tartaglia, E. M., Bamert, L., Mast, F. W., and Herzog, M. H. (2009). Human perceptual learning by mental imagery. *Curr. Biol.* 19, 2081–2085. doi: 10.1016/j.cub.2009.10.060

Varoquaux, G., Raamana, P. R., Engemann, D. A., Hoyos-Idrobo, A., Schwartz, Y., and Thirion, B. (2017). Assessing and tuning brain decoders: cross-validation, caveats, and guidelines. *Neuroimage* 145, 166–179. doi: 10.1016/j.neuroimage.2016.10.038

Velikova, S., Magnani, G., Arcari, C., Falautano, M., Franceschi, M., Comi, G., et al. (2011). Cognitive impairment and EEG background activity in adults with Down's syndrome: a topographic study. *Hum. Brain Mapp.* 32, 716–729. doi: 10.1002/hbm.21061

Vlamings, P., Jonkman, L., Van Daalen, E., Van Der Gaag, R. J., and Kemner, C. (2010). Basic abnormalities in visual processing affect face processing at an early age in autism spectrum disorder. *Biol. Psychiatry* 68, 1107–1113. doi: 10.1016/j.biopsych.2010.06.024

Vogeley, K., Bussfeld, P., Newen, A., Herrmann, S., Happé, F., Falkai, P., et al. (2001). Mind reading: neural mechanisms of theory of mind and self-perspective. *Neuroimage* 14, 170–181. doi: 10.1006/nimg.2001.0789

Wang, W., Viswanathan, S., Lee, T., and Grafton, S. T. (2016). Coupling between theta oscillations and cognitive control network during cross-modal visual and auditory attention: supramodal vs modality-specific mechanisms. *PLoS One* 11:e0158465. doi: 10.1371/journal.pone.0158465

Yang, Y. L., Deng, H. X., Xing, G. Y., Xia, X. L., and Li, H. F. (2015). Brain functional network connectivity based on a visual task: visual information processing-related brain regions are significantly activated in the task state. *Neural Regen. Res.* 10, 298–307. doi: 10.4103/1673-5374.152386

12

Abnormal Resting-State Functional Connectivity in the Whole Brain in Lifelong Premature Ejaculation Patients Based on Machine Learning Approach

Ziliang Xu[1†], Xuejuan Yang[1†], Ming Gao[2,3,4†], Lin Liu[1], Jinbo Sun[1], Peng Liu[1] and Wei Qin[1]*

[1] Engineering Research Center of Molecular and Neuro Imaging of Ministry of Education, School of Life Science and Technology, Xidian University, Xi'an, China, [2] Assisted Reproduction Center, Northwest Women's and Children's Hospital, Xi'an, China, [3] Department of Urology, Xijing Hospital, Fourth Military Medical University, Xi'an, China, [4] Department of Andrology, Xiyuan Hospital, China Academy of Chinese Medical Sciences, Beijing, China

***Correspondence:**
Wei Qin
wqin@xidian.edu.cn

† These authors have contributed equally to this work

Recent neuroimaging studies have indicated that abnormalities in brain structure and function may play an important role in the etiology of lifelong premature ejaculation (LPE). LPE patients have exhibited aberrant cortical structure, altered brain network function and abnormal brain activation in response to erotic pictures. However, it remains unclear whether resting-state whole brain functional connectivity (FC) is altered in LPE patients. Machine learning analysis has the advantage of screening the best classification features from high-throughput data (such as FC), which has the potential to identify the pathophysiological targets of disease by establishing classification indicators for patients and healthy controls (HCs). Therefore, the supported vector machine based classification model using FC as features was used in the present study to confirm the most specific FCs that distinguish LPE patients from healthy controls. After feature selection, the remained features were used to build the classification model, with an accuracy 0.85 ± 0.14, sensitivity of 0.92 ± 0.18, specificity of 0.72 ± 0.30, and recall index of 0.85 ± 0.17 across 1000 testing groups (100 times 10-folds cross validation). After that, two-sample *t*-tests with family-wise error correction were used to compare these features that occur more than 500 times during training steps between LPE patients and HCs. Four FCs, (1) between left medial part of orbital frontal cortex (mOFC) and right mOFC, (2) between the left rectus and right postcentral gyrus, (3) between the right insula and left pallidum, and (4) between the right middle part of temporal pole and right inferior part of temporal gyrus showed significant group difference. These results demonstrate that resting-state brain FC might be a discriminating feature to distinguish LPE patients from HCs. These classification features, especially the FC between bilateral mOFC, provide underlying abnormal central functional targets in LPE etiology, which offers a novel alternative target for future intervention in LPE treatment.

Keywords: lifelong premature ejaculation, feature selection, functional magnetic resonance imaging, support vector machine, functional connectivity

INTRODUCTION

In recent years, more and more neuroimaging studies have found that the etiology of sexual function dysfunction may be related to brain abnormalities, including brain structure, and functional aberrance (Zhao et al., 2015a,b; Chen et al., 2017; Jin et al., 2017; Li et al., 2018). Lifelong premature ejaculation (LPE) is one of the most common male sexual dysfunction diseases. According to the International Society for Sexual Medicine, LPE is defined as "a male sexual dysfunction characterized by ejaculation which always or nearly always occurs prior to or within about 1 min of vaginal penetration since the first sexual experience; and inability to delay ejaculation on all or nearly all vaginal penetrations; and negative personal consequences, such as distress, bother, frustration and or the avoidance of sexual intimacy (Althof et al., 2014)." Although selective serotonin reuptake inhibitors have been found to produce a side effect of delayed ejaculation in the treatment of depression and have gradually become the first-line drug for clinical treatment of premature ejaculation (PE) (Giuliano and Clement, 2012), the pathophysiological mechanisms of LPE remain unclear. As early as 10 years ago, neuroimaging studies demonstrated that the brain is involved in ejaculation behavior (Holstege et al., 2003; Georgiadis et al., 2007); however, evidence regarding to the role of the brain in the etiology of LPE remains limited, especially at the supraspinal level.

In Zhang et al. (2017), the first neuroimaging study of brain changes in LPE patients was conducted. Subsequently, there have been a few studies reporting brain structural and functional abnormalities in LPE, including by our group. These studies have shown that LPE patients have increased cortical thickness and possible improved sensory ascending conduction efficiency (Guo et al., 2017; Gao et al., 2018), and abnormal brain function either in resting state or during erotic picture stimulation (Zhang et al., 2017; Lu et al., 2018; Yang et al., 2018), which have provided new evidence for the neurobiological etiology of LPE. Recently, machine learning methods have also been used in the analysis of high-throughput brain imaging data to obtain more disease-specific imaging features. For example, classifiers based on brain structure or brain function features have been used to distinguish psychiatric patients from healthy people, to distinguish different subtypes of patients, and to predict remission and non-remission when evaluating therapeutic effects (Fu et al., 2008; Grotegerd et al., 2014; Redlich et al., 2016; Du et al., 2018). These classification features offer useful insight for detecting the biological mechanisms of diseases. Interestingly, a recent study investigating the brain mechanism of venous erectile dysfunction used machine learning classification to distinguish patients from healthy controls, and revealed more various white matter-derived indices that might underlie imaging targets related to the neurobiological etiology of venous erectile dysfunction (Li et al., 2018).

Therefore, in the present study, we aimed to use a machine learning method to classify LPE patients from healthy subjects based on high-throughput resting brain functional connectivity (FC) data, in effort to find the most specific discriminating indicators between LPE patients and healthy controls. We believe our results provide novel information for understanding the neurobiological mechanism of LPE.

MATERIALS AND METHODS

Participants

Sixty male adults non-medicated PE patients and sixty male non-drug-using healthy controls (HCs) were recruited in our study. LPE was diagnosed according to the International Society for Sexual Medicine's guidelines for the diagnosis and treatment of premature ejaculation (Althof et al., 2010). All participants underwent history taking and physical examination. Each patient had an intravaginal ejaculatory latency time (IELT) within 1 min. The premature ejaculation diagnostic tool (PEDT) score of each LPE patient was >11, but <5 for each control. The International Index of Erectile Function score was no less than 21 for all subjects. Participants were excluded if they met any of the following criteria: (1) had a history of alcohol or drug abuse, (2) had a history of psychiatric or neurologic diseases, (3) having a history of head trauma, and (4) had any contra-indication to MRI scanning.

According to the selection standards above, 45 PE patients and 40 HCs were included in the current study. Written informed consent was obtained from all study participants. Research procedures were approved by the ethical committee of the Northwest Women's and Children's Hospital in China, and were conducted in accordance with the Code of Ethics of the World Medical Association (Declaration of Helsinki).

Imaging Data Acquisition

All subjects underwent a series of image scanning using a 3T GE MR750 scanner at the Department of Radiology, Xijing Hospital, the Fourth Military Medical University, Xi'an, China. A standard 8-channel head coil was used together with a restraining foam pad to minimize head motion and diminish scanner noise. Resting-state functional images were acquired with a single-shot gradient recalled echo planar imaging sequence. (TR/TE: 2000 ms/30 ms, field of view: 240×240 mm^2, matrix size: 64×64, flip angle: 90°, in-plane resolution: 3.75×3.75 mm^2, slice thickness: 3.5 mm with no gaps, 45 axial slices). For each subject, a total of 210 volumes were acquired. High resolution T1-weighted images were collected with a volumetric three-dimensional spoiled gradient recall sequence (TR/TE: 8.2 ms/3.18 ms, field of view: 256×256 mm^2, matrix size: 512×512, flip angle = 9°, in-plane resolution: 0.5×0.5 mm^2, slice thickness = 1 mm, 196 sagittal slices). During the resting scanning, subjects were instructed to keep their eyes open and to not think about anything.

Imaging Data Preprocessing

Functional image preprocessing was carried out using CONN software[1]. Briefly, after excluding the first five images to ensure the signal had reached equilibrium, functional images were corrected for head motion and temporal differences. A participant was excluded if any translation or rotation parameters in subject's data set exceeded $\pm$ 1 mm or $\pm$ 1°,

[1] http://web.mit.edu/swg/software.htm

respectively. After this step, 39 patients and 30 HCs remained. After that, outlier detection was performed. Next, the corrected functional images were coregistered to each subject's T1 image without reslicing the image. After that, T1 images were normalized to the Montreal Neurological Institute (MNI) space, which generated a transformed matrix from native space to MNI space. Functional images were then transformed to the MNI space using this matrix and resampled at $2 \times 2 \times 2$ mm^3. Finally, all images were smoothed with a 6-mm full width at half maximum Gaussian kernel.

To remove spurious sources of variance, time series of each brain voxel were performed by the following steps: (1) linear detrending; (2) regressing out the six head motion parameters and their first-level derivative, the averaged cerebrospinal fluid and white matter signals, and the scrubbing signal from the time series generated by the functional outlier detection (ART-based identification of scans for scrubbing) process in CONN; (3) 0.01–0.1 Hz band-pass filtering.

After data preprocessing, time series of each region of interest (ROI) were extracted as the average time series across all voxels in that ROI based on the Anatomical Automatic Labeling (AAL) cortical and subcortical atlas (Tzourio-Mazoyer et al., 2002). In this step, 90 ROI time series were extracted. Finally, the FC coefficient (e.g., Pearson's correlation coefficient) between each pair of these 90 time series was calculated, which resulted in 4005 edges for each subject for subsequent analysis.

Features Selection and Classification Model

Ten-folds cross validation (CV) was used to assess the reliability of the classification model. Briefly, 69 subjects were randomly separated into 10 groups. Each time, one group in turn was used as a testing group and the other nine groups were used as training group.

Firstly, two sample T-test was used as the first step to preliminarily select features from the 4005 edges in training group. The edges with a p-value less than P_0 were selected as initial features. After that, we used a 10-folds CV based Least Absolute Shrinkage and Selection Operator (CV-LASSO) method to further select features. Briefly, subjects in training group were again randomly separated into 10 groups. Each time, one group in turn was excluded from the dataset, and the LASSO (Sauerbrei et al., 2007) method with mean of square error (MSE) as the cost function was used on the remaining nine groups to narrow down the initial features into the most important features according to the MSE+1SE criteria (Sauerbrei et al., 2007). This step was repeated 10 times, which resulted in 10 different groups of selected features. Finally, the edges that were included in the selected feature group at least N times (i.e., occurring N times) were selected as LASSO features for further analysis. Next, the linear supported vector machine (LSVM) method was used to construct the classification model based on LASSO features in training group, which was implemented using *libsvm* software[2]. The accuracy, sensitivity, specificity and recall indices of the constructed model were calculated using testing group.

All these steps above were repeated 10 times. As for the setting of P_0, N, and the cost parameter c in libsvm, we used grid-search method to find them. These parameters were set at a group of specific values when the accuracy index of the constructed classification model achieved the maximum. The P_0 was set from 0.025 to 0.2 with a step of 0.025 and including 0.001, 0.005, and 0.01. The N was set from 1 to 10 with a step of 1. The c was set from 0.1 to 2 with a step of 0.1.

To avoid the random group effect, we repeated the 10-folds CV 100 times. For each time, a new random group was split. The mean ± standard deviation of each index across the 1000 testing groups (10×100) was used to assess the performance and stability of the constructed model. Finally, 1000 times permutation test (group label permutation) was performed to check if our results were significantly different from random label. **Figure 1** illustrates the framework of our study.

[2]https://www.csie.ntu.edu.tw/~cjlin/libsvm/

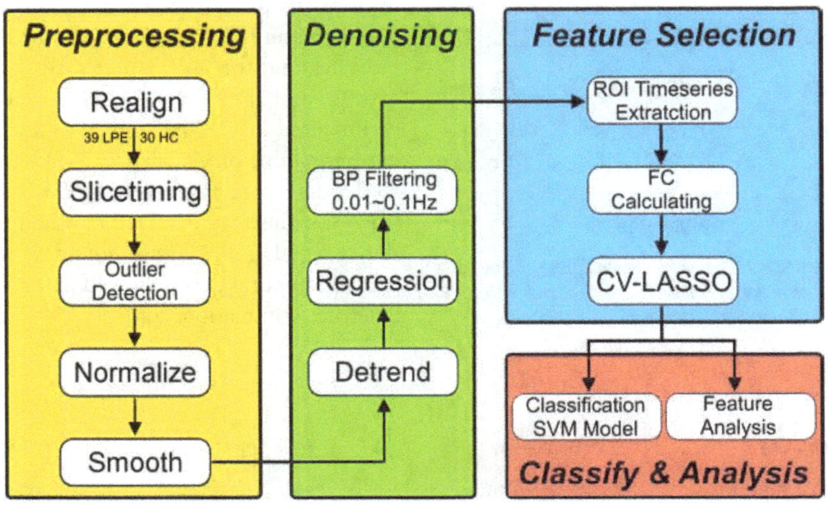

FIGURE 1 | The framework of study procedure.

RESULTS

Clinical and Demographic Characteristics

Clinical and demographic characteristics of the subjects are shown in **Table 1**. The PEDT scores of LPE patients were significantly higher than those of HCs, and the IELT of LPE patients was dramatically shorter than that of HCs.

Classification

The 100 times 10-fold CV results of the model were shown in **Table 2**. The accuracy, sensitivity, specificity and recall indices of the classification model were 0.8490 ± 0.1401, 0.9238 ± 0.1817, 0.7250 ± 0.3038, and 0.8506 ± 0.1740, respectively. **Figure 2B** displays the receiver operating characteristic curve (ROC) of the classification model, and the AUC was 0.8047. **Figure 3** shows the permutation test results of our constructed classification model. Together, these results demonstrate the stability of our classification model and the reliability of our method.

After counting the occurring time of each LASSO feature in 100 times 10-fold CV, 5 LASSO features with occurring time larger than 500 were finally selected as the most important features in classification, which involved brain regions in the frontal, temporal and limbic lobes (**Table 3**), since we believed that features which occurring time less than 500 were to a large extent relied on the specific splitting group. **Figure 2A** gives the spatial distribution of these 5 LASSO features.

DISCUSSION

By using a machine learning classification method to assess resting-state brain function in LPE patients, the present study screened 9.042 (average across every training step during 100 times 10-folds CV) out of 4005 FC features to construct the optimal classifier, which could separate patients from healthy people with an accuracy of 0.85. These FC features are mainly distributed in some areas in the frontal, temporal, and parietal cortex, and limbic system. Compared with previous studies, our results provide more novel FC-derived indicators through a strategy of classification research to understand the potential abnormalities of brain function in LPE patients.

The classification algorithm in machine learning is useful for exploring the best classification features from high-throughput information, in which multivariate decoding algorithms like supported vector machine are trained on a portion of the data by weighting all connections in order to separate the known clinical status from HCs, rather than testing each connection independently for group differences. The whole brain functional connections belong to a high-throughput data set, in which there are more than 4000 FCs in the whole brain when the human brain is divided into 90 ROIs. In our present study, through CV-LASSO dimension reduction method, we have obtained a classifier with a relatively high accuracy to individually distinguish LPE patients from HCs. This machine learning-based classification approach based on resting-state FC has previously been used to distinguish patients with brain disorders from HCs, and responders from non-responders in clinical drug or invention trials (van Waarde et al., 2015; Sarpal et al., 2016; Arbabshirani et al., 2017; Plaschke et al., 2017). Therefore, the features based on the resting-state FC in our present study may be biomarkers that allow the classification of individual LPE patients.

Among the five selected features which occur more than 500 times in training step during 100 times 10-fold CV, the connections between bilateral mOFC had the highest weight according to our results. OFC has been implicated in ejaculation control. A previous positron emission tomography study has reported a remarkable decrease of regional cerebral blood flow throughout the prefrontal cortex during ejaculation in male volunteers (Holstege et al., 2003; Georgiadis et al., 2007). Our previous study has also found abnormal prefrontal control function in LPE patients by using classical inhibitory control tasks, and reduced FC between the inferior frontal cortex and the frontal pole was found in LPE patients (Yang et al., 2018). Together with the present results that the synchronized activity of the mirror symmetric OFC had absolute superiority in discriminating LPE patients from the healthy controls, it further indicates that the OFC is likely closely involved in the etiology of LPE, and the OFC-related inhibitory control function may be impaired in LPE patients, which might cause the loss of the inhibitory tone on ejaculation in LPE patients.

Besides, most of the other FC related regions in the current study were also reported to be related to male sexual physiology. Zhang et al. (2017) have found that the insula and middle part of temporal gyrus showed abnormal activation in response to erotic stimulation, and also had aberrant regional activity

TABLE 1 | Clinical and demographic characteristics.

	HC (*n* = 30)	LPE (*n* = 39)	*P*-value
Age (years)	31.33 ± 2.77	30.52 ± 5.06	0.44
PEDT score	0.80 ± 1.40	17.50 ± 1.96	<0.0001
IIEF-5 score	24.5 ± 0.63	24.29 ± 0.47	0.17
IELT (min)	644.00 ± 366.47	37.02 ± 16.75	<0.0001

Data were presented as mean ± SD. HC, healthy control; IELT, intravaginal ejaculatory latency time; IIEF-5, International Index of Erectile Function-5; LPE, lifelong premature ejaculation; PEDT, Premature ejaculation diagnostic tool.

TABLE 2 | Performance information of classification model.

	Accuracy	Sensitivity	Specificity	Recall	AUC
	0.8490 ± 0.1401	0.9238 ± 0.1817	0.7250 ± 0.3038	0.8506 ± 0.1740	0.8047
Permutation	< 0.001	–	–	–	< 0.001

AUC, area under the curve; Permutation, 1000 Permutation test.

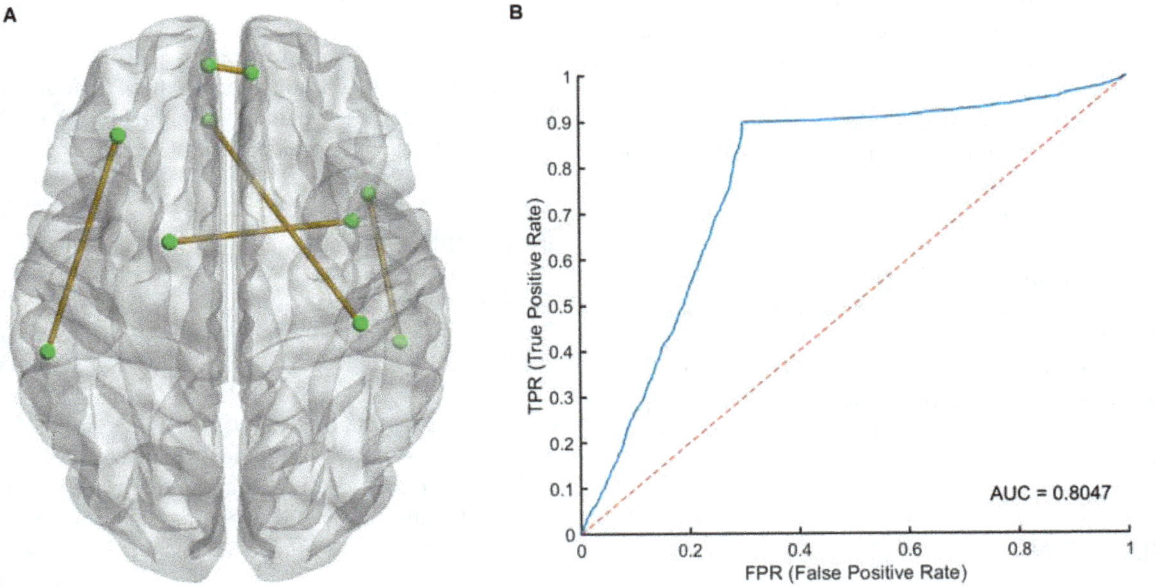

FIGURE 2 | (A) The spatial distribution of five selected LASSO features and **(B)** the receiver operating characteristic (ROC) curve of the classification model. LASSO, least absolute shrinkage and selection operator.

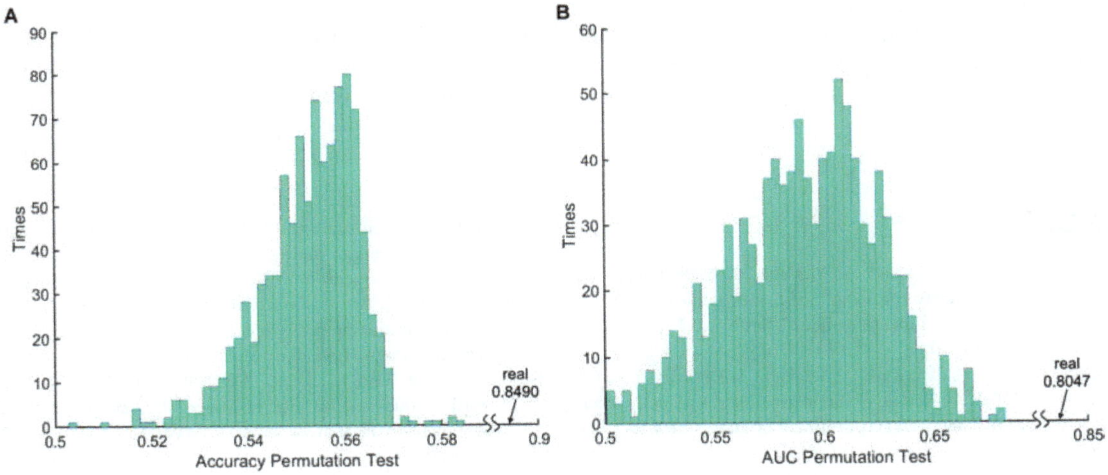

FIGURE 3 | The 1000 times permutation test results of **(A)** classification model accuracy index and **(B)** area under curve (AUC).

TABLE 3 | Detailed information of five selected LASSO features.

Edge		Weight
HC>PE		
Frontal_Med_Orb_L	Frontal_Med_Orb_R	0.4874
Rectus_L	Postcentral_R	0.0020
Insula_R	Pallidum_L	0.1270
HC<PE		
Frontal_Mid_L	SupraMarginal_L	0.1370
Temporal_Pole_Mid_R	Temporal_Inf_R	0.2466

Frontal_Med_Orb, medial part of orbital frontal cortex; Frontal_Mid, middle part of frontal cortex; Temporal_Pole_Mid, middle part of temporal pole; Temporal_Inf, inferior part of temporal gyrus; L for left and R for right; LASSO, absolute shrinkage and selection operator.

and FC during resting state in LPE patients. By using cerebral cortical thickness measurements, we once reported widespread cortical thickening in the orbitofrontal, middle frontal, and supramarginal gyrus in LPE patients (Guo et al., 2017). A recent fMRI study detected the resting-state FC density in LPE patients, which found that anterior cingulate cortex, insula, and precuneus had increased long-range FC density in LPE patients compared to healthy controls (Lu et al., 2018). Although the role of gyrus rectus and postcentral gyrus in LPE has not been reported yet, the gyrus rectus is located in the medial orbital gyrus and plays an inhibition role in sexual arousal (Stoleru et al., 2012), and sensory stimuli from penis could induce Rolandic opercula area and postcentral gyrus activation (Stoleru et al., 2012).

So, despite our results were derived from a data-driven method, these classification features that are involved in ejaculation and other sexual behaviors extend our knowledge of the central pathophysiology in LPE patients.

There are several limitations in the current study. We only included LPE patients without secondary PE patients. So, we do not know if our classifier was specific to LPE or trans-disease subtypes across all PE patients. Further research is necessary to include more subtypes of PE patients for classification studies. In addition, other than FC, brain gray matter and white matter structure have often been used as classification indicators. Li et al. (2018) have used white matter indicators to successfully distinguish venous erectile dysfunction patients from HCs. These measures were not included in the present study, but multimodal brain imaging information should be used in future classification studies of PE.

CONCLUSION

By using machine learning analysis, this study identified potential neuroimaging markers based on resting-state whole brain FC that could distinguish LPE patients from HCs. These classification features provide novel information for explaining the central mechanisms of LPE, and further emphasize the potential functional abnormalities of the central inhibitory control network and sexual-related regions in LPE patients.

AUTHOR CONTRIBUTIONS

JS, PL, XY, and WQ contributed to the conception and design. LL contributed to the acquisition of data. ZX and XY contributed to the data analysis and manuscript writing. XY, LL, and ZX contributed to the interpretation of the results.

FUNDING

This study was financially supported by National Basic Research Program of China under grant nos. 2015CB856403 and 2014CB543203, the Science and Technology Projects of Xi'an, China under grant no. 201809170CX11JC12, the National Natural Science Foundation of China under grant nos. 81471811 and 81471738, the Development Funds of Shaanxi Science and Technology Agency of China under grant no. 2018SF/091, Shaanxi Health and Family Planning Commission Foundation of China for Youths under grant no. 2016E04, and Xi'an Science and Technology Development Funds of China under grant no. 2016052SF/YX08.

ACKNOWLEDGMENTS

We thank Lesley McCollum, Ph.D., from Liwen Bianji, Edanz Editing China (www.liwenbianji.cn/ac), for editing the English text of a draft of this manuscript.

REFERENCES

Althof, S. E., Abdo, C. H., Dean, J., Hackett, G., McCabe, M., McMahon, C. G., et al. (2010). International society for sexual medicine's guidelines for the diagnosis and treatment of premature ejaculation. *J. Sex. Med.* 7, 2947–2969. doi: 10.1111/j.1743-6109.2010.01975.x

Althof, S. E., McMahon, C. G., Waldinger, M. D., Serefoglu, E. C., Shindel, A. W., Adaikan, P. G., et al. (2014). An update of the international society of sexual medicine's guidelines for the diagnosis and treatment of premature ejaculation (PE). *J. Sex. Med.* 11, 1392–1422. doi: 10.1111/jsm.12504

Arbabshirani, M. R., Plis, S., Sui, J., and Calhoun, V. D. (2017). Single subject prediction of brain disorders in neuroimaging: promises and pitfalls. *Neuroimage* 145(Pt B), 137–165. doi: 10.1016/j.neuroimage.2016.02.079

Chen, J., Chen, Y., Chen, G., Dai, Y., Yao, Z., and Lu, Q. (2017). Altered brain networks in psychogenic erectile dysfunction: a resting-state fMRI study. *Andrology* 5, 1073–1081. doi: 10.1111/andr.12411

Du, Y., Fu, Z., and Calhoun, V. D. (2018). Classification and prediction of brain disorders using functional connectivity: promising but challenging. *Front. Neurosci.* 12:525. doi: 10.3389/fnins.2018.00525

Fu, C. H., Mourao-Miranda, J., Costafreda, S. G., Khanna, A., Marquand, A. F., Williams, S. C., et al. (2008). Pattern classification of sad facial processing: toward the development of neurobiological markers in depression. *Biol. Psychiatry* 63, 656–662. doi: 10.1016/j.biopsych.2007.08.020

Gao, M., Yang, X., Liu, L., Fei, N., Xi, Y., Guo, F., et al. (2018). Abnormal white matter microstructure in lifelong premature ejaculation patients identified by tract-based spatial statistical analysis. *J. Sex. Med.* 15, 1272–1279. doi: 10.1016/j.jsxm.2018.07.012

Georgiadis, J. R., Reinders, A. A., Van der Graaf, F. H., Paans, A. M., and Kortekaas, R. (2007). Brain activation during human male ejaculation revisited. *Neuroreport* 18, 553–557. doi: 10.1097/wnr.0b013e3280b10bfe

Giuliano, F., and Clement, P. (2012). Pharmacology for the treatment of premature ejaculation. *Pharmacol. Rev.* 64, 621–644. doi: 10.1124/pr.111.004952

Grotegerd, D., Stuhrmann, A., Kugel, H., Schmidt, S., Redlich, R., Zwanzger, P., et al. (2014). Amygdala excitability to subliminally presented emotional faces distinguishes unipolar and bipolar depression: an fMRI and pattern classification study. *Hum. Brain Mapp.* 35, 2995–3007. doi: 10.1002/hbm.22380

Guo, F., Xi, Y. B., Gao, M., Liu, L., Fei, N. B., Qin, W., et al. (2017). Alterations in cortical thickness in nonmedicated premature ejaculation patients: a morphometric MRI study. *J. Magn. Reson. Imaging* 47, 656–662. doi: 10.1002/jmri.25808

Holstege, G., Georgiadis, J. R., Paans, A. M., Meiners, L. C., van der Graaf, F. H., and Reinders, A. A. (2003). Brain activation during human male ejaculation. *J. Neurosci.* 23, 9185–9193. doi: 10.1523/jneurosci.23-27-09185.2003

Jin, C., Guan, M., Dong, M., Wu, J., He, Z., Chen, X., et al. (2017). Aberrant baseline brain activity in psychogenic erectile dysfunction patients: a resting state fMRI study. *Brain Imaging Behav.* 12, 1393–1404. doi: 10.1007/s11682-017-9805-9

Li, L., Fan, W., Li, J., Li, Q., Wang, J., Fan, Y., et al. (2018). Abnormal brain structure as a potential biomarker for venous erectile dysfunction: evidence from multimodal MRI and machine learning. *Eur. Radiol.* 28, 3789–3800. doi: 10.1007/s00330-018-5365-7

Lu, J., Zhang, X., Wang, H., Qing, Z., Han, P., Li, M., et al. (2018). Short- and long-range synergism disorders in lifelong premature ejaculation evaluated using the functional connectivity density and network property. *Neuroimage Clin.* 19, 607–615. doi: 10.1016/j.nicl.2018.05.025

Plaschke, R. N., Cieslik, E. C., Muller, V. I., Hoffstaedter, F., Plachti, A., Varikuti, D. P., et al. (2017). On the integrity of functional brain networks in schizophrenia, Parkinson's disease, and advanced age: evidence from connectivity-based single-subject classification. *Hum. Brain Mapp.* 38, 5845–5858. doi: 10.1002/hbm.23763

Redlich, R., Opel, N., Grotegerd, D., Dohm, K., Zaremba, D., Burger, C., et al.

(2016). Prediction of individual response to electroconvulsive therapy via machine learning on structural magnetic resonance imaging data. *JAMA Psychiatry* 73, 557–564. doi: 10.1001/jamapsychiatry.2016.0316

Sarpal, D. K., Argyelan, M., Robinson, D. G., Szeszko, P. R., Karlsgodt, K. H., John, M., et al. (2016). Baseline striatal functional connectivity as a predictor of response to antipsychotic drug treatment. *Am. J. Psychiatry* 173, 69–77. doi: 10.1176/appi.ajp.2015.14121571

Sauerbrei, W., Royston, P., and Binder, H. (2007). Selection of important variables and determination of functional form for continuous predictors in multivariable model building. *Stat. Med.* 26, 5512–5528. doi: 10.1002/sim.3148

Stoleru, S., Fonteille, V., Cornelis, C., Joyal, C., and Moulier, V. (2012). Functional neuroimaging studies of sexual arousal and orgasm in healthy men and women: a review and meta-analysis. *Neurosci. Biobehav. Rev.* 36, 1481–1509. doi: 10.1016/j.neubiorev.2012.03.006

Tzourio-Mazoyer, N., Landeau, B., Papathanassiou, D., Crivello, F., Etard, O., Delcroix, N., et al. (2002). Automated anatomical labeling of activations in SPM using a macroscopic anatomical parcellation of the MNI MRI single-subject brain. *Neuroimage* 15, 273–289. doi: 10.1006/nimg.2001.0978

van Waarde, J. A., Scholte, H. S., van Oudheusden, L. J., Verwey, B., Denys, D., and van Wingen, G. A. (2015). A functional MRI marker may predict the outcome of electroconvulsive therapy in severe and treatment-resistant depression. *Mol. Psychiatry* 20, 609–614. doi: 10.1038/mp.2014.78

Yang, X., Gao, M., Zhang, L., Liu, L., Liu, P., Sun, J., et al. (2018). Central neural correlates during inhibitory control in lifelong premature ejaculation patients. *Front. Hum. Neurosci.* 12:206. doi: 10.3389/fnhum.2018.00206

Zhang, B., Lu, J., Xia, J., Wang, F., Li, W., Chen, F., et al. (2017). Functional insights into aberrant brain responses and integration in patients with lifelong premature ejaculation. *Sci. Rep.* 7:460. doi: 10.1038/s41598-017-00421-3

Zhao, L., Guan, M., Zhang, X., Karama, S., Khundrakpam, B., Wang, M., et al. (2015a). Structural insights into aberrant cortical morphometry and network organization in psychogenic erectile dysfunction. *Hum. Brain Mapp.* 36, 4469–4482. doi: 10.1002/hbm.22925

Zhao, L., Guan, M., Zhu, X., Karama, S., Khundrakpam, B., Wang, M., et al. (2015b). Aberrant topological patterns of structural cortical networks in psychogenic erectile dysfunction. *Front. Hum. Neurosci.* 9:675. doi: 10.3389/fnhum.2015.00675

13

Potential Mechanism for HIV-Associated Depression: Upregulation of Serotonin Transporters in SIV-Infected Macaques Detected by 11C-DASB PET

Swati Shah[1], Sanhita Sinharay[1], Kenta Matsuda[2], William Schreiber-Stainthorp[1], Siva Muthusamy[1], Dianne Lee[1], Paul Wakim[3], Vanessa Hirsch[2], Avindra Nath[4], Michele Di Mascio[5] and Dima A. Hammoud[1]*

[1] Center for Infectious Disease Imaging (CIDI), Radiology and Imaging Sciences,Clinical Center, National Institutes of Health (NIH), Bethesda, MD, United States, [2] Laboratory of Molecular Microbiology, National Institute of Allergy and Infectious Diseases (NIAID), NIH, Bethesda, MD, United States, [3] Biostatistics and Clinical Epidemiology Service, Clinical Center, NIH, Bethesda, MD, United States, [4] National Institute of Neurological Disorder and Stroke (NINDS), NIH, Bethesda, MD, United States, [5] AIDS Imaging Research Section, Division of Clinical Research, NIAID, NIH, Rockville, MD, United States

***Correspondence:**
Dima A. Hammoud
hammoudd@cc.nih.gov

Purpose: Increased incidence of depression in HIV+ patients is associated with lower adherence to treatment and increased morbidity/mortality. One possible underlying pathophysiology is serotonergic dysfunction. In this study, we used an animal model of HIV, the SIV-infected macaque, to longitudinally image serotonin transporter (SERT) expression before and after inoculation, using 11C-DASB (SERT ligand) PET imaging.

Methods: We infected seven rhesus macaques with a neurovirulent SIV strain and imaged them at baseline and multiple time points after inoculation (group A). Pyrosequencing methylation analysis of the SERT promoter region was performed. We also measured SERT mRNA/protein in brain single-cell suspensions from another group (group B) of SIV-infected animals ($n = 13$).

Results: Despite some animals showing early fluctuations, 86% of our group A animals eventually showed a net increase in midbrain/thalamus binding potential (BP_{ND}) over the course of their disease (mean increased binding between last time point and baseline = 30.2% and 32.2%, respectively). Repeated-measures mixed-model analysis showed infection duration to be predictive of midbrain BP_{ND} ($p = 0.039$). Thalamic BP_{ND} was statistically significantly associated with multiple CSF cytokines ($P < 0.05$). There was higher SERT protein levels in the second group (group B) of SIV-infected animals with SIV encephalitis (SIVE) compared to those without SIVE ($p = 0.014$). There were no longitudinal changes in SERT gene promoter region percentage methylation between baselines and last time points in group A animals.

Conclusion: Upregulated SERT leading to lower synaptic levels of serotonin is a possible mechanism of depression in HIV+ patients, and extrapolating our conclusions from SIV to HIV should be sought using translational human studies.

Keywords: HIV, SIV, depression, serotonin transporter, PET

INTRODUCTION

Despite mounting evidence of higher depression rates in HIV-positive (HIV+) individuals compared to seronegative controls and associated increased morbidity and mortality (1), there is limited literature targeting the underlying mechanisms of depressive disorders in HIV. In one paper, the levels of serotonin transporter (SERT) mRNA in the peripheral blood mononuclear cells (PBMCs) of SHIV-infected rhesus macaques were significantly reduced compared to control animals, suggesting that SERT expression might be affected in HIV (2). In another study, disruption of cytoskeletal genes and dysregulation of somatostatin were found to be part of the pathologic process of major depressive disorder (MDD) in the setting of HIV (3). Tryptophan metabolism dysregulation is also suspected to play a role (4, 5).

The only previous positron emission tomography (PET) study targeting SERT in the setting of HIV depression demonstrated generally lower 11C-DASB (radioactive ligand targeting SERT) binding in HIV+ patients compared to healthy controls. Depressed HIV+ patients, however, showed higher 11C-DASB binding than non-depressed patients, suggesting SERT upregulation in the depressed group and possible abnormal serotonergic transmission in HIV-associated depression (6). No other similar cross-sectional or longitudinal PET studies have been performed to date.

In the current study, we used PET and 11C-DASB to assess SERT binding in an HIV animal model, the SIV-infected macaque, at baseline and at different intervals after inoculation with a neurotropic SIV strain (SIVsm804E) to determine the natural history of serotonergic dysregulation in relation to serum and CSF markers of SIV infection. We correlated our findings with clinical and laboratory markers of SIV infection and performed a detailed analysis of the SERT gene promoter region methylation changes between baseline and the last time point to assess any potential epigenetic effects on gene expression. Based on previous literature describing *in vitro* and *in vivo* interactions between various cytokines (e.g., IL-1, IL-6, IL-10, TNFα, and IFNγ) and SERT expression (7–12), we specifically correlated 11C-DASB binding with levels of various CSF cytokines.

METHODS AND MATERIALS

Subjects

All procedures were performed in accordance with the recommendations of the *Guide for the Care and Use of Laboratory Animals*. The study was approved by the Animal Care and Use Committee of the National Institutes of Allergy and Infectious Diseases (NIAID), National Institutes of Health (NIH).

Fifty Indian rhesus macaques (*Macaca mulatta*) were genotyped for Trim5α. Seven animals were found to have the Q/Q genotype (group A, **Supplementary Table 1S**) and thus were selected for this study, as they are known to have increased susceptibility to development of neurological disease (13–15). All animals were inoculated intravenously with 500 $TCID_{50}$ (50% tissue culture infective doses) of SIVsm804E (14). The selected animals included five females and two males (mean baseline age = 3.7 years). Five out of seven animals (SIV #1, 2, 3, 4, and 7) progressed soon after inoculation (mean = 14.6 weeks, "rapid progressors") and were rescued with treatment (daily subcutaneous injections of tenofovir (PMPA; 20 mg/kg) and emtricitabine (FTC; 30 mg/kg) with raltegravir (20 mg/kg) mixed with food twice per day). Two of the rapid progressors succumbed to the disease despite treatment (SIV #4 and 7), while the others responded to treatment and survived. The two "slow progressors" (SIV #5 and 6) did not show symptoms until 87 and 91 weeks after inoculation, respectively. On development of symptoms, one slow progressor (SIV #6) responded to treatment, while the other subject (SIV #5) developed a presumed opportunistic infection and had to be excluded.

Treatment was eventually discontinued, and the surviving animals (one slow and three rapid progressors) were allowed to progress to a chronic infectious stage prior to necropsy. The last imaging time point, however, did not always correspond to the survival of the animals, due to logistical considerations. Details of group A animals' imaging and disease progression are included in **Table 1S**.

We also evaluated whole-brain cell suspensions obtained from a separate group of SIV-infected monkeys (group B, n = 13), of which only six animals showed neurological symptoms and were found to have neuropathology consistent with SIVE, as described earlier (16).

Magnetic Resonance Imaging

All subjects underwent magnetic resonance (MR) imaging using a 3T Achieva Philips scanner (Philips Healthcare, Best, Netherlands) and a three-dimensional (3-D) MPRAGE sequence with the following parameters: repetition time = 7.77 ms, echo time = 3.45 ms, echo train length = 128, flip angle = 9°, number of excitations = 1, field of view = 12 × 12 cm, matrix = 256 × 256, and slice thickness = 0.5 mm. Baseline and follow-up MR scanning was performed within a few days of every PET session to rule out structural abnormalities that could affect the PET results.

For both the MRI and PET studies, the animals were anesthetized using a combination of ketamine (~0.1 ml/kg) and propofol (0.2 mg/kg/min). The concentrations of various anesthetics as well as the timing of administration with respect to imaging were kept constant across the studies. Over the entire imaging session, the animals were carefully monitored for changes in body temperature, spO_2, and heart and respiratory rates.

PET Imaging

PET images were acquired on a CPS/CTI High Resolution Research Tomograph (HRRT), head-only camera (17). Prior to radiotracer injection, a 6-min transmission scan was obtained for calculation of attenuation correction maps. 11C-DASB was synthesized as previously described (18). Following intravenous bolus administration of 11C-DASB (mean injected dose = 5.67 ± 0.61 mCi), a dynamic 120-min-long emission scan was acquired using a 50-frame protocol. PET scans were reconstructed using the ordered subsets expectation maximization (OSEM) algorithm, in a 31 × 31 cm field of view and 256 × 256 pixel matrix with pixel size of 1.2 × 1.2 mm. PET frames were corrected for radioactive decay. The image frames were then co-registered to each animal's structural MRI image using Pmod 3.7 software (PMOD Technologies LLC, Zurich, Switzerland). There was a minimum gap of 5 weeks between consecutive PET scans in the same animals (range of 5–38 weeks).

PET Data Analysis

The reconstructed PET images were first co-registered to their respective MR images using rigid body transformation. Volumes of interest (VOIs) were selected based on a monkey brain template overlaid on the MR images and readjusted manually as necessary. One set of VOIs (for the midbrain, thalamus, caudate, and putamen) adjusted for the baseline study was reapplied on follow-up MRI scans to maintain consistency in measurements. One VOI was also selected in the cerebellar cortex, avoiding the cerebellar white matter and cerebellar vermis, to be used as a reference region (19). The outcome measure in our study was SERT binding potential normalized to non-displaceable tissue radioligand (BP_{ND}), measured using a simplified reference tissue model (SRTM) (20) with the cerebellar cortex as a reference region (19). Although VOIs were drawn in the midbrain, thalamus, caudate, and putamen, only thalamic and midbrain values were used for statistical analysis due to their relevance to disease pathophysiology. Mean voxel BP_{ND} values for each VOI were extracted from the scans and compared over time. Parametric maps were generated using the Pixel-wise modeling tool (PXMOD) in PMOD.

We performed a total of 27 PET scans on the 7 macaques, including 7 baseline and a total of 20 follow-up scans (**Table 1S**).

Specimen Collection

Cytokine/Chemokine Level Measurements in the CSF

Cytokine/chemokine levels in the CSF were obtained to assess the potential relationship between CSF neuroinflammatory markers and SERT expression levels as assessed by PET imaging. Concentrations of MCP-1, TNFα, IFNγ, IL-1ra, IL-2, IL-6, IL-8, IL-10, IL-18, GCSF, sCD40L, and VEGF were measured in the CSF of five infected animals within a few days of each PET scan, using a bead-based multiplex assay (EMD Millipore). The assay was performed according to the manufacturer's instructions. The assay plates were read on the Bio-plex 200 System (Bio-Rad).

PBMC Collection

We collected blood specimens from our animals (group A) corresponding to their imaging sessions in order to assess viral load, cell counts (flow cytometry), and peripheral SERT mRNA and to evaluate for potential peripheral epigenetic changes corresponding to changes in SERT expression. Blood collected was used for PBMC isolation using Ficoll. The PBMCs were re-suspended in cell freezing medium at 10 million cells/vial and stored in liquid nitrogen until needed. DNA/RNA was isolated from the cells using the ZR-Duet DNA/RNA Miniprep kit (Zymo Research) as per the manufacturer's instructions for downstream applications.

Preparation of Whole-Brain Cell Suspensions

Due to our small sample number of imaged animals and since the brain tissues of those animals could not be used for detailed PCR and Western analysis of SERT expression, we decided to evaluate another group of animals that were similarly infected and assessed for development of SIV encephalitis in another study (16). Whole-brain single-cell suspensions had already been obtained from a separate group of SIV-infected monkeys (group B, n = 13). Following saline perfusion of the animals, fresh brain tissues were collected from the frontal, parietal, and temporal lobes, the cerebellum, and the midbrain during necropsy. Multiple pieces of brain tissue from each region were then homogenized and pooled to obtain a cell suspension representative of the whole brain (14). RNA was extracted from these samples using the RNeasy Lipid Tissue Mini Kit from Qiagen. Protein lysates were obtained by re-suspending the cells in cold RIPA buffer with protease inhibitors (Roche). The samples were then vortexed and centrifuged at 14,000 rpm for 30 min at 4°C to remove debris.

Specimen Analysis

Flow Cytometry

Absolute blood CD3, CD4, and CD8 T-cell counts as well as % Ki67 in CD4 and CD8 T-cells were measured as previously described (14).

qPCR

qPCR was performed to assess SERT mRNA levels in PBMCs derived from group A animals, in order to evaluate for potential peripheral changes of SERT transcription after inoculation. qPCR was also performed to assess SERT mRNA levels in whole-brain single-cell suspensions from group B animals, in order to correlate with the incidence of SIV encephalitis. cDNA was synthesized using the RT^2 First Strand (Qiagen). The qPCR assay was set up using RT^2 SYBR Green qPCR Mastermix (Qiagen) to measure SERT (Qiagen) and normalized to *rpl13a* (Qiagen). The plates were run on the CFX96 real-time qPCR system (Bio-Rad). For data analysis, we calculated fold change using the comparative C_T method as previously described (21).

Western Blotting

Western blotting was performed to assess SERT protein levels in whole-brain single-cell suspensions from group B animals. Protein lysates from whole-brain cell suspensions (group B) were used for Western blotting as previously described (22). The primary antibodies used were SERT (Abcam) at 1:300 and GAPDH (CST) at 1:1,000 dilutions. The secondary antibody, goat anti-rabbit (Jackson), was used at 1:50,000. ImageJ was used to quantify the band intensities from scanned blots. Results are shown as fold change with respect to the average of animals with no SIVE.

Epigenetic (Methylation) Analysis

Pyrosequencing analysis was performed for the promoter region of the *SLC6A4* gene by Qiagen (GmbH Hilden, Germany) on DNA from group A animals, sampled at baseline and multiple time points between inoculation and euthanasia. Briefly, DNA extracted from the PBMCs of macaques (n = 7) was used for bisulfite conversion using the Epitect Fast Bisulfite Conversion Kit (Qiagen). The promoter region of *SLC6A4* was amplified from 20 ng of treated DNA using the primers (TAGAGTTAGGAGGGGAGGGAT) and (ACACCAACAAACCCCTAT). This was followed by sequencing using the primer (AGGAGGGGAGGGATT) with PyroMarkQ24 Advanced (Qiagen). A total of nine CpG islands were analyzed in the promoter region.

To assess global methylation changes, a Methylated CpG Island Recovery Assay (MIRA) was used as previously described (23). The assay enriches methylated CpG islands based on high-affinity interactions to methyl-binding protein complexes using the MethylCollector Ultra Kit (ActiveMotif). PBMC DNA of group A (n = 7) macaques (baseline and last time points) were used and sequenced using the Illumina Platform (NIH Intramural Sequencing Center). Data analysis was done by Acura Science (Iowa, USA). FASTQC was used for quality control of the sequencing data. Reads were aligned to the rhesus reference genome (Ensembl release 88). Methylation peaks were subsequently identified using MACS2. Differential methylation analysis was performed as before (24). Peak "summits"—i.e., the single points representing the center point of the peaks—located within 600 bp were grouped together and then merged (extended peaks) using a locally developed Perl script. Normalized counts for each extended peak were calculated as total count in this region divided by the length of the extended peak and then by the number of reads mapped in the sample. Differentially methylated regions (DMRs) were defined as extended peaks with large fold changes (>1.5) in normalized counts, and only DMRs covered by five or more reads in the samples being compared were considered. Each DMR was annotated into the following categories: exon, intron, transcription start site (TSS), promoter (−1 kb and +100 bp of a gene's TSS), 5' UTR, 3' UTR, intergenic, and non-coding.

Statistical Analysis

Statistical analysis was performed using SAS, version 9.4 (SAS Institute, NC, USA), and Prism (GraphPad, version 7.01).

Longitudinal changes of midbrain and thalamus BP_{ND} values were plotted for every animal, and the percentages of differential binding between the last time point and baseline were calculated. Repeated-measures mixed models were used to predict 11C-DASB BP_{ND} in the midbrain and thalamus of group A animals, based on CSF VL, plasma VL, the duration of infection, CD4, CD3, CD8 T-cell counts, and % Ki67 in CD4 and CD8 T-cells. CSF concentrations of MCP-1, IL-1ra, IL-2, IL-6, IL-10, IL-18, GCSF, sCD40L, and VEGF were available for five animals and were included as potential predictors. Each measurement was first included individually in a statistical model as an explanatory variable, with BP_{ND} as the response variable. We then included all measurements in one model to assess combined relationship with BP_{ND}. A mixed model was fit to the data because of the repeated-measures nature of the data. Several variance-covariance matrix structures were considered for each model, and the one with lowest Bayesian information criterion (BIC) was applied. Model-fit diagnostics were examined to check whether model assumptions were met. Because this is an exploratory study with a relatively small sample size, no multiple-comparisons adjustment was used (all reported p-values are unadjusted).

For group B animals, we compared the fold increase in SERT protein and mRNA of SIVE (n = 6) vs. non-SIVE animals (n = 7) using the Mann–Whitney test.

All data are represented as mean ± SD except for group B qPCR and Western results, which are displayed as median values ± interquartile range (IQR).

RESULTS

PET Imaging Analysis

Mean BP_{ND} values in the selected VOIs were highest in the midbrain, followed by the thalamus, caudate/putamen, and cerebellum, which is similar to reported postmortem SERT densities (25). Even though SIV involves the whole brain, including the cerebellum, the lack of specific uptake in the cerebellar cortex still warrants its use as a reference region (20, 26).

We concentrated on two high-binding regions, the midbrain and thalamus, due to their relevance to disease pathophysiology. Regional midbrain BP_{ND} values at 5–10 weeks after inoculation increased in four animals (16–38%) and decreased in two animals (22–26%). One animal did not show substantial change. Over the course of disease, six out of seven subjects showed a net increase in midbrain BP_{ND} values at the last time point compared to baseline (range: 7.1–72.4%), while one subject showed a minimal decrease (−2.6%) (**Figure 1**). The average change in all seven animals was an increase of 30.2% ± 25.8% over the course of disease.

Thalamic BP_{ND} values at 5–10 weeks after inoculation increased in five animals and decreased in two animals. Over the course of disease, all animals showed a net increase in BP_{ND} at the last time point (32.2% ± 21.1%), although in one animal, the increase was minimal (3.8%) (**Figure 1**).

A repeated-measures mixed-model analysis taking into account all the measured time points showed that among the selected variables, duration of infection correlated positively with 11C-DASB midbrain BP_{ND} (p = 0.039), with a positive trend also observed between duration of infection and thalamic BP_{ND} (p = 0.081). Neither treatment initiation nor interruption had a

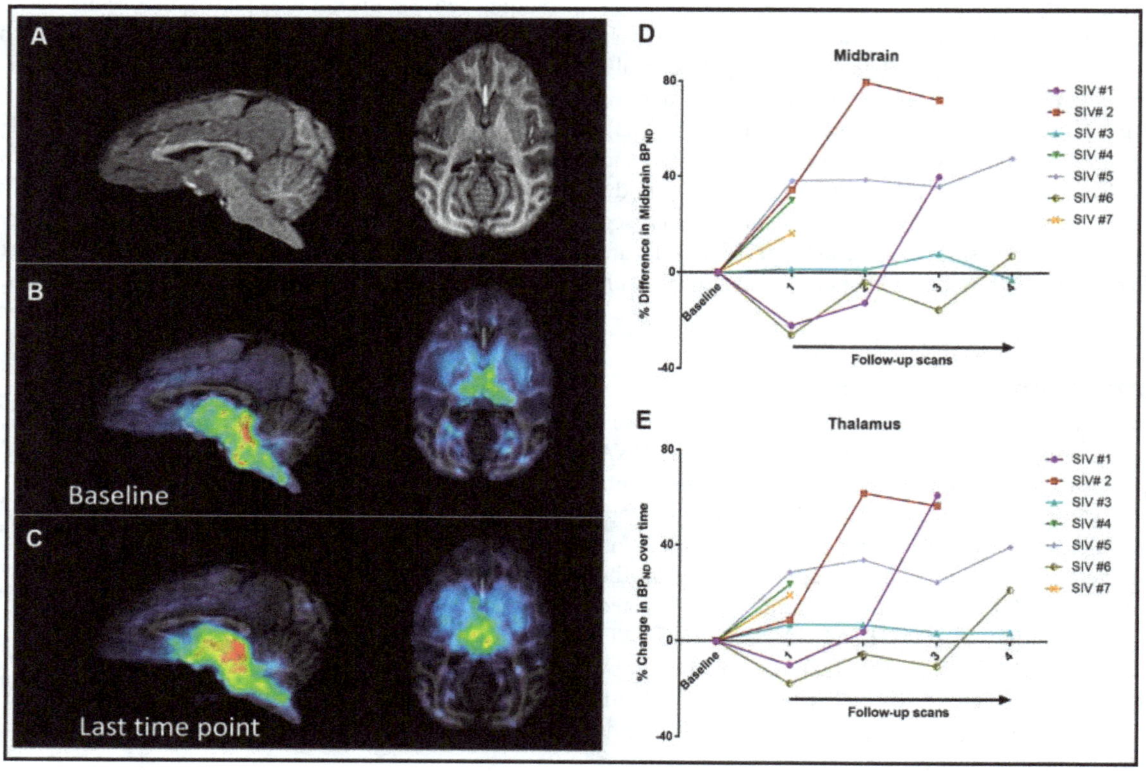

FIGURE 1 | Sagittal and axial brain MRI images **(A)** as well as parametric maps of 11C-DASB BP_{ND} at baseline **(B)** and last time point **(C)** of SIV #4. Increased BP_{ND} can be detected visually at the last time point compared to baseline. Changes in BP_{ND} over the course of disease in all seven animals in the midbrain **(D)** and thalamus **(E)**.

consistent effect on BP_{ND} (**Figure 2**). There were no significant correlations between BP_{ND} and CD4, CD3, CD8 T-cell counts, or % Ki67 in CD4 or % Ki67 in CD8 T-cell counts.

Cytokine/Chemokine Measurements

CSF cytokine analysis showed an increase in MCP-1, TNFα, IFNγ, IL-1Ra, IL-2, IL-6, IL-8, IL-10, Il-12, and IL-18 concentrations after inoculation in all animals, which corresponded to a concomitant increase in CSF VL. In four treated animals, cytokine levels decreased after treatment and rebounded after interruption of treatment, as expected.

There were significant positive correlations between CSF levels of MCP-1, IL-1Ra, IL-6, IL-8, IL-10, and IL-18 and thalamic BP_{ND} ($p = 0.002$, 0.003, 0.035, 0.013, 0.023, and 0.014, respectively). No significant correlations between CSF cytokines and midbrain BP_{ND} were found.

Expression of SERT in the Periphery and the Brain

Group A Animals

The expression of SERT mRNA in PBMCs was very low across all samples and undetectable in one animal (SIV #3). It increased slightly in three out of six animals at the last time point compared to baseline (**Figure 3B**).

Group B Animals

SERT protein levels in whole-brain lysates of group B animals were compared between infected animals that showed neurological symptoms associated with the development of SIVE ($n = 6$) and a group that was infected but did not display neurological dysfunction ($n = 7$). The values were normalized to the average of animals with no SIVE. Expression of mRNA normalized to a housekeeping gene (*rpl13A*) was also compared between SIVE ($n = 6$) and non-SIVE animals ($n = 7$), with data represented as fold increase with respect to the average of non-SIVE animals. There was no significant change in SERT mRNA expression (average increase = 1.24-fold, $p = 0.55$); however, there was a significant increase in SERT protein expression (average increase = 3.35-fold, $p = 0.014$) (**Figure 4**).

Epigenetic (Methylation) Analysis

To assess whether the observed increases in SERT expression were mediated by epigenetic regulation, our pyrosequencing analysis was focused on evaluating the percent methylation of 9 CpG islands closest to the TSS of the *SLC6A4* (SERT) gene, isolated from PBMC DNA of seven macaques taken at various time intervals starting with baseline and continuing until the terminal time point. In each case, the percent methylation was less than 5%, indicating there was hardly any methylation in the promoter region of SERT (**Supplementary Table 1S**). We did

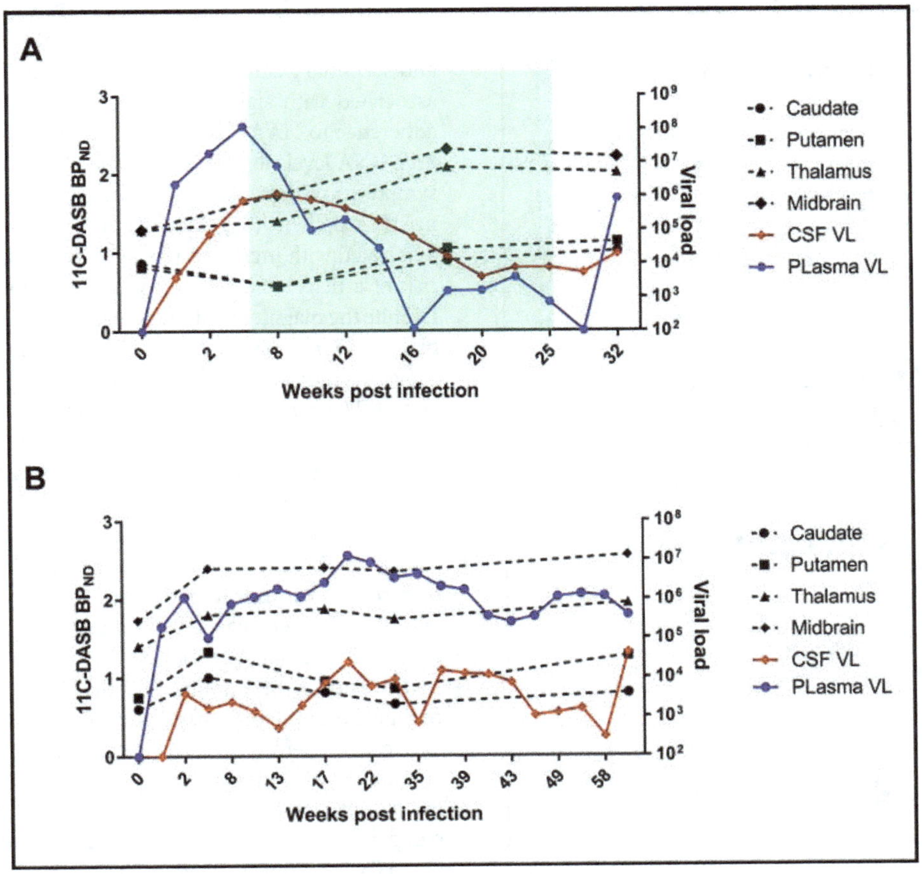

FIGURE 2 | Examples of changes of BP_{ND} values at different time points with respect to CSF and plasma VL changes in one fast progressor, SIV #2 **(A)**, and one slow progressor, SIV #5 **(B)**. The green shadow in **(A)** reflects the duration of antiretroviral treatment.

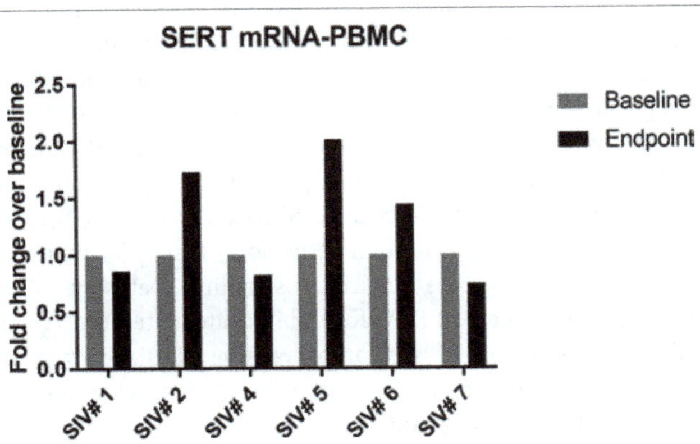

FIGURE 3 | Change in SERT mRNA levels in PBMCs of infected animals (group A) between baseline and last time point; 50% of the animals showed slight increase in SERT mRNA compared to baseline values.

not find any appreciable change in percent methylation between baseline and multiple time points after inoculation.

The MIRA-seq analysis of the whole genome was done to identify potential epigenetic modifications to other upstream factors that could affect SERT expression and trafficking. Methylated CpG islands across the entire genome were assessed for differentially methylated regions (DMR). An average of 91.4% of the reads were mapped back to the genome. Based on the differential methylation analysis obtained for the baseline and the last time point, fold change was calculated, and only genes that met the cutoff of >1.5 (hypermethylated) and <0.5 (hypomethylated) were considered. In five out of the seven animals, the promoter region (−350 to −390 from TSS) of the transcription factor deformed epidermal autoregulatory factor-1 (*DEAF1*) was differentially methylated. *DEAF1* was hypermethylated in three animals at the last time point compared to baseline, with a fold change (FC) range of 1.6–2.2. On the other hand, *DEAF1* was slightly hypomethylated in one animal that succumbed to the disease very early on (FC = 0.4) and another animal that survived and was treated (FC = 0.7). There were no consistent methylation peaks captured for two animals in the *DEAF*1 promoter region, though we saw some peaks in the intragenic regions at the terminal time point.

DISCUSSION

Using 11C-DASB high-resolution PET imaging, we have documented longitudinal *in vivo* increases in SERT expression

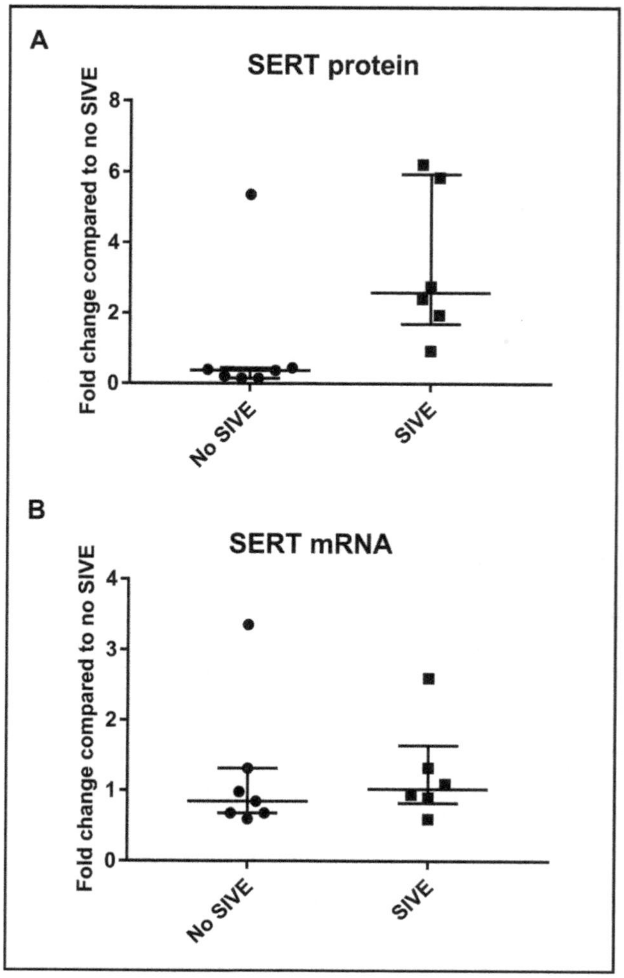

FIGURE 4 | Western blotting and qPCR results in group B animals (whole-brain lysates). **(A)** Fold change in protein levels of SIVE compared to non-SIVE animals. **(B)** Fold change in mRNA expression of SIVE compared to non-SIVE animals. Median and interquartile range values are shown (* = $p < 0.05$; n.s. = non-significant).

in 85% of SIV-infected macaques when we compared baseline BP_{ND} levels to multiple time points between inoculation and euthanasia. In a mixed-effect analysis model, midbrain BP_{ND} values for 11C-DASB correlated significantly with duration of infection, although we did not find significant correlations to CSF/plasma VL or various T-cell counts. There were also significant positive correlations between thalamic BP_{ND} and CSF levels of MCP-1, IL-6, IL-8, and IL-18, cytokines with pro-inflammatory properties, as well as IL-1Ra and IL-10, both anti-inflammatory cytokines. Our imaging data were further supported by findings of increased SERT protein levels in another set of SIV-infected animals with symptoms of SIVE compared to asymptomatic infected animals.

Higher frequency of depression has been repeatedly documented in HIV+ compared to HIV-negative (HIV-) subjects: a 2001 meta-analysis found the frequency of MDD to be nearly two times higher in HIV+ subjects (27), with more recent work confirming that figure (1, 28, 29). Beyond the psychological toll of depression in HIV+ subjects, the ramifications extend to its impact on survival, mainly through its effect on treatment adherence (30) and secondary control of the infection: untreated depression was associated with significantly decreased odds of achieving >90% adherence to HAART and significantly lower odds of controlling HIV RNA levels to <500 copies/ml (31). In another study, somatic symptoms of depression were associated with shortened survival in HIV+ patients (32). More recently, depression was found to be associated with increased risk of missing appointments, increased risk of a detectable viral load, and a doubled mortality rate (1). Despite the magnitude of the problem, the mechanisms underlying higher depression rates in HIV remain poorly understood. Previous studies suggested disturbances of tryptophan metabolism and SERT expression both *in vitro* and *in vivo* (2, 4–6). The only previous imaging study assessing the serotonergic system in HIV showed higher 11C-DASB BP_{ND} in depressed compared to non-depressed HIV+ patients (6).

Upregulation of SERT reflected by increased 11C-DASB BP_{ND} values has been described in subjects with MDD and bipolar disease (33), Parkinson's patients with depression (34), and patients with highly negativistic dysfunctional attitudes (35), among others. A possible explanation for depressive symptomatology in the setting of upregulated SERT is exaggerated serotonin reuptake into the presynaptic neurons, which subsequently leads to decreased serotonin levels in the synapse.

Our current results are not consistent with previous work where we found generally decreased 11C-DASB binding in HIV+ patients compared to controls (6). Those subjects, however, had been infected with HIV for a much longer period of time than our animals, which could have resulted in neuronal loss. Interestingly, the depressed HIV+ patients in that study showed higher 11C-DASB binding than non-depressed subjects, pointing towards a connection between SERT expression and depressive symptomatology.

What could be the cause of increased SERT expression in SIV/HIV? There is a large body of literature describing interactions between various cytokines (e.g., IL-1, IL-6, IL-10, TNFα, and IFNγ) and SERT expression, both *in vitro* and *in vivo* (7–12). For example, TNFα was found to enhance the transport capacity of SERT-specific serotonin uptake in primary astrocytes, consistent with prior observation of an increase in SERT mRNA levels (10). This seemed to be mediated through activation of the p38 mitogen-activated protein kinase (MAPK) signaling pathway, since pre-treatment with a p38 MAPK inhibitor attenuated the TNFα-mediated stimulation of serotonin transport (10). In support of this potential interaction, we have found significant positive correlations between thalamic BP_{ND} and CSF levels of multiple pro-inflammatory and anti-inflammatory cytokines. Interestingly, the cytokine correlations with the midbrain BP_{ND} were not significant. The reason for this discrepancy is unclear, although similar findings have been previously reported by another group where only thalamic and not midbrain SERT availability was correlated with IL-10 in bipolar disorder (11). One possible explanation is that thalamic neurons are in closer contact with the CSF and thus could be more affected by CSF cytokines (36).

Another connection between HIV and SERT upregulation could be through the production of SIV/HIV viral proteins. In mice, a single exposure to Tat in the brain was enough to induce brain cytokine signaling that resulted in depressive-like behavior (37). In a paper by Fu et al., Tat increased the expression of SERT in organotypic hippocampal slice cultures, an effect that was attenuated by pre-treatment with SB 202190, a p38 MAPK inhibitor (38). Prolonged exposure to viral proteins in our animals could therefore have contributed to increased SERT expression over time.

We hypothesized that the changes we observed in our SIV-infected monkeys could also be a result of epigenetic modulation. Epigenetic modifications induced by HIV have been previously described, especially related to accelerated aging and viral latency (39–41). On the other hand, depression in general and changes in SERT expression specifically have been found to be associated with epigenetic modifications, especially changes in DNA methylation (42–45). In our evaluation of SERT gene methylation, however, we did not find significant changes in methylation of SERT promoter between the pre-infected and latest time point in our imaged animals. Looking for potential interactive epigenetic changes upstream from SERT throughout the whole genome, we found one gene, *DEAF1*, which seemed to be differentially methylated in five out of the seven animals. DEAF1 regulates the transcription of multiple genes and has been implicated in type 1 diabetes (46), cancer (47), and IFNβ production (48). It is interesting to note that, since increased IFNβ secretion can restrict HIV viral replication and spreading (49, 50), the silencing of *DEAF1* can confer a significant advantage in maintaining the potency of infection. Additionally, a separate function of DEAF1 is to act as a repressor of serotonin receptor subtype 1A (5-HT1A) in non-neuronal and presynaptic raphe cells (51–53) and an enhancer of 5-HT1A in other neuronal cells (54). Therefore, hypermethylation of *DEAF1* could potentially reduce its availability to repress 5-HT1A autoreceptor expression, which in turn is linked to depression (55, 56). Multiple reports have shown that dysregulation of 5-HT1A function can have a secondary effect on SERT expression: Bose et al. showed that presynaptic 5-HT1A expression is related to SERT density in specific regions of the brain (57), while another study used autoradiography to demonstrate a concomitant decrease of SERT expression in the basal ganglia, thalamus, and cortical regions of 5-HT1A knockout mice (58). SIV-induced epigenetic alterations to DEAF1 expression could thus possibly play a role in the perceived changes in SERT expression. However, our current findings do not support a definite role, and further work is needed to better elucidate the interplay between DEAF1 signaling and SERT expression. Additionally, our results do not preclude the effect of other epigenetic and non-epigenetic mechanisms on SERT expression.

Our study is limited by a relatively small size number of SIV-infected monkeys. As such, our results should be interpreted with caution, as this is an exploratory study. We also did not have fresh brain tissue from the imaged animals to systematically assess SERT mRNA and protein levels in correlation with 11C-DASB binding. Most importantly, we did not collect neuropsychological or behavioral measures of depression in the animals, mainly because there is no clear consensus on what constitutes depressive-like behavior in animals compared to humans and because in our animals, the presence of a severe infectious process confounds the detection of subtle psychiatric manifestations. Even though we did not have control animals followed over the same period of time, we have used longitudinal imaging with each animal acting as its own control. We do not believe that scanning-related stress could have affected our results, since the scans were separated by a minimum gap of 5 weeks (range: 5–38 weeks). Finally, we have not looked for methylation changes in the brains of the infected animals, but rather, in the periphery, which allowed us to perform a longitudinal assessment. It has been previously shown, however, that there is a significant correlation between the methylation levels in the brain and peripheral blood (59).

In conclusion, we have identified increased expression of SERT in six out of seven SIV-infected monkeys using *in vivo* PET imaging, which correlated with duration of infection in the midbrain. The change in expression in the thalamus also correlated with pro- and anti-inflammatory cytokine activity in the CSF. Although we did not find direct methylation changes involving the SERT promoter gene to explain our results, scouring of the whole-genome methylation status resulted in a potential connection between a differentially methylated gene, *DEAF1*, and upregulated SERT expression. Whether this connection will prove to be widespread is unclear, and the possibility of other epigenetic factors affecting SERT expression in SIV cannot be ruled out. Extending our conclusions from SIV to HIV needs further confirmation with translational HIV human studies. More work is also needed to better understand the connection between SERT upregulation and depression symptomatology.

AUTHOR CONTRIBUTIONS

DH, KM, DL, VH, AN, and MDM conceived of and designed the study. DH, SSh, SSi, WS-S, KM, SM, and DL evaluated the study subjects and/or collected and analyzed the data. DH and PW performed the statistical analysis. All authors participated in drafting the article and/or revising it critically for intellectual content and gave final approval of the submitted manuscript.

FUNDING

Funding for this study was provided in part by the intramural research program of the National Institute of Allergy and Infectious Diseases (NIAID), National Institutes of Health (NIH), and by the Center for Infectious Disease Imaging (CIDI), Clinical Center, NIH. This project has also been funded in part with federal funds from the National Cancer Institute, NIH, under contract no. HHSN261200800001E. The content of this publication does not necessarily reflect the views or policies of the Department of Health and Human

Services, nor does the mentioning of trade names, commercial products, or organizations imply endorsement by the U.S. government.

ACKNOWLEDGMENTS

The authors wish to thank the veterinary and animal care staff of the NIAID for supporting the non-human primates used in this study, Merck for providing raltegravir, and Gilead for providing tenofovir and emtricitabine.

SUPPLEMENTARY MATERIAL

TABLE 1S | Characteristics of group A animals.

TABLE 2S | Characteristics of group B animals.

TABLE 3S | Percent methylation of 9 CpG islands closest to the transcription start site (TSS) of the *SLC6A4* (SERT) gene from PBMC DNA of 7 macaques collected at various time intervals starting with baseline (before inoculation) up to the terminal point.

REFERENCES

Pence BW, Mills JC, Bengtson AM, Gaynes BN, Breger TL, Cook RL, et al. Association of increased chronicity of depression with HIV appointment attendance, treatment failure, and mortality among HIV-infected adults in the United States. *JAMA Psychiatry* (2018) 75(4):379–85. doi: 10.1001/jamapsychiatry.2017.4726

Yu K, Qiu CL, Yang GB, Zong CM, Xing H, Shao Y, et al. Alteration of serotonin transporter messenger RNA level in the peripheral blood mononuclear cells from simian/human immunodeficiency virus infected Chinese rhesus macaques (Macaca mulatta). *Brain Behav Immun* (2010) 24:298–305. doi: 10.1016/j.bbi.2009.10.008

Everall IP, Salaria S, Atkinson JH, Young C, Corbeil J, Grant I, et al. Diminished somatostatin gene expression in individuals with HIV and major depressive disorder. *Neurology* (2006) 67:1867–9. doi: 10.1212/01.wnl.0000244436.04036.a2

Eriksson T, Lidberg L. Decreased plasma ratio of tryptophan to competing large neutral amino acids in human immunodefi cy virus type 1 infected subjects: possible implications for development of neuro- psychiatric disorders. *J Neural Transm* (1996) 103:157–64. doi: 10.1007/ BF01292624

Longatti P, Perin A, Comai S, Bertazzo A, Rizzo V, Costa CV, et al. A study of tryptophan metabolism *via* serotonin in ventricular cerebrospinal fluid in HIV-1 infection using a neuroendoscopic technique. *Curr HIV Res* (2007) 5:267–72. doi: 10.2174/157016207780077020

Hammoud DA, Endres CJ, Hammond E, Uzuner O, Brown A, Nath A, et al. Imaging serotonergic transmission with [11C]DASB-PET in depressed and non-depressed patients infected with HIV. *Neuroimage* (2010) 49:2588–95. doi: 10.1016/j.neuroimage.2009.10.037

Su S, Zhao J, Bremner JD, Miller AH, Tang W, Bouzyk M, et al. Serotonin transporter gene, depressive symptoms, and interleukin-6. *Circ Cardiovasc Genet* (2009) 2:614–20. doi: 10.1161/CIRCGENETICS.109.870386

Couch Y, Anthony DC, Dolgov O, Revischin A, Festoff B, Santos AI, et al. Microglial activation, increased TNF and SERT expression in the prefrontal cortex define stress-altered behaviour in mice susceptible to anhedonia. *Brain Behav Immun* (2013) 29:136–46. doi: 10.1016/j.bbi.2012.12.017

Latorre E, Mendoza C, Matheus N, Castro M, Grasa L, Mesonero JE, et al. IL-10 modulates serotonin transporter activity and molecular expression in intestinal epithelial cells. *Cytokine* (2013) 61:778–4. doi: 10.1016/j.cyto.2013.01.012

Malynn S, Campos-Torres A, Moynagh P, Haase J. The pro-inflammatory cytokine TNF-alpha regulates the activity and expression of the serotonin transporter (SERT) in astrocytes. *Neurochem Res* (2013) 38:694–704. doi: 10.1007/s11064-012-0967-y

Hsu JW, Lirng JF, Wang SJ, Lin CL, Yang KC, Liao MH, et al. Association of thalamic serotonin transporter and interleukin-10 in bipolar I disorder: a SPECT study. *Bipolar Disord* (2014) 16:241–8. doi: 10.1111/bdi.12164

Chou YH, Hsieh WC, Chen LC, Lirng JF, Wang SJ. Association between the serotonin transporter and cytokines: implications for the pathophysiology of bipolar disorder. *J Affect Disord* (2016) 191:29–35. doi: 10.1016/j.jad.2015.10.056

Wu F, Kirmaier A, Goeken R, Ourmanov I, Hall L, Morgan JS, et al. TRIM5 alpha drives SIVsmm evolution in rhesus macaques. *PLoS Pathog* (2013) 9:e1003577. doi: 10.1371/journal.ppat.1003577

Matsuda K, Dang Q, Brown CR, Keele BF, Wu F, Ourmanov I, et al. Characterization of simian immunodeficiency virus (SIV) that induces SIV encephalitis in rhesus macaques with high frequency: role of TRIM5 and major histocompatibility complex genotypes and early entry to the brain. *J Virol* (2014) 88:13201–11. doi: 10.1128/JVI.01996-14

Wu F, Ourmanov I, Riddick N, Matsuda K, Whitted S, Plishka RJ, et al. TRIM5alpha restriction affects clinical outcome and disease progression in simian immunodeficiency virus-infected rhesus macaques. *J Virol* (2015) 89:2233–40. doi: 10.1128/JVI.02978-14

Matsuda K, Riddick NE, Lee CA, Puryear SB, Wu F, Whitted S, et al. A SIV molecular clone that targets the CNS and induces neuroAIDS in rhesus macaques. *PLoS Pathog* (2017) 13:e1006538. doi: 10.1371/journal.ppat.1006538

Wienhard K, Schmand M, Casey ME, Baker K, Bao J, Eriksson L, et al. The ECAT HRRT: performance and first clinical application of the new High Resolution Research Tomograph. *Nucl Sci IEE ETrans* (2002) 49:104–10. doi: 10.1109/TNS.2002.998689

Wilson AA, Ginovart N, Hussey D, Meyer J, Houle S. In vitro and *in vivo* characterisation of [11C]-DASB: a probe for *in vivo* measurements of the serotonin transporter by positron emission tomography. *Nucl Med Biol* (2002) 29:509–15. doi: 10.1016/S0969-8051(02)00316-5

Meyer JH, Wilson AA, Ginovart N, Houle S. Misunderstandings about how to choose a reference region. *Biol Psychiatry* (2007) 61:1314. author reply 1314–1315. doi: 10.1016/j.biopsych.2006.06.007

Lammertsma AA, Hume SP. Simplified reference tissue model for PET receptor studies. *Neuroimage* (1996) 4:153–8. doi: 10.1006/nimg.1996.0066

Schmittgen TD, Livak KJ. Analyzing real-time PCR data by the comparative C(T) method. *Nat Protoc* (2008) 3:1101–8. doi: 10.1038/nprot. 2008.73

Shah S, Bohsali A, Ahlbrand SE, Srinivasan L, Rathinam VA, Vogel SN, et al. Cutting edge: *Mycobacterium tuberculosis* but not nonvirulent mycobacteria inhibits IFN-beta and AIM2 inflammasome-dependent IL-1beta production *via* its ESX-1 secretion system. *J Immunol* (2013) 191:3514–8. doi: 10.4049/jimmunol.1301331

Jung M, Kadam S, Xiong W, Rauch TA, Jin SG, Pfeifer GP. MIRA-seq for DNA methylation analysis of CpG islands. *Epigenomics* (2015) 7:695–706. doi: 10.2217/epi.15.33

Li X, Baker-Andresen D, Zhao Q, Marshall V, Bredy TW. Methyl CpG binding domain ultra-sequencing: a novel method for identifying inter-individual and cell-type-specific variation in DNA methylation. *Genes Brain Behav* (2014) 13:721–31. doi: 10.1111/gbb.12150

Varnas K, Halldin C, Hall H. Autoradiographic distribution of serotonin transporters and receptor subtypes in human brain. *Hum Brain Mapp* (2004) 22:246–60. doi: 10.1002/hbm.20035

Meyer JH. Imaging the serotonin transporter during major depressive disorder and antidepressant treatment. *J Psychiatry Neurosci* (2007) 32:86–102.

Ciesla JA, Roberts JE. Meta-analysis of the relationship between HIV infection and risk for depressive disorders. *Am J Psychiatry* (2001) 158:725- 30. doi: 10.1176/appi.ajp.158.5.725

Arseniou S, Arvaniti A, Samakouri M. HIV infection and depression. *Psychiatry Clin Neurosci* (2014) 68:96–109. doi: 10.1111/pcn.12097

Mills JC, Pence BW, Todd JV, Bengtson AM, Breger TL, Edmonds A, et al. Cumulative burden of depression and all-cause mortality in women living with HIV. *Clin Infect Dis* (2018) 67(10):1575–81. doi: 10.1093/cid/ciy264

Yoo-Jeong M, Waldrop-Valverde D, Mccoy K, Ownby RL. A structural equation model of HIV-related symptoms, depressive symptoms, and medication adherence. *J HIV AIDS* (2016) 2(3):1–15. doi: 10.16966/2380-5536.123

Horberg MA, Silverberg MJ, Hurley LB, Towner WJ, Klein DB, Bersoff-Matcha S, et al. Effects of depression and selective serotonin reuptake inhibitor use on adherence to highly active antiretroviral therapy and on clinical outcomes in HIV-infected patients. *J Acquir Immune Defic Syndr* (2008) 47:384–90. doi: 10.1097/QAI.0b013e318160d53e

Farinpour R, Miller EN, Satz P, Selnes OA, Cohen BA, Becker JT, et al. Psychosocial risk factors of HIV morbidity and mortality: findings from the Multicenter AIDS Cohort Study (MACS). *J Clin Exp Neuropsychol* (2003) 25:654–70. doi: 10.1076/jcen.25.5.654.14577

Cannon DM, Ichise M, Rollis D, Klaver JM, Gandhi SK, Charney DS, et al. Elevated serotonin transporter binding in major depressive disorder assessed using positron emission tomography and [11C]DASB; comparison with bipolar disorder. *Biol Psychiatry* (2007) 62:870–7. doi: 10.1016/j.biopsych.2007.03.016

Boileau I, Warsh JJ, Guttman M, Saint-Cyr JA, Mccluskey T, Rusjan P, et al. Elevated serotonin transporter binding in depressed patients with Parkinson's disease: a preliminary PET study with [11C]DASB. *Mov Disord* (2008) 23:1776–80. doi: 10.1002/mds.22212

Meyer JH, Houle S, Sagrati S, Carella A, Hussey DF, Ginovart N, et al. Brain serotonin transporter binding potential measured with carbon 11–labeled DASB positron emission tomography: effects of major depressive episodes and severity of dysfunctional attitudes. *Arch Gen Psychiatry* (2004) 61:1271–9. doi: 10.1001/archpsyc.61.12.1271

Zhang LC, Zeng YM, Ting J, Cao JP, Wang MS. The distributions and signaling directions of the cerebrospinal fluid contacting neurons in the parenchyma of a rat brain. *Brain Res* (2003) 989:1–8. doi: 10.1016/S0006-8993(03)03123-8

Lawson MA, Kelley KW, Dantzer R. Intracerebroventricular administration of HIV-1 Tat induces brain cytokine and indoleamine 2,3-dioxygenase expression: a possible mechanism for AIDS comorbid depression. *Brain Behav Immun* (2011) 25:1569–75. doi: 10.1016/j.bbi.2011.05.006

Fu X, Lawson MA, Kelley KW, Dantzer R. HIV-1 Tat activates indoleamine 2,3 dioxygenase in murine organotypic hippocampal slice cultures in a p38 mitogen-activated protein kinase–dependent manner. *J Neuroinflammation* (2011) 8:88. doi: 10.1186/1742-2094-8-88

Abdel-Hameed EA, Ji H, Shata MT. HIV-induced epigenetic alterations in host cells. *Adv Exp Med Biol* (2016) 879:27–38. doi: 10.1007/ 978-3-319-24738-0_2

Levine AJ, Quach A, Moore DJ, Achim CL, Soontornniyomkij V, Masliah E, et al. Accelerated epigenetic aging in brain is associated with pre-mortem HIV-associated neurocognitive disorders. *J Neurovirol* (2016) 22:366–75. doi: 10.1007/s13365-015-0406-3

Nelson KN, Hui Q, Rimland D, Xu K, Freiberg MS, Justice AC, et al. Identification of HIV infection-related DNA methylation sites and advanced epigenetic aging in HIV-positive, treatment-naive U.S. veterans. *Aids* (2017) 31:571–5. doi: 10.1097/QAD.0000000000001360

Nikolova YS, Hariri AR. Can we observe epigenetic effects on human brain function? *Trends Cogn Sci* (2015) 19:366–73. doi: 10.1016/j.tics.2015.05.003

Kader F, Ghai M, Maharaj L. The effects of DNA methylation on human psychology. *Behav Brain Res* (2017) 346:47–65. doi: 10.1016/j.bbr.2017.12.004

Schneider I, Kugel H, Redlich R, Grotegerd D, Burger C, Burkner PC, et al. Association of serotonin transporter gene AluJb methylation with major depression, amygdala responsiveness, 5-HTTLPR/rs25531 polymorphism, and stress. *Neuropsychopharmacology* (2017) 43(6):1308–16. doi: 10.1038/npp.2017.273

Uchida S, Yamagata H, Seki T, Watanabe Y. Epigenetic mechanisms of major depression: targeting neuronal plasticity. *Psychiatry Clin Neurosci* (2017) 72(4):212–27. doi: 10.1111/pcn.12621

Yip L, Su L, Sheng D, Chang P, Atkinson M, Czesak M, et al. Deaf1 isoforms control the expression of genes encoding peripheral tissue antigens in the pancreatic lymph nodes during type 1 diabetes. *Nat Immunol* (2009) 10:1026–33. doi: 10.1038/ni.1773

Barker HE, Smyth GK, Wettenhall J, Ward TA, Bath ML, Lindeman GJ, et al. Deaf-1 regulates epithelial cell proliferation and side-branching in the mammary gland. *BMC Dev Biol* (2008) 8:94. doi: 10.1186/ 1471-213X-8-94

Ordureau A, Enesa K, Nanda S, Le Francois B, Peggie M, Prescott A, et al. DEAF1 is a Pellino1-interacting protein required for interferon production by Sendai virus and double-stranded RNA. *J Biol Chem* (2013) 288:24569–80. doi: 10.1074/jbc.M113.479550

Barr SD, Smiley JR, Bushman FD. The interferon response inhibits HIV particle production by induction of TRIM22. *PLoS Pathog* (2008) 4:e1000007. doi: 10.1371/journal.ppat.1000007

Yan N, Regalado-Magdos AD, Stiggelbout B, Lee-Kirsch MA, Lieberman J. The cytosolic exonuclease TREX1 inhibits the innate immune response to human immunodeficiency virus type 1. *Nat Immunol* (2010) 11:1005–13. doi: 10.1038/ni.1941

Michelson RJ, Collard MW, Ziemba AJ, Persinger J, Bartholomew B, Huggenvik JI. Nuclear DEAF-1-related (NUDR) protein contains a novel DNA binding domain and represses transcription of the heterogeneous nuclear ribonucleoprotein A2/B1 promoter. *J Biol Chem* (1999) 274:30510– 9. doi: 10.1074/jbc.274.43.30510

Lemonde S, Turecki G, Bakish D, Du L, Hrdina PD, Bown CD, et al. Impaired repression at a 5-hydroxytryptamine 1A receptor gene polymorphism associated with major depression and suicide. *J Neurosci* (2003) 23:8788–99. doi: 10.1523/JNEUROSCI.23-25-08788.2003

Szewczyk B, Albert PR, Burns AM, Czesak M, Overholser JC, Jurjus GJ, et al. Gender-specifi decrease in NUDR and 5-HT1A receptor proteins in the prefrontal cortex of subjects with major depressive disorder. *Int J Neuropsychopharmacol* (2009) 12:155–68. doi: 10.1017/S1461145708009012

Czesak M, Lemonde S, Peterson EA, Rogaeva A, Albert PR. Cell-specific repressor or enhancer activities of Deaf-1 at a serotonin 1A receptor gene polymorphism. *J Neurosci* (2006) 26:1864–71. doi: 10.1523/JNEUROSCI.2643-05.2006

Drevets WC, Thase ME, Moses-Kolko EL, Price J, Frank E, Kupfer DJ, et al. Serotonin-1A receptor imaging in recurrent depression: replication and literature review. *Nucl Med Biol* (2007) 34:865–77. doi: 10.1016/j.nucmedbio.2007.06.008

Boldrini M, Underwood MD, Mann JJ, Arango V. Serotonin-1A autoreceptor binding in the dorsal raphe nucleus of depressed suicides. *J Psychiatr Res* (2008) 42:433–42. doi: 10.1016/j.jpsychires.2007.05.004

Bose SK, Mehta MA, Selvaraj S, Howes OD, Hinz R, Rabiner EA, et al. Presynaptic 5-HT1A is related to 5-HTT receptor density in the human brain. *Neuropsychopharmacology* (2011) 36:2258–65. doi: 10.1038/npp.2011.113

Ase AR, Reader TA, Hen R, Riad M, Descarries L. Regional changes in density of serotonin transporter in the brain of 5-HT1A and 5-HT1B knockout mice, and of serotonin innervation in the 5-HT1B knockout. *J Neurochem* (2001) 78:619–30. doi: 10.1046/j.1471-4159.2001.00437.x

Tylee DS, Kawaguchi DM, Glatt SJ. On the outside, looking in: a review and evaluation of the comparability of blood and brain "-omes". *Am J Med Genet B Neuropsychiatr Genet* (2013) 162b:595–603. doi: 10.1002/ajmg.b.32150

14

Characterizing Whole Brain Temporal Variation of Functional Connectivity via Zero and First Order Derivatives of Sliding Window Correlations

Flor A. Espinoza[1,2], Victor M. Vergara[1,2], Eswar Damaraju[1,2], Kyle G. Henke[1,3], Ashkan Faghiri[1,2,4], Jessica A. Turner[2,5], Aysenil A. Belger[6], Judith M. Ford[7,8], Sarah C. McEwen[9,10], Daniel H. Mathalon[7,8], Bryon A. Mueller[11], Steven G. Potkin[12], Adrian Preda[12], Jatin G. Vaidya[13], Theo G. M. van Erp[14,15] and Vince D. Calhoun[1,2,4,5]*

[1] Mind Research Network, Albuquerque, NM, United States, [2] Tri-Institutional Center for Translational Research in Neuroimaging and Data Science (TReNDS), Georgia State University, Georgia Institute of Technology, Emory University, Atlanta, GA, United States, [3] Department of Mathematics and Statistics, The University of New Mexico, Albuquerque, NM, United States, [4] Department of Electrical and Computer Engineering, The University of New Mexico, Albuquerque, NM, United States, [5] Department of Psychology and Neuroscience, Georgia State University, Atlanta, GA, United States, [6] Department of Psychiatry, University of North Carolina at Chapel Hill, Chapel Hill, NC, United States, [7] Department of Psychiatry, University of California, San Francisco, San Francisco, CA, United States, [8] San Francisco VA Medical Center, San Francisco, CA, United States, [9] Pacific Neuroscience Institute, Santa Monica, CA, United States, [10] John Wayne Cancer Institute, Department of Translational Neurosciences and Neurotherapeutics, Santa Monica, CA, United States, [11] Department of Psychiatry, University of Minnesota, Minneapolis, MN, United States, [12] Department of Psychiatry and Human Behavior, University of California, Irvine, Irvine, CA, United States, [13] Department of Psychiatry, The University of Iowa, Iowa City, IA, United States, [14] Clinical Translational Neuroscience Laboratory, Department of Psychiatry and Human Behavior, University of California, Irvine, Irvine, CA, United States, [15] Center for the Neurobiology of Learning and Memory, University of California, Irvine, Irvine, CA, United States

***Correspondence:**
Flor A. Espinoza
yoyy75@gmail.com

Brain functional connectivity has been shown to change over time during resting state fMRI experiments. Close examination of temporal changes have revealed a small set of whole-brain connectivity patterns called dynamic states. Dynamic functional network connectivity (dFNC) studies have demonstrated that it is possible to replicate the dynamic states across several resting state experiments. However, estimation of states and their temporal dynamicity still suffers from noisy and imperfect estimations. In regular dFNC implementations, states are estimated by comparing connectivity patterns through the data without considering time, in other words only zero order changes are examined. In this work we propose a method that includes first order variations of dFNC in the searching scheme of dynamic connectivity patterns. Our approach, referred to as temporal variation of functional network connectivity (tvFNC), estimates the derivative of dFNC, and then searches for reoccurring patterns of concurrent dFNC states and their derivatives. The tvFNC method is first validated using a simulated dataset and then applied to a resting-state fMRI sample including healthy controls (HC) and schizophrenia (SZ) patients and compared to the standard dFNC approach. Our dynamic approach reveals extra patterns in the connectivity derivatives complementing the already reported state patterns. State derivatives consist of additional information about increment and decrement of connectivity among brain networks not observed by the original dFNC method. The tvFNC shows more sensitivity than regular dFNC by uncovering additional FNC differences between the HC and SZ groups in each state. In summary, the tvFNC method provides a new and enhanced approach to examine time-varying functional connectivity.

Keywords: functional network connectivity, group independent component analysis, windowed correlation, derivatives, resting state fMRI

INTRODUCTION

Connectivity studies have uncovered a complex functional organization of brain connectome thanks to the use of functional magnetic resonance imaging (fMRI) (Fox et al., 2005; Power et al., 2011). The existence of disease-related abnormalities in the human connectome brings progress toward the use of fMRI acquisition in the clinical setting (Fox et al., 2010). As with any biological system, the brain connectome does not function in a static manner. Researchers have recognized the importance of developing techniques to characterize dynamic features embedded in the connectome dynamics (Hutchison et al., 2013; Saggar et al., 2018). Although one of the most basic measures of dynamicity is the derivative, this feature is underexplored in the context of functional connectivity. This limitation is related to the fact that functional connectivity is linked to the phase between neuronal activations (Yaesoubi et al., 2015). Study of the phase dynamics is more difficult to characterize than the dynamics of the actual activations. This work fills the gap by focusing on the derivative as a measure of the instantaneous variation of brain connectivity.

Functional connectivity measures the level of co-activation of fMRI time-series from anatomically separated brain regions (Friston et al., 1993). Previous connectivity studies considered functional connectivity to remain constant during the scan duration (Allen et al., 2011; Espinoza et al., 2018). Recent studies applying the dynamic FNC method (dFNC) have demonstrated that temporal functional network connectivity (FNC) analysis (i.e., co-activation between covarying networks estimated via independent component analysis) can uncover reoccurring connectivity patterns at resting state or during task performances. Their results also indicate that brain connectivity patterns iterate through time and show smooth variations of connectivity (Allen et al., 2014; Calhoun et al., 2014; Damaraju et al., 2014; Rashid et al., 2014; Espinoza et al., 2019). The dFNC method provides a way to explore temporally transient changes in the functional connectivity among brain networks using sliding windows to compute FNC across time (Sakoğlu et al., 2010; Allen et al., 2014). Among the limitations of the dFNC method, is the lack of justification for the reporting of very similar connectivity states identified by k-means clustering algorithm. At glance, the similar states can be combined into one state without taking into account the states temporal behavior. In this work, we aim to improve the ability of the dFNC method to characterize connectivity dynamics by including derivatives of windowed FNC in the identification of reoccurring states of connectivity.

Our approach referred to as temporal variation of functional network connectivity (tvFNC) is validated with a simulated data sample, and then applied to a resting-state fMRI sample formed by healthy controls (HC) and schizophrenia (SZ) patients that was previously analyzed with the original dFNC method (Damaraju et al., 2014). Among our goals were: to extend time-varying FNC states characterization by including the first derivatives of the windowed FNC; to provide complement states differentiation by including their derivatives information; to expose group differences not captured by the current dFNC method.

METHODS

Static Functional Network Connectivity

Static FNC (sFNC) analysis is based on the assumption that functional connectivity, defined as statistical dependence among N number of fMRI time-courses does not change during scanning time. Currently available connectivity measures include correlations (Rodgers and Nicewander, 1988), coherence (Chang and Glover, 2010; Yaesoubi et al., 2015) and mutual information (Gomez-Verdejo et al., 2012; Wang et al., 2015) among others. In this study, functional connectivity is measured via the Pearson's pairwise correlation, which is the most widely used approach to date (Allen et al., 2011; Espinoza et al., 2018). Correlations between each pair of time-courses generates a FNC vector with $N^*(N-1)/2$ unique FNC values. The FNC vector is then represented by an NxN symmetric FNC matrix (**Figure 1A**).

Dynamic Functional Network Connectivity

The dFNC analysis is an extension of sFNC, developed to capture time-varying FNC. In this method each time-course is discretized into a set of time domains using the sliding windowed approach (Sakoğlu et al., 2010; Allen et al., 2014). Then, in each time-windowed domain a FNC vector is calculated. This procedure generates a discrete sequence of windowed FNC (wFNC) vectors that are then represented by wFNC matrices (**Figure 1B**) describing connectivity behavior across time (Sakoğlu et al., 2010; Allen et al., 2014; Damaraju et al., 2014; Rashid et al., 2014; Espinoza et al., 2019). Subjects' dFNC data is formed by all wFNC vectors, and is referred to as the zero order derivatives of the sliding window correlations. In summary, the dFNC method pipeline is as follows, for all subjects compute sliding windowed correlations (wFNC); form dFNC data by stacking time-wise all subjects' dFNC data; run clustering analysis on dFNC data to identify reoccurring connectivity states.

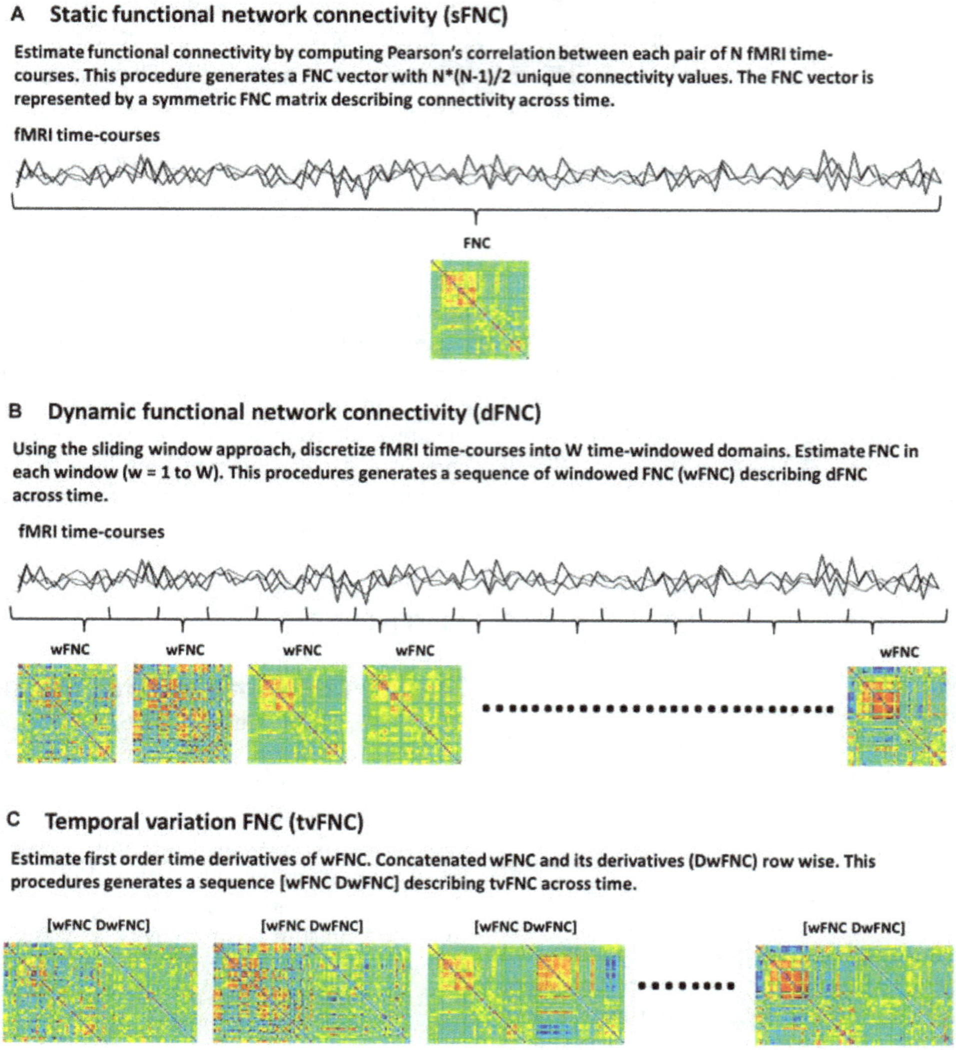

FIGURE 1 | Functional network connectivity (FNC) subject's data, **(A)** Static FNC, **(B)** Dynamic FNC, and **(C)** Temporal variation of FNC.

Temporal Variation of Functional Network Connectivity

The tvFNC analysis is an extension of dFNC, aiming to improve state classification by including wFNC derivatives in the clustering step. First order time derivatives of wFNC vectors are computed using finite difference approximations. For each subject, the discrete derivative of the first wFNC was estimated using the forward difference formula, $Dw_1FNC = w_2FNC - w_1FNC$. The discrete derivatives of the interior wFNC were estimated using central difference formula, $Dw_iFNC = (w_{i+1}FNC - w_{i-1}FNC)/2$, for $i = 2$ to $W-1$, where W is the number of windows. Lastly, the discrete derivative of the last wFNC was estimated using the backward difference formula, $Dw_WFNC = w_WFNC - w_{W-1}FNC$. Subjects' DdFNC data is formed by all wFNC derivatives, and is referred to as the first order derivatives of the sliding window correlations.

The tvFNC method pipeline is as follows, for all subjects (1) compute dFNC data (sliding windowed correlations wFNC); (2) estimate DdFNC data (derivatives of sliding windowed correlations DwFNC); (3) concatenate row wise zero and first order windowed correlations [wFNC and DwFNC] divided by their corresponding standard deviations (**Figure 1C**). The tvFNC data is formed by stacking time-wise all subjects [dFNC and DdFNC] data, and is referred to as the zero and first order derivatives of the sliding window correlations; (4) run clustering analysis on all subjects' tvFNC data to identify reoccurring connectivity states and their derivatives patterns.

Clustering Analysis

In both methods dFNC and tvFNC, time-varying connectivity is captured by performing k-means clustering analysis, assigning all subjects' temporal FNC data into a selected number of clusters representing distinct functional connectivity states. The clustering algorithm selection is based on previous connectivity studies that successfully applied k-means algorithm to identify reoccurring patterns of connectivity within and between subjects across time (Allen et al., 2014; Calhoun et al., 2014; Damaraju et al., 2014; Rashid et al., 2014; Faghiri et al., 2018; Vergara et al., 2018; Espinoza et al., 2019). We refer to Allen et al. (2014), Damaraju et al. (2014), and Abrol et al. (2017) for details on k-means clustering validation. The k-means clustering algorithm is applied to the temporal FNC data with the number of clusters ranging from 1 to K along with the Elbow criterion to identify the optimal number of clusters referred to as states. The optimal number of clusters is selected from the Elbow criterion cluster index results. The cluster index is defined as the ratio between the sums of the within-cluster sums of point-to-centroid distances to the sums of all the distances from each point to every centroid (Allen et al., 2014).

Simulated Data

The simulated data was designed to show the tvFNC method for a given a number of subjects S, and their corresponding N number of fMRI time-courses. For simplicity, we considered $N = 12$ and generated tvFNC data for $S = 300$ subjects. For simulation purposes, the subjects were divided into five groups with the same number of individuals in each group. For each subject, a time-varying sequence of 136 wFNC vectors describing subjects' dFNC behavior during scan duration was created. The number of windows, $W = 136$ was chosen to match the one obtained in the dFNC analysis of the selected fMRI data sample. Each simulated FNC and wFNC vectors contains 66 [=N*(N−1)/2)] unique FNC pairs. Subjects' dFNC data sets were created using three distinct connectivity patterns referred to as FNC seeds plus perturbation seeds created using random noise and white Gaussian noise ($\sigma = 0.003$). The first FNC seed shows a pattern with positive connectivity in the upper left block. The second FNC seed shows a pattern with positive connectivity in the lower right block. The third FNC seed shows a pattern with positive connectivity in the upper right and lower left blocks. FNC seed patterns are shown in **Figure 2A**. The perturbation seeds were chosen to be the first derivatives of the FNC seeds. These derivatives were tailored to have unique patterns simulating subject specific differences existing in real data. FNC seed derivatives patterns are shown in **Figure 2B**.

The simulation is initialized by setting the first window to the seed pattern plus noise: w_1FNC = FNC seed. Windowed FNC vectors are then simulated by using the recursive equation: $w_{i+1}\text{FNC} = w_i\text{FNC} \pm \text{DFNC seed} + N(0,\sigma)$, $i = 1$ to $W-1$. The symbol $\pm$ indicates that DFNC seed was added in some subjects, but subtracted in others. The recurrent equation was applied only to generate dFNC data from seeds 1 and 2. Dynamic FNC data generated from the third FNC seed did not include the derivative term DFNC seed. This way we covered the cases where states can have different derivative patterns across time (derivatives could go in opposite directions) and where there are no significant derivative changes. Next, first order time DdFNC of simulated data were computed, and tvFNC data was formed as previously explained. Then, the k-means clustering algorithm was applied to each simulated temporal FNC set ([dFNC] and [dFNC DdFNC]) with the number of clusters ranging from 1 to 10 along with the Elbow criterion to identify the optimal number of clusters. The simulations were repeated one hundred times and mean values of cluster index were computed.

Resting State fMRI Data

Data Sample

The resting state functional magnetic resonance imaging (fMRI) data used in this study was taken from the Functional Imaging Biomedical Informatics Research Network (FBIRN) Phase III study. Participants (healthy controls and patients) were recruited in seven sites across the United States. Participants' information and scan collection was approved by all seven sites' institutional review boards (IRB). The sample is formed by a total of 314 participants. The cohort includes 163 healthy controls (117 males, 46 females; average age 36.9 years) and 151 age- and gender matched patients with SZ (114 males, 37 females; average age 37.8 years).

Data Acquisition

All participants provided written informed consent before scanning. Resting-state fMRI scans were collected at seven sites using a 3T Siemens Tim Trio System scanner in six locations and a 3T General Electric Discovery MR750 scanner in one location. Participants were asked to lay still, stay awake and keep their eyes closed during the whole scan duration. In all sites, T2*-weighted gradient-echo echo-planar images (EPIs) were acquired with the following parameters: voxel size = $3.4375 \times 3.4375 \times 4.0$ mm^3, repetition time (TR) = 2 s, eco time (TE) = 30 ms, flip angle (FA) = 77 degrees, field of view (FOV) = 220×220 mm (64×64 matrix), slice thickness = 4 mm, gap = 1 mm, number of slices = 32 sequential ascending slices. Scans lasted 5:4 min, a total of 162 volumes of echo planar imaging BOLD fMRI were collected.

Data Pre-processing, Group Independent Component Analysis, and Post-processing

Detail information of selected rsfMRI scans quality control, pre-processing, group independent component analysis (GICA), and post-processing can be found in Damaraju et al. (2014). In summary, functional images were preprocessed using custom written Matlab scripts along with three available toolboxes, Analysis of Functional NeuroImages (AFNI)[1], Spatial Parametric Mapping (SPM)[2], and Group ICA/IVA of fMRI Toolbox (GIFT)[3]. Rigid body motion correction was performed using INRIalign (Freire and Mangin, 2001). Resting-state fMRI scans were spatially normalized to the Montreal Neurological Institute (MNI) space (Friston, 1995), resliced to 3 mm x 3 mm x 3 mm voxels, and smoothed using a Gaussian kernel with a full-width at half maximum (FWHM) of 6 mm. Lastly, each voxel time-course was variance normalized completing the data preprocess step. Participants (HC and SZ) whole brain functional parcellation was obtained by applying the spatial GICA algorithm implemented in the GIFT toolbox (Calhoun et al., 2001; Correa et al., 2005) to the preprocessed fMRI data. Spatial GICA is an

---

[1] http://mialab.mrn.org/software/gift/

[2] https://afni.nimh.nih.gov/

[3] http://www.fil.ion.ucl.ac.uk/spm/

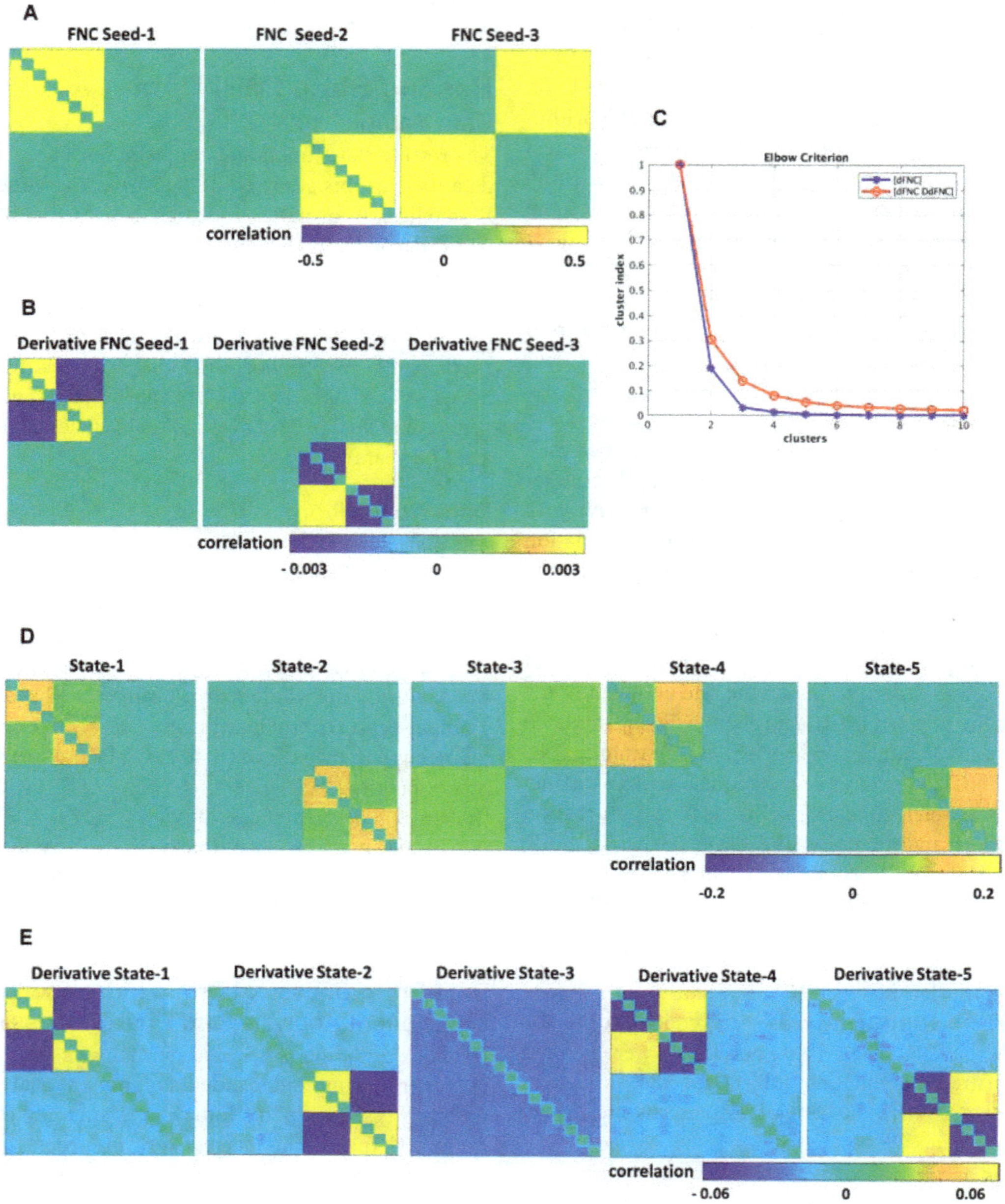

FIGURE 2 | Simulated data, **(A)** FNC seeds, **(B)** derivatives of FNC seeds, **(C)** Elbow criterion results for dFNC and tvFNC methods, panels **(D,E)** show FNC states and their derivatives choosing optimal number of clusters = 5.

extension of spatial ICA, which decomposes all subjects' fMRI data into linear mixtures of maximally spatially independent components and provides their unique time-course profiles. One hundred independent components (ICs) representing whole brain functional parcellation were obtained using principal component analysis (Rachakonda et al., 2016) and the infomax algorithm (Bell and Sejnowski, 1995). Subjects' ICs anatomical brain regions referred as spatial maps and their corresponding time-courses were obtained using the spatiotemporal regression back reconstruction approach (Calhoun et al., 2001; Erhardt et al., 2011). Out of the 100 ICs that were estimated, $N = 47$ ICs were identified as meaningful resting state networks (RSNs) by evaluating the ratio of high to low frequency power in the spectra of components, as well as whether peak activations took place in gray matter (Meda et al., 2008; Robinson et al., 2009; Allen et al., 2011). Post-processing of the selected 47 RSNs time-courses included: detrending and despiking using 3DDespike, filtering using a fifth-order Butterworth low-pass filter with a high frequency cutoff of 0.15 Hz, and variance normalization.

Estimation of dFNC and tvFNC Data

Whole brain dFNC is computed by obtaining a sequence of time domains for each of the selected 47 RSNs time-courses using the tapered sliding window approach (Allen et al., 2014).

A total of 136 widows (W = 136) were obtained using a rectangular window width of 22 TRs (=44 s, TR = 2 s) convolved with a Gaussian of sigma 3 TRs, and sliding in one TR step until covering the whole time domain. Then, for each subject's windows 1 to 136, FNC among the RSN windowed time-courses was calculated generating a discrete sequence of wFNC vectors containing 1081 [=N*(N−1)/2] unique FNC pairs. Each wFNC vector is then represented by a full covariance matrix named wFNC and/or dFNC matrix. Since time-courses of short length may have insufficient information to characterize full covariance matrices, the graphical LASSO algorithm (Friedman et al., 2008) was used to overcome this limitation. Covariance matrices were estimated from regularized inverse covariance matrices (Smith et al., 2011). A penalty on the L1 norm of the precision matrix was applied to enforce sparsity. The cross-validation scheme for estimating covariance with graphical lasso framework is as follows: For each subject, a random windowed data is chosen and rest of the subject's windowed data is considered as unseen data. The regularization parameter defined as the optimum hyperparameter lambda (among a set of lambda values selected *a priori*) that maximizes the log likelihood of the unseen data is chosen. This process is repeated for few randomly chosen windows of the subject and the mean lambda across the repetitions is then used for estimating covariance for all of the windows of that subject. Overall 42,704 (=314 participants times 136 wFNC) dFNC matrices were obtained representing subjects' FNC as a function of time. To account for nuisance effects, subjects' dFNC data (zero order sliding windowed correlations) were Fisher z transformed, and residualized with respect to age, gender and multi-site (Damaraju et al., 2014). Next, time derivatives of the dFNC data were computed (first order derivatives of sliding windowed correlations). Lastly, tvFNC data was formed as previously explained.

Clustering of dFNC and tvFNC Data

The dFNC data was represented by five FNC states using the K-means clustering algorithm along with the correlation distance metric. The optimal number of states/clusters k = 5 was identifying using the elbow criterion of the cluster index (Damaraju et al., 2014). To be able to compare our results to the dFNC results, the tvFNC data was clustered with the same cluster algorithm, number of clusters and distance metric. Connectivity dynamism was assessed by two measures computed from the clustering results (1) mean dwell time and (2) fraction time. Mean dwell time provides an average time an individual spend in each state before changing to another state, and fraction time provides a percentage of total time an individual spend in each state.

Group Differences

Group differences in tvFNC between HC and SZ subjects were tested using two sample t-tests and results were corrected for multiple comparisons applying false discovery rate threshold at a significant level of $q < 0.05$. Group differences were tested for connectivity dynamism on the clustering measures, mean dwell time and fraction time; and for FNC states on all FNC pairs. In each state, first we identified subjects with at least one tvFNC element ([wFNC DwFNC]) in that state. Then, the median of all identified tvFNC elements was calculated as the subject state contribution. Therefore, the number of subjects in each state is not fixed. Next, we separate subjects' states' median FNC as states FNC and their corresponding derivatives. Lastly, SZ-HC group differences were tested in each state and their corresponding derivatives for each FNC pair.

RESULTS

Simulated dFNC Data

Simulations were designed to extend three original FNC states (**Figure 2A**) into five states (**Figure 2D**). Dynamically, the first two states show two patterns of positive and negative derivatives, and the last state show small connectivity changes across time (**Figure 2E**). From the Elbow plot **Figure 2C**, we can observe that the dFNC method shows a sharp decay in the cluster index from two to three clusters. This result could imply that three could be selected as the optimal number of clusters/states. However, we can notice no changes in the cluster index for the number of clusters bigger than five. In other words, this data can be well represented by five clusters. On the other hand, the tvFNC method shows smooth cluster index decay from two to five clusters and small decline for the higher number of clusters. The tvFNC clustering results with the optimal number of clusters, k = 5 are shown in **Figure 2D** (states) and **Figure 2E** (states derivatives). These results show that the inclusion of a derivative pattern in the simulation allowed for a clearer identification of similar clusters with different temporal behavior.

The tvFNC method supports the identification of very similar states capturing different temporal behavior not shown in the dFNC method. The absence of derivatives in the clustering estimation resulted in a poor differentiation of similar states even at small noise perturbations. As in the simulation, clustering of real data analyzed in the next subsection can also benefit from the extra information provided by the derivatives.

Resting State fMRI Data

Functional classification of the selected 47 RSNs is based on anatomy and brain functioning. The 47 RSNs were grouped into seven functional domains: sub-cortical [(SC), 5 RSNs]; auditory [(AUD), 2 RSNs]; visual [(VIS), 11 RSNs]; sensorimotor [(SM), 6 RSNs]; attention/cognitive control [(CC), 13 RSNs]; default mode network [(DMN), 8 RSNs]; cerebellar [(CB), 2RSNs]. Table 1 in Damaraju et al. (2014) of the 47 RSNs along with their Brodmann area numbers, number of voxels in each components cluster, component numbers and peak activation coordinates x, y, and z. **Figure 3** depicts the spatial maps of the 47 RSNs grouped by seven functional domains.

Temporal Variation of Functional Network Connectivity Characterization

Using sliding-window and k-means clustering whole brain temporal variation of FNC during scan duration were represented by five connectivity states. **Figure 4** displays the centroids of the five states broke down as FNC states 1–5

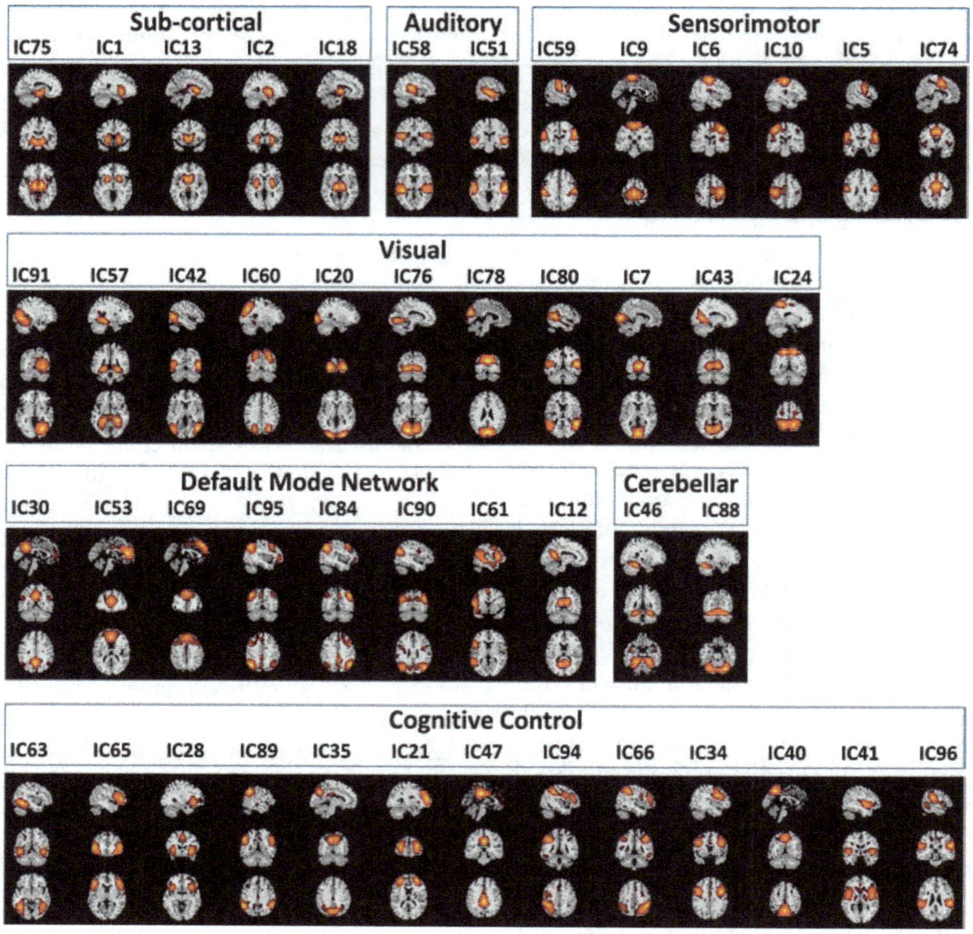

FIGURE 3 | Spatial Maps and their corresponding independent component numbers of the 47 selected resting state networks group into seven domains subcortical (SC), auditory (AUD), sensorimotor (SM), visual (VIS), default mode network (DMN), cerebellar (CB), and cognitive control (CC).

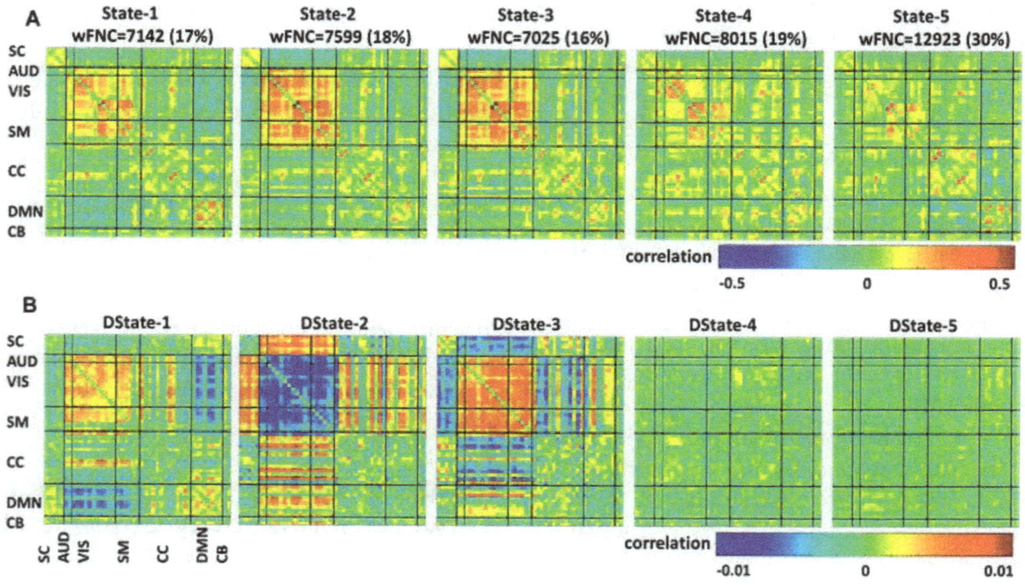

FIGURE 4 | Functional network connectivity states **(A)** and their derivatives **(B)**.

(first row) and their corresponding derivatives (second row); the total number of wFNC in each state along with its equivalent percent frequency in parenthesis is also listed. States numbering was assigned based on the order of clustering formation. States' FNC pattern description is presented in descend order based on their wFNC frequency distribution.

State 5, the one with the higher frequency distribution (30% wFNC) shows weak connectivity overall. This state displays mostly negative correlations between domains and positive correlations within visual, cognitive control and default mode domains. The derivative of State 5 is represented by an unstructured weak connectivity pattern. Small positive and negative correlation values display a mix of increasing and decreasing connectivity.

State 4, the one with the second higher frequency distribution (19% wFNC) shows slightly stronger connectivity than State 5, with higher within- and between connectivity modularity in the visual and sensorimotor domains. The derivative of State 4 is represented by a similar unstructured weak connectivity as the derivative of State 5. In addition, this state derivative displays more pronounced positive correlation values between cognitive control and visual domain can be observed.

State 2, the one with the third higher frequency distribution (18% wFNC) shows a more structured connectivity pattern compared to States 4 and 5. This state captures stronger positive correlations within the visual and sensorimotor domains, and between most RSNs from the auditory, visual, and sensorimotor domains, and a few components from the cognitive control and default mode domains. We can also observe notable negative correlations between the subcortical domain and the auditory, visual, and sensorimotor domains. The derivative of State 2 is represented by a well-structured connectivity pattern displaying increase and/or decrease in connectivity within and between domains. We can observe that the marked positive and negative FNC captured in State 2 has negative and positive derivatives. These results imply that (1) there is noticeable decrease in connectivity within the visual domain and between the auditory, visual, sensorimotor and a few components from the cognitive control domains. (2) There is noticeable increase in connectivity between the subcortical, auditory, sensorimotor and some components from the cognitive control and default mode domains.

State 1, the one with the second lowest frequency distribution (17% wFNC) shows weaker connectivity patterns than States 2 and 3. This state also shows noticeable positive correlations between RSNs from the default mode domain. In addition, we can observe slightly stronger negative correlations between the auditory, visual, sensorimotor, and default node domains. The derivative of State 1 is represented by weaker connectivity pattern in comparison to the derivative of State 3.

We can observe that most of the pronounced positive and negative FNC captured in State 1 has positive and negative derivatives. These results imply that (1) there is a noticeable increase in connectivity within the visual domain and between the auditory, visual, sensorimotor and a few components from the cognitive control domains. (2) There is a noticeable decrease in connectivity between the auditory, visual, and default mode domains. Also we can observe weaker decrease in connectivity between the subcortical, cognitive control, and cerebellar and the rest of domains.

State 3, the one with the lowest frequency distribution (16% wFNC) shows very similar connectivity patterns as State 2. However, the derivative of State 3 is represented by a well-structured connectivity pattern very different than the derivative of State 2. The derivative of State 3 seems like the complement of the derivative of State 2 displaying increase and/or decrease in connectivity within and between domains. We can observe that the marked positive and negative FNC captured in State 3 has positive and negative derivatives. These results imply that (1) there is a noticeable increase in connectivity within the visual domain and between the auditory, visual, sensorimotor and a few components from the cognitive control and default node domains. (2) There is a noticeable decrease in connectivity between the subcortical, auditory, sensorimotor and some components from the cognitive control and default mode domains.

Figure 5 depicts the FNC states (A) and their derivative (B) centroids separated by groups HC (first row) and SZ (second row). The total number of subjects in each state is listed in parenthesis. The HC and SZ group FNC states 1–5 and their derivatives patterns are very similar to those shown in **Figure 4.** State 1, the fourth state in the wFNC percent frequency rank contains the highest number of subjects [N = 254, HC = 127, and SZ = 127]. It is followed by State 5 [N = 236, HC = 109, and SZ = 127], the number one in the wFNC percent frequency rank. The HC FNC states show slightly higher positive and negative connectivity patterns than SZ states.

Schizophrenia and Healthy Control Group Differences in Temporal Variation of Functional Network Connectivity

All presented results were corrected for multiple testing. From **Figure 6** we can observe that HC individuals spend significantly more time in States 2 and 3. These states show stronger within- and between-connectivity in the auditory, visual, and sensorimotor domains compared to the other states. On the other hand, SZ individuals spend more time in State 5 (a state displaying weakly connectivity between RSNs from all domains). The t- and p-values are listed in **Table 1**.

Figure 7 depicts the significant connectivity differences between SZ and HC subjects in states 1–5 (**Figure 7A**, first row) and in the states derivatives (**Figure 7B**, second row). From **Figure 7A**, showing FNC group differences in states 1–3 we can observe that compared to HC, SZ patients showed higher connectivity between a RSN from the subcortical domain [thalamus (IC18)] and RSNS from the auditory [superior temporal (IC58) and middle temporal gyrus (IC51)], visual [lingual gyrus (IC91), parahippocampal gyrus IC(57), middle temporal gyrus(IC42), middle frontal gyrus (IC20), cuneus (IC78), middle temporal gyrus (IC80), cuneus IC(7), superior parietal lobule (IC24)], and sensorimotor [medial frontal gyrus (IC9), right post-central gyrus (IC6)] domains. We can also notice less pronounced connectivity between RSNs from the

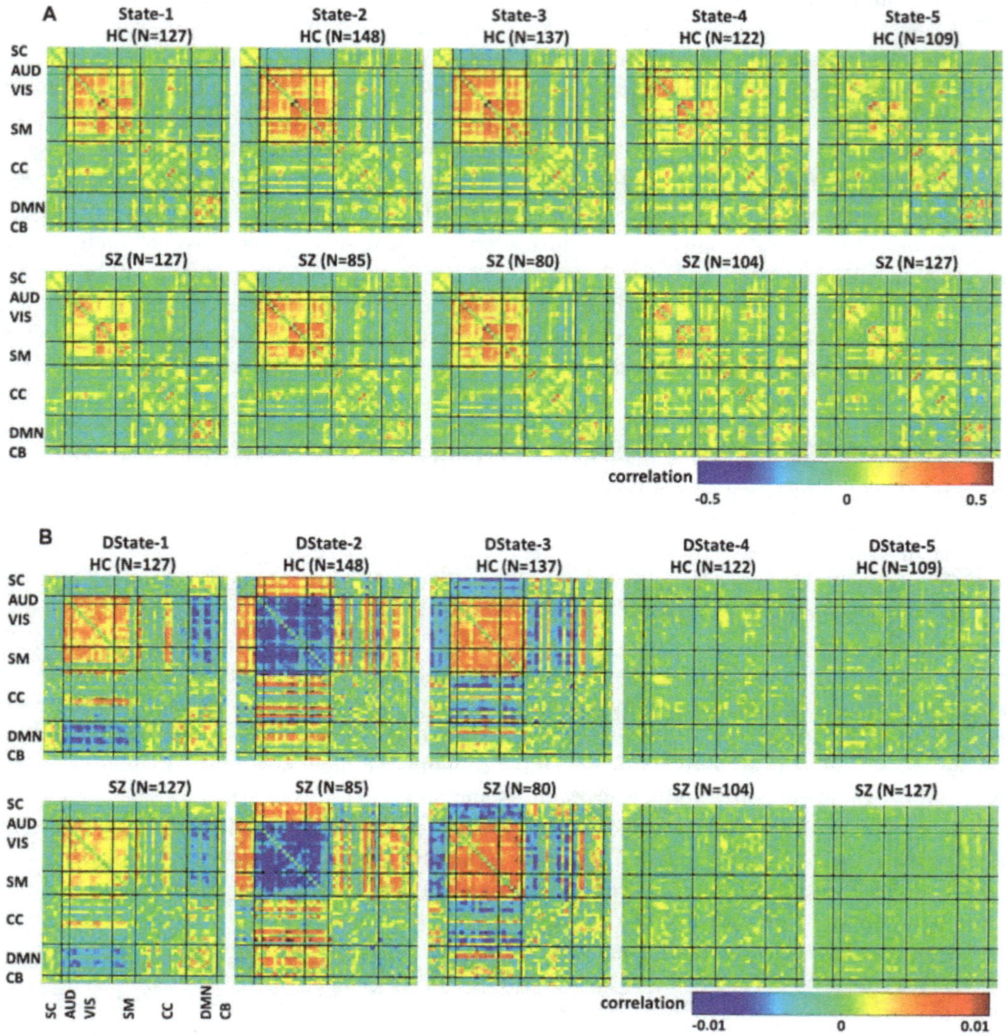

FIGURE 5 | Healthy control (HC) and schizophrenia (SZ) participants' functional Network connectivity states **(A)** and their derivatives **(B)**.

subcortical domain and RSNs from the auditory, visual, cognitive control, and cerebellar domains in State 1; between RSNs from the subcortical and cerebellar domains and RSNs from the other domains in States 2 and 3; between subcortical, auditory, visual, cognitive control, default mode, and cerebellar domains in State 4. On the other hand, compared to SZ, HC showed higher within connectivity in the visual, sensorimotor, cognitive control domains; and among the subcortical, auditory, sensorimotor and the rest of domains. From **Figure 7B**, we can observe FNC group differences between SZ and HC in the derivatives of states 1–3. No significant differences in the derivatives of states 4 and 5 were found. Compared to HC, SZ subjects showed higher increase in derivatives in State 1 between inferior parietal lobe (IC96, CC) and precentral gyrus (IC5, SM), middle frontal gyrus (IC21, CC); and between cingulate gyrus (IC47, CC) and anterior cingulate gyrus (IC53, DMN); in State 2 between inferior frontal gyrus (IC34, CC) and thalamus (IC18, SC), and middle frontal gyrus (IC69, DMN) and post-central gyrus (IC6, SM); and in State 3 between middle temporal gyrus (IC80, VIS), and thalamus (IC18, SC).

DISCUSSION

In this work we have presented the tvFNC method which is an extension of the current dFNC approach to include the first derivative of the time dependent FNC patterns in the overall analysis. We found that time derivatives exhibits their own clustering patterns. The inclusion of the derivative information was useful for the clustering procedure to find an accurate clustering partition.

Clustering and tvFNC

Simulated data showed that the identification of occurring connectivity patterns performed by clustering analysis can benefit from using the first derivative information to support the existence of similar patterns with different temporal behavior. We

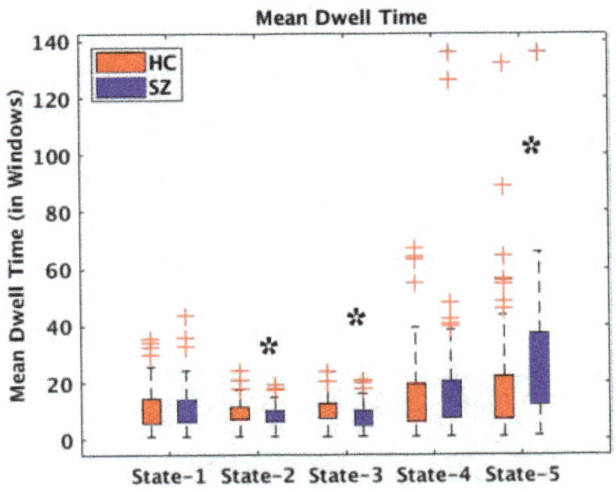

FIGURE 6 | Bar plots displaying mean dwell times in States 1–5 for HC (red) and SZ (blue) participants. The states showing significant differences between the HC and SZ groups are marked with a black star (FDR-corrected results). The two test *t*- and *p*-values are listed in **Table 1**.

confirm the premise that time point information can be better described, and subsequently clustered, by using its derivative. It is not the first time that derivatives are used to improve the characterization of a time varying signal. This assumption is rooted in Taylor's theorem. Notice that due to fMRI protocols we don't really have a continuous description of the signal. In fact, the fMRI data consists of snapshots spaced in time by a predefined TR. In the current context, we are improving the discrete time estimation of the dFNC at a given time point t = n*TR by adding information of the estimated derivative DdFNC at that time point. The simulation showed that including time specific estimations of derivatives helped in recognizing the different dFNC patterns imposed in the simulation. The importance of the derivative extends to the real data where an extra set of observations can be accounted for.

Dynamic FNC was captured by five connectivity states that reoccurred over time supporting previous finding that whole-brain functional connectivity is not stationary (Allen et al., 2014; Damaraju et al., 2014; Rashid et al., 2014; Faghiri et al., 2018; Espinoza et al., 2019). In addition, the dFNC states' time derivatives provide a measure that is sensitive to dFNC changes over a period of time. These tvFNC results are also in line with previous resting state studies results examining functional disruptions in SZ. For instance, the five dFNC states identified in this study are very similar to those identified by Damaraju and collaborators (Damaraju et al., 2014). In that study, the optimum number of clusters representing connectivity states was selected using the Elbow criterion. Based on this approach, five states were obtained to describe FNC over time. It can be observed in both, **Figure 4** here and in Damaraju et al., that States 2 and 3 are very similar. From just looking at the dFNC states results, it can be inferred that the number of FNC states can be reduced from five to four. However, the derivative patterns observed using the tvFNC method complements the results from the dFNC approach, validating the previously obtained FNC states and providing additional support for states separation. A clear state differentiation is observed from the FNC derivatives of States 2 and 3 which display different connectivity patterns, **Figure 4B**.

Another important observation to make is that the connectivity patterns of States 2 and 3 derivatives seem to complement each other. For example, from **Figure 4** we observe that the derivative of State 2 shows decreasing connectivity among auditory, visual and sensorimotor domains while the derivative of State 3, shows increasing connectivity among these domains. On the other hand, the derivative of State 2 shows increasing connectivity among subcortical, auditory, visual, and sensorimotor domains while the derivative of State 3 shows decreasing connectivity among these domains. Overall, both states derivatives values are very close to zero showing almost constant (very small temporal variations) connectivity over time.

TABLE 1 | Two *t*-test mean dwell time and fraction time results showing Healthy control (HC) and Schizophrenia (SZ) differences in each state.

	State-1	State-2	State-3	State-4	State-5
Mean dwell time					
p-value	0.6984	0.0278*	0.0058*	0.3811	9.88*e* − 05*
t-Value	−0.3880	2.2134	2.7899	−0.8776	−3.9618
Fraction time					
p-value	0.1089	0.0006*	3.22*e* − 07	0.9943	9.98*e* − 10*
t-Value	−1.6088	3.4697	5.2759	−0.0072	−6.3690

The FDR corrected p-values showing significant differences between HC and SZ are marked with a star.

HC Versus SZ

In terms of dynamism, HC changed states more than SZ subjects did. These changes were measured by computing the fraction time (FT) spend in states for the two groups. Compared to HC, SZ individuals spend significant more time in State 5, a state showing weakly dFNC and almost constant behavior over time. Lower degree of functional connectivity and reduced in modularity in SZ was also reported by Lynall et al. (2010), Yu et al. (2011), and Damaraju et al. (2014). The tvFNC analysis captured group differences in all five states. It also uncovered significant group differences in States 4 and 5 not previously captured (Damaraju et al., 2014). **Figure 7** shows SZ individuals with lower connectivity than HC in states where the connectivity is already weak (States 4 and 5). These two states might be visualized as a valley or a point in time where the general connectivity lowers then rises. Since there is no significant difference in the derivatives of States 4 and 5, we can argue that spending more time in the weak states (just as SZ subjects do) allows reaching lower connectivity. On the contrary, HC dwelling is shorter and the connectivity does not reach the same minimum value. This new observation shows extra evidence that derivatives gives new refinements in the analysis. With respect to States 1, 2, and 3, **Figure 7A** shows hyperconnectivity in SZ between the subcortical (thalamus) and RSNs from the auditory, visual and sensorimotor domains. Hypoconnectivity between (1) subcortical and cognitive control and default mode domains; (2) default mode and cognitive

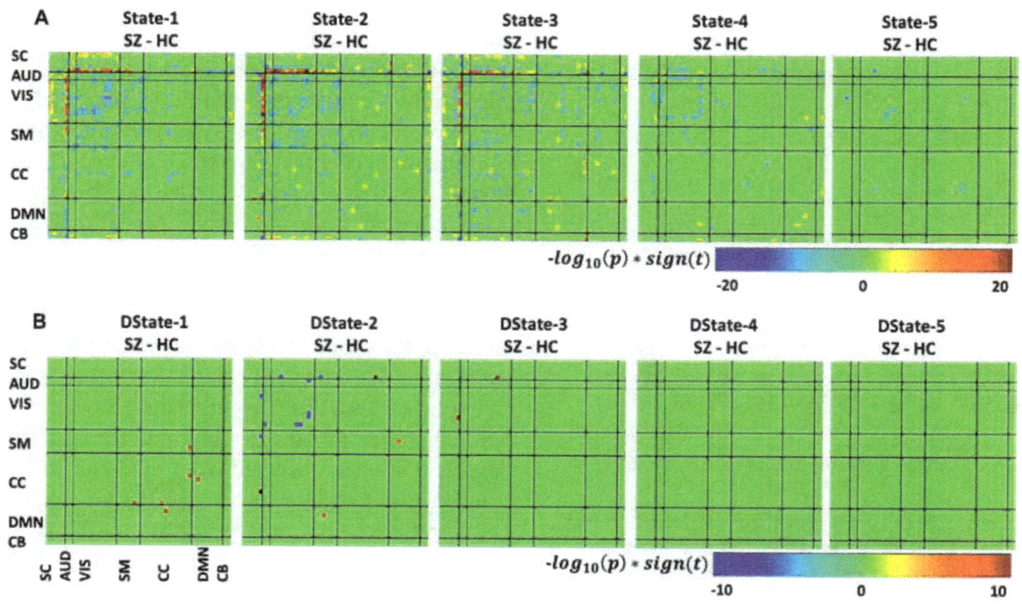

FIGURE 7 | Two t-test results showing states **(A)** and derivatives **(B)** connectivity differences between the SZ and HC groups, FDR corrected results threshold at a $q < 0.05$.

control domains; and (3) cerebellar and auditory, visual and sensorimotor, cognitive control domains is also observed. These states (1, 2, and 3) suffer more sudden and faster changes, thus the dynamics are different than States 4 and 5. Note that, a similar pattern of hypoconnectivity within auditory and visual domains can be seen in all five states which is consistent with the disconnection hypothesis (Friston et al., 2016). Results seem in higher agreement with the disconnection hypothesis since some dFNC has slower dynamicity as seen in **Figures 5B, 6** where some derivatives exhibit lower magnitudes in SZ.

In a compensatory manner, thalamic connectivity is stronger in SZ as it is the main characteristic shared by states 1, 2, and 3. Although this observation seems contrary to Friston's disconnection hypothesis, it is not a rare observation. Resting-state fMRI studies have reported SZ thalamic hyperconnectivity with sensorimotor cortices, whole brain (Woodward et al., 2012; Damaraju et al., 2014; Rashid et al., 2014) and seed-based (Woodward et al., 2012; Anticevic et al., 2014). To counterbalance the previous statement, we must point out that thalamic hyperconnectivity pertain to states with short dwelling while larger dwelling states characterizes the absence of this hyperconnectivity (see **Figures 5, 6**). However, sensorial hypoconnectivity (auditory, visual and sensorimotor) can be found in all states, thus present 100 % of the time.

The novel contributions of this work are the differences in dynamicity, as measured using the derivatives of dFNC. **Figure 7B** displays states derivative differences' between SZ and HC. Group differences were captured in three out of the five states among six domains. Compared to HC, SZ subjects showed higher increase in derivatives in State 1 between inferior parietal lobe and, precentral gyrus and middle frontal gyrus; and cingulate gyrus and anterior cingulate gyrus. In State 2 between inferior frontal gyrus and thalamus; and middle frontal gyrus and post-central gyrus. In State 3 between middle temporal gyrus and thalamus. Despite these increments in variation, the connectivity strength was not different for the mentioned IC pairs in States 2 and 3. This can be observed by comparing the mentioned derivatives in **Figure 5B** with the connectivity in **Figure 5A**. This observation is not consistent since we could expect that higher derivatives would help increasing the magnitude of connectivity. Since this was not the case, we can conclude that the aggregated effect of the increased derivatives was not coherent or not strong enough to produce a consistent difference in connectivity. However, the observation points to a more rapid connectivity fluctuation in CC and DMN brain areas pointing to possible causes of cognitive deficiencies known to occur in schizophrenia (Schaefer et al., 2013).

Limitations and Future Directions

Among the limitations to be consider in this work: Functional connectivity is measured as the Pearson correlation between fMRI time-courses, and this lower order statistic provided significant results. Higher order statistics, such as mutual information, could be considered in future work to extend this analysis. The calculation of dFNC data requires a window length selection. The selected windowed size should be able to capture functional connectivity variability in small time domains (Sakoğlu et al., 2010). Following this recommendation, a fixed window size of 22 TR (=44 s) similar to the one used in Damaraju et al. (2014) was selected. Future work should evaluate state derivative changes over range of window sizes. Another limitation lies on the scan duration. This resting state fMRI data was collected for 5.4 min, a longer scanning time may uncover the identification of critical time points where FNC states reaches stationary behavior.

AUTHOR CONTRIBUTIONS

FE, VV, and VC designed the methods and carried out the study. VV and AF helped to refine the data simulations. FE, ED, and KH carried out the data analysis. JT, AB, JF, SM, DM, BM, SP, AP, JV, and TvE collected the data. FE wrote the first draft of the manuscript. All authors contributed to the manuscript revision, read, and approved its final version.

FUNDING

This work was supported by grants from the National Institutes of Health (R01EB020407, P20GM103472, and P30GM122734) and the National Science Foundation (1539067).

REFERENCES

Abrol, A., Damaraju, E., Miller, R. L., Stephen, J. M., Claus, E. D., Mayer, A. R., et al. (2017). Replicability of time-varying connectivity patterns in large resting state fMRI samples. *Neuroimage* 163, 160–176. doi: 10.1016/j.neuroimage.2017.09.020

Allen, E. A., Damaraju, E., Plis, S. M., Erhardt, E. B., Eichele, T., and Calhoun, V. D. (2014). Tracking whole-brain connectivity dynamics in the resting state. *Cereb. Cortex* 24, 663–676. doi: 10.1093/cercor/bhs352

Allen, E. A., Erhardt, E. B., Damaraju, E., Gruner, W., Segall, J. M., Silva, R. F., et al. (2011). A baseline for the multivariate comparison of resting-state networks. *Front. Syst. Neurosci.* 5:2. doi: 10.3389/fnsys.2011.00002

Anticevic, A., Cole, M. W., Repovs, G., Murray, J. D., Brumbaugh, M. S., Winkler, A. M., et al. (2014). Characterizing thalamo-cortical disturbances in schizophrenia and bipolar illness. *Cereb. Cortex* 24, 3116–3130. doi: 10.1093/cercor/bht165

Bell, A. J., and Sejnowski, T. J. (1995). An information-maximization approach to blind separation and blind deconvolution. *Neural Comput.* 7, 1129–1159. doi: 10.1162/neco.1995.7.6.1129

Calhoun, V. D., Adali, T., Pearlson, G. D., and Pekar, J. J. (2001). A method for making group inferences from functional MRI data using independent component analysis. *Hum. Brain Map.* 14, 140–151. doi: 10.1002/hbm.1048

Calhoun, V. D., Miller, R., Pearlson, G., and Adalı, T. (2014). The chronnectome: time-varying connectivity networks as the next frontier in fMRI data discovery. *Neuron* 84, 262–274. doi: 10.1016/j.neuron.2014.10.015

Chang, C., and Glover, G. H. (2010). Time-frequency dynamics of resting-state brain connectivity measured with fMRI. *Neuroimage* 50, 81–98. doi: 10.1016/j.neuroimage.2009.12.011

Correa, N., Adali, T., Li, Y. O., and Calhoun, V. D. (2005). "Comparison of blind source separation algorithms for FMRI using a new Matlab toolbox: Gift," in *IEEE International Conference on Acoustics, Speech, and Signal Processing, ICASSP*, Philadelphia, PA, 401–404.

Damaraju, E., Allen, E. A., Belger, A., Ford, J. M., McEwen, S., Mathalon, D. H., et al. (2014). Dynamic functional connectivity analysis reveals transient states of dysconnectivity in schizophrenia. *Neuroimage. Clin.* 5, 298–308. doi: 10.1016/j.nicl.2014.07.003

Erhardt, E. B., Rachakonda, S., Bedrick, E. J., Allen, E. A., Adali, T., and Calhoun, V. D. (2011). Comparison of multi-subject ICA methods for analysis of fMRI data. *Hum. Brain Mapp.* 32, 2075–2095. doi: 10.1002/hbm.21170

Espinoza, F. A., Liu, J., Ciarochi, J., Turner, J. A., Vergara, V. M., Caprihan, A., et al. (2019). Dynamic functional network connectivity in Huntington's disease and its associations with motor and cognitive measures. *Hum. Brain Mapp.* 40, 1955–1968. doi: 10.1002/hbm.24504

Espinoza, F. A., Turner, J. A., Vergara, V. M., Miller, R. L., Mennigen, E., Liu, J., et al. (2018). Whole-brain connectivity in a large study of Huntington's disease gene mutation carriers and healthy controls. *Brain Connect.* 8, 166–178. doi: 10.1089/brain.2017.0538

Faghiri, A., Stephen, J. M., Wang, Y. P., Wilson, T. W., and Calhoun, V. D. (2018). Changing brain connectivity dynamics: from early childhood to adulthood. *Hum. Brain Mapp.* 39, 1108–1117. doi: 10.1002/hbm.23896

Fox, M. D., Greicius, M., Fox, M., and Greicius, M. (2010). Clinical applications of resting state functional connectivity. *Front. Syst. Neurosci.* 4:19. doi: 10.3389/fnsys.2010.00019

Fox, M. D., Snyder, A. Z., Vincent, J. L., Corbetta, M., Van Essen, D. C., and Raichle, M. E. (2005). The human brain is intrinsically organized into dynamic, anticorrelated functional networks. *Proc. Natl. Acad. Sci. U.S.A.* 102, 9673–9678. doi: 10.1073/pnas.0504136102

Freire, L., and Mangin, J. F. (2001). Motion correction algorithms may create spurious brain activations in the absence of subject motion. *Neuroimage* 14, 709–722. doi: 10.1006/nimg.2001.0869

Friedman, J., Hastie, T., and Tibshirani, R. (2008). Sparse inverse covariance estimation with the graphical lasso. *Biostatistics* 9, 432–441. doi: 10.1093/biostatistics/kxm045

Friston, K. (1995). *Spatial Normalisation: A New Approach.* San Antonio, TX: Presented at the BrainMap '95 UTHSC.

Friston, K., Brown, H. R., Siemerkus, J., and Stephan, K. E. (2016). The dysconnection hypothesis (2016). *Schizophr. Res.* 176, 83–94. doi: 10.1016/j.schres.2016.07.014

Friston, K. J., Frith, C. D., Liddle, P. F., and Frackowiak, R. S. (1993). Functional connectivity: the principal-component analysis of large (PET) data sets. *J. Cereb. Blood Flow Metab.* 13, 5–14. doi: 10.1038/jcbfm.1993.4

Gomez-Verdejo, V., Martinez-Ramon, M., Florensa-Vila, J., and Oliviero, A. (2012). Analysis of fMRI time series with mutual information. *Med. Image Anal.* 16, 451–458. doi: 10.1016/j.media.2011.11.002

Hutchison, R. M., Womelsdorf, T., Allen, E. A., Bandettini, P. A., Calhoun, V. D., Corbetta, M., et al. (2013). Dynamic functional connectivity: promise, issues, and interpretations. *Neuroimage* 80, 360–378. doi: 10.1016/j.neuroimage.2013.05.079

Lynall, M. E., Bassett, D. S., Kerwin, R., McKenna, P. J., Kitzbichler, M., Muller, U., et al. (2010). Functional connectivity and brain networks in schizophrenia. *J. Neurosci.* 30, 9477–9487. doi: 10.1523/JNEUROSCI.0333-10.2010

Meda, S. A., Giuliani, N. R., Calhoun, V. D., Jagannathan, K., Schretlen, D. J., Pulver, A., et al. (2008). A large scale (N = 400) investigation of gray matter differences in schizophrenia using optimized voxel-based morphometry. *Schizophr. Res.* 101, 95–105. doi: 10.1016/j.schres.2008.02.007

Power, J. D., Cohen, A. L., Nelson, S. M., Wig, G. S., Barnes, K. A., Church, J. A., et al. (2011). Functional network organization of the human brain. *Neuron* 72, 665–678.

Rachakonda, S., Silva, R. F., Liu, J., and Calhoun, V. D. (2016). Memory efficient PCA methods for large group ICA. *Front. Neurosci.* 10:17. doi: 10.3389/fnins.2016.00017

Rashid, B., Damaraju, E., Pearlson, G. D., and Calhoun, V. D. (2014). Dynamic connectivity states estimated from resting fMRI Identify differences among Schizophrenia, bipolar disorder, and healthy control subjects. *Front. Hum. Neurosci.* 8:897. doi: 10.3389/fnhum.2014.00897

Robinson, S., Basso, G., Soldati, N., Sailer, U., Jovicich, J., Bruzzone, L., et al. (2009). A resting state network in the motor control circuit of the basal ganglia. *BMC Neurosci.* 10:137. doi: 10.1186/1471-2202-10-137

Rodgers, J. L., and Nicewander, W. A. (1988). Thirteen ways to look at the correlation coefficient. *Am. Stat.* 42, 59–66. doi: 10.1080/00031305.1988.10475524

Saggar, M., Sporns, O., Gonzalez-Castillo, J., Bandettini, P. A., Carlsson, G., Glover, G., et al. (2018). Towards a new approach to reveal dynamical organization of the brain using topological data analysis. *Nat. Commun.* 9:1399. doi: 10.1038/s41467-018-03664-4

Sakoğlu, Ü, Pearlson, G. D., Kiehl, K. A., Wang, Y. M., Michael, A. M., and Calhoun, V. D. (2010). A method for evaluating dynamic functional network connectivity and task-modulation: application to schizophrenia. *MAGMA* 23, 351–366. doi: 10.1007/s10334-010-0197-8

Schaefer, J., Giangrande, E., Weinberger, D. R., and Dickinson, D. (2013). The global cognitive impairment in schizophrenia: consistent over decades and around the world. *Schizophr. Res.* 150, 42–50. doi: 10.1016/j.schres.2013.07.00

Smith, S. M., Miller, K. L., Salimi-Khorshidi, G., Webster, M., Beckmann, C. F., Nichols, T. E., et al. (2011). Network modelling methods for FMRI. *Neuroimage* 54, 875–891. doi: 10.1016/j.neuroimage.2010.08.063

Vergara, V. M., Mayer, A. R., Kiehl, K. A., and Calhoun, V. D. (2018). Dynamic functional network connectivity discriminates mild traumatic brain injury through machine learning. *Neuroimage Clin.* 19, 30–37. doi: 10.1016/j.nicl.2018.03.017

Wang, Z., Alahmadi, A., Zhu, D., and Li, T. T. (2015). "Brain Functional Connectivity Analysis Using Mutual Information," in *Proceedings of the 2015 IEEE Global Conference on Signal and Information Processing (Globalsip)*, Orlando, FL, 542–546.

Woodward, N. D., Karbasforoushan, H., and Heckers, S. (2012). Thalamocortical dysconnectivity in schizophrenia. *Am. J. Psychiatry* 169, 1092–1099. doi: 10.1176/appi.ajp.2012.12010056

Yaesoubi, M., Allen, E. A., Miller, R. L., and Calhoun, V. D. (2015). Dynamic coherence analysis of resting fMRI data to jointly capture state-based phase, frequency, and time-domain information. *Neuroimage* 120, 133–142. doi: 10.1016/j.neuroimage.2015.07.002

Yu, Q., Plis, S. M., Erhardt, E. B., Allen, E. A., Sui, J., Kiehl, K. A., et al. (2011). Modular organization of functional network connectivity in healthy controls and patients with schizophrenia during the resting state. *Front. Syst. Neurosci.* 5:103. doi: 10.3389/fnsys.2011.00103

15

A Comparative Atlas-Based Recognition of Mild Cognitive Impairment with Voxel-Based Morphometry

Zhuqing Long[1,2†], Jinchang Huang[3†], Bo Li[4,5], Zuojia Li[1], Zihao Li[1], Hongwen Chen[1] and Bin Jing[2*]*

[1] Medical Apparatus and Equipment Deployment, Nanfang Hospital, Southern Medical University, Guangzhou, China, [2] School of Biomedical Engineering, Capital Medical University, Beijing, China, [3] Department of Acupuncture and Minimally Invasive Oncology, Beijing University of Chinese Medicine Third Affiliated Hospital, Beijing, China, [4] Department of Traditional Chinese Medicine, Beijing Chest Hospital, Capital Medical University, Beijing, China, [5] Beijing Tuberculosis and Thoracic Tumor Research Institute, Beijing, China

***Correspondence:**
Hongwen Chen
chw47922@126.com
Bin Jing
bjing@ccmu.edu.cn

†These authors have contributed equally to this work

An accurate and reliable brain partition atlas is vital to quantitatively investigate the structural and functional abnormalities in mild cognitive impairment (MCI), generally considered to be a prodromal phase of Alzheimer's disease. In this paper, we proposed an automated structural classification method to identify MCI from healthy controls (HC) and investigated whether the classification performance was dependent on the brain parcellation schemes, including Automated Anatomical Labeling (AAL-90) atlas, Brainnetome (BN-246) atlas, and AAL-1024 atlas. In detail, structural magnetic resonance imaging (sMRI) data of 69 MCI patients and 63 HC matched well on gender, age, and education level were collected and analyzed with voxel-based morphometry method first, then the volume features of every region of interest (ROI) belonging to the above-mentioned three atlases were calculated and compared between MCI and HC groups, respectively. At last, the abnormal volume features were selected as the classification features for a proposed support vector machine based identification method. After the leave-one-out cross-validation to estimate the classification performance, our results reported accuracies of 83, 92, and 89% with AAL-90, BN-246, and AAL-1024 atlas, respectively, suggesting that future studies should pay more attention to the selection of brain partition schemes in the atlas-based studies. Furthermore, the consistent atrophic brain regions among three atlases were predominately located at bilateral hippocampus, bilateral parahippocampal, bilateral amygdala, bilateral cingulate gyrus, left angular gyrus, right superior frontal gyrus, right middle frontal gyrus, left inferior frontal gyrus, and left precentral gyrus.

Keywords: mild cognitive impairment, brain parcellation, automated anatomical labeling atlas, brainnetome atlas, voxel-based morphometry

INTRODUCTION

Mild cognitive impairment (MCI), which represents the transition state between normal aging and the early changes related to Alzheimer's disease (AD) (Han et al., 2011; Wang et al., 2015; Khazaee et al., 2016, 2017), is characterized by intellectual and cognitive deficits, memory complaints, and behavioral disturbances (Zhang et al., 2012; Beheshti et al., 2017), and generally regarded as a prodromal phase of AD (Long et al., 2018). Overall, the prevalence of MCI in the elderly is 19%, and nearly half of them will evolve to AD within 3 to 5 years (Long et al., 2016). Increasing attention from neurologists, neuroscientists, and neuroradiologists has been paid to MCI due that early intervention before irreversible brain tissue damage is crucial for efficient AD treatments (Davatzikos et al., 2008a). Therefore, accurate MCI identification methodologies that could serve as non-invasive surrogates for these pathologic examinations are desperately needed, which may provide additional insights into the clinical diagnosis of MCI.

Structural magnetic resonance imaging (sMRI) has been prevalently utilized to characterize differences in shape and neuroanatomical configuration in MCI and AD because it could provide visualization of the macroscopic tissue atrophy caused by the cellular changes underlying MCI and AD (Desikan et al., 2009). By analyzing the sMRI data with voxel-based morphometry (VBM) method, which is utilized to assess the structure of the whole brain with voxel-by-voxel comparisons between groups in an anatomically unbiased way (Ashburner and Friston, 2000), many prior studies found that the atrophic brain regions mainly lay in the medial temporal lobe containing hippocampus, parahippocampal, and amygdala in MCI and AD (Baron et al., 2001; Hirata et al., 2005). In addition, some studies employed sMRI data to identify MCI or AD from healthy controls (HC) by extracting structural characteristics such as voxel-wise volume (Fan et al., 2007; Davatzikos et al., 2008a,b; Klöppel et al., 2008; Magnin et al., 2009; Beheshti and Demirel, 2016) and vertex-based cortical thickness (Lerch et al., 2008; Eskildsen et al., 2013; Dimitriadis et al., 2018), and the classifying accuracies varied largely from 58% to 100%, which indicated that the discriminative diagnoses of MCI and AD with sMRI data need to be continued.

From the previous voxel-based MCI or AD discrimination studies, these studies could be roughly classified into two categories, data-driven adaptive characteristic extraction methods (Misra et al., 2009; Davatzikos et al., 2011) and atlas-based partition characteristic extraction methods with a predefined brain atlas (Cuingnet et al., 2011; Cho et al., 2012; Liu et al., 2015). The former method was not easy to interpret anatomically because each region of interest (ROI) obtained from the input data may involve in many anatomical regions simultaneously. In contrast, the latter could better extract the classification features with a good anatomical interpretability. At present, the automated anatomical labeling (AAL-90) atlas is the most popular atlas, which has been widely employed to identify kinds of psychological disorders in recent years (Dai et al., 2012; Wee et al., 2012; Zeng et al., 2012). Besides, some other atlases were also proposed, such as AAL-1024 atlas (Zhang et al., 2011; Wu et al., 2013) and the novel connectional architecture based brainnetome (BN-246) atlas (Fan et al., 2016). Different brain atlases lead to different partitions in terms of the number of regions and the size and location of these regions in the brain (Asim et al., 2018). Till now, few studies compared the classification performance with different atlases (Mesrob et al., 2009; Ota et al., 2014, 2015; Asim et al., 2018), and no study has utilized the BN-246 atlas to identify MCI from HC subjects with structural data. Moreover, it remains unknown whether BN-246 atlas would perform better compared with the two above-mentioned atlases in identifying MCI patients from HC subjects. Also, it is intriguing whether better accuracy could be acquired by using the shared features extracted from three atlases.

In this paper, we proposed an automated classification method to identify MCI from HC and aimed to investigate whether the classification performance was dependent upon the brain parcellation schemes. To accomplish this goal, we first analyzed the sMRI data with VBM analysis, and then the volume features of every ROI in the above-mentioned three atlases were calculated and compared between MCI and HC groups, respectively. At last, these volumes of abnormal ROIs and the overlapping brain regions in three atlases were adopted as the classification features for the proposed support vector machine (SVM) based classification algorithm, respectively, and the leave-one-out cross-validation (LOOCV) was used to estimate the classification performance.

MATERIALS AND METHODS

Participants

Sixty-nine MCI patients and 63 HC participated in this study, and all participants have not taken any medication that may influence cognition function. All MCI patients were diagnosed by two experienced neurologists, and the detailed inclusion criteria for MCI patients included: (1) memory complaint, confirmed by patient-self or family members; (2) objective memory impairment, adjusted for education and age; (3) normal or near normal activities of daily living; (4) normal or near-normal performance on cognitive function; (5) clinical dementia rating (CDR) score equals 0.5; (6) without dementia according to DSM-IV (Diagnostic and Statistical Manual of Mental Disorders, 4th edition, revised). The 63 HC matched well with MCI patients on gender, age, and education level, and the detailed inclusion criteria for HC included: (1) no nervous system diseases that could cause cognitive function impairment, such as Parkinson's disease, depression, encephalitis, and brain tumors; (2) no history of psychosis or congenital mental growth retardation; (3) no medication conditions that may interfere with cognitive performance; (4) no visible vascular lesions on sMRI; (5) no history of stroke or dependence on alcohol; (6) no other systemic diseases that cause cognitive impairment, such as syphilis, severe anemia, and HIV. All participants underwent a standardized clinical assessment protocol including mini-mental state exam (MMSE), CDR, and Auditory Verbal Learning Test. Written informed consent forms were obtained from all participants, and this study was approved by the medical research ethics committee of Nanfang Hospital affiliated to Southern Medical University. The detailed demographics and clinical characteristics of all participants were presented in **Table 1**.

Data Acquisition

All participants were scanned on a 3.0-Tesla Siemens scanner with 8-channel radio frequency coil at Nangfang hospital.

TABLE 1 | Participants' demographic and clinical characteristics.

Characteristics	MCI	HC	*P*-values
Gender (M/F)	69(30/39)	63(27/36)	0.94#
Age (years)	66.64 ± 7.70	64.22 ± 7.38	0.07*
Education (years)	9.75 ± 4.37	9.35 ± 4.20	0.59*
CDR	0.5	0	0*
MMSE	23.03 ± 3.10	27.92 ± 1.58	< 0.001*
AVLT-immediate recall	8.22 ± 2.54	13.48 ± 3.02	< 0.001*
AVLT-delay recall	3.68 ± 3.16	10.27 ± 2.57	< 0.001*
AVLT-recognition	6.49 ± 3.50	11.71 ± 2.32	< 0.001*

*Values are mean ± SD unless the SD was not calculated. M, male; F, female. CDR, Clinical Dementia Rating scale; MMSE, Mini-Mental State Examination; AVLT, Auditory Verbal Learning Test. #The P-value was obtained by Chi-square test. *The P-values were obtained by two-sample two-tailed t-test.*

Sagittal structural images for all participants were collected using a magnetization prepared rapid gradient echo (MPRAGE) three-dimensional T1-weighted sequence with the following parameters: repetition time (TR) = 1900 ms, echo time (TE) = 2.2 ms, flip angle (FA) = 9°, inversion time (TI) = 900 ms, matrix = 256 × 256, number of slices = 176, thickness = 1.0 mm, and voxel size = 1 × 1 × 1 mm^3.

Image Analysis

All sMRI data were performed with the VBM toolbox (VBM8[1]) implemented in SPM8 according to the following steps: First, the T1-weighted images were checked by two experienced neuroradiologists, and no obvious abnormalities or artifacts were observed in all subjects. Then all images were segmented into gray matter, white matter, and cerebrospinal fluid (CSF) by utilizing the "New-segment" routine in SPM8. Next, all the segmented images were normalized into the Montreal Neurological Institute (MNI) space using the high-dimensional DARTEL normalization algorithm, and the normalized images were modulated with Jacobian matrices to preserve the actual amounts of a tissue class within each voxel. At last, the modulated images were smoothed with an 8-mm full width at half-maximum Gaussian kernel.

Feature Calculations and Selections Under Three Atlases

The processed sMRI images were utilized to extract the volume features for identifying MCI from HC with three different brain parcellation atlases: AAL-90, BN-246, and AAL-1024 atlas (**Figure 1**). The AAL-90 atlas, which was generated from 27 high resolution T1-weighted images of a young male (Tzouriomazoyer et al., 2002), partitions the whole cerebral cortex into 90 ROIs (without cerebellum) (Dai et al., 2012; Khazaee et al., 2016). The newly built BN-246 atlas, which was generated based on anatomical connections, divides the whole cerebral cortex into 210 cortical and 36 subcortical subregions (Fan et al., 2016). The AAL-1024 atlas, which is generated by subdividing each region of the low resolution AAL-90 atlas into a set of subregions, partitions the whole cerebral cortex into 1024 ROIs, and every ROI of AAL-1024 atlas has approximately identical size (Wu et al., 2013).

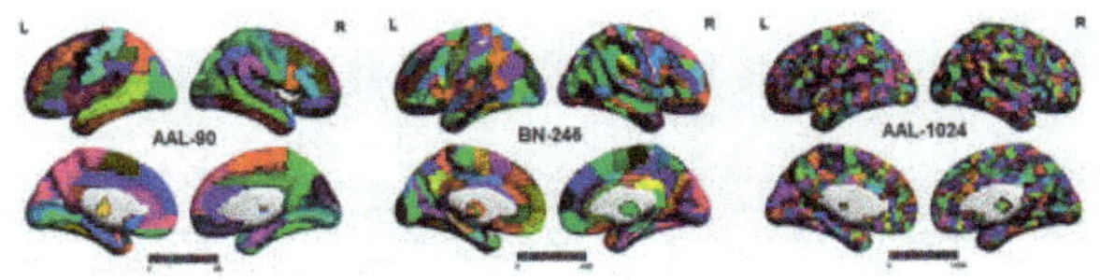

FIGURE 1 | The three atlases including AAL-90 atlas, BN-246 atlas, and AAL-1024 atlas.

According to the above-mentioned three different parcellation schemes, the volume of each ROI was calculated for all subjects by using the MATLAB program[2], and the extracted volume features of all subjects in three atlases were served as the candidate features, respectively. Given some features were redundant and irrelevant for classification; it is desirable to select out the discriminative features to improve the classification performance. Several previous studies have demonstrated that properly reducing the number of features can not only improve the performance of the classifier but also speed up the computation (Dosenbach et al., 2010; Dai et al., 2012). Therefore, two-sample two-tailed t-test was performed on the candidate features of three atlases, respectively, to determine the significantly different features ($P < 0.01$, uncorrected) as the classification features. Besides, a Fisher score method was also used for feature selection (Khazaee et al., 2016), and the selected features with this method were consistent with two-sample two-tailed t-test. The Fisher score criteria for each feature is defined as:

$$FS = \frac{n_1(m_1 - m)^2 + n_2(m_2 - m)^2}{n_1\sigma_1^2 + n_2\sigma_1^2} \quad (1)$$

Here n_1 and n_2 represent the number of samples on each group, m_1 and m_2 represent the respective mean value of the feature, m represents the mean value of the total features, and σ_1^2 and σ_1^2 represent the respective variances. At last, it is worth noting that the feature selection process was only carried out on the training set of each LOOCV fold, which can reduce the overfitting of the classifier.

SVM-Based Classification Method

The SVM algorithm conceptually implements the idea that the classification features are nonlinearly mapped into a high dimensional feature space where a hyperplane with maximum margin is created to separate the two-group data (Magnin et al., 2009). The SVM algorithm has been widely utilized in neuroimaging studies for its powerful classification performance as well as the simplicity of its theory and implementation (Moradi et al., 2015). In this paper, the LibSVM toolbox[3] was used to implement the classification.

The radial basis function (RBF) defined as $(X, X_i) \rightarrow K(X, X_i) = e^{\gamma|X-X_i|^2}$ was adopted as the kernel function. Besides, in order to improve the classification performance, a grid-search

[1] http://dbm.neuro.uni-jena.de/vbm.html

[2] http://www.cs.ucl.ac.uk/staff/G.Ridgway/vbm/get_totals.m

[3] http://www.csie.ntu.edu.tw/~cjlin/libsvm

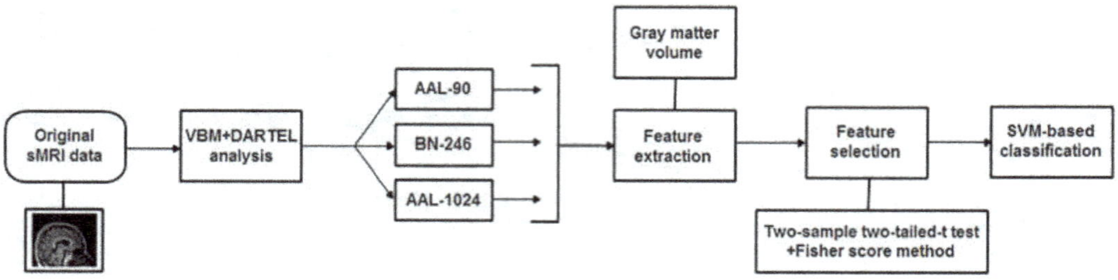

FIGURE 2 | The flowchart of the proposed method for MCI discrimination.

method was utilized to optimize two parameters: γ, the width of the RBF, and C, the penalty parameter of the error term, which adjusts the importance of the separation error in the creation of hyperplane. In this paper, the ranges of these two parameters were $\gamma = 2^{-8}, 2^{-7.5}, ..., 2^{8}$ and $C = 2^{-8}, 2^{-7.5}, ..., 2^{8}$. In detail, the optimal two parameters of γ and C were determined with an internal LOOCV that was only performed on selected features of the training data. The set of parameters obtained the best performance in the internal LOOCV were utilized to train the classification algorithm. In addition, by applying an external LOOCV, the performance of classification method was estimated with the accuracy, sensitivity and specificity, which represent the correctly classified rate of all samples, MCI patients and HC, respectively. It is worth noting that the feature selections and parameter optimization process were only performed on the training set, which could avoid the overfitting of the classifier. In addition, the flowchart of the proposed method for MCI discrimination was shown in **Figure 2**.

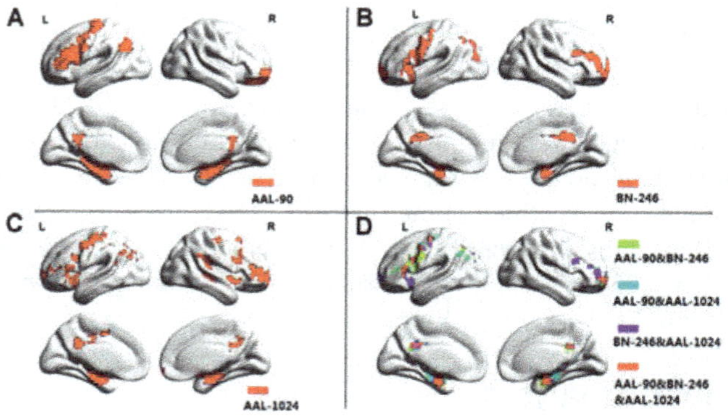

FIGURE 3 | The atrophic brain regions in three atlases, respectively. **(A)** The abnormal brain regions in AAL-90; **(B)** the abnormal brain regions in BN-246; **(C)** the abnormal brain regions in AAL-1024; **(D)** the overlapping abnormal regions among atlases.

RESULTS

Between-Group Differences in Gray Matter Volumes

Figure 3 showed the ROIs with reliable and discriminative powers during classification process, namely, the features retained more than 125 (132 × 95%, 132 is the total number of cross validation) times in the whole LOOCV process were displayed in the brain mappings. The overlapping abnormal brain regions in three atlases were predominantly located at bilateral hippocampus, bilateral parahippocampal, bilateral amygdala, bilateral cingulate gyrus, left angular gyrus, right superior frontal gyrus, right middle frontal gyrus, left inferior frontal gyrus, and left precentral gyrus. Besides, the Fisher score values of the abnormal ROIs in these atlases were shown in **Figure 4**.

Classification Performances Under Three Atlases

When adopting the AAL-90 atlas, a correct classification rate of 83%, a sensitivity of 85%, and a specificity of 81% were obtained. When adopting the BN-246 atlas, a correct classification rate of 92%, a sensitivity of 90%, and a specificity of 94% were obtained. When adopting the AAL-1024 atlas, a correct classification rate of 89%, a sensitivity of 91%, and a specificity of 87% were obtained. When using the volume features of the overlapping abnormal brain regions in three atlases, an accuracy rate was 86%, and sensitivity of 81%, and a specificity of 90% were obtained. The detailed results were summarized in **Table 2**. Besides, four receiver operating characteristics (ROC) curves were obtained (**Figure 5**), and the areas under ROC curves (AUCs) with AAL-90, BN-246, AAL-1024 atlas and the overlapping brain regions were 0.89, 0.95 and 0.92, and 0.90, respectively.

DISCUSSION

This study focused on comparing the classification performance of identifying MCI patients from HC subjects with VBM under three widely used brain atlases, and found that the performance varied in different brain atlases. The best recognition performance was obtained by BN-246 atlas with an accuracy of 92%, indicating a powerful discriminative ability for MCI patients.

In this paper, a RBF kernel function that could deal with the nonlinear relationship between features and labels was adopted to improve the classification performance (Hsu et al., 2003). The grid search method, which has a high learning accuracy and could be implemented with parallel processing, was utilized to optimize the two parameters of SVM, and

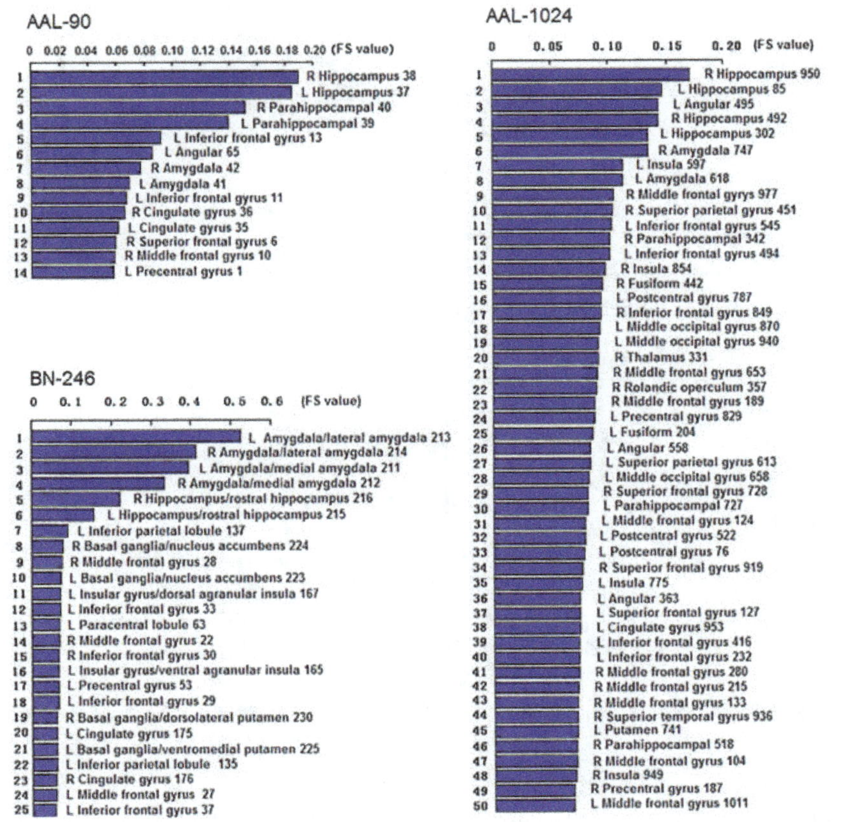

FIGURE 4 | The Fisher score values of the discriminative features in AAL-90, BN-246, and AAL-1024, respectively (The number of the discriminative features in AAL-1024 atlas was 93, and only the prior 50 features were displayed).

it could also improve the classification performance. Besides, considering the feature selections and parameters optimization process were only constrained on the training set of each LOOCV fold, which could reduce the overfitting of the classifier. Thus, the improved accuracies we obtained may be unlikely the inflated accuracies due to overfitting. In addition, the total 90, 246, and 1024 features with parameters optimization were also tested for classification, respectively, and the accuracies without feature selection were all less than 70%, which were significantly lower than that with feature selection. Besides, when using the proposed method to identify MCI patients by extracting the volume features of the overlapping abnormal brain regions in three atlases, the accuracy was 86%. To our best knowledge, it is the first time to classify MCI patients from HC subjects by using the overlapping brain regions in three different atlases. Furthermore, the linear kernel based SVM method and the logistic regression classifier were also applied to the same data to identify MCI patients, and the former classifier achieved accuracies of 80%, 91%, and 87% with AAL-90, BN-246, and AAL-1024 atlas, respectively, and the latter one acquired accuracies of 70, 84, and 76% with AAL-90, BN-246, and AAL-1024 atlas, respectively, suggesting that the RBF kernel based SVM method performed better than these two classifiers and the BN-246 atlas could persistently provide more effective information in identifying MCI patients. Moreover, to validate whether the between-group differences and the performance were stable, the re-sampling based permutation test was performed, which was similar with some previous studies to testify the stability of the between-group differences and classification performance (Magnin et al., 2009; Awate et al., 2016; Awate et al., 2017). In detail, 75% random selected subjects of each group were used to determine the abnormal features and then to train the proposed classification method, then the remaining 25% participants were utilized to estimate the classification accuracy. The above-mentioned processes were repeated 1000 times, and the final accuracies were estimated with the mean of the 1000 re-samplings. The probability of each feature selected in permutation test was defined as the selected times of the feature in the whole process divided by the re-sampling times, and the probability

TABLE 2 | The classification performance of the proposed method on three atlases.

Three atlases	Accuracy	Sensitivity	Specificity
AAL-90	83%	85%	81%
BN-246	92%	90%	94%
AAL-1024	89%	91%	87%
The overlapping regions	86%	81%	90%

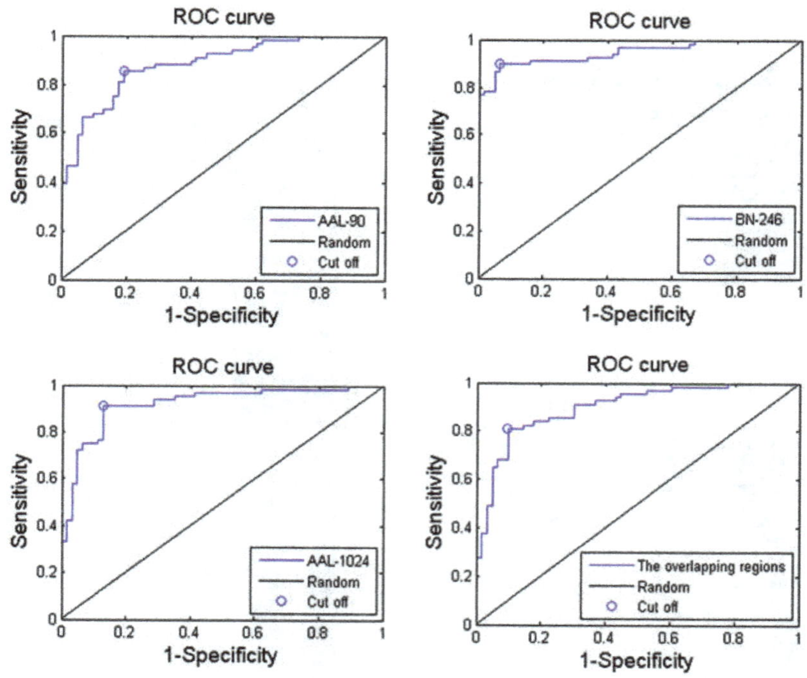

FIGURE 5 | Three ROC curves of the proposed MCI identification method with AAL-90, BN-246, AAL-1024 atlas, and the overlapping abnormal regions, respectively.

mappings of these selected features were shown in **Figure 6**. We found that the frequently selected regions in the whole permutation test were consistent with our proposed method. Besides, the accuracies distributions of the permutation test in three atlases were shown in **Figure 7**, and the final mean accuracies were 82.58, 92.52, and 87.60% with AAL-90, BN-246, and AAL-1024 atlas, respectively, which again demonstrated that our results were stable. At last, the atrophic brain regions in MCI detected by VBM procedure in our study were consistent with many previous VBM studies (Hirata et al., 2005; Hämäläinen et al., 2007; Matsuda, 2013), including hippocampus and parahippocampal, etc. The correspondence indicated the validity of the MRI data and the method of VBM analysis.

In our previous study (Jing et al., 2017), the AAL-90 and AAL-1024 atlas were utilized to make a comparison in identifying major depressive disorder from HC using the functional characteristic, and the AAL-1024 obtained better performance than the AAL-90 atlas. In addition, considering the newly built BN-246 atlas contains both functional and structural connectivity information, thus these three atlases were simultaneously selected in this paper. Through comparing the classification results among them, we found that the BN-246 atlas obtained the best recognition rate than AAL-90 and AAL-1024 atlas. The main reasons for resulting in a considerable disparity in the classification performance may be attributed to the differences between atlases. The AAL-1024 atlas is generated from AAL-90 atlas, and therefore a comparison between BN-246 atlas and AAL-90 atlas is essential for the interpretation of the differences in classification performance.

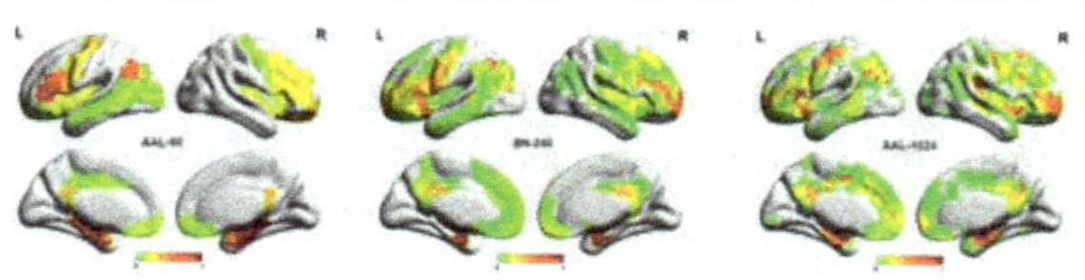

FIGURE 6 | The probability mappings of the selected abnormal features in permutation test with three different atlases.

Brain atlases could be classified into two categories: single-subject topological atlases and population-based probabilistic atlases (Cabezas et al., 2011; Arslan et al., 2017). The AAL-90 atlas is a single-subject atlas generated from a young male (Tzouriomazoyer et al., 2002), whereas the BN-246 is a probabilistic atlas based on 40 MRI data of healthy adults (Fan et al., 2016). This difference might be the major factor resulting in the discrepant classification performance. Namely, no single brain could represent the population due to the neuroanatomical variability across individuals (Devlin and Poldrack, 2007). In addition, the AAL-90 atlas has been found with some other problems such as anatomical variation and methodological limitation. Regarding to the anatomical variation, the AAL-90 atlas displays an atypical rightward asymmetry of planum temporale (PT) that is a triangular structure located on the superior temporal gyrus, and the PT that is involved in mediating sensorimotor control processing has extensive connections to other brain regions (Zheng, 2009). A previous study found microanatomical changes in cortical minicolumn organization of the association cortex in the PT in MCI and AD (Chance

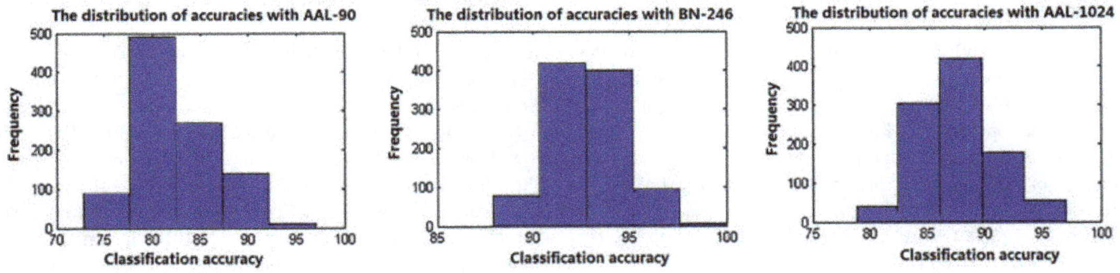

FIGURE 7 | The classification accuracies distributions of the permutation test with three different atlases.

et al., 2011), and another previous VBM study also found the early atrophic changes in superior temporal gyrus in AD (Karas et al., 2004). In terms of methodological limitation, the AAL-90 atlas was originally intended to provide a standard reference of anatomical location for functional neuroimaging studies with low spatial resolution (Tzouriomazoyer et al., 2002). However, the partition pattern of AAL-90 does not match the cytoarchitectonic borders well in most cases due that the sulcal and gyral patterns are extremely variable (Amunts et al., 2007). Therefore, the single-subject AAL-90 atlas could not well represent the partition pattern of human brain. Regarding to BN-246 atlas, this atlas partitioned the human brain into distinct subregions based on local structural connectivity architecture, namely, the BN-246 atlas is created by identifying subregions that are maximally homogeneous internally and maximally different from each other in terms of their structural connections (Fan et al., 2016). To some extent, the BN-246 atlas not only confirmed some differentiation from early cytoarchitectonic mappings but also revealed many anatomical subdivisions which were not described previously (Fan et al., 2016). In addition, it is worth noting that although BN-246 atlas showed better classification performance than AAL-90 and AAL-1024 atlas, the BN-246 atlas might not be the best choice, and future neuroimaging studies should pay more attention to the choice of brain parcellation atlases in atlas-based studies.

Another factor that may affect the recognition performance is the number of ROIs in three atlases. Different numbers of ROIs resulted in distinct feature vectors, and the variation in topological patterns of feature vectors corresponded to diverse hyperplanes in feature space, which naturally brought about the discrepancies in the classification performance. In this paper, the performance of AAL-1024 was better than AAL-90 atlas, which may be attributed to the reason that the AAL-1024 atlas could detect more fine abnormalities due to a more subtle parcellation scheme compared to AAL-90 atlas. At last, we found that the Fisher Score value of the volume features with BN-246 was significantly bigger than that of AAL-90 and AAL-1024, which complementarily supported the fact that the BN-246 atlas would obtain the best classification performance in the identification of MCI.

Two issues need to be addressed in this paper. First, some other brain atlases exist in the area of neuroimaging study nowadays, and these atlases could also be utilized to investigate the brain abnormalities affected by atrophy in MCI patients. Second, all the selected atlases in this study did not include cerebellum which may provide some contribution for discriminating MCI patients from HC, and future identification studies could adopt some cerebellum-included atlases to identify MCI patients.

AUTHOR CONTRIBUTIONS

ZhL and JH made substantial contributions to the conception, design, analysis, and interpretation of data and drafted the manuscript. BJ and ZhL made contributions to the revision of the manuscript. BL, ZuL, and ZiL made contributions to the conception, design, and revision of figures. ZhL and HC made contributions to the data acquisition. BJ and HC, the corresponding authors, made contributions to conception and interpretation of data and determined the final version to be submitted for publishing. All authors read and approved the final manuscript.

FUNDING

BJ was supported by the Beijing Natural Science Foundation (No. 7174282) and the Basic and Clinical Cooperative Research Program of Capital Medical University (16JL25, 17JL36, and 17JL62).

ACKNOWLEDGMENTS

Thank you very much for all editors and reviewers for our manuscript.

REFERENCES

Amunts, K., Schleicher, A. K., and Zilles, K. (2007). Cytoarchitecture of the cerebral cortex–more than localization. *Neuroimage* 37, 1061–1065. doi: 10.1016/j.neuroimage.2007.02.037

Arslan, S., Ktena, S. I., Makropoulos, A., Robinson, E. C., Rueckert, D., and Parisot, S. (2017). Human brain mapping: a systematic comparison of parcellation methods for the human cerebral cortex. *Neuroimage* 170, 5–30. doi: 10.1016/j.neuroimage.2017.04.014

Ashburner, J., and Friston, K. J. (2000). Voxel based morphometry. *Neuroimage* 11, 805–821. doi: 10.1006/nimg.2000.0582

Asim, Y., Raza, B., Malik, A. K., Rathore, S., Hussain, L., and Iftikhar, M. A. (2018). A multi-modal, multi-atlas-based approach for Alzheimer detection via machine learning. *Int. J. Imaging Syst. Technol.* 28, 113–123. doi: 10.1002/ima.22263

Awate, S. P., Leahy, R. M., and Joshi, A. A. (2016). Riemannian statistical analysis of cortical geometry with robustness to partial homology and misalignment. *Med. Image Comput. Comput. Assist. Interv.* 9900, 237–246. doi: 10.1007/978-3-319-46720-7_28

Awate, S. P., Leahy, R. M., and Joshi, A. A. (2017). Kernel methods for riemannian analysis of robust descriptors of the cerebral cortex. *Inf. Process. Med. Imaging* 10265, 28–40. doi: 10.1007/978-3-319-59050-9_3

Baron, J. C., Chételat, G., Desgranges, B., Perchey, G., Landeau, B., de la Sayette, V., et al. (2001). In vivo mapping of gray matter loss with voxel-based morphometry in mild Alzheimer's disease. *Neuroimage* 14, 298–309. doi: 10.1006/nimg.2001.0848

Beheshti, I., and Demirel, H. (2016). Feature-ranking-based Alzheimer's disease classification from structural MRI. *Magn. Reson. Imaging* 34, 252–263. doi: 10.1016/j.mri.2015.11.009

Beheshti, I., Demirel, H., Matsuda, H., and Alzheimer's Disease Neuroimaging Initiative (2017). Classification of Alzheimer's disease and prediction of mild cognitive impairment-to-Alzheimer's conversion from structural magnetic resource imaging using feature ranking and a genetic algorithm. *Comput. Biol. Med.* 83, 109–119. doi: 10.1016/j.compbiomed.2017.02.011

Cabezas, M., Oliver, A., Lladó, X., Freixenet, J., and Cuadra, M. B. (2011). A review of atlas-based segmentation for magnetic resonance brain images. *Comput. Methods Programs Biomed.* 104, e158–e177. doi: 10.1016/j.cmpb.2011.07.015

Chance, S. A., Clover, L., Cousijn, H., Currah, L., Pettingill, R., and Esiri, M. M. (2011). Microanatomical correlates of cognitive ability and decline: normal ageing, MCI, and Alzheimer's disease. *Cereb. Cortex* 21, 1870–1878. doi: 10.1093/cercor/bhq264

Cho, Y., Seong, J. K., Jeong, Y., Shin, S. Y., and Alzheimer's Disease Neuroimaging Initiative. (2012). Individual subject classification for Alzheimer's disease based on incremental learning using a spatial frequency representation of cortical thickness data. *Neuroimage* 59, 2217–2230. doi: 10.1016/j.neuroimage.2011.09.085

Cuingnet, R., Gerardin, E., Tessieras, J., Auzias, G., Lehéricy, S., Habert, M. O., et al. (2011). Automatic classification of patients with Alzheimer's disease from structural MRI: a comparison of ten methods using the ADNI database. *Neuroimage* 56, 766–781. doi: 10.1016/j.neuroimage.2010.06.013

Dai, Z., Yan, C., Wang, Z., Wang, J., Xia, M., Li, K., et al. (2012). Discriminative analysis of early Alzheimer's disease using multi-modal imaging and multi-level characterization with multi-classifier (M3). *Neuroimage* 59, 2187–2195. doi: 10.1016/j.neuroimage.2011.10.003

Davatzikos, C., Bhatt, P., Shaw, L. M., Batmanghelich, K. N., and Trojanowski, J. Q. (2011). Prediction of MCI to AD conversion, via MRI, CSF biomarkers, pattern classification. *Neurobiol. Aging* 32, e19–e27. doi: 10.1016/j.neurobiolaging.2010.05.023

Davatzikos, C., Fan, Y., Wu, X., Shen, D., and Resnick, S. M. (2008a). Detection of prodromal Alzheimer's disease via pattern classification of magnetic resonance imaging. *Neurobiol. Aging* 29, 514–523. doi: 10.1016/j.neurobiolaging.2006.11.010

Davatzikos, C., Resnick, S. M., Wu, X., Parmpi, P., and Clark, C. M. (2008b). Individual patient diagnosis of AD and FTD via high-dimensional pattern classification of MRI. *Neuroimage* 41, 1220–1227. doi: 10.1016/j.neuroimage.2008.03.050

Desikan, R. S., Cabral, H. J., Hess, C. P., Dillon, W. P., Glastonbury, C. M., Weiner, M. W., et al. (2009). Automated MRI measures identify individuals with mild cognitive impairment and Alzheimer's disease. *Brain* 132, 2048–2057. doi: 10.1093/brain/awp123

Devlin, J. T., and Poldrack, R. A. (2007). In praise of tedious anatomy. *Neuroimage* 37, 1033–1041. doi: 10.1016/j.neuroimage.2006.09.055

Dimitriadis, S. I., Liparas, D., Tsolaki, M. N., and Alzheimer's Disease Neuroimaging Initiative. (2018). Random forest feature selection, fusion and ensemble strategy: combining multiple morphological MRI measures to discriminate among healthy elderly, MCI, cMCI and alzheimer's disease patients: from the alzheimer's disease neuroimaging initiative (ADNI) database. *J. Neurosci. Method* 302, 14–23. doi: 10.1016/j.jneumeth.2017.12.010

Dosenbach, N. U., Nardos, B., Cohen, A. L., Fair, D. A., Power, J. D., Church, J. A., et al. (2010). Prediction of individual brain maturity using fMRI. *Science* 329, 1358–1361. doi: 10.1126/science.1194144

Eskildsen, S. F., Coupé, P., García-Lorenzo, D., Fonov, V., Pruessner, J. C., Collins, D. L., et al. (2013). Prediction of Alzheimer's disease in subjects with mild cognitive impairment from the ADNI cohort using patterns of cortical thinning. *Neuroimage* 65, 511–521. doi: 10.1016/j.neuroimage.2012.09.058

Fan, L., Li, H., Zhuo, J., Zhang, Y., Wang, J., Chen, L., et al. (2016). The human brainnetome Atlas: a new brain atlas based on connectional architecture. *Cereb. Cortex* 26, 3508–3526. doi: 10.1093/cercor/bhw157

Fan, Y., Rao, H., Hurt, H., Giannetta, J., Korczykowski, M., Shera, D., et al. (2007). Multivariate examination of brain abnormality using both structural and functional MRI. *Neuroimage* 36, 1189–1199. doi: 10.1016/j.neuroimage.2007.04.009

Hämäläinen, A., Tervo, S., Grau-Olivares, M., Niskanen, E., Pennanen, C., Huuskonen, J., et al. (2007). Voxel-based morphometry to detect brain atrophy in progressive mild cognitive impairment. *Neuroimage* 37, 1122–1131. doi: 10.1016/j.neuroimage.2007.06.016

Han, Y., Wang, J., Zhao, Z., Min, B., Lu, J., Li, K., et al. (2011). Frequency-dependent changes in the amplitude of low-frequency fluctuations in amnestic mild cognitive impairment: a resting-state fMRI study. *Neuroimage* 55, 287–295. doi: 10.1016/j.neuroimage.2010.11.059

Hirata, Y., Matsuda, H., Nemoto, K., Ohnishi, T., Hirao, K., Yamashita, F., et al. (2005). Voxel-based morphometry to discriminate early Alzheimer's disease from controls. *Neurosci. Lett.* 382, 269–274. doi: 10.1016/j.neulet.2005.03.038

Hsu, C. W., Chang, C. C., and Lin, C. J. (2003). *A Practical Guide to Support Vector Classification*. Taipei: National Taiwan University.

Jing, B., Long, Z., Liu, H., Yan, H., Dong, J., Mo, X., et al. (2017). Identifying current and remitted major depressive disorder with the Hurst exponent: a comparative study on two automated anatomical labeling atlases. *Oncotarget* 8, 90452–90464. doi: 10.18632/oncotarget.19860

Karas, G. B., Scheltens, P., Rombouts, S. A., Visser, P. J., van, Schijndel RA, Fox, N. C., et al. (2004). Global and local gray matter loss in mild cognitive impairment and Alzheimer's disease. *Neuroimage* 23, 708–716. doi: 10.1016/j.neuroimage.2004.07.006

Khazaee, A., Ebrahimzadeh, A., and Babajani-Feremi, A. (2016). Application of advanced machine learning methods on resting-state fMRI network for identification of mild cognitive impairment and Alzheimer's disease. *Brain Imaging Behav.* 10, 799–817. doi: 10.1007/s11682-015-9448-7

Khazaee, A., Ebrahimzadeh, A., and Babajani-Feremi, A. (2017). Classification of patients with MCI and AD from healthy controls using directed graph measures of resting-state fMRI. *Behav. Brain Res.* 322, 339–350. doi: 10.1016/j.bbr.2016.06.043

Klöppel, S., Stonnington, C. M., Chu, C., Draganski, B., Scahill, R. I., Rohrer, J. D., et al. (2008). Automatic classification of MR scans in Alzheimer's disease. *Brain* 131, 681–689. doi: 10.1093/brain/awm319

Lerch, J. P., Pruessner, J., Zijdenbos, A. P., Collins, D. L., Teipel, S. J., Hampel, H., et al. (2008). Automated cortical thickness measurements from MRI can accurately separate Alzheimer's patients from normal elderly controls. *Neurobiol. Aging* 29, 23–30. doi: 10.1016/j.neurobiolaging.2006.09.013

Liu, M., Zhang, D., and Shen, D. (2015). View-centralized multi-atlas classification for Alzheimer's disease diagnosis. *Hum. Brain Mapp.* 36, 1847–1865. doi: 10.1002/hbm.22741

Long, Z., Jing, B., Guo, R., Li, B., Cui, F., Wang, T., et al. (2018). A brainnetome Atlas based mild cognitive impairment identification using hurst exponent. *Front. Aging Neurosci* 10:103. doi: 10.3389/fnagi.2018.00103

Long, Z., Jing, B., Yan, H., Dong, J., Liu, H., Mo, X., et al. (2016). A support vector machine-based method to identify mild cognitive impairment with multi-level characteristics of magnetic resonance imaging. *Neuroscience* 331, 169–176. doi: 10.1016/j.neuroscience.2016.06.025

Magnin, B., Mesrob, L., Kinkingnéhun, S., Pélégrini-Issac, M., Colliot, O., Sarazin, M., et al. (2009). Support vector machine-based classification of Alzheimer's disease from whole-brain anatomical MRI. *Neuroradiology* 51, 73–83. doi: 10.1007/s00234-008-0463-x

Matsuda, H. (2013). Voxel-based morphometry of brain MRI in normal aging and alzheimer's disease. *Aging Dis.* 4, 29–37.

Mesrob, L., Magnin, B., Colliot, O., Sarazin, M., Hahn-Barma, V., Dubois, B., et al. (2009). Identification of atrophy patterns in alzheimer's disease based on SVM feature selection and anatomical parcellation. *Annals of the BMVA* 7, 1–9.

Misra, C., Fan, Y., and Davatzikos, C. (2009). Baseline and longitudinal patterns of brain atrophy in MCI patients, and their use in prediction of short-term conversion to AD: results from ADNI. *Neuroimage* 44, 1415–1422. doi: 10.1016/j.neuroimage.2008.10.031

Moradi, E., Pepe, A., Gaser, C., Huttunen, H., Tohka, J., and Alzheimer's Disease Neuroimaging Initiative. (2015). Machine learning framework for early MRI-based Alzheimer's conversion prediction in MCI subjects. *Neuroimage* 104, 398–412. doi: 10.1016/j.neuroimage.2014.10.002

Ota, K., Oishi, N., Ito, K., Fukuyama, H., and Sead-J Study Group. (2014). A comparison of three brain atlases for MCI prediction. *J. Neurosci. Methods* 221, 139–150. doi: 10.1016/j.jneumeth.2013.10.003

Ota, K., Oishi, N., Ito, K., Fukuyama, H., Sead-J Study Group, and Alzheimer's Disease Neuroimaging Initiative. (2015). Effects of imaging modalities, brain atlases and feature selection on prediction of Alzheimer's disease. *J. Neurosci. Methods* 256, 168–183. doi: 10.1016/j.jneumeth.2015.08.020

Tzourio-Mazoyer, N., Landeau, B., Papathanassiou, D., Crivello, F., Etard, O., Delcroix, N., et al. (2002). Automated anatomical labeling of activations in SPM using a macroscopic anatomical parcellation of the MNI MRI single-subject brain. *Neuroimage* 15, 273–289. doi: 10.1006/nimg.2001.0978

Wang, Y., Zhao, X., Xu, S., Yu, L., Wang, L., Song, M., et al. (2015). Using Regional Homogeneity to Reveal Altered Spontaneous Activity in Patients with Mild Cognitive Impairment. *BioMed Res. Int.* 2015, 807093. doi: 10.1155/2015/807093

Wee, C. Y., Yap, P. T., Zhang, D., Denny, K., Browndyke, J. N., Potter, G. G., et al. (2012). Identification of MCI individuals using structural and functional connectivity networks. *Neuroimage* 59, 2045–2056. doi: 10.1016/j.neuroimage.2011.10.015

Wu, G. R., Stramaglia, S., Chen, H., Liao, W., and Marinazzo, D. (2013). Mapping the voxel-wise effective connectome in resting state FMRI. *PLoS One* 8:e73670. doi: 10.1371/journal.pone.0073670

Zeng, L. L., Shen, H., Liu, L., Wang, L., Li, B., Fang, P., et al. (2012). Identifying major depression using whole-brain functional connectivity: a multivariate pattern analysis. *Brain* 135, 1497–1507. doi: 10.1093/brain/aws059

Zhang, Z., Liao, W., Chen, H., Mantini, D., Ding, J. R., Xu, Q., et al. (2011). Altered functional-structural coupling of large-scale brain networks in idiopathic generalized epilepsy. *Brain* 134, 2912–2928. doi: 10.1093/brain/awr223

Zhang, Z., Liu, Y., Jiang, T., Zhou, B., An, N., Dai, H., et al. (2012). Altered spontaneous activity in Alzheimer's disease and mild cognitive impairment revealed by Regional Homogeneity. *Neuroimage* 59, 1429–1440. doi: 10.1016/j.neuroimage.2011.08.049

Zheng, Z. Z. (2009). The functional specialization of the planum temporale. *J. Neurophysiol* 102, 3079–3081. doi: 10.1152/jn.00434.2009

16

Unraveling Diagnostic Biomarkers of Schizophrenia Through Structure-Revealing Fusion of Multi-Modal Neuroimaging Data

Evrim Acar[1], Carla Schenker[1], Yuri Levin-Schwartz[2], Vince D. Calhoun[3,4] and Tülay Adali[5]*

[1] Machine Intelligence Department, Simula Metropolitan Center for Digital Engineering, Oslo, Norway, [2] Department of Environmental Medicine and Public Health, Icahn School of Medicine at Mount Sinai, New York, NY, United States, [3] The Mind Research Network, Albuquerque, NM, United States, [4] Department of Electrical and Computer Engineering, University of New Mexico, Albuquerque, NM, United States, [5] Department of Computer Science and Electrical Engineering, University of Maryland Baltimore County, Baltimore, MD, United States

Correspondence:
Evrim Acar
evrim@simula.no

Fusing complementary information from different modalities can lead to the discovery of more accurate diagnostic biomarkers for psychiatric disorders. However, biomarker discovery through data fusion is challenging since it requires extracting interpretable and reproducible patterns from data sets, consisting of shared/unshared patterns and of different orders. For example, multi-channel electroencephalography (EEG) signals from multiple subjects can be represented as a third-order tensor with modes: subject, time, and channel, while functional magnetic resonance imaging (fMRI) data may be in the form of subject by voxel matrices. Traditional data fusion methods rearrange higher-order tensors, such as EEG, as matrices to use matrix factorization-based approaches. In contrast, fusion methods based on coupled matrix and tensor factorizations (CMTF) exploit the potential multi-way structure of higher-order tensors. The CMTF approach has been shown to capture underlying patterns more accurately without imposing strong constraints on the latent neural patterns, i.e., biomarkers. In this paper, EEG, fMRI, and structural MRI (sMRI) data collected during an auditory oddball task (AOD) from a group of subjects consisting of patients with schizophrenia and healthy controls, are arranged as matrices and higher-order tensors coupled along the subject mode, and jointly analyzed using structure-revealing CMTF methods [also known as advanced CMTF (ACMTF)] focusing on unique identification of underlying patterns in the presence of shared/unshared patterns. We demonstrate that joint analysis of the EEG tensor and fMRI matrix using ACMTF reveals significant and biologically meaningful components in terms of differentiating between patients with schizophrenia and healthy controls while also providing spatial patterns with high resolution and improving the clustering performance compared to the analysis of only the EEG tensor. We also show that these patterns are reproducible, and study reproducibility for different model parameters. In comparison to the joint independent component analysis (jICA) data fusion approach, ACMTF provides easier interpretation of EEG data by revealing a single summary map of the topography for each component. Furthermore, fusion of sMRI data with EEG and fMRI through an ACMTF model provides structural patterns; however, we also show that when fusing data sets from multiple modalities, hence of very different nature, preprocessing plays a crucial role.

Keywords: EEG, fMRI, sMRI, schizophrenia, structural/functional biomarkers, coupled matrix/tensor factorization, ICA

1. INTRODUCTION

Multiple neuroimaging techniques provide complementary views of neural structure and function. For instance, one of the most commonly used neuroimaging methods, electroencephalography (EEG), measures the electrical activity with high temporal but low spatial resolution, while functional magnetic resonance imaging (fMRI) records the changes in the blood flow with high spatial but low temporal resolution (Bunge and Kahn, 2009; Uludag and Roebroeck, 2014). Therefore, joint analysis of signals from multiple neuroimaging modalities is of interest in order to better understand neural activity and to discover reliable diagnostic biomarkers for psychiatric disorders, such as schizophrenia (Daunizeau et al., 2009; Sui et al., 2012, 2018; Dahne et al., 2015; Liu et al., 2015).

With the advances in technology, vast amounts of neuroimaging data has been generated; however, data mining or signal processing methods so far have limited success in terms of finding reliable diagnostic imaging biomarkers for many psychiatric disorders (Sui et al., 2012; Takahashi and Suzuki, 2018). One of the reasons for this limited success has been the fact that data fusion is a particularly challenging task when the goal is to extract reproducible and interpretable patterns. Data from different sources consists of both shared (or common) and unshared (or distinct) underlying patterns (Alter et al., 2003; Daunizeau et al., 2009; Lock et al., 2013; Uludag and Roebroeck, 2014), and even the definition of "sharedness" is a topic of current research (Farias et al., 2016; Smilde et al., 2017). Furthermore, data sets from different modalities may be of different orders, such as multi-channel EEG signals from multiple subjects can be represented in the form of a third-order tensor with modes: subject, time, and channel, while fMRI data is often represented as a subject by voxel matrix (**Figure 1**). Similar challenges have been observed in other disciplines targeting biomarker discovery as well, e.g., in joint analysis of omics data (Acar et al., 2015), where the ultimate goal is to discover significant metabolites, genes, etc. as potential biomarkers.

The common approaches for fusion of multi-modal neuroimaging data are based on matrix factorizations, such as joint independent component analysis (jICA) (Calhoun et al., 2006b), parallel ICA (Calhoun et al., 2009) and independent vector analysis (IVA)-based techniques (Adali et al., 2015a), where signals from multiple modalities are represented as matrices, e.g., fMRI data in the form of a subject by voxel matrix, and EEG signals as a subject by time matrix (Adali et al., 2015a). Matrix factorization-based fusion methods require additional constraints to recover patterns uniquely (Alter et al., 2003; Klami et al., 2013; Lock et al., 2013; Adali et al., 2015a) and a

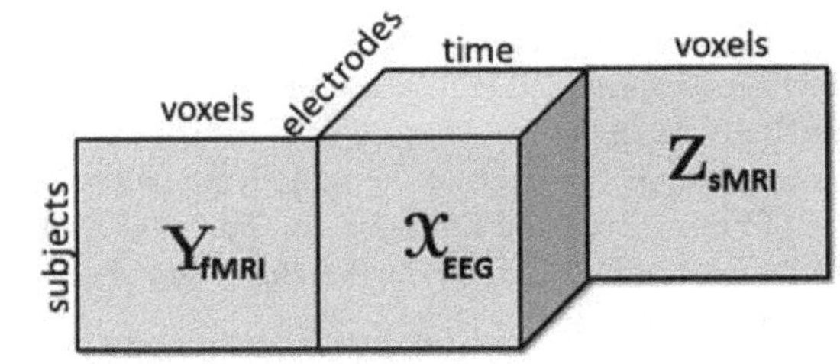

FIGURE 1 | A third-order tensor representing multi-channel EEG signals is coupled with fMRI and sMRI data in the form of matrices in the subject mode.

common practice in neuroscience is to assume that extracted patterns (i.e., biomarkers, or spatial/temporal patterns) are statistically independent. Drawbacks of the traditional methods are 2-fold: (i) in the presence of multi-channel EEG signals, which can naturally be represented as a third-order tensor, data is either matricized in the form of a subject by time-channel matrix (Swinnen et al., 2014) or only the signal from a single channel is analyzed (Adali et al., 2015a), ignoring the potential multilinear structure of multi-channel EEG signals, (ii) statistical independence might be a too strong constraint to impose on the patterns; therefore, methods may fail to capture the true patterns (Acar et al., 2015).

In contrast, coupled matrix and tensor factorizations (CMTF), introduced more recently, have proven useful in terms of addressing the drawbacks of matrix factorization-based fusion methods by jointly analyzing data sets in the form of matrices and higher-order tensors without imposing constraints on the components when the higher-order tensors have a defined multilinear structure (Acar et al., 2015). CMTF-based approaches factorize higher-order tensors using a tensor factorization model while simultaneously factorizing the data sets in the form of matrices, and enable the exploration of the potential multilinear structure inherent to, for instance, multi-channel EEG signals. Previously, analyzing multi-channel EEG signals using tensor factorizations has shown promising performance in terms of capturing spatial, spectral and temporal signatures of epileptic seizures (Acar et al., 2007; De Vos et al., 2007) as well as providing better understanding of brain activity patterns (Möcks, 1988; Miwakeichi et al., 2004; Mørup et al., 2007), see also (Cong et al., 2015) for a review. Another review (Hunyadi et al., 2017) discusses the studies making use of tensor factorizations to analyze EEG and fMRI signals, with a particular focus on epilepsy. Therefore, recent studies analyzing neuroimaging signals from multiple modalities have arranged neuroimaging data sets as higher-order tensors, and used CMTF-type methods to jointly analyze, e.g., EEG and magnetoencephalography (Becker et al., 2012; Naskovska et al., 2017) (both arranged as higher-order tensors), EEG and electro-ocular artifacts (Rivet et al., 2015) (both arranged as higher-order tensors), and EEG and fMRI (Karahan et al., 2015; Hunyadi et al., 2016; Eyndhoven et al., 2017) in the form of a matrix coupled with a third-order tensor, or as coupled higher-order tensors as in Chatzichristos et al. (2018), or arranged multiple diffusion tensor imaging modalities as a third-order tensor and coupled that with gray matter maps (Groves et al., 2011). However, when jointly analyzing a matrix coupled with a higher-order tensor, CMTF-based methods assuming that coupled data sets have only shared components, may fail to capture the underlying patterns in the presence of both shared and unshared components (Acar et al., 2014; Lathauwer and Kofidis, 2017); therefore, they are not ideal for biomarker discovery.

In this paper, we use a CMTF-based approach to jointly analyze neuroimaging signals from multiple modalities, more specifically, fMRI, sMRI and EEG data, collected during an auditory oddball (AOD) task from a group of subjects consisting of patients with schizophrenia and healthy controls with the goal of unraveling potential diagnostic biomarkers for schizophrenia. To the best of our knowledge, this is the first comprehensive study of a CMTF-based method for biomarker discovery for a psychiatric disorder discussing both strengths and limitations of the proposed framework, building onto our preliminary results in Acar et al. (2017a,b). Furthermore, due to the reproducibility and uniqueness requirements of such an application, we use a structure-revealing CMTF model, known as the advanced CMTF (ACMTF) model (Acar et al., 2014), to estimate weights of the components in each modality in order to identify shared/unshared components and quantify the contribution from each modality. Our preliminary studies have shown the promise of the ACMTF model in terms of capturing neural patterns that can differentiate between patients with schizophrenia and healthy controls by jointly analyzing EEG-fMRI signals (Acar et al., 2017b) and EEG-fMRI-sMRI data (Acar et al., 2017a); however, those two studies used only a subset of electrodes, making it difficult to evaluate the added value of each modality in terms of biomarker discovery. Also, in this paper, we include an additional metric to study the additive value of each modality, and evaluate the performance of the models in terms of clustering subjects from different groups, whereas the previous studies only used the interpretation and statistical significance of extracted patterns in terms of differentiating between groups. Clustering results complement univariate statistical significance tests and show whether combinations of potential biomarkers provide meaningful clusters. We show that EEG analysis using a CP [also known as Canonical Decomposition (CANDECOMP) and Parallel Factor Analysis (PARAFAC)] tensor model and joint analysis of EEG, fMRI as well as EEG, fMRI and sMRI reveal statistically significant and biologically meaningful components in terms of differentiating between patients with schizophrenia and healthy controls. In comparison to the results when only the EEG data is analyzed, the incorporation of fMRI signals results in clearer spatial maps and better clustering performance. With the incorporation of sMRI, we obtain structural patterns in addition to temporal and spatial patterns of functional activity without degrading the clustering performance. ACMTF models with different parameter settings have been compared, and based on detailed experiments, we observe that ACMTF consistently reveals similar significant patterns, which provide a concise summary of the topography, while being sensitive to certain parameters for uniqueness.

2. MATERIALS AND METHODS

2.1. Background

In this section, we briefly discuss the CP tensor model as well as structure-revealing CMTF and jICA models. Let the third-order tensor $\mathcal{X} \in \mathbb{R}^{I \times J \times K}$ with modes subject, time, and electrode, and matrices $\mathbf{Y} \in \mathbb{R}^{I \times M}$ (subject by voxel) and $\mathbf{Z} \in \mathbb{R}^{I \times L}$ (subject by voxel), represent multi-channel EEG, fMRI, and sMRI data, respectively (as in **Figure 1**).

2.1.1. CANDECOMP/PARAFAC (CP)

The CP model (Carroll and Chang, 1970; Harshman, 1970), also referred to as the canonical polyadic decomposition (Hitchcock, 1927), is one of the most popular tensor factorization models. It is considered as one of the extensions of the matrix singular value decomposition (SVD) to higher-order tensors ($N \geq 3$) and represents the tensor as a sum of rank-one tensors, i.e., rank-one components. For a third-order tensor $\mathcal{X} \in \mathbb{R}^{I \times J \times K}$, the R-component CP model is defined as

$$\mathcal{X} \approx \hat{\mathcal{X}} = [\![\lambda; \mathbf{A}, \mathbf{B}, \mathbf{C}]\!] = \sum_{r=1}^{R} \lambda_r \mathbf{a}_r \circ \mathbf{b}_r \circ \mathbf{c}_r,$$

where $\circ$ indicates the vector outer product. The vectors from the rank-one components are collected in the factor matrices $\mathbf{A} \in \mathbb{R}^{I \times R} = [\mathbf{a}_1 \ldots \mathbf{a}_R]$, $\mathbf{B} \in \mathbb{R}^{J \times R} = [\mathbf{b}_1 \ldots \mathbf{b}_R]$ and $\mathbf{C} \in \mathbb{R}^{K \times R} = [\mathbf{c}_1 \ldots \mathbf{c}_R]$. In this definition, columns of all factor matrices are assumed to be normalized to unit 2-norm and the norms are absorbed in the vector $\lambda \in \mathbb{R}^{R \times 1}$. For the third-order tensor $\mathcal{X}$ consisting of the EEG data, the factor matrices $\mathbf{A}, \mathbf{B}$ and $\mathbf{C}$ correspond to the extracted factor vectors in the subject, time and electrode modes, respectively. By modeling $\mathcal{X}$ using a CP model, we assume that component r models a brain activity with temporal and spatial patterns represented by $\mathbf{b}_r$ and $\mathbf{c}_r$. Multi-channel EEG signals from each subject are a linear mixture of these R brain activities mixed using subject-specific weights. The CP model is also known as a topographic components model (Möcks, 1988). Note that the terms factor and *component* are used interchangeably throughout the paper, and refer to the rank-one matrices and/or higher-order rank-one tensors.

In contrast to matrix factorizations, the CP model of higher order tensors is unique up to scaling and permutation under mild conditions (Kruskal, 1977; Sidiropoulos and Bro, 2000), without the need to impose additional constraints.

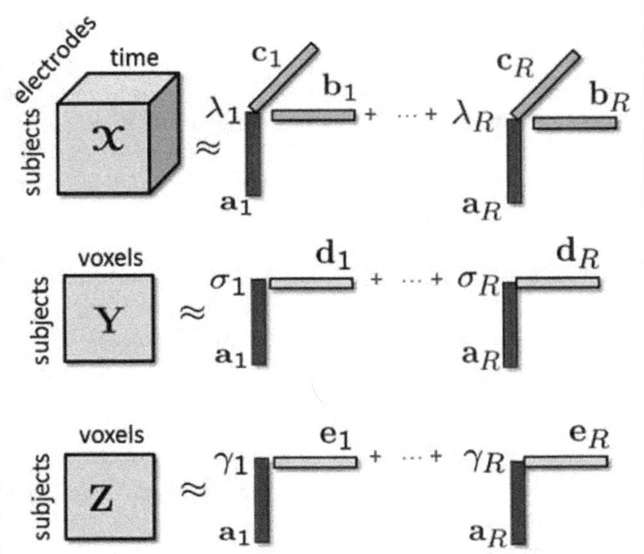

FIGURE 2 | Modeling of tensor $\mathcal{X}$ coupled with matrices **Y** and **Z** in the subject mode using a structure-revealing CMTF model.

2.1.2. Structure-Revealing Coupled Matrix and Tensor Factorizations

Given the third-order tensor $\mathcal{X}$ coupled with matrices **Y** and **Z** in the subject mode we can jointly factorize them using a structure-revealing CMTF model (a.k.a. ACMTF) (Acar et al., 2014) that fits a CP model to tensor $\mathcal{X}$ and factorizes matrices **Y** and **Z** in such a way that the factor matrix extracted from the common mode, i.e., subject, is the same in the factorizations of all data sets. An R-component ACMTF model minimizes the following objective function:

$$f(\lambda, \Sigma, \Gamma, \mathbf{A}, \mathbf{B}, \mathbf{C}, \mathbf{D}, \mathbf{E}) = \| \mathcal{X} - [\![\lambda; \mathbf{A}, \mathbf{B}, \mathbf{C}]\!] \|^2 + \| \mathbf{Y} - \mathbf{A}\Sigma\mathbf{D}^\mathsf{T} \|^2 + \| \mathbf{Z} - \mathbf{A}\Gamma\mathbf{E}^\mathsf{T} \|^2 + \beta \| \lambda \|_1 + \beta \| \sigma \|_1 + \beta \| \gamma \|_1, \quad (1)$$

where the columns of factor matrices have unit norm, i.e., $\| \mathbf{a}_r \| = \| \mathbf{b}_r \| = \| \mathbf{c}_r \| = \| \mathbf{d}_r \| = \| \mathbf{e}_r \| = 1$ for $r = 1, \ldots, R$. $\lambda, \sigma, \gamma \in \mathbb{R}^{R\times 1}$ are the weights of rank-one terms in $\mathcal{X}$, **Y**, and **Z**, respectively. $\Sigma, \Gamma \in \mathbb{R}^{R\times R}$ are diagonal matrices with entries of σ and γ on the diagonal. $\mathbf{D} \in \mathbb{R}^{M\times R}$ and $\mathbf{E} \in \mathbb{R}^{L\times R}$ correspond to factor matrices in the voxel mode in fMRI and sMRI. $\| . \|$ denotes the Frobenius norm for matrices/higher-order tensors, and the 2-norm for vectors. $\| . \|_1$ denotes the 1-norm of a vector, i.e., $\| \mathbf{x} \|_1 = \sum_{r=1}^{R} |x_r|$ and $\beta > 0$ is a penalty parameter. Imposing penalties on the weights in Equation (1) sparsifies the weights so that unshared components have weights close to 0 in some data sets. The model is illustrated in **Figure 2**. By jointly analyzing neuroimaging data using an ACMTF model, we assume that each component extracted from $\mathcal{X}$ models a brain activity with certain temporal ($\mathbf{b}_r$) and spatial ($\mathbf{c}_r$) signatures, and the corresponding component in **Y** models related brain activity with higher spatial resolution using $\mathbf{d}_r$ while the component in **Z** provides information about the tissue type at a very high spatial resolution using $\mathbf{e}_r$. Since the same factor matrix **A** is extracted from the subject mode from all data sets, subject-specific coefficients in all modalities are assumed to be the same. The ACMTF model inherits uniqueness from CP (Sorensen and De Lathauwer, 2015), as long as all factors are shared, and provides reproducible and interpretable factors. Note that, in the presence of both shared/unshared components, 1-norm penalties on the weights help to obtain unique solutions, which has been so far only shown experimentally (Acar et al., 2014).

2.1.3. Joint ICA

An alternative approach to jointly analyze $\mathcal{X}$, **Y** and **Z** is to use a matrix factorization-based fusion approach by matricizing $\mathcal{X}$ in the subject mode as a subject by time–electrode matrix denoted as $\mathbf{X}_{(1)}$. Joint ICA (Calhoun et al., 2006b) concatenates matrices representing the data from different modalities and models the constructed matrix using an ICA model as follows:

$$[\mathbf{X}_{(1)}\ \mathbf{Y}\ \mathbf{Z}] = \mathbf{AS} \quad (2)$$

where, for an R-component ICA model, $\mathbf{A} \in \mathbb{R}^{I\times R}$ corresponds to the mixing matrix, similar to the factor matrix in Equation (1), and $\mathbf{S} \in \mathbb{R}^{R\times(JK+M+L)}$ represents the source signals. Note that subject covariations across all data sets, i.e., modalities, are assumed to be the same in jICA as in ACMTF, since the same mixing matrix is shared across the data sets. However, in this case the model does not include an adaptive estimation of contributions from each modality as in ACMTF, and though this can be captured to a degree within the weights from the estimated components from each modality, it represents a more constrained model. The rows of **S** corresponding to patterns of brain activity are assumed to be statistically independent.

2.2. Experiments

We make use of EEG, fMRI, and sMRI data collected from patients with schizophrenia and healthy controls to show the use of ACMTF models to discover potential diagnostic biomarkers for schizophrenia. Our experiments focus on joint analysis of EEG and fMRI data, and discuss the effect of different modeling choices, i.e., number of components (R), the penalty parameter (β), preprocessing, and use of subsets of electrodes. We also discuss the performance of ACMTF in comparison with jICA. Furthermore, the analysis of only EEG signals and joint analysis of EEG, fMRI, and sMRI have been studied to show the information gain with each modality and potential issues due to the use of additional modalities.

2.2.1. Data

The participants in this study were recruited through advertisements, presentations at local universities, and word-of-mouth. The 32 participants provided written and informed IRB-approved consent at Hartford Hospital. The participants were compensated for their participation. Patients met the criteria for schizophrenia as defined in the DSM-IV on the basis of a SCID diagnosis as well as a review of their case file (First et al., 2002b). The healthy participants were screened to ensure that they were free from DSM-IV Axis I or Axis II psychopathology, as assessed using the SCID (First et al., 2002a) prior to their inclusion in the study. Exclusion criteria for the healthy participants also included a history of psychosis in any first-degree relatives. This was assessed through an interview. The participants in both groups had self-reported normal hearing and were able to perform the AOD task successfully in the trial sessions prior to scanning.

The EEG, fMRI and sMRI data were separately collected from 21 healthy controls and 11 patients with schizophrenia during an auditory oddball task (AOD), where subjects pressed a button when they detected an infrequent target sound within a series of auditory stimuli. The details of the AOD task used in this work have been published previously (Kiehl et al., 2005). The task consisted of two runs of 244 pseudo-randomly distributed stimuli each, following an initial practice block of 10 trails to ensure that the participants understood the instructions. The stimuli were three different types of tones: a standard stimulus (1,000 Hz tone, probability = 0.8), a target stimulus (1,500 Hz tone, probability = 0.1), and novel stimuli (non-repeating random digital noises, such as tone sweeps or whistles, probability = 0.1). Each auditory stimulus was presented for 200 ms with an inter-stimulus interval of 2,000 ms. The intervals between the non-standard stimuli consisted of 3–5 standard stimuli (approximately 8–12 s) (Kiehl et al., 2005). Two scans were performed, each lasting approximately 9 min. Thus, the total duration of the scan lasted approximately 18 min.

2.2.2. Data Preprocessing

For the fMRI data, task-related spatial activity maps for each subject were computed by the general linear model-based regression approach using the statistical parametric mapping toolbox (SPM2)[1]. The fMRI preprocessing pipeline used for this data has been described previously (Calhoun et al., 2006a). More precisely, for each subject, each image in the scan was realigned using the INRIalign algorithm (Freire and Mangin, 2001). The aligned data was then normalized into Montreal Neurological Institute (MNI) space and spatially smoothed with a $10 \times 10 \times 12$ mm^3 full width at half maximum (FWHM) Gaussian kernel. The normalized data was then subsampled to $3 \times 3 \times 3$ mm, thus resulting in brain volumes of dimensions $53 \times 63 \times 46$ voxels. The data for each subject was then analyzed through a multivariate regression where the regressors are formed from the auditory stimuli, their temporal derivatives, and an intercept. The regressors for the auditory stimuli are formed by modeling the stimuli as delta functions convolved with the default SPM2 hemodynamic response function. We use the regression coefficients (beta-values) corresponding to the target tone as the feature for these analyses (Calhoun et al., 2006a). By making use of these features and removing voxels not corresponding to brain regions, we constructed a matrix of 32 subjects by 60,186 voxels representing the fMRI signals.

The details of the preprocessing pipeline used for the EEG data have been previously published in Calhoun et al. (2006b). Briefly, the EEG channels were amplified (20,000 gain) with a passband between 0.01 and 100 Hz. The signals were digitized at a rate of 500 samples per second. The EEG data was then preprocessed using ICA to remove any ocular artifacts (Jung et al., 2000). The data were then filtered with a 20 Hz low-pass filter in order to reduce electromyographic activity. EEG epochs from -115 to 788 ms (451 time points) around stimulus onsets were used for the event-related potentials (ERP). ERP were formed only from those trials in which the subjects correctly identified the target stimulus (Calhoun et al., 2006b). Out of 64 electrodes in total, we used 62 electrodes by excluding the two corresponding to vertical and horizontal electrooculography (EOG) electrodes. Multi-channel EEG signals were then arranged as a third-order tensor: 32 subjects by 451 time samples by 62 electrodes. In order to assess the modeling assumptions, we also used a subset of electrodes, i.e., AF3, AF4, Fz, T7, C3, Cz, C4, T8, Pz, PO3, PO, and in that case, formed a third-order tensor with 11 electrodes as in (Acar et al., 2017a,b). This subset of electrodes was determined with the goal of selecting a small set of electrodes that would record the relevant functional activity related to the AOD task. The selected subset includes electrodes from the frontal, motor and parietal areas that are expected to be involved in the motor and auditory responses as well as the planning stage for the given task.

For the sMRI data, we computed probabilistically segmented gray matter images for each subject and by using these features formed a matrix of 32 subjects by 306,640 voxels. The details of the sMRI preprocessing pipeline have also been presented previously in Calhoun et al. (2006a). The image files were first normalized using a 12 parameter affine model to the 152 average T_1 MNI template. The images were next segmented into gray matter, white matter, and cerebrospinal fluid. Then the segmentation was smoothed with an 8-mm FWHM Gaussian kernel and the segments were then averaged to create the gray matter, white matter, and cerebrospinal fluid templates. Each subject's segmented T_1 images were then normalized to the customized gray matter templates. Then, for each subject, the warped T_1 images were segmented into gray matter, white matter, and cerebrospinal fluid maps using a model clustering algorithm resulting in probabilistic segmentations of gray matter (Ashburner and Friston, 2000). Finally, the resulting gray matter images were smoothed with a 12-mm FWHM Gaussian kernel (Good et al., 2001).

2.2.3. Experimental Setting

Before the analysis, we centered the third-order EEG tensor across the time mode, and scaled within the subject mode by dividing each horizontal slice by its standard deviation (see Bro and Smilde, 2003 for further details on preprocessing of higher-order tensors). The fMRI and sMRI data were also preprocessed by centering each row (subject-wise) and dividing each row by its standard deviation. When fitting the ACMTF model, each data set was also divided by its Frobenius norm to give equal importance to the approximation of each data set.

In order to demonstrate the information gained by the addition of each modality and sensitivity of the fusion approach to various modeling choices, the following experiments are carried out:

[1] https://www.fil.ion.ucl.ac.uk/spm/

- Individual analysis of the EEG tensor using a CP model,
- Joint analysis of the EEG tensor coupled with fMRI using an ACMTF model (i) by leaving out signals from one subject at a time, (ii) for 11-electrode vs. 62-electrode case, (iii) in comparison with jICA, (iv) with different number of components, R, (v) with different sparsity penalty parameters, β, (vi) with/without additional centering across the subject mode.
- Joint analysis of the EEG tensor coupled with fMRI and sMRI using an ACMTF model.

The CP model is fit using CP-OPT (Acar et al., 2011) from the Tensor Toolbox version 2.5[2] using the non-linear conjugate gradient algorithm (NCG). For the ACMTF model, we use ACMTF-OPT (Acar et al., 2014) from the CMTF Toolbox version 1.1[3], also using NCG to fit the model. Multiple random initializations are used to fit the models, and the solution corresponding to the minimum function value is reported. Furthermore, the ACMTF model is experimentally validated to be unique by obtaining the same minimum function value[4] a number of times and checking the uniqueness of model parameters, i.e., factor matrices and weights of the components (up to permutation)[5]. For jICA, we unfold the EEG tensor in the subject mode forming a matrix of 32 subjects × 27,962 (time-electrodes), and concatenate the resulting matrix with the fMRI matrix. The concatenated matrix is decomposed using an ICA algorithm based on entropy bound minimization (ICA-EBM)[6] (Li and Adali, 2010), which makes use of a flexible density model that is a better fit to data formed by concatenating signals from different modalities (Adali et al., 2015a). We fit the model using multiple random initializations and report the most stable run determined by a minimum spanning tree-based approach (Du et al., 2016).

2.3. Performance Evaluation

The performance is assessed both qualitatively and quantitatively. The qualitative assessment relies on the interpretation of the extracted temporal and spatial patterns as well as comparisons with the previous findings in the literature on schizophrenia. For the quantitative assessment, we perform the following:

- Two-sample t-test: Since the ultimate goal of any factorization of this data is the discovery of latent factors that can differentiate between patients with schizophrenia and healthy controls, we can quantify the performance of a method based on its ability to produce factors that can provide such a differentiation. With the assumption of unequal variance for the healthy control and patient groups, a two-sample t-test is applied on each column of the factor matrix extracted from the subject mode, which is of size 32 by R. Out of R columns, those that have subject mode vectors that are statistically significant, i.e., with p-values < 0.05, are identified and corresponding temporal and spatial patterns are reported as potential biomarkers.
- Clustering: Subjects are clustered into two groups based on the factor matrix corresponding to the subject mode using k-means clustering, where k-means is performed 100 times with different initializations and the most consistent cluster assignments are used. Unlike the t-test based approach that is performed on each column individually, clustering is performed on all possible combinations of the columns of the factor matrix and the performance of the best combination is reported. Therefore, this approach provides a more global view of the discriminatory power of the resulting factorization than the t-test based approach. The clustering performance is assessed in terms of accuracy and F_1-score, where F_1-score $= \frac{2\text{Precision}\times\text{Recall}}{\text{Precision}+\text{Recall}}$. Precision and Recall are defined as Precision $= \frac{\#\text{ of true positives}}{\#\text{ of true positives}+\#\text{ of false positives}}$ and Recall $= \frac{\#\text{ of true positives}}{\#\text{ of true positives}+\#\text{ of false negatives}}$, and a patient being clustered as a patient is considered a true-positive.

When assessing different modeling choices, we also report the model fit defined as:

$$\text{Fit} = 100 \times \left(1 - \frac{\| \mathbf{X} - \widehat{\mathbf{X}} \|^2}{\| \mathbf{X} \|^2}\right),$$

where $\mathbf{X}$ stands for the raw data (e.g., EEG tensor or fMRI/sMRI matrix), and $\widehat{\mathbf{X}}$ denotes the model. A fit of 100% means that the data is fully explained by the model. The fit shows whether the model explains the data well and indicates the unexplained part left in the residuals. Also, the change in model fit for different number of components shows whether there is a significant gain, in terms of explaining the remaining part in the residuals, by adding more components.

Finally, we compare the similarity of the significant components extracted by different models using a similarity score called the factor match score (FMS). The FMS of component k from two models $\hat{\mathcal{X}}^{(1)}$ and $\hat{\mathcal{X}}^{(2)}$ of the EEG tensor $\mathcal{X}$ is defined as

$$\text{FMS}_k(\hat{\mathcal{X}}^{(1)}, \hat{\mathcal{X}}^{(2)}) = \frac{|\mathbf{a}_k^{(1)^{\mathsf{T}}} \mathbf{a}_k^{(2)}|}{\left\| \mathbf{a}_k^{(1)} \right\| \left\| \mathbf{a}_k^{(2)} \right\|} \times \frac{|\mathbf{b}_k^{(1)^{\mathsf{T}}} \mathbf{b}_k^{(2)}|}{\left\| \mathbf{b}_k^{(1)} \right\| \left\| \mathbf{b}_k^{(2)} \right\|} \times \frac{|\mathbf{c}_k^{(1)^{\mathsf{T}}} \mathbf{c}_k^{(2)}|}{\left\| \mathbf{c}_k^{(1)} \right\| \left\| \mathbf{c}_k^{(2)} \right\|},$$

and from two models $\widehat{\mathbf{Y}}^{(1)}, \widehat{\mathbf{Y}}^{(2)}$ of the fMRI matrix $\mathbf{Y}$ as

$$\text{FMS}_k(\widehat{\mathbf{Y}}^{(1)}, \widehat{\mathbf{Y}}^{(2)}) = \frac{|\mathbf{a}_k^{(1)^{\mathsf{T}}} \mathbf{a}_k^{(2)}|}{\left\| \mathbf{a}_k^{(1)} \right\| \left\| \mathbf{a}_k^{(2)} \right\|} \times \frac{|\mathbf{d}_k^{(1)^{\mathsf{T}}} \mathbf{d}_k^{(2)}|}{\left\| \mathbf{d}_k^{(1)} \right\| \left\| \mathbf{d}_k^{(2)} \right\|},$$

where $\mathbf{a}_k^{(i)}, \mathbf{b}_k^{(i)}, \mathbf{c}_k^{(i)}, \mathbf{d}_k^{(i)}$ correspond to the kth column of the factor matrix corresponding to subject, time, electrode, and voxel mode of the ith model, respectively, after finding the best matching factors for the two models. When components are compared for the models with mismatching dimensions, such as number of subjects or number of electrodes, the mismatching dimension is omitted in the product. An FMS close to one implies similarity of the compared components, while very different components

[2] http://www.sandia.gov/tgkolda/TensorToolbox/
[3] http://www.models.life.ku.dk/joda/CMTF_Toolbox
[4] Up to the sixth decimal place.
[5] Depending on the difficulty of the problem, 160-200 random initializations are used to check for uniqueness.
[6] The ICA-EBM code is available at http://mlsp.umbc.edu/ica_ebm.html.

will have an FMS close to zero. FMS is used to quantify the reproducibility of the extracted patterns in addition to qualitative interpretations based on the plots.

For visualization of the extracted components, patterns from fMRI and sMRI voxel modes are plotted as z-maps, thresholded at $|z| \geq 2.7$, where red indicates an increase in controls over patients and blue indicates an increase in patients over controls. This threshold value was selected after considering several alternatives in order to aid in the visual interpretation of the components. Patterns extracted from the electrode mode of the EEG tensor are plotted using the topoplot function from the EEGLAB v13.6.5b (Delorme and Makeig, 2004).

3. RESULTS

3.1. Individual Analysis of the EEG Tensor Using a CP Model

As shown in **Figure 3**, the CP model of the EEG data in the form of a subject by time by electrode tensor constructed using 62 electrodes has captured significant components in terms of differentiating healthy controls and patients with schizophrenia. The model is fit using $R = 3$ components, and reveals factor matrices $\mathbf{A} \in \mathbb{R}^{32\times3}$, $\mathbf{B} \in \mathbb{R}^{451\times3}$, and $\mathbf{C} \in \mathbb{R}^{62\times3}$ corresponding to subject, time, and electrode modes, respectively. The fit of the model is 62% indicating that using only three components a major part of the data can be explained. The t-tests performed on the columns of $\mathbf{A}$ indicate that all three components are significant. The first component, whose factor vectors in time and electrode modes are represented in **Figure 3A**, corresponds to the third positive peak (P3) and is heavily weighted by central electrodes. The second component with the factor vectors in time and electrode modes represented in **Figure 3B**, refers to the N1-P2 as well as the N2-P3 transitions and is heavily weighted by central and parietal electrodes. The third component with the factor vectors in time and electrode modes represented in **Figure 3C**, refers to the N2 as well as a negative peak after P3 and is heavily weighted by frontal and central electrodes. CP models with different number of components have been fitted to the data as well but those either revealed fewer components with less significance or are degenerate, i.e., a CP model with that many components is not an appropriate model for the data (see Kolda and Bader, 2009 for more on degeneracy). **Table 1** shows that subjects can be clustered into two groups with 81% accuracy using the factor matrix $\mathbf{A}$. Note that clustering performance is similar to the one achieved using the CP model of a tensor constructed using only a subset of electrodes indicating that the assumption of same subject coefficients and temporal patterns across all electrodes is not decreasing the performance. This also may indicate that the additional electrodes are not providing much added information beyond that which is contained by a subset of the electrodes.

3.2. Joint Analysis of EEG and fMRI

Shown in **Figure 4**, the joint analysis of the EEG tensor and fMRI matrix using an ACMTF model has revealed significant components in terms of differentiating between healthy controls and patients while also providing spatial patterns in much higher resolution and improving the clustering performance compared with the CP model of the EEG tensor. The 10-component ACMTF model extracts factor matrices $\mathbf{A} \in \mathbb{R}^{32\times10}$, $\mathbf{B} \in \mathbb{R}^{451\times10}$, $\mathbf{C} \in \mathbb{R}^{62\times10}$, and $\mathbf{D} \in \mathbb{R}^{60186\times10}$ corresponding to subject, time, electrode, and voxel modes, respectively, as well as weights of the components in EEG ($\lambda \in \mathbb{R}^{10\times1}$) and fMRI ($\sigma \in \mathbb{R}^{10\times1}$). The sparsity penalty parameter is set to $\beta = 10^{-3}$. The fit is 79% and 65% for EEG and fMRI, respectively, indicating that the extracted factors, which have high weights in both data sets indicating shared factors, account for a large part of both data sets. The t-test on the columns of $\mathbf{A}$ reveals that out of ten components, only two, components 1 and 9, are statistically significant. **Figures 4A,B** illustrate the factor vectors of the two significant factors in time ($\mathbf{b}_r$), electrode ($\mathbf{c}_r$) and voxel ($\mathbf{d}_r$) modes. **Figure 4C** shows component weights in each data set. From **Figure 4**, we see that though both significant components have a contribution from both EEG and fMRI, the contribution from EEG to each of these components is greater. This means that the discriminatory information plays a larger part in the EEG data than it does in fMRI (see Acar et al., 2014 for further information on how to interpret the weights of the components). Note that the statistical significance of the components and weights of components are different concepts. Statistical significance is determined based on a two-sample t-test on the columns of the factor matrix in the subject mode and indicates whether a component can be considered to be significant in terms of separating patients and controls. On the other hand, the weight of a component indicates how much that component contributes to the model fit. Therefore, a component with a high weight may not be statistically significant in terms of distinguishing between patients and controls.

The first component, whose factor vectors in the time, electrode, and voxel modes are shown in **Figure 4A**, is similar to the component shown in **Figure 3C**, and refers to the P2-N2 transition as well as the P3 peak and is heavily weighted by the frontal and central electrodes. A similar activation pattern is seen in the positive activations in the fMRI, though with greater spatial resolution. The second component, with the factor vectors in time, electrode, and voxel modes shown in **Figure 4B**, shares some similarity with the component shown in **Figure 3A**, since both are related to the P3 peak but this component is more heavily weighted by the frontal electrodes. The fMRI part in **Figure 4B** indicates a decrease in activation of controls vs. patients in parts of the anterior sensorimotor cortex. We should note that there are some similarities between the areas highlighted in the topographic maps and the regions highlighted in the fMRI. The areas of increased activation of controls over patients in the fMRI, namely frontal and sensorimotor, generally correspond to the greatest weights in the topographic maps. Similar components have been found previously in other analyses of similar data (Acar et al., 2017b), thus increasing our confidence in the results. In comparison to the individual analysis of the EEG tensor, the clustering performance is also much higher, i.e., 88% accuracy and F_1 score of 0.82, as shown in **Table 1**. This indicates that the ACMTF reveals more discriminatory factors through the inclusion of complementary information from the fMRI.

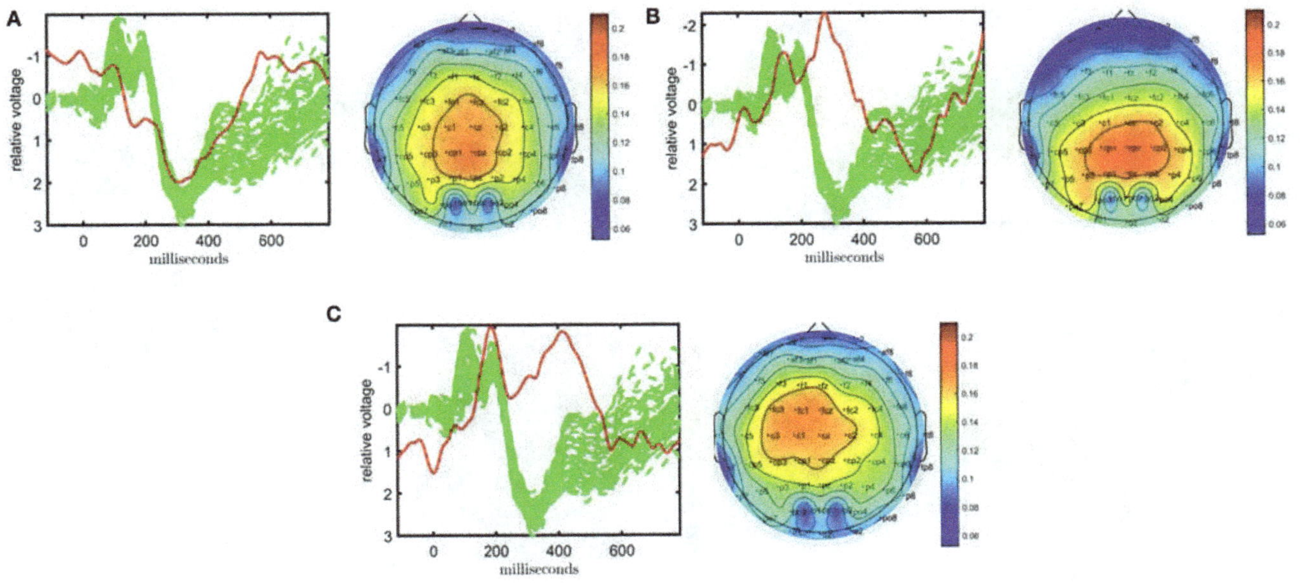

FIGURE 3 | Temporal and spatial patterns from the statistically significant components of the CP model. **(A)** Component 1 corresponds to the P3 peak mainly represented by central electrodes, **(B)** Component 2 refers to the N1-P2 as well as N2-P3 transitions, with high contributions from central and parietal electrodes, **(C)** Component 3 refers to the N2 as well as a negative peak after P3, heavily weighted by frontal and central electrodes. The corresponding p-values are 2.1×10^{-3}, 1.6×10^{-2}, 1.4×10^{-4}, respectively. Columns of the factor matrix in the time mode are in red while green plots show signals from individual electrodes averaged across all subjects.

TABLE 1 | Performance in terms of clustering for different modeling values as well as the factor match scores in comparison to the 10-component ACMTF model (no centering, 62 electrodes).

						FMS			
				Clustering performance		Component A		Component B	
	R	Centering	Number of electrodes	Accuracy (%)	F_1-score	EEG	fMRI	EEG	fMRI
EEG (CP)	3	No	11	78	0.76				
	3	No	62	81	0.79				
EEG–fMRI (ACMTF)	10	No	11	91	0.87	0.82	0.73	0.80	0.72
	10	No	62	88	0.82	1.00	1.00	1.00	1.00
	11	No	62	88	0.80	0.95	0.92	0.65	0.61
	12	No	62	91	0.86	0.93	0.89	0.56	0.61
	9	Yes	62	88	0.78	0.82	0.80	0.64	0.56
	10	Yes	62	91	0.88	0.85	0.81	0.57	0.57
	11	Yes	62	91	0.87	0.84	0.81	0.69	0.55
	12	Yes	62	88	0.78	0.66	0.63	0.65	0.57
EEG–fMRI (jICA)	10	No	62	84	0.74				
	15	No	62	82	0.70				
	20	No	62	91	0.84				
EEG–fMRI–sMRI (ACMTF)	10	No	62	84	0.71	0.93	0.86	0.87	0.84
	10	Yes	62	91	0.87	0.78	0.73	0.68	0.60
	15	Yes	62	91	0.86	–	–	0.66	0.58

3.2.1. Sensitivity Analyses

3.2.1.1. Leave-one-out

The patterns captured in different modes using an ACMTF model are reproducible in case of changes in data sets. In order to evaluate the consistency of the results to changes in the original data, we leave out one subject at a time and fit the ACMTF model using the same parameters (i.e., $R = 10, \beta = 10^{-3}$). In other words, we construct 32 different EEG-fMRI data set pairs (with 31 subjects) and compare the significant factors extracted using the ACMTF model of each pair with the model derived using 32 subjects. **Table 2** shows that average FMS for component 1 (**Figure 4A**), which is the most significant factor, is 0.98 for

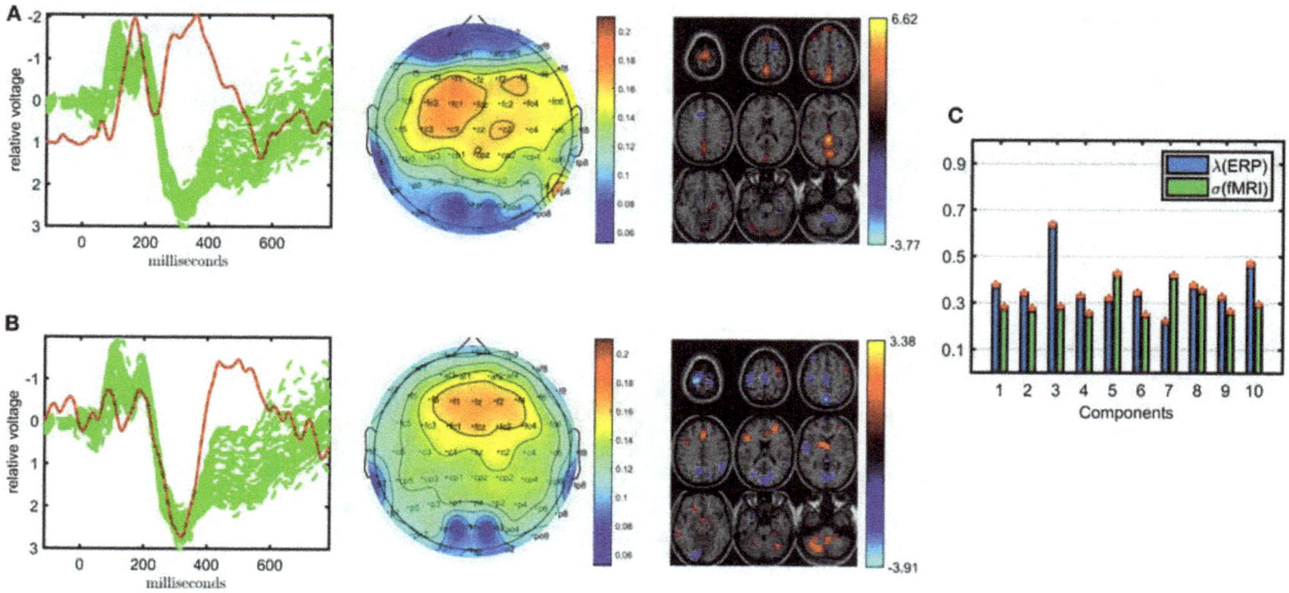

FIGURE 4 | Temporal and spatial patterns from the statistically significant components of the ACMTF model of the EEG tensor with 62 electrodes and fMRI data, with $R = 10$. **(A)** Component 1 refers to the P2-N2 transition as well as the P3 peak, heavily weighted by the frontal and central electrodes in the EEG, and the fMRI shows increased activation of controls over patients in the sensorimotor cortex, **(B)** component 9 is related to the P3 peak, heavily weighted by the frontal electrodes in the EEG and the fMRI indicates a decrease in activation of controls vs. patients in some regions of the sensorimotor cortex and parietal lobe, **(C)** weights of the components in each data set. The corresponding p-values are 6.2×10^{-3}, 1.9×10^{-2}, respectively. Columns of the factor matrix in the time mode are in red while green plots show signals from individual electrodes averaged across all subjects.

EEG and 0.95 for fMRI indicating close to exact recovery of the same patterns. Average FMS for the less significant component, i.e., component 9 (**Figure 4B**), is around 0.90 indicating similar patterns. Furthermore, the average clustering performance is the same as the performance of the original model estimated using data from 32 subjects.

3.2.1.2. 11 electrodes vs. 62 electrodes

When jointly analyzing EEG and fMRI, ACMTF achieves a slightly better performance using a subset of electrodes from certain regions of interest during the construction of the EEG tensor than the case where all 62 electrodes are used to construct the tensor. In our preliminary studies (Acar et al., 2017b), we observed similar components when comparing the 11-electrode case with 62-electrode case while achieving higher statistical significance and better interpretability using 11 electrodes. These observations are also supported by our findings in this study on a slightly different set of subjects (38 subjects in Acar et al., 2017b vs. 32 subjects in this paper). **Figure 5** illustrates the factor vectors, in the time and voxel modes, of the two most significant components, captured by a 10-component ACMTF model of the EEG tensor with 11 electrodes and fMRI data[7]. The fit is 80% and 65% for EEG and fMRI, respectively. As previously observed, both components have higher significance thus indicating that the additional electrodes are not contributing much additional discriminatory information compared with the original 11 electrodes. This may also be related to the fact that the most contributing electrodes to the components in **Figure 4** are the electrodes that are part of the set of 11 electrodes. The first component, shown in **Figure 5A**, is similar to the component shown in **Figure 4A** and refers to P2-N2 transition as well as the P3 peak though with more parietal activation in the fMRI. The second component, with the factor vectors in time and voxel modes shown in **Figure 5B**, is similar to the component shown in **Figure 4B** and refers to the P3 peak though has more parietal activation in the fMRI, similar to the default mode network. When significant components from 11- and 62-electrode cases are compared, FMS is 0.82 for EEG (excluding the electrode mode) and 0.73 for fMRI for the component given in **Figure 4A**, and 0.80 for EEG and 0.72 for fMRI for **Figure 4B**. These scores indicate that components are similar to some extent but are not identical. **Table 1** indicates slightly higher clustering performance for the 11-electrode case. To summarize, considering that there is minimal difference in performance beyond a slight increase in significance, and that the factors are similar, using all electrodes is preferable to choosing a subset of electrodes, as the latter requires prior knowledge about the functionally relevant electrodes to select and may also introduce a bias by targeting specific regions.

3.2.1.3. ACMTF vs. JICA

The traditional fusion approach jICA can also capture components that can differentiate between healthy controls and patients; however, jICA provides less interpretable patterns. For jICA, the EEG tensor unfolded in the subject mode is

[7] *T*-tests reveal, in total, four statistically significant components for this model. However, the other two components, not illustrated in **Figure 5**, are less significant and have lower FMS values.

TABLE 2 | Leave-one-out sensitivity analysis: average values (standard deviation) of FMS, clustering performance and fit of the models built on data sets with 31 subjects.

FMS				Clustering performance		Fit (%)	
Component A		Component B		Accuracy (%)	F_1-score	EEG	fMRI
EEG	fMRI	EEG	fMRI				
0.98 (0.05)	0.95 (0.09)	0.92 (0.16)	0.90 (0.16)	87.7 (2.4)	0.81 (0.04)	79.5 (0.4)	65.6 (0.3)

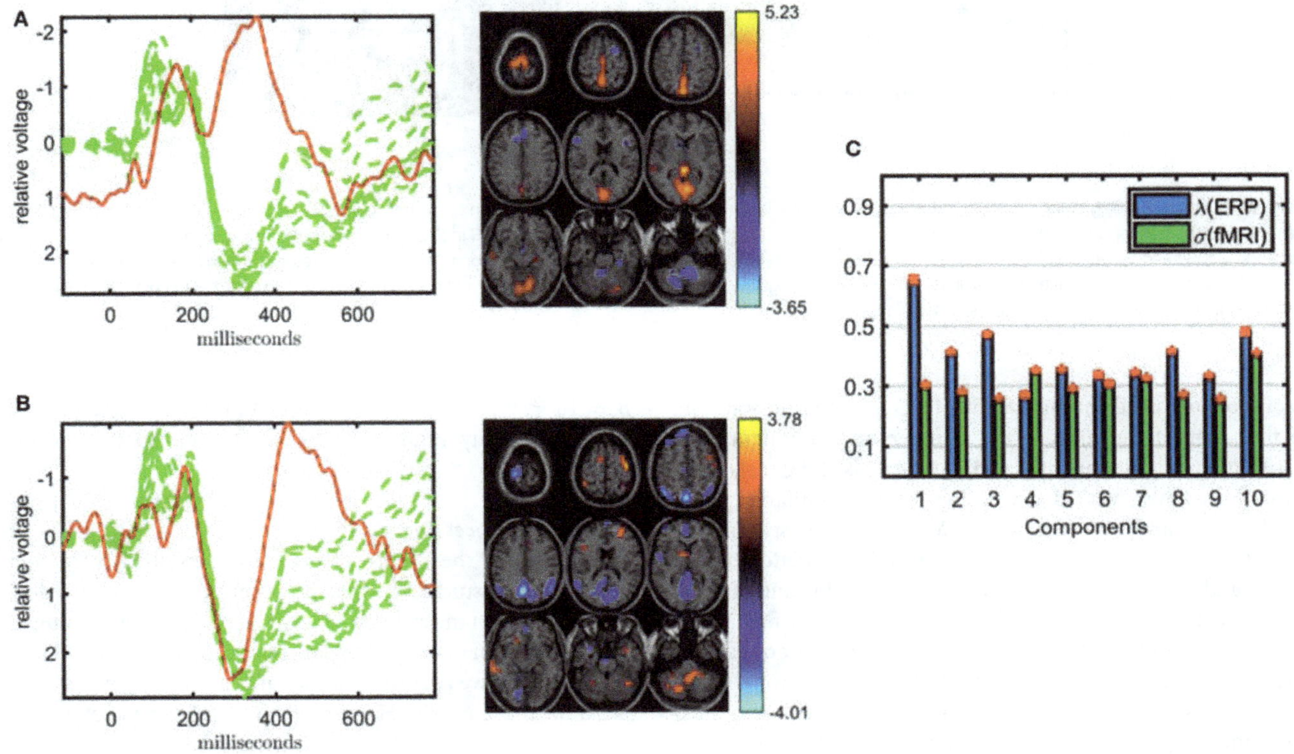

FIGURE 5 | Temporal and spatial patterns from the statistically significant components of the ACMTF model of the EEG tensor with 11 electrodes and fMRI data, with $R = 10$. **(A)** Component 10 corresponds to the P2-N2 transition as well as the P3 peak in the EEG with an increase in sensorimotor and parietal activation of controls over patients in the fMRI, **(B)** component 5 refers to the P3 peak with a decrease in default mode activity of controls vs. patients in the fMRI, **(C)** weights of the components in each data set. The corresponding p-values are 4.3×10^{-3}, 8.0×10^{-3}, respectively. Columns of the factor matrix in the time mode are in red while green plots show signals from individual electrodes averaged across all subjects.

concatenated with the fMRI data resulting in a 32 (subject) by 88,148 (time × electrode-voxel) matrix. When this matrix is modeled using jICA with $R = 10, 15, 20$ components, the 10-component model reveals a single component that may be considered statistically significant but the p-value is 0.05. The 15-component model reveals a more significant component as illustrated in **Figure 6**. JICA captures neither a single temporal pattern for all electrodes nor a spatial pattern for all time points, making the interpretation of the components more difficult. In order to provide insight into the topology, spatial patterns as in ACMTF can be computed *post hoc* from the analysis, e.g., by using peak value of each channel to construct a spatial map for each component (Liu et al., 2009); however, that comes with additional assumptions and does not reveal the underlying patterns as naturally as a tensor factorization-based approach. The component, whose source signals corresponding to the time and voxel parts are shown in **Figure 6**, is related to the P2-N2 and N2-P3 transition and the fMRI map includes the expected temporal lobe and default mode regions. We should note that using a 20-component model, a component similar to the one in **Figure 6** is captured, indicating that jICA has some stability in regards to the value of R. **Table 1** shows that while the clustering performance of jICA is lower compared with ACMTF models of EEG and fMRI data sets for $R = 10$ and $R = 15$, it is similar for $R = 20$, indicating that methods with different assumptions may perform the best with different number of components.

3.2.1.4. Parameter selection

The ACMTF model is sensitive to two parameters, i.e., the number of components, R, and the sparsity penalty parameter, β. So far, R and β are set to $R = 10$ and $\beta = 10^{-3}$. In order to probe the effect of the model order, R, we have increased the number

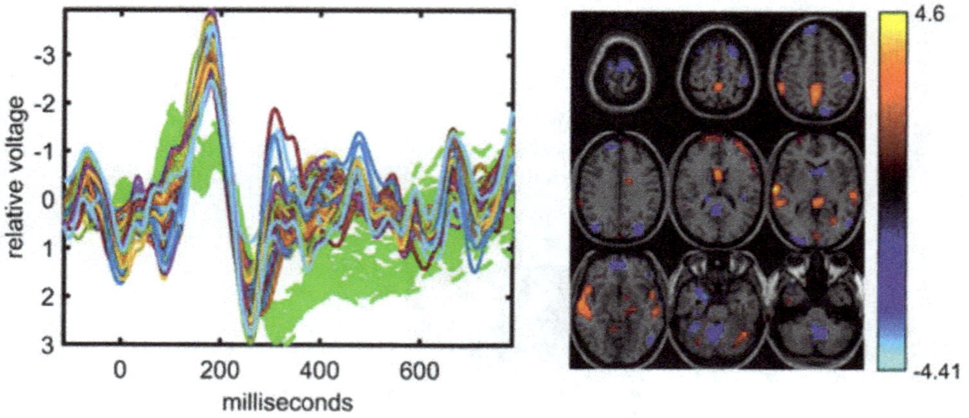

FIGURE 6 | The statistically significant component captured by the jICA model fitted to the concatenation of the unfolded EEG tensor (with 62 electrodes) and fMRI, with $R = 15$. The corresponding p-value is 5.2×10^{-3}. Parts of $\mathbf{s}_r$, i.e., rth column of the source matrix $\mathbf{S}$ in Equation (2), corresponding to the time samples for each electrode in EEG and voxels in fMRI are plotted. The EEG part is related to the P2-N2 and N2-P3 transitions. The fMRI indicates some increased activation in the temporal lobe of controls vs. patients as well as some posterior cingulate representing the default mode network. In the EEG plot, green dashed plots show signals from individual electrodes averaged across all subjects.

of components until the model fails to give a unique solution. We find that as we increase the number of components, the most significant component (i.e., **Figure 4A**) is still consistently captured; however, with a decreasing level of similarity. With both $R = 11$ and $R = 12$, the ACMTF model is still unique and reveals significant components that can differentiate between patients and healthy controls. The fit is 81% for EEG and 68% for fMRI with $R = 11$ while 82% for EEG and 70% for fMRI with $R = 12$, indicating that additional components do not explain much additional information. **Table 1** shows that a component with a FMS score around 0.90 when compared with the most significant component in a 10-component model (**Figure 4A**) has been revealed by both models. The less significant component (**Figure 4B**), on the other hand, has limited similarity of around FMS 0.60 with the captured components. The clustering performance for both $R = 11$ and $R = 12$ is similar to that of $R = 10$. **Figure S1** illustrates the factor vectors, in the time, electrode, and voxel modes, of the significant components captured by the ACMTF model with $R = 12$ components. When R is increased any further, we cannot obtain a unique solution.

The sensitivity of an ACMTF model to different values of β has been studied in Acar et al. (2014) using simulated data sets, and it has been shown that in the presence of both shared and unshared components, small values, such as $\beta = 10^{-3}$ or $\beta = 10^{-4}$ are effective in terms of uniquely recovering the underlying patterns. For $\beta = 0$, which corresponds to a CMTF model, the model fails to give a unique solution in the presence of unshared components (Acar et al., 2014). For larger values, such as $\beta = 10^{-2}$, it is still possible to find the true solution but the algorithm is very sensitive to the initialization. When EEG and fMRI data sets are jointly analyzed using a 10-component model, weights of the components shown in **Figure 4C** indicate that all components are shared. However, even in the presence of only shared components, $\beta = 10^{-4}$ fails to give a unique solution, which is due to the fact that without an effective sparsity penalty term, the model can become degenerate. For $\beta = 10^{-2}$, it is not possible to reach to the same function values even with many random initializations due to the sensitivity to initialization.

3.2.1.5. Preprocessing

In addition to the preprocessing steps described in section 2, in data fusion studies, further preprocessing may be needed, in particular, when the average behavior across subjects accounts for a large variation in one of the data sets vs. the other. SMRI is such a data set and we perform additional centering when we include sMRI in the analysis. Here, when we only consider the joint analysis of EEG and fMRI, an additional centering step across the subjects mode does not affect the clustering performance of the ACMTF model and the significant component in **Figure 4A** has also been captured with FMS between 0.80 and 0.85 (for different number of components $R = 9, 10, 11$) as shown in **Table 1**. FMS drops for $R = 12$. The less significant component (**Figure 4B**), on the other hand, is also estimated, but with FMS within the range 0.55–0.69. **Figure S2** illustrates the significant components captured by an ACMTF model with $R = 12$ components. It is important to note that in this case, despite the low FMS values, temporal and spatial patterns are similar to the ones observed in **Figure 4** and the interpretation of these two components is the same.

3.3. Joint Analysis of EEG, fMRI, and sMRI

Inclusion of the sMRI data introduces several issues highlighting challenges in data fusion, in particular, preprocessing. If a joint analysis of EEG, fMRI, and sMRI data is carried out using an ACMTF model after the preprocessing steps described in section 2.2.3, the model has two statistically significant components in terms of differentiating healthy controls and patients. **Figure 7** illustrates the temporal patterns as well as functional/structural spatial patterns revealed by the significant components. Both components are similar to the components shown in **Figure 4** with FMS values between 0.84 and 0.93 as given in **Table 1** as well

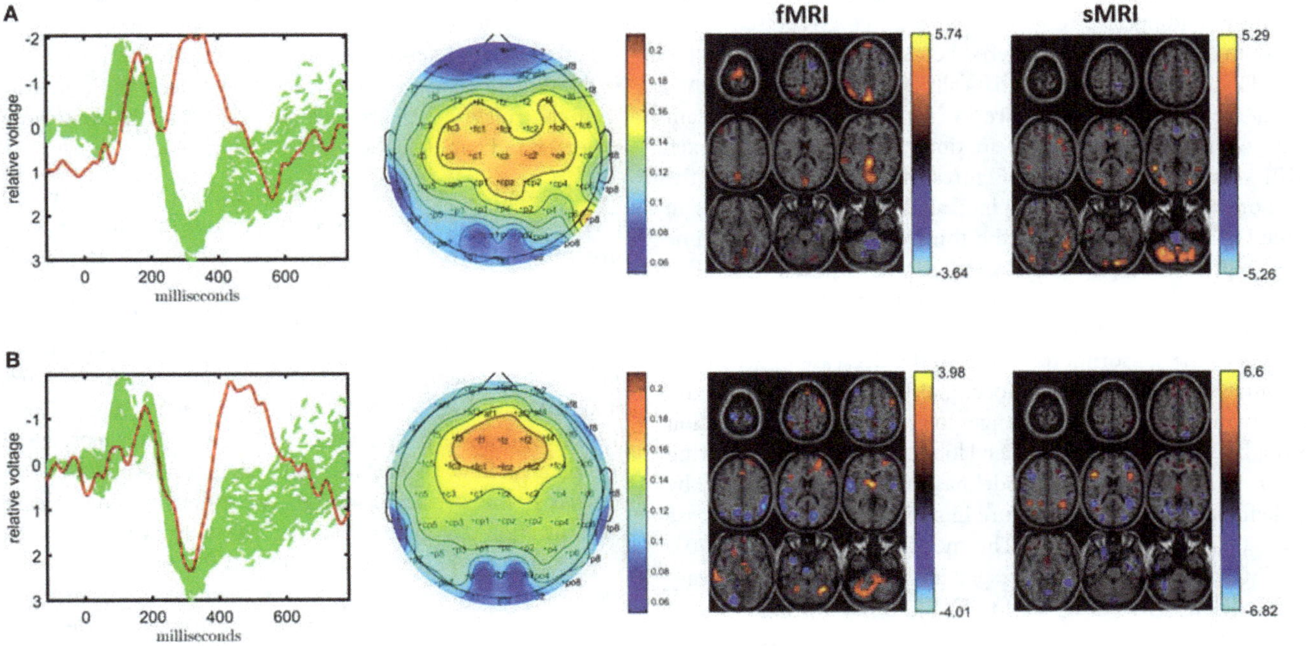

FIGURE 7 | Temporal and spatial patterns from the statistically significant components of the ACMTF model of the EEG tensor with 62 electrodes, fMRI and sMRI data, with $R = 10$. **(A)** Component 10 refers to the P2-N2 transition as well as the P3 peak, heavily weighted by the frontal and central electrodes in the EEG, an increase in sensorimotor and parietal activation of controls over patients in the fMRI, and an increase in concentration of gray matter in controls over patients in sections of the parietal lobe and cerebellum in the sMRI, **(B)** component 6 corresponds to the P3 peak heavily weighted the frontal electrodes in the EEG, the fMRI indicates a decrease in activation of controls vs. patients in some regions of the sensorimotor cortex and parietal lobe, and increases in gray matter for controls over patients in multiple portions of the frontal and parietal lobes in the sMRI. The corresponding p-values are 8.0×10^{-3}, 4.0×10^{-3}, respectively. Columns of the factor matrix in the time mode are in red while green plots show signals from individual electrodes averaged across all subjects.

as components shown in **Figure 3**. However, now information from the two functional modalities, EEG and fMRI, has been combined with information from the structural modality, sMRI. In **Figure 7A**, the sMRI portion of the component shows an increase in concentration of gray matter in controls over patients in sections of the parietal lobe and cerebellum. In **Figure 7B**, the sMRI portion of the component shows increases in gray matter for controls over patients in multiple portions of the frontal and parietal lobes. Overall these components are similar to components found previously in other analyses of data from the same subjects but with 11 electrodes (Acar et al., 2017a).

Weights of the components, shown in **Figure 8**, indicate that sMRI does not contribute much to the significant components. In most components the weights of the components in the sMRI are low, indicating potentially unshared factors. However, a closer look at the model reveals that the model fit is 97% for sMRI, while it is 79% for EEG and 64% for fMRI (see **Figure S3** for the singular value spectrum of each data set), and components with high weights in sMRI are mainly modeling the average structure across subjects with highly correlated components, i.e., the correlation of component vector in the voxel mode is 0.95 for components 1 and 5. Therefore, data sets must be centered across the subject mode to incorporate information other than the mean from sMRI into the analysis. Furthermore, as a result of including components from sMRI, which do not differentiate between the groups, we also observe a drop in the clustering performance in **Table 1**. Note that the clustering performance is based on all possible combinations of the columns of the factor matrix in the subject mode. However, we do note that the significance of both components have increased, thus indicating

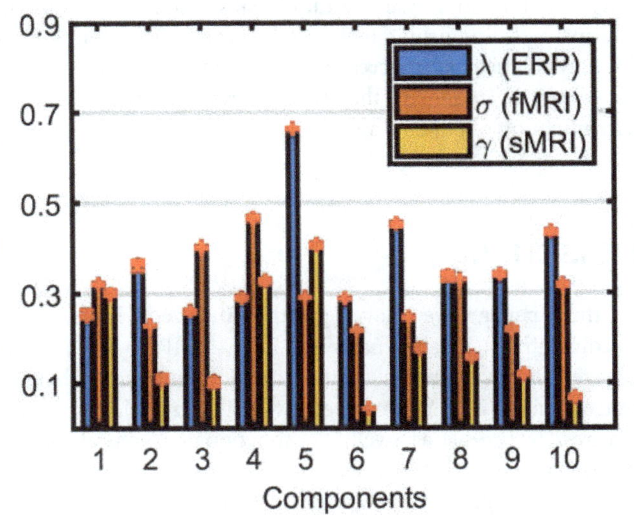

FIGURE 8 | Weights of the components in EEG, fMRI, and sMRI extracted by the ACMTF model of the EEG tensor with 62 electrodes, fMRI and sMRI data, with $R = 10$ and no additional centering across the subject mode.

that there is additional discriminatory information that the sMRI is providing.

When all data sets are centered across the subject mode, the ACMTF model has three statistically significant components, which are illustrated in **Figure S4**. The two most significant ones, with the factor vectors in time, electrode, fMRI voxel, sMRI voxel modes shown in **Figures S4A,B**, are similar to the components in **Figure 4**, also indicated by the FMS values in **Table 1**. The factor vector of the third component in the time mode represents the N2 peak as well as the P3 peak in the EEG. The topographic map indicates activation in the parietal lobe, while the fMRI part shows increased activation of controls over patients in the sensorimotor cortex and a decrease in activation of controls vs. patients in the occipital lobe. The sMRI portion of the component indicates changes to gray matter concentration throughout the frontal and parietal lobes. Note that the clustering performance of the overall model has improved significantly by modeling more relevant structure in sMRI compared to the case where there is no centering. The model fit is 69, 47, and 70% for EEG, fMRI, and sMRI, respectively. In order to increase the model fits, in particular for fMRI, when we increase the number of components to $R = 15$, a unique model can still be obtained with model fits 78, 64, and 79% for EEG, fMRI, and sMRI, respectively. In that case, however, only a single statistically significant component (p-value=1.4×10^{-4}) that is similar to **Figure 4B**, is captured. The clustering performance of the 15-component ACMTF model is similar to the 10-component case. These observations indicate that the model is consistent to some degree across models with different numbers of components, by still revealing one of the significant components. The additional components explain some of the remaining information in the data sets but do not reveal any additional significant components in terms of distinguishing between the groups. The results show that they still help with increasing the significance of the relevant component by modeling the structure not contributing to the discrimination of patients and controls.

4. DISCUSSION

In this paper, we have jointly analyzed multi-modal neuroimaging signals, namely, EEG, fMRI, and sMRI, collected from patients with schizophrenia and healthy controls, using a structure-revealing CMTF model. The model captures temporal as well as functional/structural spatial patterns that can differentiate between patients and healthy controls. Compared to traditional fusion approaches, such as jICA, the structure-revealing CMTF model enables us to exploit the multilinear structure of multi-channel EEG signals providing both interpretable patterns and improved uniqueness properties without imposing additional constraints on the extracted patterns. Through joint analysis of EEG, and fMRI, the following temporal and spatial patterns are identified as potential biomarkers:

- Pattern 1: The temporal part referring to the P2-N2 transition as well as the P3 peak, and the functional spatial part showing increased activation of controls over patients in the sensorimotor cortex.
- Pattern 2: The temporal part referring to the P3 peak, and the functional spatial part indicating a decrease in activation of controls vs. patients in some regions of the sensorimotor cortex and parietal lobe.

The biomarkers that are extracted using the ACMTF model correspond to signals observed in previous investigations of the structural and functional impacts of schizophrenia. The EEG signals are similar to those observed in previous schizophrenia research (Calhoun et al., 2010; Kayser et al., 2010). Additionally, the regions in spatial patterns have also been shown to be affected in patients with schizophrenia previously (Schroder et al., 1999; Wolf et al., 2008; Minzenberg et al., 2009). Through the incorporation of the sMRI data, these patterns have been complemented with the following structural spatial parts: (i) Pattern 1, the structural spatial part indicating an increase in concentration of gray matter in controls over patients in sections of the parietal lobe and cerebellum. (ii) Pattern 2, the structural spatial part showing increases in gray matter for controls over patients in multiple portions of the frontal and parietal lobes. All three regions have been shown to be impacted in patients with schizophrenia (Shenton et al., 2010; Olabi et al., 2011; Brent et al., 2013; Lungu et al., 2013). These patterns are reproducible and have been revealed even in the case of changes in data sets, as we have illustrated by leaving out data from one subject at a time and in our preliminary studies on a slightly different set of subjects (Acar et al., 2017b) and using a subset of electrodes (Acar et al., 2017a).

Any method targeting biomarker discovery must capture the underlying patterns corresponding to the potential biomarkers uniquely; therefore, in this paper, we have used the structure-revealing CMTF model that focuses on unique identification of underlying patterns when jointly analyzing multi-modal data sets with shared and unshared factors, rather than other CMTF methods that have proved useful in missing data estimation applications (where uniqueness of underlying patterns is not of interest) (Zheng et al., 2010; Ermis et al., 2015). In addition to the patterns interpreted as potential biomarkers, the structure-revealing CMTF model also reveals weights of the patterns that can be used to identify shared/unshared patterns in each data set and quantify the contribution from each data set. In joint analysis of EEG and fMRI, all components, including the statistically significant components differentiating between patients and controls, correspond to shared components. Similarly, in joint analysis of EEG, fMRI, and sMRI, as long as necessary preprocessing steps, such as centering are carried out as discussed in section 3.3, all components are shared among three modalities as shown in **Figure S5**.

The structure-revealing CMTF model relies on the hard coupling assumption, i.e., the factor vectors in the coupled (e.g., subject) mode are exactly the same in different modalities for the shared factors. That is a strong assumption, which may be relaxed using soft coupling approaches (Seichepine et al., 2013; Farias et al., 2016), e.g., having different factor matrices in the coupled mode and penalizing the distance between the factor matrices based on various norms, as in Rivet et al. (2015) when jointly analyzing EEG and electro-ocular artifacts, or as in Chatzichristos et al. (2018) when jointly analyzing EEG and raw fMRI signals. However, a hard coupling-based approach may be preferable in noisy cases (Adali et al., 2015b). Therefore, whether or not it is a limitation is an open research question.

One potential drawback of the structure-revealing CMTF model is sensitivity to its parameters, i.e., the number of components, R, and the sparsity penalty parameter, β. Despite the sensitivity, we have consistently observed similar statistically significant patterns for different number of components, as shown in **Table 1** in terms of FMS values. Note that FMS takes into account every entry in the factor vectors (i.e., many voxels in the fMRI) and it is rather a strict measure. Therefore, we have observed that even for lower FMS values, interpretations of the captured patterns are the same visually (e.g., **Figure 4** vs. **Figure S2**). Another challenge as a result of sensitivity to model parameters is that the model must be experimentally validated to be unique. An important future research direction is to study the landscape of the optimization problem and develop ways to make the problem less sensitive to parameters as well as the initialization. A theoretical understanding of the uniqueness properties of the structure-revealing CMTF model would also significantly mitigate this challenge. Recent work on uniqueness (Lathauwer and Kofidis, 2017) of coupled matrix and tensor factorizations provides a step in this direction studying the indeterminacies in CMTF in the presence of unshared factors. Furthermore, while we have used the same sparsity penalty parameter for all data sets in this paper, in some applications, this parameter may need to be data-specific depending on the structure of each data set.

While data fusion methods are of interest in many disciplines, preprocessing steps have not been well-studied within the framework of data fusion. In this paper, we have shown that while centering across the subject mode does not affect the joint analysis of EEG and fMRI data, it has a dramatic effect when the sMRI data is incorporated, and the interpretation of the component weights changes significantly. In addition to such preprocessing steps, there are further steps that should be carefully incorporated to data fusion methods, such as outlier removal, residual analysis, which may also enable better tools for selecting the number of components.

This paper is a systematic study of the structure-revealing CMTF model for biomarker discovery but with limited number of subjects. In order to see the real promise of the method as a biomarker discovery approach and assess the validity of the potential biomarkers for schizophrenia, joint analysis of EEG, fMRI, and sMRI signals must be carried out on a larger set of subjects and also including patients with different neurological disorders. There are increasingly more studies exploiting the multilinear structure of different neuroimaging signals (Andersen and Rayens, 2004; Davidson et al., 2013; He et al., 2014; Ferdowsi et al., 2015; Madsen et al., 2017; Chatzichristos et al., 2018, 2019; Williams et al., 2018), and understanding the advantages and limitations of CMTF-based approaches, that can exploit those multilinear structures, is crucial as the fusion of multimodal neuroimaging data holds promise to enhance biomarker discovery.

AUTHOR CONTRIBUTIONS

EA and TA conceived the project. EA, YL-S, and TA designed the experiments. EA and CS performed the data analysis. YL-S, TA, and VC interpreted the extracted patterns. EA, CS, YL-S, and TA were involved in the preparation of the manuscript. All authors have given approval to the final version of the manuscript.

FUNDING

This work has been funded in part by the following grants: NSF-CCF 1618551, NSF-NCS 1631838, NIH-NIBIB R01EB005846, and NIH-T32 HD049311.

REFERENCES

Acar, E., Bingol, C. A., Bingol, H., Bro, R., and Yener, B. (2007). Multiway analysis of epilepsy tensors. *Bioinformatics.* 23, i10–i18. doi: 10.1093/bioinformatics/btm210

Acar, E., Bro, R., and Smilde, A. K. (2015). Data fusion in metabolomics using coupled matrix and tensor factorizations. *Proc. IEEE.* 103, 1602–1620. doi: 10.1109/JPROC.2015.2438719

Acar, E., Dunlavy, D. M., and Kolda, T. G. (2011). A scalable optimization approach for fitting canonical tensor decompositions. *J. Chemometr.* 25, 67–86. doi: 10.1002/cem.1335

Acar, E., Levin-Schwartz, Y., Calhoun, V., and Adali, T. (2017a). "ACMTF for fusion of multi-modal neuroimaging data and identification of biomarkers," in *Eusipco'17: Proceedings of the 25th European Signal Processing Conference* (Kos), 673–677. doi: 10.23919/EUSIPCO.2017.8081286

Acar, E., Levin-Schwartz, Y., Calhoun, V. D., and Adali, T. (2017b). "Tensor-based fusion of EEG and FMRI to understand neurological changes in schizophrenia," in *ISCAS '17: Proceedings of IEEE International Symposium on Circuits and Systems* (Baltimore, MD), 314–317. doi: 10.1109/ISCAS.2017.8050303

Acar, E., Papalexakis, E. E., Gurdeniz, G., Rasmussen, M. A., Lawaetz, A. J., Nilsson, M., et al. (2014). Structure-revealing data fusion. *BMC Bioinform.* 15:239. doi: 10.1186/1471-2105-15-239

Adali, T., Schwartz, Y. L., and Calhoun, V. D. (2015a). Multimodal data fusion using source separation: application to medical imaging. *Proc. IEEE.* 103, 1494–1506. doi: 10.1109/JPROC.2015.2461601

Adali, T., Schwartz, Y. L., and Calhoun, V. D. (2015b). Multimodal data fusion using source separation: two effective models based on ica and iva and their properties. *Proc. IEEE.* 103, 1478–1493. doi: 10.1109/JPROC.2015.2461624

Alter, O., Brown, P. O., and Botstein, D. (2003). Generalized singular value decomposition for comparative analysis of genome-scale expression data sets of two different organisms. *PNAS.* 100, 3351–3356. doi: 10.1073/pnas.0530258100

Andersen, A. H., and Rayens, W. S. (2004). Structure-seeking multilinear methods for the analysis of fMRI data. *Neuroimage.* 22, 728–739. doi: 10.1016/j.neuroimage.2004.02.026

Ashburner, J., and Friston, K. J. (2000). Voxel-based morphometry–the methods. *Neuroimage.* 11, 805 - 821. doi: 10.1006/nimg.2000.0582

Becker, H., Comon, P., and Albera, L. (2012). "Tensor-based processing of combined EEG/MEG data," in *Eusipco'12: Proceedings of the 20th European Signal Processing Conference* (Bucharest), 275–279.

Brent, B. K., Thermenos, H. W., Keshavan, M. S., and Seidman, L. J. (2013). Gray matter alterations in schizophrenia high-risk youth and early-onset schizophrenia. *Child Adolesc. Psychiatr. Clin. N. Am.* 22, 689–714. doi: 10.1016/j.chc.2013.06.003

Bro, R., and Smilde, A. K. (2003). Centering and scaling in component analysis. *J. Chemometr.* 17, 16–33. doi: 10.1002/cem.773

Bunge, S. A., and Kahn, I. (2009). Cognition: an overview of neuroimaging techniques. *Encyc. Neurosci.* 2, 1063–1067. doi: 10.1016/B978-008045046-9.00298-9

Calhoun, V., Adali, T., Giuliani, N., Pekar, J., Kiehl, K., and Pearlson, G. (2006a). Method for multimodal analysis of independent source differences in schizophrenia: combining gray matter structural and auditory oddball functional data. *Hum. Brain Mapp.* 27, 47–62. doi: 10.1002/hbm.20166

Calhoun, V., Adali, T., Pearlson, G., and Kiehl, K. (2006b). Neuronal chronometry of target detection: fusion of hemodynamic and event-related potential data. *Neuroimage.* 30, 544–553. doi: 10.1016/j.neuroimage.2005.08.060

Calhoun, V., Wu, L., Kiehl, K., Eichele, T., and Pearlson, G. (2010). Aberrant processing of deviant stimuli in schizophrenia revealed by fusion of FMRI and EEG data. *Acta Neuropsychiatr.* 22, 127–138. doi: 10.1111/j.1601-5215.2010.00467.x

Calhoun, V. D., Liu, J., and Adali, T. (2009). A review of group ICA for fMRI data and ICA for joint inference of imaging, genetic, and ERP data. *Neuroimage.* 45, S163–S172. doi: 10.1016/j.neuroimage.2008.10.057

Carroll, J. D., and Chang, J. J. (1970). Analysis of individual differences in multidimensional scaling via an N-way generalization of "Eckart-Young" decomposition. *Psychometrika.* 35, 283–319.

Chatzichristos, C., Davies, M., Escudero, J., Kofidis, E., and Theodoridis, S. (2018). "Fusion of EEG and fMRI via soft coupled tensor decompositions," in *Eusipco'18: Proceedings of the 26th European Signal Processing Conference* (Rome). doi: 10.23919/EUSIPCO.2018.8553077

Chatzichristos, C., Kofidis, E., Morante, M., and Theodoridis, S. (2019). Blind fMRI source unmixing via higher-order tensor decompositions. *J. Neurosci. Methods.* 315, 17–47. doi: 10.1016/j.jneumeth.2018.12.007

Cong, F., Lin, Q.-H., Kuang, L.-D., Gong, X.-F., Astikainen, P., and Ristaniemi, T. (2015). Tensor decomposition of EEG signals: a brief review. *J. Neurosci. Methods.* 248, 59–69. doi: 10.1016/j.jneumeth.2015.03.018

Dahne, S., Biebmann, F., Samek, W., Haufe, S., Goltz, D., Gundlach, C., et al. (2015). Multivariate machine learning methods for fusing multimodal functional neuroimaging data. *Proc. IEEE.* 103, 1507–1530. doi: 10.1109/JPROC.2015.2425807

Daunizeau, J., Laufs, H., and Friston, K. J. (2009). "EEG–fMRI information fusion: Biophysics and data analysis," in *EEG–fMRI,* eds C. Mulert and L. Lemieux (Berlin; Heidelberg: Springer), 511–526.

Davidson, I., Gilpin, S., Carmichael, O., and Walker, P. (2013). "Network discovery via constrained tensor analysis of fMRI data," in *KDD '13: Proceedings of the 19th ACM SIGKDD International Conference on Knowledge Discovery and Data Mining* (Chicago, IL), 194–202. doi: 10.1145/2487575.2487619

De Vos, M., Vergult, A., De Lathauwer, L., De Clercq, W., Van Huffel, S., Dupont, P., et al. (2007). Canonical decomposition of ictal scalp EEG reliably detects the seizure onset zone. *Neuroimage.* 37, 844–854. doi: 10.1016/j.neuroimage.2007.04.041

Delorme, A., and Makeig, S. (2004). EEGLAB: an open source toolbox for analysis of single-trial EEG dynamics. *J. Neurosci. Methods.* 134, 9–21. doi: 10.1016/j.jneumeth.2003.10.009

Du, W., Levin-Schwartz, Y., Fu, G. D., Ma, S., Calhoun, V. D., and Adali, T. (2016). The role of diversity in complex ICA algorithms for fMRI analysis. *J. Neurosci. Methods.* 264, 129–135. doi: 10.1016/j.jneumeth.2016.03.012

Ermis, B., Acar, E., and Cemgil, A. T. (2015). Link prediction in heterogeneous data via generalized coupled tensor factorization. *Data Mining Knowl. Discov.* 29, 203–236. doi: 10.1007/s10618-013-0341-y

Eyndhoven, S. V., Hunyadi, B., De Lathauwer, L., and Van Huffel, S. (2017). "Flexible data fusion of EEG-fMRI: revealing neural-hemodynamic coupling through structured matrix-tensor factorization," in *Eusipco'17: Proceedings of the 25th European Signal Processing Conference* (Kos), 26–30. doi: 10.23919/EUSIPCO.2017.8081162

Farias, R. C., Cohen, J. E., and Comon, P. (2016). Exploring multimodal data fusion through joint decompositions with flexible couplings. *IEEE Trans. Signal Process.* 64, 4830–4844. doi: 10.1109/TSP.2016.2576425

Ferdowsi, S., Abolghasemi, V., and Sanei, S. (2015). A new informed tensor factorization approach to EEG–fMRI fusion. *J. Neurosci. Methods.* 254, 27–35. doi: 10.1016/j.jneumeth.2015.07.018

First, M. B., Spitzer, R. L., Miriam, G., and Williams, J. B. (2002a). *Structured Clinical Interview for DSM-IV: Non-Patient Edition (SCID-NP).* New York, NY: Biometrics Research, New York State Psychiatric Institute.

First, M. B., Spitzer, R. L., Miriam, G., and Williams, J. B. (2002b). *Structured Clinical Interview for DSM-IV-TR Axis I Disorders, Research Version, Patient Edition. (SCID-I/P).* New York, NY: Biometrics Research, New York State Psychiatric Institute.

Freire, L., and Mangin, J.-F. (2001). Motion correction algorithms may create spurious brain activations in the absence of subject motion. *Neuroimage.* 14, 709–722. doi: 10.1006/nimg.2001.0869

Good, C. D., Johnsrude, I. S., Ashburner, J., Henson, R. N., Friston, K. J., and Frackowiak, R. S. (2001). A voxel-based morphometric study of ageing in 465 normal adult human brains. *Neuroimage.* 14, 21–36. doi: 10.1006/nimg.2001.0786

Groves, A. R., Beckmann, C. F., Smith, S. M., and Woolrich, M. W. (2011). Linked independent component analysis for multimodal data fusion. *Neuroimage.* 54, 2198–2217. doi: 10.1016/j.neuroimage.2010.09.073

Harshman, R. A. (1970). Foundations of the PARAFAC procedure: models and conditions for an "explanatory" multi-modal factor analysis. *UCLA Working Papers Phonetics.* 16, 1–84.

He, L., Kong, X., Yu, P. S., Ragin, A. B., Hao, Z., and Yang, X. (2014). "Dusk: a dual structure-preserving kernel for supervised tensor learning with applications to neuroimages," in *SDM'14: Proceedings of the SIAM International Conference on Data Mining,* 127–135. doi: 10.1137/1.9781611973440.15

Hitchcock, F. L. (1927). The expression of a tensor or a polyadic as a sum of products. *J. Math. Phys.* 6, 164–189.

Hunyadi, B., Dupont, P., Paesschen, W. V., and Huffel, S. V. (2017). Tensor decompositions and data fusion in epileptic electroencephalography and functional magnetic resonance imaging data. *WIREs Data Mining Knowl. Discov.* 7:e1197. doi: 10.1002/widm.1197

Hunyadi, B., Paesschen, W. V., De Vos, M., and Van Huffel, S. (2016). "Fusion of electroencephalography and functional magnetic resonance imaging to explore epileptic network activity," in *Eusipco' 16: Proceedings of the 24th European Signal Processing Conference* (Budapest), 240–244. doi: 10.1109/EUSIPCO.2016.7760246

Jung, T.-P., Makeig, S., Humphries, C., Lee, T.-W., McKeown, M. J., Iragui, V., et al. (2000). Removing electroencephalographic artifacts by blind source separation. *Psychophysiology.* 37, 163–178. doi: 10.1111/1469-8986.3720163

Karahan, E., Rojas-Lopez, P. A., Bringas-Vega, M. L., Valdes-Hernandez, P. A., and Valdes-Sosa, P. A. (2015). Tensor analysis and fusion of multimodal brain images. *Proc. IEEE.* 103, 1531–1559. doi: 10.1109/JPROC.2015.2455028

Kayser, J., Tenke, C. E., Gil, R., and Bruder, G. E. (2010). ERP generator patterns in schizophrenia during tonal and phonetic oddball tasks: effects of response hand and silent count. *Clin. EEG Neurosci.* 41, 184–195. doi: 10.1177/155005941004100405

Kiehl, K. A., Stevens, M. C., Laurens, K. R., Pearlson, G., Calhoun, V. D., and Liddle, P. F. (2005). An adaptive reflexive processing model of neurocognitive function: supporting evidence from a large scale (n = 100) fmri study of an auditory oddball task. *Neuroimage.* 25, 899–915. doi: 10.1016/j.neuroimage.2004.12.035

Klami, A., Virtanen, S., and Kaski, S. (2013). Bayesian canonical correlation analysis. *J. Mach. Learn. Res.* 14, 965–1003. Available online at: http://www.jmlr.org/papers/v14/klami13a.html

Kolda, T. G., and Bader, B. W. (2009). Tensor decompositions and applications. *SIAM Rev.* 51, 455–500. doi: 10.1137/07070111X

Kruskal, J. B. (1977). Three-way arrays: rank and uniqueness of trilinear decompositions, with application to arithmetic complexity and statistics. *Linear Algebra Appl.* 18, 95–138. doi: 10.1016/0024-3795(77)90069-6

Lathauwer, L. D., and Kofidis, E. (2017). "Coupled matrix-tensor factorizations–the case of partially shared factors," in *ASILOMAR'17: Proceedings of the Asilomar Conference on Signals, Systems and Computers* (Pacific Grove, CA). doi: 10.1109/ACSSC.2017.8335436

Li, X.-L., and Adali, T. (2010). Independent component analysis by entropy bound minimization. *IEEE Trans. Signal Process.* 58, 5151–5164. doi: 10.1109/TSP.2010.2055859

Liu, J., Kiehl, K. A., Pearlson, G., Perrone-Bizzozero, N. I., Eichele, T., and Calhoun, V. D. (2009). Genetic determinants of target and novelty-related event-related potentials in the auditory oddball response. *Neuroimage.* 46, 809–816. doi: 10.1016/j.neuroimage.2009.02.045

Liu, S., Liu, S., Cai, W., Che, H., Pujol, S., Kikinis, R., et al., (2015). Multimodal neuroimaging feature learning for multiclass diagnosis of Alzheimer's disease. *IEEE Trans. Biomed. Eng.* 62, 1132–1140. doi: 10.1109/TBME.2014.2372011

Lock, E. F., Hoadley, K. A., Marron, J., and Nobel, A. B. (2013). Joint and individual variation explained (jive) for integrated analysis of multiple data types. *Ann. Appl. Stat.* 7, 523–542. doi: 10.1214/12-AOAS597

Lungu, O., Barakat, M., Laventure, S., Debas, K., Proulx, S., Luck, D., et al. (2013). The incidence and nature of cerebellar findings in schizophrenia: a quantitative review of fMRI literature. *Schizophr. Bull.* 39, 797–806. doi: 10.1093/schbul/sbr193

Madsen, K. H., Churchill, N. W., and Mørup, M. (2017). Quantifying functional connectivity in multi-subject fMRI data using component models. *Hum. Brain Mapp.* 38, 882–899. doi: 10.1002/hbm.23425

Minzenberg, M. J., Laird, A. R., Thelen, S., Carter, C. S., and Glahn, D. C. (2009). Meta-analysis of 41 functional neuroimaging studies of executive function in schizophrenia. *Arch. Gen. Psychiatry.* 66, 811–822. doi: 10.1001/archgenpsychiatry.2009.91

Miwakeichi, F., Martínez-Montes, E., Valdés-Sosa, P. A., Nishiyama, N., Mizuhara, H., and Yamaguchi, Y. (2004). Decomposing EEG data into space-time-frequency components using parallel factor analysis. *Neuroimage.* 22, 1035–1045. doi: 10.1016/j.neuroimage.2004.03.039

Möcks, J. (1988). Topographic components model for event-related potentials and some biophysical considerations. *IEEE Trans. Biomed. Eng.* 35, 482–484.

Mørup, M., Hansen, L. K., and Arnfred, S. M. (2007). ERPWAVELAB a toolbox for multi-channel analysis of time - frequency transformed event related potentials. *J. Neurosci. Methods.* 161, 361–368. doi: 10.1016/j.jneumeth.2006.11.008

Naskovska, K., Korobkov, A. A., Haardt, M., and Haueisen, J. (2017). "Analysis of the photic driving effect via joint EEG and MEG data processing based on the coupled CP decomposition," in *Eusipco'17: Proceedings of the 25th European Signal Processing Conference* (Kos), 1325–1329. doi: 10.23919/EUSIPCO.2017.8081415

Olabi, B., Ellison-Wright, I., McIntosh, A. M., Wood, S. J., Bullmore, E., and Lawrie, S. M. (2011). Are there progressive brain changes in schizophrenia? A meta-analysis of structural magnetic resonance imaging studies. *Biol. Psychiatry.* 70, 88–96. doi: 10.1016/j.biopsych.2011.01.032

Rivet, B., Duda, M., Guerin-Dugue, A., Jutten, C., and Comon, P. (2015). "Multimodal approach to estimate the ocular movements during EEG recordings: a coupled tensor factorization method," in *EMBC'15: Proceedings of 37th Annual International Conference of the IEEE Engineering in Medicine and Biology Society* (Milan). doi: 10.1109/EMBC.2015.7319999

Schroder, J., Essig, M., Baudendistel, K., Jahn, T., Gerdsen, I., Stockert, A., et al. (1999). Motor dysfunction and sensorimotor cortex activation changes in schizophrenia: a study with functional magnetic resonance imaging. *Neuroimage.* 9, 81–87.

Seichepine, N., Essid, S., Févotte, C., and Cappé, O. (2013). "Soft nonnegative matrix co-factorization with application to multimodal speaker diarization," in *ICASSP'13: Proceedings of the IEEE Int. Conf. on Acoustics, Speech and Signal* (Vancouver, BC). doi: 10.1109/ICASSP.2013.6638316

Shenton, M. E., Whitford, T. J., and Kubicki, M. (2010). Structural neuroimaging in schizophrenia: from methods to insights to treatments. *Dialog. Clin. Neurosci.* 12, 317–332.

Sidiropoulos, N. D., and Bro, R. (2000). On the uniqueness of multilinear decomposition of N-way arrays. *J. Chemometr.* 14, 229–239. doi: 10.1002/1099-128X(200005/06)14:3<229::AID-CEM587>3.0.CO;2-N

Smilde, A. K., Mage, I., Naes, T., Hankemeier, T., Lips, M. A., Kiers, H. A., et al. (2017). Common and distinct components in data fusion. *J. Chemometr.* 31:e2900. doi: 10.1002/cem.2900

Sorensen, M., and De Lathauwer, L. (2015). Coupled canonical polyadic decompositions and (coupled) decompositions in multilinear rank $-(l_{r,n}, l_{r,n}, 1)$ terms — part i: Uniqueness. *SIAM J. Matrix Anal. Appl.* 36, 496–522. doi: 10.1137/140956853

Sui, J., Qi, S., van Erp, T. G. M., Bustillo, J., Jiang, R., Lin, D., et al. (2018). Multimodal neuromarkers in schizophrenia via cognition-guided MRI fusion. *Nat. Commun.* 9:3028. doi: 10.1038/s41467-018-05432-w

Sui, J., Yu, Q., He, H., Pearlson, G. D., and Calhoun, V. D. (2012). A selective review of multimodal fusion methods in schizophrenia. *Front. Hum. Neurosci.* 6:27. doi: 10.3389/fnhum.2012.00027

Swinnen, W., Hunyadi, B., Acar, E., Van Huffel, S., and Vos, M. D. (2014). "Incorporating higher dimensionality in joint decomposition of EEG and fMRI," in *Eusipco'14: Proceedings of the 22nd European Signal Processing Conference* (Lisbon), 121–125.

Takahashi, T., and Suzuki, M. (2018). Brain morphologic changes in early stages of psychosis: implications for clinical application and early intervention. *Psychiatry Clin. Neurosci.* 72, 556–571. doi: 10.1111/pcn.12670

Uludag, K., and Roebroeck, A. (2014). General overview on the merits of multimodal neuroimaging data fusion. *Neuroimage.* 102, 3–10. doi: 10.1016/j.neuroimage.2014.05.018

Williams, A. H., Kim, T. H., Wang, F., Vyas, S., Ryu, S. I., Shenoy, K. V., et al. (2018). Unsupervised discovery of demixed, low-dimensional neural dynamics across multiple timescales through tensor component analysis. *Neuron.* 98, 1099–1115. doi: 10.1016/j.neuron.2018.05.015

Wolf, D. H., Turetsky, B. I., Loughead, J., Elliott, M. A., Pratiwadi, R., Gur, R. E., et al. (2008). Auditory oddball fMRI in schizophrenia: association of negative symptoms with regional hypoactivation to novel distractors. *Brain Imaging Behav.* 2, 132–145. doi: 10.1007/s11682-008-9022-7

Zheng, V. W., Cao, B., Zheng, Y., Xie, X., and Yang, Q. (2010). "Collaborative filtering meets mobile recommendation: a user-centered approach," in *AAAI'10: Proceedings of the 24th Conf. on Artificial Intelligence* (Atlanta, GA), 236–241.

17

Spatial Dynamic Functional Connectivity Analysis Identifies Distinctive Biomarkers in Schizophrenia

Suchita Bhinge [1]*, Qunfang Long [1], Vince D. Calhoun [2,3] and Tülay Adali [1]

[1] Department of Computer Science and Electrical Engineering, University of Maryland Baltimore County, Baltimore, MD, United States, [2] The Mind Research Network, Albuquerque, NM, United States, [3] Department of Electrical and Computer Engineering, University of New Mexico, Albuquerque, NM, United States

****Correspondence:***
Suchita Bhinge
suchita1@umbc.edu

Dynamic functional network connectivity (dFNC) analysis is a widely-used to study associations between dynamic functional correlations and cognitive abilities. Traditional methods analyze time-varying association of different spatial networks while assuming that the spatial network itself is stationary. However, there has been very little work focused on voxelwise spatial variability. Exploiting the variability across both the temporal and spatial domains provide a more promising direction to obtain reliable dynamic functional patterns. However, methods for extracting time-varying spatio-temporal patterns from large-scale functional magnetic resonance imaging (fMRI) data present some challenges, such as degradation in performance with respect to increase in size of the data, estimation of the number of dynamic components, and the potential sensitivity of the resulting dFNCs to selection of the networks. In this work, we implement subsequent extraction of exemplars and dynamics using a constrained independent vector analysis, a data-driven method that efficiently estimates spatial and temporal dynamics from large-scale resting-state fMRI data. We explore the benefits of analyzing spatial dFNC (sdFNC) patterns over temporal dFNC (tdFNC) patterns in the context of differentiating healthy controls and patients with schizophrenia. Our results indicate that for resting-state fMRI data, sdFNC patterns were able to better classify patients and controls, and yield more distinguishing features compared with tdFNC patterns. We also estimate structured patterns of connectivity/states using sdFNC patterns, an area that has not been studied so far, and observe that sdFNC was able to successfully capture distinct information from healthy controls and patients with schizophrenia. In addition, sdFNC patterns were also able to identify functional patterns that associate with signs of paranoia and abnormalities in the patients group. We also observe that patients with schizophrenia tend to switch to or stay in a state corresponding to a hyperconnected brain network.

Keywords: prediction, dynamic functional connectivity, independent vector analysis, schizophrenia, spatio-temporal, states

1. INTRODUCTION

Dynamic functional network connectivity (dFNC) analyzes the time-varying associations among different regions of the brain and has been widely studied in order to identify correlations between functional changes and cognitive abilities (Fox et al., 2005; Chang and Glover, 2010; Sakoğlu et al., 2010). In order to identify these functional patterns of different brain regions, conventional methods identify groups of temporally coherent voxels, referred to as spatial maps, and their corresponding activation patterns, referred to as time courses (Lee et al., 2013). Followed by the estimation of time courses, a sliding window is applied on the time courses that divides it into consecutive windows and an analysis on the time points within each window is performed (Allen et al., 2014). The analysis of dFNC patterns depends on the length of the window, where the use of a longer window length increases the risk of averaging the temporal fluctuations of interest resulting in false negatives (Preti et al., 2017), and the use of a shorter window length has too few samples for a reliable computation of correlation (Hero and Rajaratnam, 2016), resulting in the temporal variations to capture spurious fluctuations and increasing the risk of false positives (Sakoğlu et al., 2010; Hutchison et al., 2013; Leonardi and Van De Ville, 2015). Previous studies have shown that a window length between 30 and 60 s successfully estimates temporal fluctuations in resting-state functional magnetic resonance imaging (fMRI) data (Preti et al., 2017), and for most cases higher window lengths do not alter the results significantly (Keilholz et al., 2013; Li et al., 2014; Liégeois et al., 2016). However, there is a lower bound in being able to capture fluctuations due to the limited number of samples, limiting the use of dFNC analysis in the temporal domain.

Conventional methods also estimate the time-varying FNC patterns of the spatial networks while assuming that the spatial network itself is stationary. However, studies have shown that changes in the FNC patterns imply changes in the spatial networks (Calhoun et al., 2008). Hence, spatio-temporal dFNC analysis relaxes the assumption of stationarity in both the spatial and temporal domain, and provides a more general framework for capturing time-varying FNC patterns (Ma et al., 2014; Kottaram et al., 2018; Kunert-Graf et al., 2018). The availability of higher number of samples in the spatial domain also guarantees reliable estimation of functional correlations (Hero and Rajaratnam, 2016), thus providing a promising direction for the use of spatial domain for dFNC analysis. However, the methods used to extract time-varying spatio-temporal patterns face few challenges. Region of interest based methods use pre-defined resting-state networks causing the estimated functional connectivity to be sensitive to network selection. Dynamic mode decomposition, a spatio-temporal modal decomposition technique, requires significant dimension reduction that may restrict the method to estimate fewer dynamic components (Kunert-Graf et al., 2018). Independent vector analysis (IVA) provides a general and flexible framework to spatio-temporal dFNC analysis and estimates window-specific time courses and spatial maps. However its performance degrades with increase in the size of the data, for a given number of samples (Bhinge et al., 2019). Hence, in this work, we use a data-driven method to jointly extract spatio-temporal patterns using the subsequent extraction of exemplar and dynamic components using constrained IVA (SED-cIVA) method (Bhinge et al., 2019), from a large-scale fMRI data acquired from 91 healthy controls and 88 patients with schizophrenia. This two-stage method preserves variability in both domains while addressing the issue with large-scale data, by using a parameter tuning technique. This parameter tuning technique adapts to the variability of each brain region separately, thus allowing accurate estimation of time-varying spatial maps and corresponding time courses.

Although exploiting variability in the spatial domain for dFNC analysis has shown better performance in terms of classification using a seed-based analysis (Kottaram et al., 2018), which is sensitive to the networks selected, the features extracted from sdFNC patterns are not explored. In this work, we explore the use of spatial domain for dFNC analysis in order to demonstrate the benefits of exploiting variability in the spatial domain and taking advantage of the large sample size in this domain, using a data-driven approach. We perform a prediction technique to compare the ability of temporal dFNC (tdFNC) patterns and sdFNC patterns to predict if a subject is a patient or a control. We also perform a joint analysis by combining the sdFNC and tdFNC patterns together in order to explore the contribution of each toward prediction and observe that the use of sdFNC patterns alone provides higher prediction accuracy than using tdFNC patterns, or a combined feature set. This shows that exploiting the variability and taking advantage of large sample size in the spatial domain provides meaningful discriminative features. We also obtain structured patterns of connectivity/states from sdFNC patterns and identify differences between patients and controls in terms of dwell time, transition matrix and fraction of time spent in each state. To the best of our knowledge, no study has been performed to identify these properties from sdFNC patterns. Our results indicate that patients tend to stay in or transition between states associated with hyperconnected brain network. We also find significant associations between the resulting functional connectivity and signs of paranoia in the patient group using sdFNC patterns.

The remainder of the paper is organized as follows. Section 2 introduces the dataset used in this work and the method used for extraction of spatio-temporal dynamic patterns. This section also discusses the prediction technique followed by the method used for estimating states. Section 3 shows the results and discusses these results. Section 4 concludes the paper.

2. MATERIALS AND METHODS

2.1. Material

We work with resting-state fMRI data is acquired from $K = 179$ subjects including 91 healthy controls (HCs) (average age: 38 ± 12) and 88 patients with schizophrenia (SZs) (average age: 37 ± 14). The dataset was obtained from the Center for Biomedical Research Excellence (COBRE) (Aine et al., 2017) and is available on the collaborative informatics and neuroimaging suite data exchange repository (https://coins.trendscenter.org/) (Scott et al., 2011). The data was obtained over the duration of

5 min with a sampling period of 2 s yielding 150 timepoints per subject. The subjects were asked to keep their eyes open during the entire scanning period. Each subject's data was pre-processed to account for motion correction, slice-time correction, spatial normalization and was slightly re-sampled to $3 \times 3 \times 3\,\text{mm}^3$ yielding $53 \times 63 \times 46$ voxels. The first 6 time points were removed to account for the T1-effect. We perform masking on each image volume to remove the non-brain voxels and flatten the result to form an observation vector of $V = 58{,}604$ voxels, giving $T = 144$ time evolving observations for each subject.

2.2. SED-cIVA

In this work, we use the SED-cIVA method to extract time-varying spatial and temporal patterns. SED-cIVA consists of two stages: the first stage extracts exemplar/informative components from all subjects and uses these components as reference signals in a sliding-window parameter-tuned cIVA framework in the second stage, to obtain the time-varying representation of these components. The idea of SED-cIVA is to extract stationary representation of the most informative resting-state networks from the given dataset, in the first stage followed by estimating the time-varying representation of these networks for each subject using a sliding-window approach. **Figure 1A** shows the flow-chart of the method.

2.2.1. Extraction of Exemplars

SED-cIVA provides flexibility in the choice of the method used to extract the exemplar components. Templates of resting-state networks of interest that are pre-defined based on extensive studies of resting-state fMRI data can be used as exemplars. Sparsity-learning methods such as dictionary learning (Varoquaux et al., 2011) or sparse ICA (Boukouvalas et al., 2017) can be used to extract more focal spatial components. One of the widely used methods for extraction of components from multiple subjects is group independent component analysis (GICA) that estimates a common subspace consisting of the most informative components across all subjects (Calhoun et al., 2001a,b). In this work, we perform GICA on all subjects to extract exemplars of resting-state networks using the group ICA for fMRI toolbox (GIFT). GICA performs a subject-level principal component analysis (PCA) to extract the signal subspace for each subject followed by a group-level PCA on the principal components (PCs) from all the subjects. In order to exploit higher order statistics, it performs independent component analysis (ICA) on the group-level PCs. We estimate the model order for each subject using the minimum description length criterion that accounts for sample dependence (Li et al., 2007) and the final order is selected as the mean (30) plus one standard deviation (5) across all subject's model orders. The dimension of the signal subspace in the subject-level PCA stage is set as 53 and the order for the group-level PCA stage is set as 35. By default, GIFT selects the subject-level PCA order (53) to be 1.5 times the final order (35). We use the entropy rate bound minimization (ERBM) algorithm (Li and Adali, 2010) to estimate the group-level independent components. ERBM is a flexible ICA algorithm that exploits multiple statistical properties of the sources such as sample dependence and higher order statistics, and provides a better estimation of fMRI sources (Long et al., 2018a). The ICA algorithm is run 10 times and the best run is selected using the minimum spanning tree approach (Du et al., 2014). Among the 35 group-level components, we visually select $N = 17$ components as exemplars, denoted as $\mathbf{d}_n$, $n = 1, \ldots, 17$, and these components are used as reference signals in the second stage.

2.2.2. Extraction of Spatial and Temporal Dynamics of Exemplars

In the second stage, time-varying representation of the exemplar components is estimated using a sliding-window IVA approach. In the sliding-window approach, each subject's data is divided into $M = 17$ windows of length $L = 16$ (32 s) with a 50% overlap. We extract time-varying spatio-temporal patterns of the exemplars by performing parameter-tuned cIVA on each subject's data. Parameter-tuned cIVA is a type of IVA that incorporates information regarding the exemplars into the IVA framework and extracts window-specific time courses and spatial maps of these exemplars. The general IVA model, for a given set of observations, can be written as $\mathbf{X}^{[m]} = \mathbf{A}^{[m]}\mathbf{S}^{[m]}, m = 1, \ldots, M$, where $\mathbf{X}^{[m]} \in \mathbb{R}^{L \times V}$ denotes the observations from window m, $\mathbf{A}^{[m]} \in \mathbb{R}^{L \times L}$ denotes the mixing matrix and the rows in $\mathbf{S}^{[m]} \in \mathbb{R}^{L \times V}$ are the latent sources. IVA estimates M demixing matrices, $\mathbf{W}^{[m]}$, such that the sources within each dataset are maximally independent and sources across dataset are maximally dependent. The cost function, written using random vector notation, is given as (Anderson et al., 2012; Adali et al., 2014),

$$\mathcal{J}_{\text{IVA}} = \sum_{l=1}^{L} \left[\sum_{m=1}^{M} \mathcal{H}\left(\hat{s}_l^{[m]}\right) - \mathcal{I}\left(\hat{\mathbf{s}}_l\right) \right] - \sum_{m=1}^{M} \log \left| \det \mathbf{W}^{[m]} \right|, \quad (1)$$

where $\mathcal{H}\left(\hat{s}_l^{[m]}\right)$ denotes the entropy of the lth source estimate for the mth dataset, and $\mathcal{I}\left(\mathbf{s}_l\right)$ denotes the mutual information of the lth source component vector (SCV) estimate, $\hat{\mathbf{s}}_l^{\mathrm{T}} = \left[\hat{s}_l^{[1]}, \ldots, \hat{s}_l^{[M]}\right]$. The optimization of Equation (1) jointly weighs the independence within the dataset through the entropy term along with the log determinant term and dependence across the datasets through the mutual information term. The dependent sources across datasets can be grouped together to form a SCV. Thus, in the SED-cIVA framework, IVA treats each window as a dataset and estimates window-specific time courses and spatial maps, and a SCV represents the time-varying representation of a spatial map. Parameter-tuned cIVA directs the estimation of the sources toward the reference components through an additional term in the IVA cost function given as,

$$\mathcal{J} = \mathcal{J}_{\text{IVA}} - \sum_{l=1}^{L} \frac{1}{2\gamma_n} \sum_{m=1}^{M} \left\{ \left[\max\{0, \mu_n^{[m]} + \gamma_n g(\hat{\mathbf{s}}_n^{[m]}, \mathbf{d}_n)\} \right]^2 - (\mu_n^{[m]})^2 \right\}, \quad (2)$$

where $\mu_n^{[m]}$ is the regularization parameter, γ_n is a positive scalar and $g(\hat{\mathbf{s}}_l^{[m]}, \mathbf{d}_n)$ is the inequality constraint function given as,

$$g(\hat{\mathbf{s}}_l^{[m]}, \mathbf{d}_n) = \rho_n - \left| \text{corr}(\hat{\mathbf{s}}_l^{[m]}, \mathbf{d}_n) \right| \leq 0. \quad (3)$$

The constraint parameter, ρ_n, controls the amount of correspondence between the exemplar, $\mathbf{d}_n$, and the estimated source, and acts as a lower bound for the amount of correlation between them. A higher value for this parameter enforces the estimated source to be exactly similar to the exemplar component, not allowing the other components to interact with the exemplar component. On the other hand, a lower value deviates the estimated source from the exemplar component causing the source to be prone to noise and other artifacts. Additionally, the interaction between an exemplar component and other components vary with respect windows and subjects, hence a fixed value for this parameter across all m and for all subjects does not allow the model to efficiently capture the variability across windows. Thus in order to capture the variability, SED-cIVA implements parameter-tuned cIVA, that adaptively selects a value from a set of possible values for ρ_n, denoted as $\mathcal{P}$, as follows,

$$\hat{\rho}_n = \arg\min_{\rho_n \in \mathcal{P}} \left[\min_{m} \left\{ \left| \rho_n - \left| \mathrm{corr}(\hat{\mathbf{s}}_l^{[m]}, \mathbf{d}_n) \right| \right| \right\}_{m=1}^{M} \right],$$
$$\mathcal{P} \in \{0.001, 0.1, \dots, 0.9\} \quad (4)$$

This updates computes $g(\hat{\mathbf{s}}_l^{[m]}, \mathbf{d}_n)$ for all m and for each value in set $\mathcal{P}$ and selects the highest value of ρ_n from set $\mathcal{P}$ that satisfies the condition in Equation (3) for all windows. From Equation (3), we observe that $\rho_n \leq \left|\mathrm{corr}(\hat{\mathbf{s}}_l^{[m]}, \mathbf{d}_n)\right|$, allowing ρ_n to be between 0 and 1. Thus, we define the set $\mathcal{P}$ as the possible values between 0 and 1. Hence, parameter-tuned cIVA selects the highest lower bound using Equation (4) and adaptively tunes itself with respect to each exemplar component, allowing the method to capture variability across windows. The use of exemplars also guides the solution toward the optimal solution addressing the issue of large-scale data that is observed in regular IVA, and relaxes the independence assumption of IVA (Bhinge et al., 2017). Hence SED-cIVA effectively captures variability of the exemplars across windows and subjects.

In parameter-tuned cIVA, we constrain one source at a time, $\hat{\mathbf{s}}_1^{[m]}$, to one of the exemplar components, $\mathbf{d}_n$, whereas the rest of the sources, $\hat{\mathbf{s}}_l^{[m]}$, $l = 2, \dots, L$, are unconstrained. For each $\mathbf{d}_n$, we obtain 10 solutions using parameter-tuned cIVA with $\gamma_n = 3, n = 1, \dots, N$, using the IVA-L-SOS algorithm for different random initializations and select the most consistent run using the method described in Long et al. (2018b). IVA-L-SOS is a type of IVA algorithm that assumes the sources are multivariate Laplacian distributed and exploits second order statistics (SOS) (Bhinge et al., 2019). This algorithm provides a better match to the properties of fMRI sources, since fMRI sources are in general expected to have a super-Gaussian distribution, like Laplacian (Calhoun and Adali, 2012), and are correlated across windows. The estimated sources corresponding to the constrained exemplars from the consistent run are denoted as $\mathbf{y}_n^{[m,k]}$, $n = 1, \dots, N$, $m = 1, \dots, M$, $k = 1, \dots, K$, whereas the corresponding time courses are denoted as $\mathbf{a}_n^{[m,k]}$.

2.3. Post-processing

SED-cIVA estimates time-varying spatial components and corresponding time courses for each exemplars that are further used to compute spatial and temporal dFNC matrices. The time courses at each window are further processed to remove quadratic, linear and cubic trends, and low-pass filtered with a cutoff frequency of 0.15 Hz (Allen et al., 2014). The tdFNC matrix at the mth time window for the kth subject is denoted as $R^{[m,k]}$. Each element in $R^{[m,k]}$ is obtained by computing the Pearson's correlation coefficient between each pair of the time courses in that time window, $r_{ij}^{[m,k]} = \mathrm{corr}\left(\mathbf{a}_i^{[m,k]}, \mathbf{a}_j^{[m,k]}\right)$, $i, j = 1, \dots, N$. Similarly sdFNC matrices are obtained by computing the Pearson's correlation coefficient between each pair of spatial maps at each time window. The correlation can be interpreted as the similarity in the activated sources in the spatial maps. Although IVA, like ICA, estimates spatial maps that are maximally independent within a time window, it also groups together the voxels that have a similar activation pattern (Calhoun and de Lacy, 2017). Hence, if in a time window two sources have a similar activation pattern these sources would be estimated as a single spatial map. Hence, we would expect a high correlation between the estimated spatial maps of the corresponding constrained sources. These matrices are further used to classify subjects as patients or controls, and to obtain spatial and temporal FC states. The post-analysis steps are shown in **Figure 1B**.

2.4. Prediction Technique

In order to study how informative the spatial and temporal dFNC features are, we evaluate the predictability of these features in terms of predicting if a subject is a patient or a control. Note that the aim of this experiment is to observe potential advantages of sdFNC features and not the actual prediction accuracy, hence we use a simpler Naïve Bayes classifier that does not require tuning of parameters. The flowchart for the prediction technique is shown in **Figure 2**. We obtain 1,000 independent Monte-Carlo subsamplings of the data. In each subsampling, subjects from HC and SZ group are divided into training and testing sets, where each training group consists of 75 randomly sampled subjects from the HC and the SZ group ($K_{\mathrm{train}} = 150$). The remaining subjects form the testing set ($K_{\mathrm{test}} = 29$). We then obtain $K_{\mathrm{train}} \times M$ observations of $N(N-1)/2$ dimensional features from the tdFNC/sdFNC matrices. In order to select the distinguishing features from the $N(N-1)/2$ features, we perform a two-sample t-test on the features from the HC and SZ group as shown in **Figure 2B**. Features that demonstrate significant difference ($p < 0.05$) are used in further stages. The indices of the significant features are recorded and used in the testing stage. This feature selection is done separately for tdFNC and sdFNC matrices. The selected features are clustered into C clusters, where in this experiment we vary the number of clusters from 3 to 30. For training the Naïve Bayes classifier, we obtain the probability of each state for the HC group and SZ group, $p^g(C_i)$, $g = \{\mathrm{HC}, \mathrm{SZ}\}$. In the testing stage, the features that indicated significant difference in the training stage were selected and each observation from a test subject is assigned a state with maximum Pearson's correlation between the observation and the cluster centroid. We then obtain the probability of each state using $p^{[k]}(C_i) = n_i^{[k]}/M$, $i = 1, \dots, C$ and use the test feature vector to predict the class of the subject. A test subject is assigned

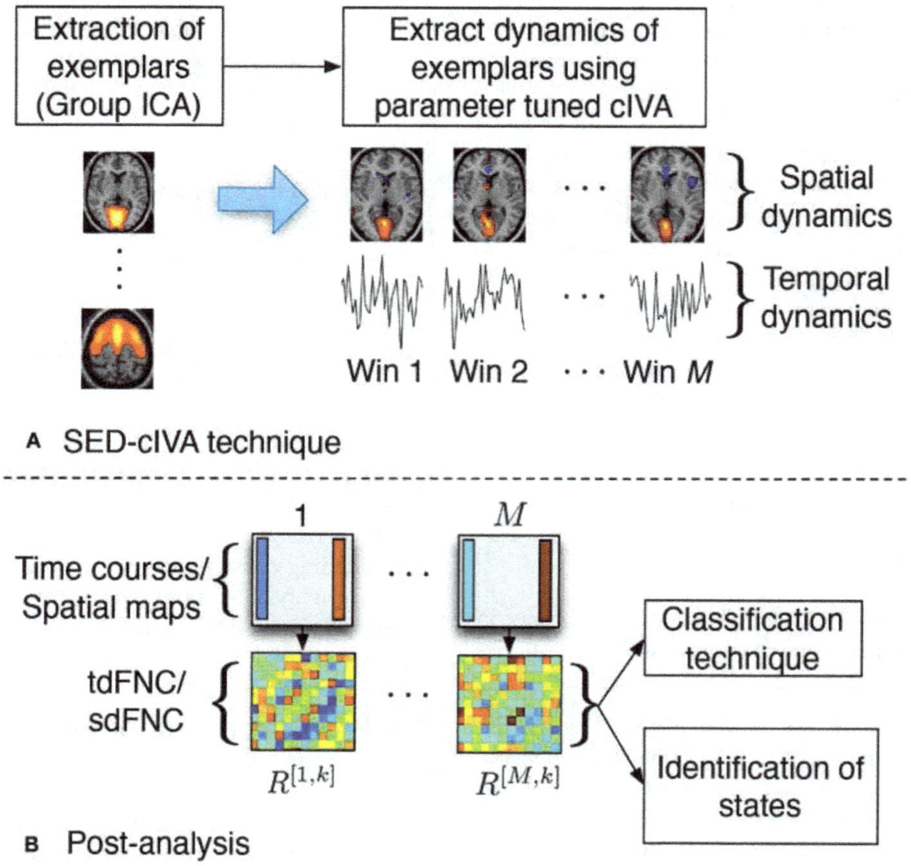

FIGURE 1 | (A) SED-cIVA technique consists of two stages. In the first stage exemplars of resting-state networks are extracted using GICA. In the second stage, these exemplars are used as reference signals in a sliding-window cIVA framework to extract their spatial and temporal dynamics. **(B)** Spatial or temporal dFNC matrices are obtained at each time window by computing the Pearson's correlation coefficient between each pair of spatial maps or time course, respectively. These matrices are further used to classify subject as a patient or a control, and also to identify states.

to HC or SZ group using the following rule,

$$\hat{y} = \arg \max_{g=\{\mathrm{HC},\mathrm{SZ}\}} p(g) \prod_{i=1}^{C} [p^g(C_i)]^{n_i} \qquad (5)$$

where n_i denotes the number of occurrences of state i in the test subject. Steps (B–D) from **Figure 2** are performed for each sub-sampling of the data.

For the joint analysis of spatio-temporal features, the sdFNC and tdFNC features selected after the two-sample t-test on these feature sets separately, are concatenated in the feature dimension to study the effect of combining the two feature sets on prediction accuracy. We compare the results from the combined feature set with the results from using sdFNC and tdFNC feature set alone. **Table 1** provides some inferences regarding the comparison results. Let Q_S denote the prediction accuracy obtained using sdFNC matrices, Q_T denote the prediction accuracy obtained using tdFNC matrices and Q_{ST} denote the prediction accuracy obtained using the combined feature set. We can say that if the prediction accuracy increases after combining the sdFNC and tdFNC features, both feature sets provide unique discriminative features, whereas if the prediction accuracy using sdFNC features is greater than Q_{ST}, then tdFNC provide non-discriminative features, hindering the classification performance.

2.5. Identification of States

Recent studies have shown that fluctuations in the brain networks in resting-state are not random but exhibit structured patterns that vary over time (Cribben et al., 2012; Allen et al., 2014; Yang et al., 2014). In this study, we obtain these structured patterns or states using sdFNC matrices. In the first step toward identifying the states, we flatten the upper diagonal part of each correlation matrix, $R^{[m,k]}$, to obtain a feature vector of dimension $N(N-1)/2$ yielding MK observations. For each subject, the standard deviation across the feature dimension is computed and a subset of FNC matrices are selected corresponding to the maximum standard deviation as subject exemplars. Thus the subject exemplars represent the features that are more informative, alternatively those with higher variability. Further k-means clustering is performed to cluster these subject exemplars into C clusters using Pearson's correlation coefficient as the distance measure. The centroids resulting from clustering the

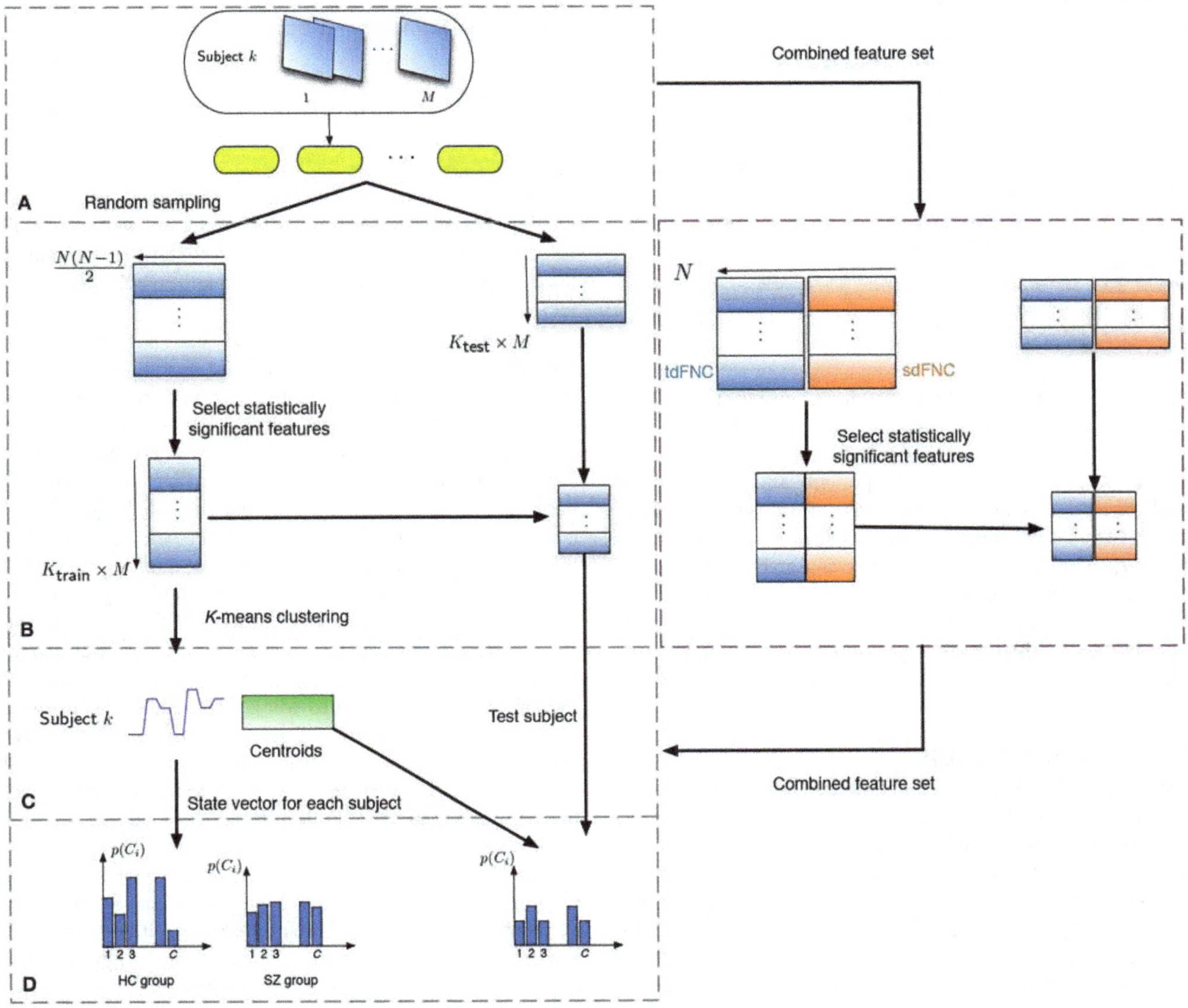

FIGURE 2 | Flowchart to obtain the features for prediction. **(A)** The subjects are divided into training and testing set, where the training set consists of 150 subjects, 75 from the HC and SZ group each. The remaining 29 subjects form the testing set. **(B)** Each tdFNC/sdFNC matrix is flattened to a row and the distinguishing features are extracted using a two-sample t-test. The indices of the distinguishing features are recorded and used to select the corresponding features in the testing stage. In the combined feature set for joint analysis, the flattened features from both domains are concatenated in the feature dimension and similar steps are performed. **(C)** The selected features from the training set are clustered into C clusters using K-means clustering to obtain the centroids and the state vector for each subject. **(D)** The probability of occurrence of each state is computed for the HC and SZ group separately. For the testing stage the state vector for each subject is obtained using the centroids from the training stage and probability of occurrence for each state is computed.

subject exemplars are used as initial points to cluster the entire observation set. This two-step clustering process is performed in order to obtain a robust solution. The performance of k-means clustering assigns a cluster or state index to each observation resulting in a state vector for each subject. The state vector thus represents the evolution of the states over time. This vector is further analyzed to obtain the transition matrix, dwell time and fraction of time spent for each state and for each subject. The transition matrix denotes the number of transitions from state i to state j, $i,j = \{1, \ldots, C\}$, the dwell time denotes the amount of time a subject remains in a particular state, and fraction of time spent denotes the probability of occurrence of a state.

3. RESULTS AND DISCUSSION

The 17 components selected as exemplars after performing GICA are shown in **Figure 3**. These components are divided into 8 domains: auditory (AUD), sensorimotor (SM), frontal (FRO), fronto-parietal (FP), parietal (PAR), visual (VIS), default mode network (DMN) and cerebellum (CB). The PAR domain comprise three networks: PAR1, PAR2, and PAR3, corresponding to their peak activation located in the primary somatosensory cortex, supramarginal gyrus and somatosensory association cortex, respectively. The DMN domain consists of one component corresponding to

TABLE 1 | Inferences about predictability of sdFNC, tdFNC, and combined feature set.

$Q_{ST} > Q_S, Q_T$	sdFNC and tdFNC yield unique discriminative features jointly contributing to classify subjects
$Q_{ST} < Q_S, Q_T$	sdFNC and tdFNC both yield non-discriminative features that are unable to classify subjects
Q_S or $Q_T > Q_{ST} >$ Q_T or Q_S	tdFNC or sdFNC yield non-discriminative features affecting the prediction
$Q_{ST} = Q_S$ or Q_T	tdFNC or sdFNC are not providing additional information to classify subjects

Q_S denotes the prediction accuracy obtained using sdFNC matrices, Q_T denotes the prediction accuracy obtained using tdFNC matrices and Q_{ST} denotes the prediction accuracy obtained using the combined feature set.

posterior DMN, one component corresponding to anterior DMN (ADMN), one DIC network and one insular (INS) component. The DIC component shows a network of a de-activated posterior DMN component and an activated central executive network and right fronto-insular (INS) network. The VIS domain comprise two networks: VIS1 and VIS2, corresponding to their peak activation situated in the lateral and medial visual cortex, respectively. The FRO domain comprise two networks: FRO1 and FRO2 corresponding to their peak activation in the frontal cortex located anterior to the premotor cortex and dorsolateral prefrontal cortex, respectively.

3.1. Prediction Results

The average prediction accuracies computed across 1,000 Monte Carlo subsamplings, using the sdFNC, tdFNC and combined feature set for different number of clusters is shown in **Figure 4**. **Figure 4A** shows the result for the HC group and **Figure 4B** shows the result for the SZ group. In order to test if the prediction accuracies computed using sdFNC and tdFNC features are significantly different from the combined feature set, we perform a permutation test using a two-sample t-test as the hypothesis test. The results indicate that the prediction accuracy computed using sdFNC features is significantly higher than the one computed using tdFNC and the combined feature set for the SZ group for different number of clusters. This suggests the use of tdFNC features yield non-discriminative features that degrade the prediction performance for the SZ group. For the HC group, the prediction accuracy computed using sdFNC features is higher than the one computed using tdFNC features and equal to the combined feature set for the SZ group for different number of clusters. This suggests that the tdFNC features are not providing additional information to classify subjects as controls.

We also compute the sensitivity and specificity of the prediction model obtained using sdFNC and tdFNC features. The true positives (TP) denote the percentage of SZ subjects that are correctly identified as SZ, true negatives (TN) denote the percentage of HC subjects that are correctly identified as HC, false negatives (FN) denote the percentage of SZ subjects incorrectly identified as HC, and false positives (FP) denote the percentage of HC subjects incorrectly identified as SZ. Sensitivity and specificity for each Monte Carlo subsampling is computed as follows,

$$\text{Sensitivity} = \frac{\text{TP}}{\text{TP} + \text{FN}}, \quad \text{Specificity} = \frac{\text{TN}}{\text{TN} + \text{FP}}.$$

Figure 5 shows the results of these measures computed for sdFNC and tdFNC features. Sensitivity and specificity values are higher using sdFNC features compared with the tdFNC features. A higher sensitivity for sdFNC features indicates that these features are better able to identify SZ subjects than HC subjects.

In order to test for differences between the prediction accuracies using sdFNC and tdFNC features, and between the HC group and the SZ group, we perform a permutation test between these groups using a two-sample t-test as a hypothesis test. The distribution plots of the accuracies and the permutation test results are shown in **Figure 6**. The permutation test result indicates that the sdFNC features yield a significantly higher prediction accuracy when compared with tdFNC features, providing evidence that exploiting variability in the spatial domain yields meaningful distinguishing information. The average prediction accuracy using tdFNC features is around 50%, which is equivalent to providing random guesses regarding the class of a subject. This provides additional evidence that tdFNC features are not providing any additional information as compared to a random classifier. The permutation test result between the HC and the SZ group indicates a significantly higher prediction accuracy for the SZ group using sdFNC features. Since the feature used in this technique is the probability of occurrence of each state, we can infer that patients with schizophrenia tend to stay or transition to a certain group of states more often than healthy controls. A natural question is the identification of these predictable states and their differences with respect to states associated to a healthy group of subjects. In the next section we discuss the results obtained from the state-based analysis using the sdFNC matrices and identify the states that are associated with the patients and controls group.

3.2. Analysis of States

We identify six distinct states using both temporal and spatial FNC matrices using the method described in section 2.5. The number of clusters is estimated as six using the silhouette criterion. We also compute the optimal number of clusters using other criteria available in the group ICA for fMRI toolbox. The estimated values are in the range 2–10, with the median value being six. Hence, we choose the final values as six for the optimal number of clusters. The group-specific states and features that demonstrate significant differences between HC and SZ group using sdFNC matrices are shown in **Figure 7A**. The significantly different features within each state were identified by performing a permutation test between the HC group and the SZ group. The group-specific states show differences in the level of connectivity between pairs of components, which are reflected in the third row of **Figure 7A** that shows differences between the HC and SZ group. The parietal component has high positive connectivity with the auditory, sensorimotor and frontal

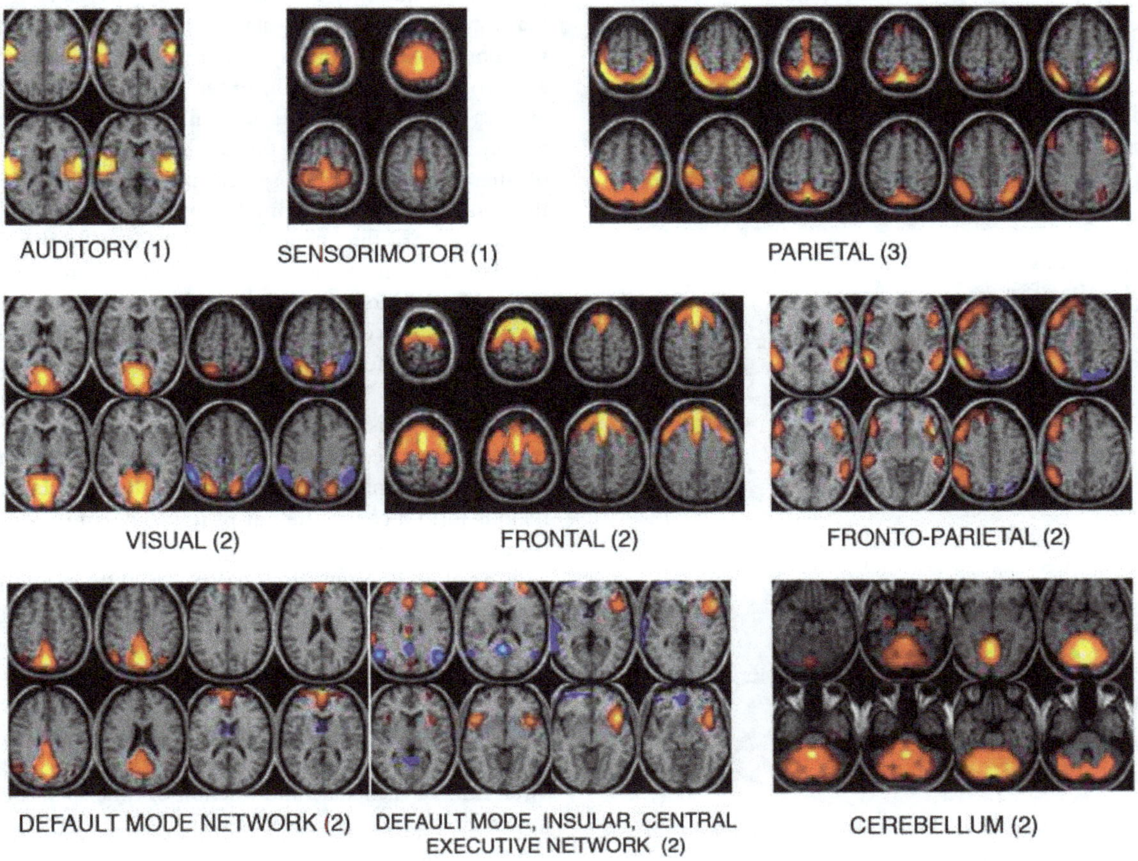

FIGURE 3 | The 17 components selected are divided into 8 domains: auditory (AUD), sensorimotor (SM), frontal (FRO), fronto-parietal (FP), parietal (PAR), visual (VIS), default mode network (DMN), and cerebellum (CB). The DMN domain includes spatial maps consisting the anterior, posterior DMN, central executive network and insular (INS) components. The number indicated next to each domain name is number of components belonging to that domain.

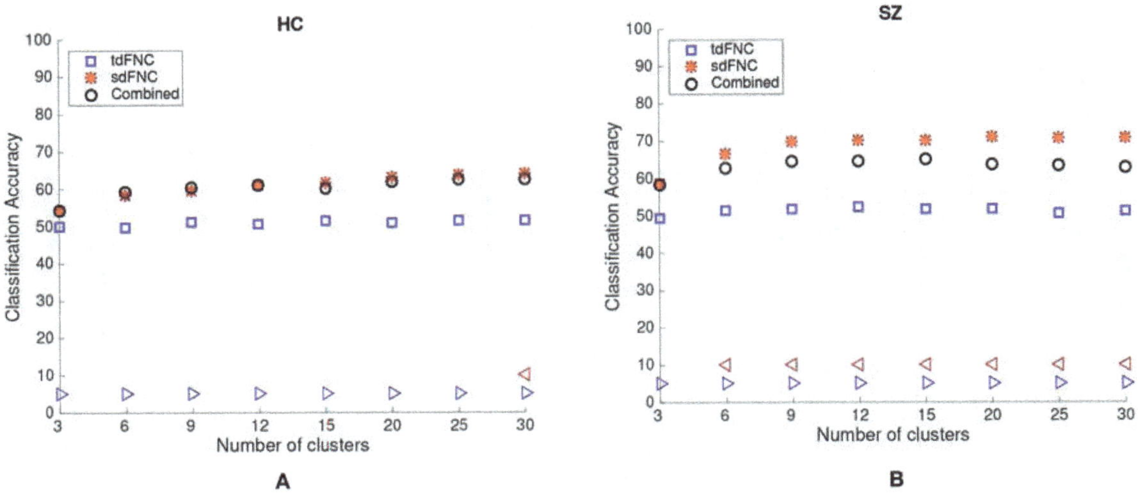

FIGURE 4 | Average prediction accuracy computed over 1,000 independent Monte-Carlo samplings using tdFNC, sdFNC and combined features for **(A)** HC group and **(B)** SZ group. A blue triangle denotes significant difference between tdFNC result and combined feature set result, whereas a read triangle denotes significant difference between sdFNC result and combined feature set result. A triangle pointing left, "◁," indicates the prediction accuracy of tdFNC/sdFNC is greater than the combined feature set result, whereas a triangle pointing right, "▷," indicates the prediction accuracy of tdFNC/sdFNC is less than the combined feature set result.

components in all states and indicates simultaneous activation of these regions. The parietal lobe plays a vital role in processing sensory information such as touch, sound and vision, which is obtained from different parts of the body. A subject in the scanner is exposed to scanner noise and hence the brain is involved in processing the auditory information, causing activation of parietal and auditory components. The parietal component also plays a role in receiving signals from sensory organs, which is then passed to motor-related regions, such as sensorimotor and frontal components, in order to control the body posture. Since a subject is asked to lay still in the scanner, the subject is focusing on balancing his/her body, causing the activation of these regions. An observed positive correlation between the sensorimotor and frontal component provides additional support toward the hypothesis. Cerebellum on the other hand, receives the sensory information from different parts of the body. Hence, a high negative correlation between the parietal and cerebellum component indicates simultaneous deactivation of one component while the other is active, suggesting a process of first receiving and then processing the sensory information. This might also help explain the observed negative correlation between cerebellum and motor-related components. These connections are observed in all states, indicating that these regions form a central hub at resting-state and play a vital role resting-state fMRI data.

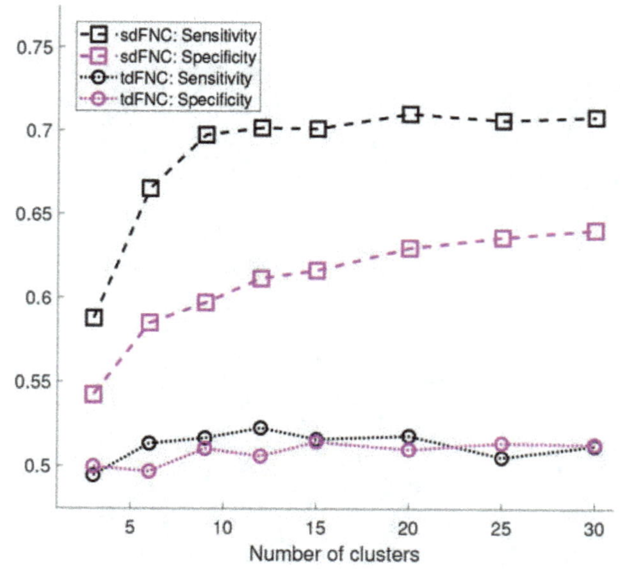

FIGURE 5 | Sensitivity and specificity of the prediction model trained using sdFNC and tdFNC features. The sensitivity and specificity values are averaged over 1,000 Monte Carlo subsamplings. The results indicate that sensitivity and specificity is higher using sdFNC features compared with the tdFNC features. A higher sensitivity for sdFNC indicates a better prediction ability of these features to correctly identify SZ subjects.

We obtain the transition matrix, dwell times and fraction of time spent in each state for each subject as described in section 2.5. For each transition pair $\{i,j\}$, $i,j = 1,\ldots,6$, we perform a permutation test to identify differences between the HC and the SZ group. Each significantly different pair denotes that one group transitioned from state i to j more frequently than the other group. Similarly, we perform a permutation test on the mean dwell time of each state and fraction of time spent in each state to test for differences between HC and SZ group. The results for transition matrices (TM), mean dwell time (MDT) and fraction of time spent (FR) are shown in **Figures 7B–D**, respectively. The transition matrix indicates that healthy controls tend to stay in State 1 more frequently, whereas patients with schizophrenia tend to transition more frequently from State 3 to State 4 and

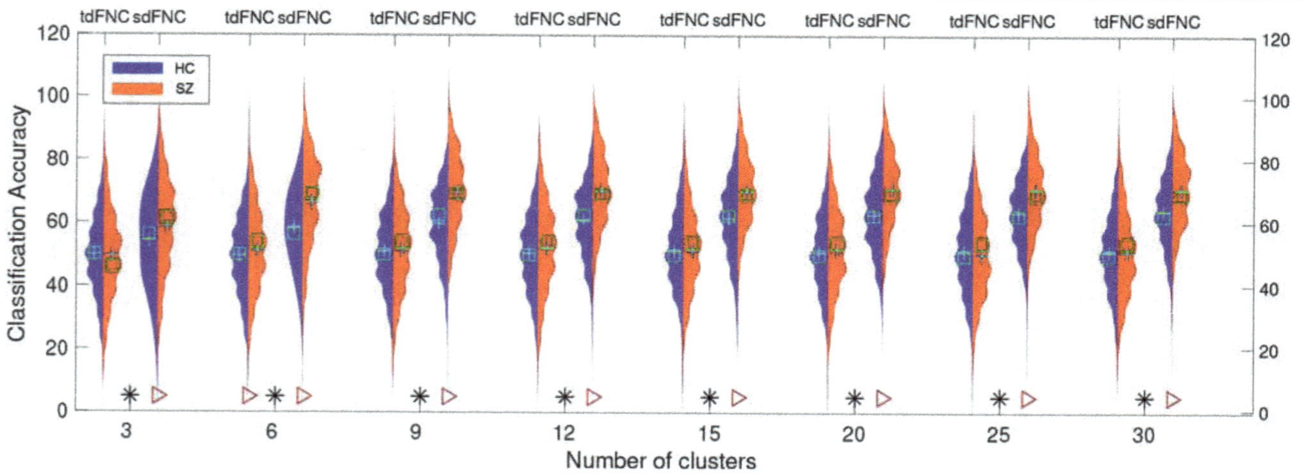

FIGURE 6 | Predictability results using Naïve Bayes classifier. Red color indicates the histogram of prediction accuracies obtained for the SZ group whereas blue indicates the histogram of prediction accuracies for the HC group. X-axis denotes the number of clusters, C used to cluster the features from tdFNC/sdFNC graphs. The green "+" sign denotes the mean value and "□" sign indicates the median value. The markers at the bottom show results from a permutation test to test for statistical differences ($p < 0.05$, corrected). A "*" denotes the accuracies are significantly higher using sdFNC features compared with tdFNC features. A "▷" denotes higher prediction accuracy for SZ group. We observe a higher prediction accuracy using sdFNC features and a significantly higher accuracy for the patients group, for different number of clusters.

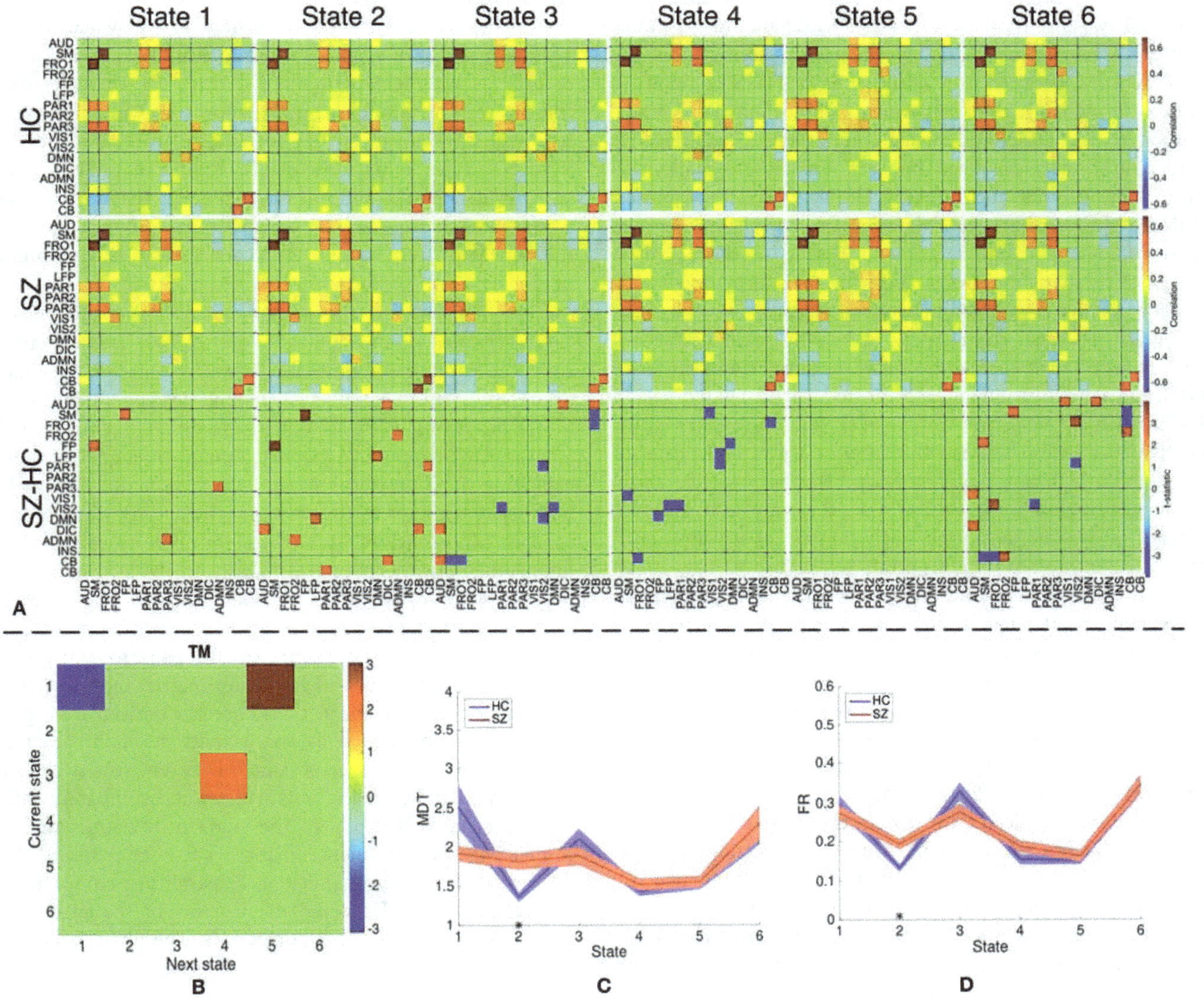

FIGURE 7 | (A) The top two rows shows the group-specific states obtained using sdFNC matrices. The bottom row corresponds to the features that demonstrated significant difference ($p < 0.05$, corrected) between HC and SZ group. Red indicates higher value for SZ whereas blue indicates higher value for HC. **(B)** Transition matrix (TM) with each element in the matrix showing transitions that are significantly ($p < 0.05$, corrected) different. Blue indicates HCs transitioned more frequently from current state to next state whereas red indicates SZs transitioned more frequently from current state to next state. **(C)** Mean dwell time of each state for the HC and SZ group. **(D)** Fraction of time spent (FR) in each state by the HC group and SZ group. Results indicate that SZ subjects tend to transition more frequently from State 3 to State 4 whereas those obtained using dsFNC graphs indicate that SZ subjects transition more frequently from State 1 to State 5. We also observe that SZ subjects tend to stay more in State 2.

State 1 to State 5. State 3 and 4 differ in the level of positive correlation between cerebellum and auditory component, insular and parietal component, visual and parietal component and anterior DMN and visual component, whereas State 1 and 5 differ in the level of positive correlation within the visual network, and between the cerebellum and visual component. These states also differ in the level of negative correlation between the cerebellum and left fronto-parietal component. These connections are also observed in State 2 where patients demonstrate a significantly higher mean dwell time and fraction of time spent compared to controls. Hence patients with schizophrenia tend to reside in or switch to a state that has high positive correlation within the visual network and between the anterior DMN and frontal component, visual and parietal component, anterior DMN and frontal component, and cerebellum and visual component. The patients group also tend to reside in or switch to a state that has high negative correlation between the cerebellum and left fronto-parietal component. This suggests that patients with schizophrenia are associated to a hyperconnected brain network and studies have shown their tendency to engage more brain regions than healthy controls (Ma et al., 2011; Ćurčić-Blake et al., 2015; Walther et al., 2017).

Since patients with schizophrenia demonstrate a significantly high mean dwell time and fraction of time spent in State 2, and controls show a high (although not significant) mean dwell time in State 1, we discuss these two states in detail. State 2 differs from State 1 in terms of high positive correlation within the visual network, between frontal and anterior DMN component, cerebellum and parietal component, cerebellum and visual component, and DMN and insular component. A high negative correlation is also observed between the frontal and visual component, parietal and anterior DMN, DMN and anterior DMN. As discussed above, a high negative correlation between parietal and cerebellum component is due to the cognitive process of receiving and processing sensory information one at a time, a positive correlation between these components in State 2 suggests abnormal connectivity. A healthy brain has shown evidence of positive correlation between anterior and posterior DMN, and a deactivation in DMN due to an activated INS region (Sridharan et al., 2008; Nekovarova et al., 2014). However a high negative correlation between the anterior DMN and posterior DMN, and a high positive correlation between posterior DMN and insular region in State 2 of the SZ group also provides evidence of dysfunction in the DMN domain of schizophrenia, which is a common trait in this group (Nekovarova et al., 2014). A high positive correlation between anterior DMN and frontal component might suggest the activation of both region due to their role in social behavior and impulse control. Patients with schizophrenia are known to have paranoia traits, causing them to be constantly aware of the surroundings and prone to impulse control disorder. This causes hyperactivity in the DMN and frontal components of schizophrenic patients (Fusar-Poli et al., 2011; Guo et al., 2017; Zhou et al., 2019). The bottom row of **Figure 7** indicates the connections that demonstrated significant difference ($p < 0.05$, corrected) between the HC and SZ group. High absolute connectivity is SZ group is indicated by red while high absolute connectivity in the HC group is indicated by blue. State 2 shows most connections that have significantly high absolute correlation in the SZ group. Patients exhibit high correlation between the cerebellum and parietal component, posterior and anterior DMN component, posterior DMN and left fronto-parietal, auditory and DIC component, and cerebellum and DIC network. A significantly high correlation between these components in the SZ group suggest a hyperconnected DMN, which is a common trait of patients with schizophrenia (Garrity et al., 2007; Whitfield-Gabrieli et al., 2009). A significantly higher connectivity between the anterior DMN and frontal component, and parietal and cerebellum component provides additional support to the hypothesis of paranoia and abnormal behavior in schizophrenia patients.

4. CONCLUSION AND FUTURE WORK

Dynamic functional connectivity analysis is widely studied in the temporal domain. However there are also substantial dynamics present in the spatial variability across networks, an understudied area. In this work, we explore the benefits of exploiting the variability in the spatial domain using a prediction technique. Our results indicate that for resting-state fMRI data, the use of spatial dFNC matrices provides meaningful distinguishing characteristics from healthy controls and patients with schizophrenia. We also observe a higher prediction accuracy for the patients group compared with healthy controls, indicating that patients are more likely to stay in or switch among a particular group of states. We also identify the states associated to patients with schizophrenia and study the characteristics of these states. Our results indicate that patients with schizophrenia tend to stay in or switch to a state corresponding to a hyperconnected brain network. In additional, sdFNC features show evidence of significant association of spatial networks to a measure of paranoia in schizophrenia group, highlighting the benefit of the proposed approach as a possible biomarker of illness.

The higher predictability of the sdFNC features and its ability to capture discriminating features, enables the analysis of dFNC in the spatial domain, and leads to a number of future directions. A study to compare different sliding window lengths can be applied to identify a range of lengths suitable for capturing dFNC patterns in the spatial domain. Due to large number of samples in this domain, the sliding window length can be reduced below 30 s as well, in order to capture highly fluctuating networks of interest. This study would not have been possible with conventional methods that use time courses to study dFNC patterns, due to limited number of samples. In this study we identified states from sdFNC patterns and obtained state-based metrics such as transition matrix, mean dwell time and fraction of time spent. Other metrics derived from graph-theoretical analysis such as connectivity strength, modularity and centrality can also be obtained. Different robust clustering approaches can be used to obtain states and compared with the method used in this paper. The study of dynamic functional connectivity is prominent during resting-state during which the neuronal activity is under no constraint as compared with task-related fMRI. However, the benefits of spatial dynamics can be explored under task-constraints. The main focus of this paper is to determine the power of the spatial dynamic features and not achieving a high classification accuracy. Hence, we use a simple Naïve Bayes classifier for predicting the subject class, which ensures that the classification rates would be as independent as possible from the tuning of classifier parameters. However, the prediction accuracy can be improved by using complex classifiers such as kernel support vector machines or neural networks, e.g., a seed-based approach obtained a classification accuracy of 86.3% by using a support vector machine classifier (Kottaram et al., 2018).

AUTHOR CONTRIBUTIONS

SB contributed the primary research idea, implementation, experimentation, organization, and primary writing. QL and VC provided valuable insights toward understanding the results and helped with writing and organization. TA directed the research, identified the direction and problems to investigate, provided feedback, and helped with writing.

FUNDING

This work was supported in parts by the National Institute of Biomedical Imaging and Bioengineering under Grant R01EB020407, National Science Foundation under Grant 1631838, and National Science Foundation-Computing and Communication Foundations under Grant 1618551.

REFERENCES

Adali, T., Anderson, M., and Fu, G.-S. (2014). Diversity in independent component and vector analyses: identifiability, algorithms, and applications in medical imaging. *IEEE Sig. Process. Mag.* 31, 18–33. doi: 10.1109/MSP.2014.2300511

Aine, C., Bockholt, H., Bustillo, J., Canive, J., Caprihan, A., Gasparovic, C., et al. (2017). Multimodal neuroimaging in schizophrenia: description and dissemination. *NeuroInformatics* 15, 343–364. doi: 10.1007/s12021-017-9338-9

Allen, E. A., Damaraju, E., Plis, S. M., Erhardt, E. B., Eichele, T., and Calhoun, V. D. (2014). Tracking whole-brain connectivity dynamics in the resting state. *Cereb. Cortex* 24, 663–676. doi: 10.1093/cercor/bhs352

Anderson, M., Adali, T., and Li, X.-L. (2012). Joint blind source separation with multivariate Gaussian model: algorithms and performance analysis. *IEEE Trans. Sig. Process.* 60, 1672–1683. doi: 10.1109/TSP.2011.2181836

Bhinge, S., Long, Q., Levin-Schwartz, Y., Boukouvalas, Z., Calhoun, V. D., and Adali, T. (2017). "Non-orthogonal constrained independent vector analysis: application to data fusion," in *International Conference on Acoustics, Speech and Signal Processing (ICASSP)* (New Orleans, LA), 2666–2670.

Bhinge, S., Mowakeaa, R., Calhoun, V. D., and Adali, T. (2019). Extraction of time-varying spatio-temporal networks using parameter-tuned constrained IVA. *IEEE Trans. Med. Imaging.* 38, 1715–1725. doi: 10.1109/TMI.2019.2893651

Boukouvalas, Z., Levin-Schwartz, Y., and Adali, T. (2017). "Enhancing ICA performance by exploiting sparsity: application to FMRI analysis," in *IEEE International Conference on Acoustics, Speech and Signal Processing (ICASSP)* (New Orleans, LA: IEEE), 2532–2536.

Calhoun, V. D., and Adali, T. (2012). Multisubject independent component analysis of fMRI: a decade of intrinsic networks, default mode, and neurodiagnostic discovery. *IEEE Rev. Biomed. Eng.* 5, 60–73. doi: 10.1109/RBME.2012.2211076

Calhoun, V. D., Adali, T., Pearlson, G., and Pekar, J. (2001a). "Group ICA of functional MRI data: separability, stationarity, and inference," in *Proceedings of the International Conference on ICA and BSS San Diego, CA.* Vol. 155.

Calhoun, V. D., Adali, T., Pearlson, G. D., and Pekar, J. (2001b). A method for making group inferences from functional MRI data using independent component analysis. *Hum. Brain Mapp.* 14, 140–151. doi: 10.1002/hbm.1048

Calhoun, V. D., and de Lacy, N. (2017). Ten key observations on the analysis of resting-state functional MR imaging data using independent component analysis. *NeuroImaging Clin.* 27, 561–579. doi: 10.1016/j.nic.2017.06.012

Calhoun, V. D., Kiehl, K. A., and Pearlson, G. D. (2008). Modulation of temporally coherent brain networks estimated using ICA at rest and during cognitive tasks. *Hum. Brain Mapp.* 29, 828–838. doi: 10.1002/hbm.20581

Chang, C., and Glover, G. H. (2010). Time-frequency dynamics of resting-state brain connectivity measured with fMRI. *Neuroimage* 50, 81–98. doi: 10.1016/j.neuroimage.2009.12.011

Cribben, I., Haraldsdottir, R., Atlas, L. Y., Wager, T. D., and Lindquist, M. A. (2012). Dynamic connectivity regression: determining state-related changes in brain connectivity. *NeuroImage* 61, 907–920. doi: 10.1016/j.neuroimage.2012.03.070

Ćurčić-Blake, B., van der Meer, L., Pijnenborg, G. H., David, A. S., and Aleman, A. (2015). Insight and psychosis: functional and anatomical brain connectivity and self-reflection in Schizophrenia. *Hum. Brain Mapp.* 36, 4859–4868. doi: 10.1002/hbm.22955

Du, W., Ma, S., Fu, G.-S., Calhoun, V. D., and Adali, T. (2014). "A novel approach for assessing reliability of ICA for fMRI analysis," in *International Conference on Acoustics, Speech and Signal Processing (ICASSP)* (Florence: IEEE), 2084–2088.

Fox, M. D., Snyder, A. Z., Vincent, J. L., Corbetta, M., Van Essen, D. C., and Raichle, M. E. (2005). The human brain is intrinsically organized into dynamic, anticorrelated functional networks. *Proc. Natl. Acad. Sci. U.S.A.* 102, 9673–9678. doi: 10.1073/pnas.0504136102

Fusar-Poli, P., Howes, O., Allen, P., Broome, M., Valli, I., Asselin, M., et al. (2011). Abnormal prefrontal activation directly related to pre-synaptic striatal dopamine dysfunction in people at clinical high risk for psychosis. *Mol. Psychiatry* 16:67. doi: 10.1038/mp.2009.108

Garrity, A. G., Pearlson, G. D., McKiernan, K., Lloyd, D., Kiehl, K. A., and Calhoun, V. D. (2007). Aberrant "default mode" functional connectivity in schizophrenia. *Amer. J. Psychiatry* 164, 450–457. doi: 10.1176/ajp.2007.164.3.450

Guo, W., Liu, F., Chen, J., Wu, R., Li, L., Zhang, Z., et al. (2017). Hyperactivity of the default-mode network in first-episode, drug-naive schizophrenia at rest revealed by family-based case–control and traditional case–control designs. *Medicine* 96:e6223. doi: 10.1097/MD.0000000000006223

Hero, A. O., and Rajaratnam, B. (2016). Foundational principles for large-scale inference: illustrations through correlation mining. *Proc. IEEE* 104, 93–110. doi: 10.1109/JPROC.2015.2494178

Hutchison, R. M., Womelsdorf, T., Allen, E. A., Bandettini, P. A., Calhoun, V. D., Corbetta, M., et al. (2013). Dynamic functional connectivity: promise, issues, and interpretations. *NeuroImage* 80, 360–378. doi: 10.1016/j.neuroimage.2013.05.079

Keilholz, S. D., Magnuson, M. E., Pan, W.-J., Willis, M., and Thompson, G. J. (2013). Dynamic properties of functional connectivity in the rodent. *Brain Connect.* 3, 31–40. doi: 10.1089/brain.2012.0115

Kottaram, A., Johnston, L., Ganella, E., Pantelis, C., Kotagiri, R., and Zalesky, A. (2018). Spatio-temporal dynamics of resting-state brain networks improve single-subject prediction of schizophrenia diagnosis. *Hum. Brain Mapp.* 39, 3663–3681. doi: 10.1002/hbm.24202

Kunert-Graf, J. M., Eschenburg, K. M., Galas, D. J., Kutz, J. N., Rane, S. D., and Brunton, B. W. (2018). Extracting reproducible time-resolved resting state networks using dynamic mode decomposition. *bioRxiv* 343061. doi: 10.1101/343061

Lee, M. H., Smyser, C. D., and Shimony, J. S. (2013). Resting-state fMRI: a review of methods and clinical applications. *Amer. J. Neuroradiol.* 34, 1866–1872. doi: 10.3174/ajnr.A3263

Leonardi, N., and Van De Ville, D. (2015). On spurious and real fluctuations of dynamic functional connectivity during rest. *Neuroimage* 104, 430–436. doi: 10.1016/j.neuroimage.2014.09.007

Li, X., Zhu, D., Jiang, X., Jin, C., Zhang, X., Guo, L., et al. (2014). Dynamic functional connectomics signatures for characterization and differentiation of PTSD patients. *Hum. Brain Mapp.* 35, 1761–1778. doi: 10.1002/hbm.22290

Li, X.-L., and Adali, T. (2010). "Blind spatiotemporal separation of second and/or higher-order correlated sources by entropy rate minimization," in *International Conference on Acoustics Speech and Signal Processing (ICASSP)* (Dallas, TX: IEEE), 1934–1937.

Li, Y.-O., Adali, T., and Calhoun, V. D. (2007). Estimating the number of independent components for functional magnetic resonance imaging data. *Hum. Brain Mapp.* 28, 1251–1266. doi: 10.1002/hbm.20359

Liégeois, R., Ziegler, E., Phillips, C., Geurts, P., Gómez, F., Bahri, M. A., et al. (2016). Cerebral functional connectivity periodically (de)synchronizes with anatomical constraints. *Brain Struct. Funct.* 221, 2985–2997. doi: 10.1007/s00429-015-1083-y

Long, Q., Bhinge, S., Levin-Schwartz, Y., Boukouvalas, Z., Calhoun, V. D., and Adali, T. (2018a). The role of diversity in data-driven analysis of multi-subject fMRI data: comparison of approaches based on independence and sparsity using global performance metrics. *Hum. Brain Mapp.* 40, 489–504. doi: 10.1002/hbm.24389

Long, Q., Jia, C., Boukouvalas, Z., Gabrielson, B., Emge, D., and Adali, T. (2018b). "Consistent run selection for independent component analysis: application to fMRI analysis," in *International Conference on Acoustics, Speech and Signal Processing (ICASSP)* (Calgary, AB: IEEE), 2581–2585. doi: 10.1109/ICASSP.2018.8461646

Ma, S., Calhoun, V. D., Phlypo, R., and Adali, T. (2014). Dynamic changes of spatial functional network connectivity in healthy individuals and schizophrenia patients using independent vector analysis. *NeuroImage* 90, 196–206. doi: 10.1016/j.neuroimage.2013.12.063

Ma, S., Eichele, T., Correa, N. M., Calhoun, V. D., and Adali, T. (2011). "Hierarchical and graphical analysis of fMRI network connectivity in healthy and schizophrenic groups," in *IEEE International Symposium on Biomedical Imaging: From Nano to Macro* (Chicago, IL: IEEE), 1031–1034. doi: 10.1109/ISBI.2011.5872577

Nekovarova, T., Fajnerova, I., Horacek, J., and Spaniel, F. (2014). Bridging disparate symptoms of schizophrenia: a triple network dysfunction theory. *Front. Behav. Neurosci.* 8:171. doi: 10.3389/fnbeh.2014.00171

Preti, M. G., Bolton, T. A., and Van De Ville, D. (2017). The dynamic functional connectome: state-of-the-art and perspectives. *NeuroImage* 160, 41–54. doi: 10.1016/j.neuroimage.2016.12.061

Sakoğlu, Ü., Pearlson, G. D., Kiehl, K. A., Wang, Y. M., Michael, A. M., and Calhoun, V. D. (2010). A method for evaluating dynamic functional network connectivity and task-modulation: application to schizophrenia. *Magn. Reson. Mater. Phys. Biol. Med.* 23, 351–366. doi: 10.1007/s10334-010-0197-8

Scott, A., Courtney, W., Wood, D., De la Garza, R., Lane, S., Wang, R., et al. (2011). COINS: an innovative informatics and neuroimaging tool suite built for large heterogeneous datasets. *Front. Neuroinformatics* 5:33. doi: 10.3389/fninf.2011.00033

Sridharan, D., Levitin, D. J., and Menon, V. (2008). A critical role for the right fronto-insular cortex in switching between central-executive and default-mode networks. *Proc. Natl. Acad. Sci. U.S.A.* 105, 12569–12574. doi: 10.1073/pnas.0800005105

Varoquaux, G., Gramfort, A., Pedregosa, F., Michel, V., and Thirion, B. (2011). "Multi-subject dictionary learning to segment an atlas of brain spontaneous activity," in *Biennial International Conference on Information Processing in Medical Imaging* (Berlin; Heidelberg: Springer), 562–573.

Walther, S., Stegmayer, K., Federspiel, A., Bohlhalter, S., Wiest, R., and Viher, P. V. (2017). Aberrant hyperconnectivity in the motor system at rest is linked to motor abnormalities in schizophrenia spectrum disorders. *Schizophr. Bull.* 43, 982–992. doi: 10.1093/schbul/sbx091

Whitfield-Gabrieli, S., Thermenos, H. W., Milanovic, S., Tsuang, M. T., Faraone, S. V., McCarley, R. W., et al. (2009). Hyperactivity and hyperconnectivity of the default network in schizophrenia and in first-degree relatives of persons with schizophrenia. *Proc. Natl. Acad. Sci. U.S.A.* 106, 1279–1284. doi: 10.1073/pnas.0809141106

Yang, Z., Craddock, R. C., Margulies, D. S., Yan, C.-G., and Milham, M. P. (2014). Common intrinsic connectivity states among posteromedial cortex subdivisions: insights from analysis of temporal dynamics. *NeuroImage* 93, 124–137. doi: 10.1016/j.neuroimage.2014.02.014

Zhou, C., Yu, M., Tang, X., Wang, X., Zhang, X., Zhang, X., et al. (2019). Convergent and divergent altered patterns of default mode network in deficit and non-deficit schizophrenia. *Prog. Neuropsychopharmacol. Biol. Psychiatry* 89, 427–434. doi: 10.1016/j.pnpbp.2018.10.012

18

Connectome-Based Biomarkers Predict Subclinical Depression and Identify Abnormal Brain Connections with the Lateral Habenula and Thalamus

Yunkai Zhu[1]*, Shouliang Qi*[1,2]**, Bo Zhang*[1]*, Dianning He*[1]*, Yueyang Teng*[1,2]*, Jiani Hu*[3] *and Xinhua Wei*[4]***

[1] *Sino-Dutch Biomedical and Information Engineering School, Northeastern University, Shenyang, China,* [2] *Key Laboratory of Medical Image Computing of Northeastern University (Ministry of Education), Shenyang, China,* [3] *Department of Radiology, Wayne State University, Detroit, United States,* [4] *Department of Radiology, Guangzhou First People's Hospital, School of Medicine, South China University of Technology, Guangzhou, China*

Correspondence:
Shouliang Qi
qisl@bmie.neu.edu.cn
Xinhua Wei
weixinhua@aliyun.com

Subclinical depression (SD) has been considered as the precursor to major depressive disorder. Accurate prediction of SD and identification of its etiological origin are urgent. Bursts within the lateral habenula (LHb) drive depression in rats, but whether dysfunctional LHb is associated with SD in human is unknown. Here we develop connectome-based biomarkers which predict SD and identify dysfunctional brain regions and connections. T1 weighted images and resting-state functional MRI (fMRI) data were collected from 34 subjects with SD and 40 healthy controls (HCs). After the brain is parcellated into 48 brain regions (246 subregions) using the human Brainnetome Atlas, the functional network of each participant is constructed by calculating the correlation coefficient for the time series of fMRI signals of each pair of subregions. Initial candidates of abnormal connections are identified by the two-sample *t*-test and input into Support Vector Machine models as features. A total of 24 anatomical-region-based models, 231 sliding-window-based models, and 100 random-selection-based models are built. The performance of these models is estimated through leave-one-out cross-validation and evaluated by measures of accuracy, sensitivity, confusion matrix, receiver operating characteristic curve, and the area under the curve (AUC). After confirming the region with the highest accuracy, subregions within the thalamus and connections associated with subregions of LHb are compared. It is found that five prediction models using connections of the thalamus, posterior superior temporal sulcus, cingulate gyrus, superior parietal lobule, and superior frontal gyrus achieve an accuracy >0.9 and an AUC >0.93. Among 90 abnormal connections associated with the thalamus, the subregion of the right posterior parietal thalamus where LHb is located has the most connections (n = 18), the left subregion only has 3 connections. In SD group, 10 subregions in the thalamus have significantly different node degrees with those in the HC group, while 8 subregions have lower degrees ($p < 0.01$), including the one with LHb. These results implicate abnormal brain connections associated with the thalamus and LHb to be associated with SD. Integration of these connections by machine learning can provide connectome-based biomarkers to accurately diagnose SD.

Keywords: resting state functional MRI, brain network, subclinical depression, brain biomarker, functional connection, node degree

INTRODUCTION

On the depression severity continuum, subclinical depression (SD) is a mild condition considered to be the precursor to major depressive disorder (MDD) (1, 2). Subjects with SD are very vulnerable to depression and are apt to generate suicide ideation (3, 4). The increasingly high incidence of SD among both college students and the elderly (estimated as high as 15%) clearly demonstrates the need for intensive investigation (5–7). Unfortunately, knowledge of neural substrates of SD is incomplete, making it difficult to identify reliable diagnostic biomarkers and take preventative treatments (8).

Some dysfunctional brain regions and connections have been evaluated in order to identify new biomarkers for SD. *Via* resting state fMRI (rs-fMRI), we have previously demonstrated that the altered spontaneous neuronal activity by measurement of amplitude of low-frequency fluctuations (ALFF) and disrupted functional connectivity (FC) are implicated in SD (9–11). We also found that SD presents the increased interhemispheric FC and cortical degree centrality, as well as decreased subcortical degree centrality. These measures differentiate SD subjects from healthy controls (HCs) (10–12). SD is characterized by changed FCs between subregions of the anterior cingulate cortex (ACC), increased FC of Hb within default model network regions, and decreased FC within salience network regions (8, 13). Kaiser et al. (14) demonstrated that there exists a high correlation between the neural activity of dorsal anterior cingulate cortex (dACC) and posterior cingulate cortex (PCC) in SD subjects, indicating that SD subjects are confronted with greater difficulty of shifting out of internally directed and ruminative thinking. Dedovic et al. (15) and Petrican et al. (16) reported the weaker functional dominance in dorsal attention network (DAN) [low connectivity between the superior parietal lobule (SPL) and the frontoparietal control network].

Network neuroscience explores interactions of different neurobiological element from an integrative perspective and is capable of providing with better predictive biomarkers for brain disorders by machine learning (17, 18). Machine learning is suitable for individual-level prediction from a prospective viewpoint, and it is a potentially powerful tool for precision psychiatry (19). For example, Support Vector Machine (SVM), as a typical method of machine learning, has been widely used to identify imaging biomarkers in diseases such as schizophrenia, major depression, bipolar disorder, etc. (20). For more information on machine learning and its application in psychiatry, one can refer to the comprehensive reviews (21–24). Recently, machine learning has proved useful to build connectome-based biomarkers for autism spectrum disorder, bipolar disorder, subtypes of depression, and schizophrenia (25–28). However, not many connectome-based biomarkers have been developed for SD.

Compared with SD, MDD has received more attention and significant breakthroughs have been achieved. For example, concrete evidence has demonstrated that bursts within the lateral habenula (LHb) drive depression in rats (29). As an evolutionary conserved epithalamic structure, LHb is involved in negative motivational value and decision-making (30–33). LHb is also considered to be the pathophysiological basement of MDD (34, 35). For more details on LHb, one can refer to these recent reviews (36–38). The deep brain stimulation of LHb has been successfully used to treat patients with refractory MDD (39). These findings on MDD may provide useful clues regarding SD.

LHb has been investigated by multimodal MRI in depressive and healthy subjects, but not in subjects with SD. LHb volume measured by high-resolution T1-weighted images decreases in depression, but not in posttraumatic stress disorder or schizophrenia (40, 41). Using task-based functional MRI (fMRI), Salas et al. (42) have shown that LHb is activated in response to negative reward prediction. It is worth noting that the fMRI study on LHb has several limitations. First, the habenula volume approximately ranges from 29 to 36 mm^3 in each hemisphere based on structural MRI and postmortem measurement, which can be smaller than the voxel size of standard fMRI (40, 41, 43). The smoothing kernels [5–12 mm full width at half maximum (FWHM)] are larger in size than LHb. Second, the habenular signal is likely contaminated by adjacent structures, such as the medial dorsal thalamus or the epithalamic paraventricular nucleus (43).

Herein, connectome-based biomarkers are developed to predict subclinical depression through a machine learning algorithm and identify dysfunctional brain regions and connections. The method of predictive modeling used in our study is different with the traditional method of brain mapping (13). Predictive modeling integrates all brain data or features into a single prediction of outcome, making multiple comparisons unnecessary and increasing statistical power (18). Specifically, we parcellate the whole brain into 48 regions and 246 subregions using the latest human Brainnetome Atlas (44) and build large-scale resting-state functional brain networks using fMRI data. A two-sample t-test is used to identify initial candidate connections, and the resultant regional connections are input into SVM models as features. The performance of the predictive models is estimated by leave-one-out cross-validation. The node degree of subregions within the thalamus is compared between SD and HC groups. Connections linked with subregions of LHb are further investigated.

MATERIALS AND METHODS

Participants

All the participants were enlisted from volunteers who had undergone health screening at Guangzhou Medical University from 2012 to 2014. The Beck Depression Inventory II (BDI-II) scale is administered to evaluate the depression symptom severity. Thirty-four subjects (11 males, 23 females) with BDI-II score >13 are placed into the SD group (BDI score mean ± SD: 22.58 ± 6.92) and 40 healthy controls (21 males, 19 females) are selected to match the SD group by age, sex, and education. According to the two-sample *t*-test, there is no significant difference for the age (years) between SD and HC groups (mean ± SD: 19.91 ± 1.64 vs. 19.70 ± 0.85, $p = 0.50$), neither for the education (years) (mean ± SD: 13.18 ± 0.58 vs. 13.08 ± 0.62, $p = 0.47$). By the chi-square test, there is no significant difference for the gender ($p = 0.07$). None of the participants fulfilled the criteria for MDD based on *Diagnostic and Statistical Manual of Mental Disorders IV (DSM-IV)*. Other inclusion criteria for all participants include age ranging from 19 to 25 years, right-handedness, no visualized lesion on any MRI scans, no neurological illness, and no alcohol or drug dependence. The study is approved by the Medical Ethics Committee of Guangzhou First People's Hospital of Guangzhou Medical University and is in accordance with the 1964 Helsinki declaration and its later amendments or comparable ethical standards. All participants signed a written informed consent in accordance with the Declaration of Helsinki (2000).

MRI Imaging Data Acquisition

All MRI images were acquired using one 3-Tesla MRI scanner (Siemens, Erlangen, Germany) with an eight-channel phase-array brain coil. Foam pads and headphone were utilized to minimize the head motion and reduce noise, respectively. As in our previous studies (10–12), high-resolution T1-weighted images were obtained with a standard magnetization prepared rapid gradient echo (MP-RAGE) sequence [repetition time (TR)/echo time (TE) 2,530/2.34 ms, flip angle (FA) 7°, field of view (FOV) 256 × 224 mm, slice thickness 1.0 mm]. The resting-state fMRI data were collected by one echo-planar imaging (EPI) sequence (TR/TE 2,500/21 ms, FA 90°, FOV 200 × 200 mm, matrix 64 × 64, 42 slices without gap, voxel size 3.5 × 3.1 × 3.1 mm). The images of 200 time points were collected, and the total amount of fMRI acquisition time is 500 s. During the resting-state fMRI scan, the participants were asked to relax, to close their eyes, not to think of anything in particular, and not to fall asleep. Wakefulness of participants has been confirmed immediately after the fMRI scanning session.

Study Design and Main Procedures

The study design and procedures are schematically shown in **Figure 1**. There are six steps for this study (**Figure1A**). After the first step of image preprocessing, functional brain networks for HCs and SDs are constructed. Then two-sample *t*-tests are used to identify potential dysfunctional connections. Three methods are proposed to further select connections from previously identified candidates. These selected connections are used to train and test the predictive models of SD. After excluding confounders such as the number of connections and *p*-value, dysfunctional brain regions and connections are determined by examining the models with high predictive accuracy. Finally the emphasis is placed on the dysfunctional thalamus and LHb. Abnormal connections associated with the thalamus and its subregions, including LHb, as well as the node degree of these subregions are characterized. These six steps are described in details below.

Functional MRI Image Preprocessing

As shown in **Figure 1B**, the T1-weighted and rs-fMRI data is preprocessed using the DPARSF toolbox (http://www.restfmri.net/forum/DPARSF) (45, 46) as follows. First, the initial 20 time points of raw fMRI data are removed in order to eliminate unstable factors. Second, the time layer correction and head movement correction are carried out. Third, the brain of each subject is registered to a normative template through spatial standardization. Fourth, a band-pass filtering of 0.01–0.1 Hz and Gaussian smoothing with 6 mm FWHM are implemented.

Construction of Functional Brain Networks

The procedure for constructing functional brain networks is shown in **Figure 1C**. First, the newly developed human Brainnetome Atlas is used to parcellate the whole brain into 48 brain regions (246 subregions). This atlas is four to five times as accurate as the traditional Brodmann map and has a more objective and accurate boundary (44). Each subregion represents a node in the constructed brain network. The time course of each subregion is calculated by averaging the time course of all voxels therein. The strength of functional connection or the connection weight (W_{ij}), also identified as edge weight, is expressed as the Pearson correlation coefficient between the time courses of any two subregions (*i, j*). The correlation matrix is transformed into *Z* scores by applying Fisher's *r*-to-*Z* transformation. For each individual, a weighted undirected network is obtained in the form of a 246 × 246 adjacency matrix (*A*). Given that it is controversial for interpreting negative correlation or functional connectivity (47, 48), the normalized absolute value of the matrix is used as done in previous studies (49, 50), such that $0 \leq W_{ij} \leq 1$ for all *i* and *j*.

Node degree and edge weight are used to determine whether a brain region (or subregion) is connected or dysfunctional in SD. The node degree (k_i) refers to the number of connections that link this node to the rest of the network. For our weighted networks, the definition can be transformed as

$$k_i = {}_{j\;N}\, W_{ij} \qquad (1)$$

where W_{ij} is the strength of the connection between node *i* and node *j*, and *N* is the set of nodes in the network. The edge weight (W_{ij}) is an important measure for evaluating the alteration in the strength of a connection in SD.

Identification of Dysfunctional Connections

As shown in **Figure 1D**, two-sample *t*-tests are performed to examine significant differences between edge weight in SD and HC

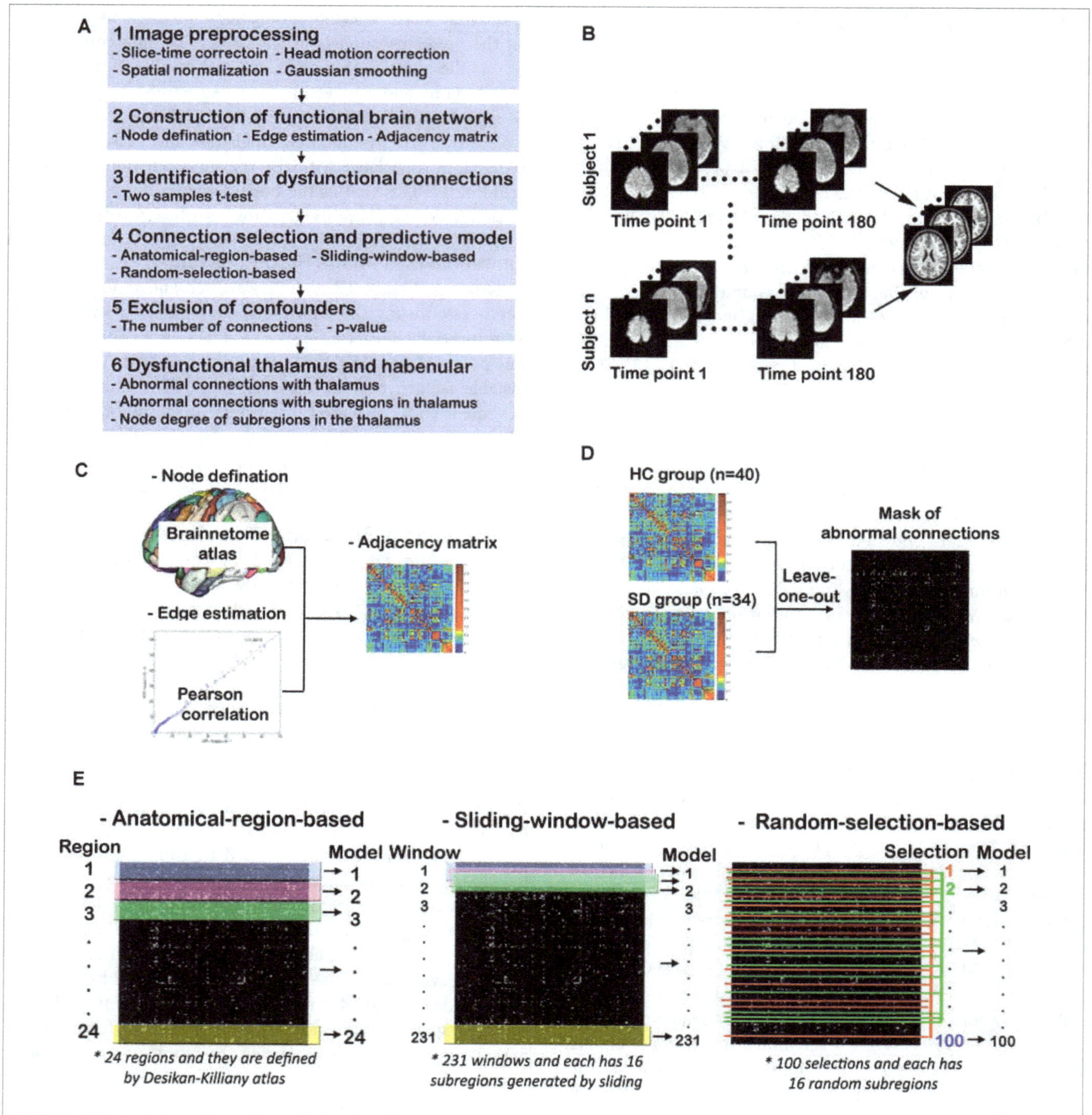

FIGURE 1 | Study design and procedures. **(A)** Overview of the study procedures; **(B)** functional MRI (fMRI) image preprocessing; **(C)** construction of functional brain networks; **(D)** identification of dysfunctional connections; **(E)** connection selection and predictive models.

groups ($p < 0.05$). For multiple comparisons, the false discovery rate (FDR) is controlled by the linear step-up procedure introduced by Benjamini and Hochberg (51). To avoid the information leakage, the two-sample *t*-test is carried out after leaving one out, not for all subjects. This step generated 74 different masks of abnormal connections. Based on each mask, the work in Connection Selection and Predictive Models is done. However, for the group study in Dysfunctional Thalamus and Lateral Habenula, the two-sample *t*-test is done for all subjects.

Connection Selection and Predictive Models

The study uses the library for support vector machines (LIBSVM) toolkit developed by Professor Lin of Taiwan University (https://www.csie.ntu.edu.tw/~cjlin/libsvm/), which integrates many functions such as kernel selection, parameter adjustment, and prediction. For the training of SVM classification model, the radial basis kernel function (RBF) is used. This kernel function provides a good classification for samples with nonlinear relationship between labels and features as expressed below.

$$K\left(x_i,x_j\right) = exp \ - \ \left\|x_i - x_j\right\|^2 \ , \ >0 \quad (2)$$

According to the recommendation from LIBSVM, the values of the optimal penalty coefficient C and the kernel function parameter γ are determined by the way of "grid-search" using cross-validation (52). After going through all the pairs of (C, γ) with $C = 2^{-5}, 2^{-3},\ldots, 2^{15}$ and $\gamma = 2^{-15}, 2^{-13},\ldots, 2^{3}$, the pair leading to the best cross-validation accuracy is found.

Three methods are proposed to select connections from identified candidates, and these selected connections are used to train and test the predictive SVM models of SD, as shown in **Figure 1E**. For the first method, the significantly altered connections associated with each brain region defined by the human Briannetome Atlas are used as input features. A total of 24 SVM models are built to predict SD, and they are named as anatomical-region-based models. The performance of these models is estimated through leave-one-out cross-validation using measures of accuracy, sensitivity, confusion matrix, receiver operating characteristic (ROC) curve, and the area under the curve (AUC). These models are ranked by accuracy. The brain regions leading to the models with an accuracy >0.90 are considered to be dysfunctional.

To determine whether models using connections associated with subregions not belonging to one specific anatomically well-defined brain region and with subregions that are anatomically nonadjacent can achieve comparable performance to the anatomical-region-based models, two more independent experiments are conducted. First, the method of sliding window with 16 subregions is employed to generate different input features and models. The reason why the number of subregions was set as 16 is that the thalamus leading to the predictive model of the highest ACC owns 16 subregions. As shown in the middle column of **Figure 1E**, to slide the window row by row throughout the adjacency matrix (246 × 246) will generate 231 windows (246 − 16 + 1 = 231). The models using the connections within each individual window as input features are named as sliding-window-based models. Second, a model is constructed using the functional connections within 16 randomly selected subregions as input features. A total of 100 similar models are generated and identified as random-selection-based models. The accuracy values of these three categories of models are compared.

Exclusion of Confounders

To estimate whether the performances of the anatomical-region-based models are dependent on the number of connections associated with the brain region and the p-value of these connections, their correlation coefficients are assessed. The distribution of connections in the model with the highest accuracy is investigated to explore whether these models with good performance are independent.

Dysfunctional Thalamus and Lateral Habenula

In order to further identify dysfunctional subregions and connections, the connections of brain regions achieving the highest predictive accuracy (thalamus) are examined. The number and p-value of connections associated with each of the 16 subregions are identified. Finally, the node degree of each subregions is compared between SD and HC groups.

RESULTS

Anatomical-Region-Based Models

The 24 anatomical-region-based models ranked by the accuracy of predicting SD are presented in **Figure 2A**. The accuracy ranges from 0.65 to 0.92. The top five models used connections associated with the regions of thalamus, posterior superior temporal sulcus, cingulate gyrus, superior parietal lobule, and superior frontal gyrus. The accuracy of each of these five models is higher than 0.90. The anatomical locations are shown in **Figure 2B**. The ROC curves and the AUC values are shown in **Figure 2C**. The cingulate model achieves the highest AUC of 0.957. The thalamus model yields the second highest AUC of 0.943. The confusion matrices of the top five anatomical-region-based models are listed in **Table 1**. For the thalamus model, 31 out of 34 subjects with SD (91.2%, also defined as sensitivity) and 37 out of 40 HCs (92.5%, also defined as specificity) are predicted accurately. The posterior superior temporal sulcus model yields the highest specificity of 95.0%, and the posterior superior temporal sulcus model yields the highest sensitivity.

Other Subregion Selection Strategies

The accuracy of the models using other subregion selection strategies is compared with that of the anatomical-region-based models, as shown in **Figure 2D**. No significant difference in accuracy is observed between the 231 sliding-window-based models and the 24 anatomical-region-based models (0.81 ± 0.06 vs. 0.80 ± 0.08). The accuracy of the 100 random-selection-based models is 0.45 ± 0.06, which is significantly lower than that of the anatomical-region-based models and the sliding-window-based models (p < 0.001). The top five anatomical-region-based models, and in particular the thalamus model, achieve extraordinarily higher accuracy, as compared with the other models. Two important features are worthy to be noted. First, the brain regions involved in the top five anatomical-region-based models are potentially dysfunctional due to SD. Second, the arbitrary anatomically adjacent subregions (obtained by the sliding window method) can generate comparable prediction accuracy with anatomically well-defined subregions (obtained by the anatomical-region-based method), but the randomly selected subregions cannot reliably predict SD.

Effect of the Number of Connections and the *p*-value

The number of connections associated with the 24 brain regions used for the predictive models of SD ranges from 52 to 240, as shown in **Figure 3A**. The top five models, which correspond to the regions of thalamus, posterior superior temporal sulcus, cingulate gyrus, superior parietal lobule, and superior frontal gyrus, have connections with the average number of 85, 120, 83,

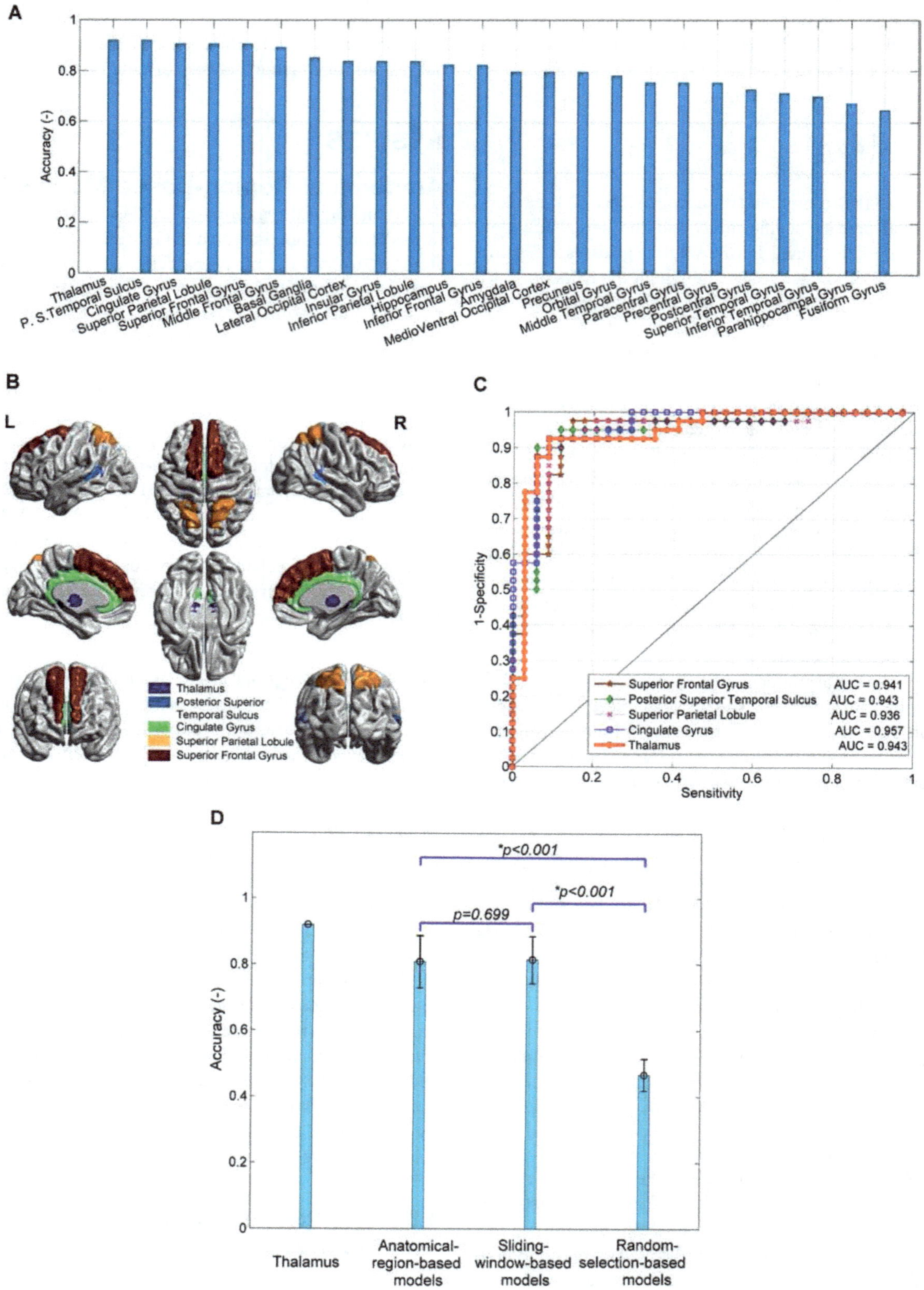

FIGURE 2 | The performances of predictive models of subclinical depression (SD) and their comparison. **(A)** The prediction accuracy of 24 anatomical-region-based models; **(B)** the brain regions leading to the top five accuracy models; **(C)** receiver operating characteristic (ROC) curves and area under the curve (AUC) of the top five models; **(D)** comparison of the accuracy of models using connections with thalamus, 24 anatomical-region-based models, 231 sliding-window-based models, and 100 random-selection-based models.

TABLE 1 | The confusion matrices of the top five anatomical-region-based models.

Model and items	Normal (gold standard)	Patient (gold standard)	Total
Thalamus model			
Predict to normal	37 (92.5%)	3 (8.8%)	40
Predict to patient	3 (7.5%)	31 (91.2%)	34
Posterior superior temporal sulcus model			
Predict to normal	36 (90.0%)	2 (5.9%)	38
Predict to patient	4 (10.0%)	**32 (94.1%)**	36
Cingulate gyrus model			
Predict to normal	37 (94.4%)	4 (11.8%)	41
Predict to patient	3 (5.6%)	30 (88.2%)	33
Superior parietal lobule model			
Predict to normal	36 (90.0%)	3 (11.1%)	39
Predict to patient	4 (10.0%)	31 (88.9%)	35
Superior frontal gyrus model			
Predict to normal	**38 (95.0%)**	5 (14.7%)	43
Predict to patient	2 (5.0%)	29 (85.3%)	31

222, and 131, respectively. **Figure 3B** shows the mean p-value of connections in individual brain regions, which ranges from 0.025 to 0.031.

The dependence of the accuracy of the predictive models on the number of connections associated within individual brain regions and the mean p-value of connections are shown in **Figure 3C**. The accuracy of the predictive models is related to the number of connection associated with brain regions ($r = 0.093$), but there is no statistical significance ($p = 0.665$). When the number of connections associated with brain regions is randomly reduced to 90, as with the thalamus, the accuracy does not increase. For instance, after reducing the number of connections in middle frontal gyrus from 229 to 90, the accuracy decreases from 0.89 to 0.70 (the mean of 100 times random samples). The accuracy of the predictive models is negatively related to the mean p-value of connections associated with brain regions without statistical significance ($r = 0.169$, $p = 0.429$). The high value of accuracy of the top five models is due to neither the large number of connections, nor the small p-value of the connections.

Dysfunctional Connections With the Thalamus

Given that the thalamus is seen as one possible dysfunctional brain region of SD, connections associated with the thalamus are investigated, as shown in **Figure 4**. The number of connections between the thalamus and precuneus, insular gyrus, paracentral gyrus, and amygdala is higher than that of the other regions (11, 8, 8, and 8, respectively). However, the number of connections between the thalamus and itself, the posterior superior temporal sulcus, cingulate gyrus, superior parietal lobule, and superior frontal gyrus is only 6, 5, 3, 4, and 4, respectively. High accuracy values of the models using connections associated with the posterior superior temporal sulcus, cingulate gyrus, superior parietal lobule, and superior frontal gyrus are independent on the thalamus. These regions may also be impacted by SD.

Subregions Within the Thalamus and Lateral Habenula

The distribution of the 90 significantly different connections associated with the thalamus among 16 subregions is shown in **Figure 5A**. There are 18 connections associated with the right posterior parietal thalamus (PPtha_r), much higher than those connected with the other regions. The significant asymmetry is observed, i.e., the right side has more connections than the left. Astonishingly, only two edges are connected to the left posterior parietal thalamus. The p-value of connections associated with PPtha_r is smaller than that of PPtha_l, as illustrated in the right part of **Figure 5A**. Based on Montreal Neurological Institute (MNI) coordinates, LHb is located in the posterior parietal thalamus (**Figure 5B**).

Node Degree of Subregions Within the Thalamus

The node degrees of 16 subregions within the thalamus are compared between SD and HC groups, as shown in **Figure 6**. Significant difference is found for 10 subregions. For eight subregions, the node degree of SD is significantly smaller than that of HC. The node degree of subregions on the right is higher than that of subregions on the left, for both SD and HC groups.

DISCUSSIONS

Sophisticated connectome-based brain biomarkers permit the association of brain measures with both subjective experiences and objective behaviors, leading to a reconceptualization of diagnoses of mental illness. Herein, we have built several reliable brain biomarkers (>0.9 accuracy) that predict SD using abnormal functional connections as input features and SVM as the machine learning algorithm. We have found dysfunctional brain regions, especially the thalamus and LHb, which may be the etiological origin of SD. We have observed a reduction of the node degree for the right LHb in SD, but not for the left. The significance of these findings and the related advantages of this methodology are interpreted and discussed in the following subsections.

Reliable Biomarkers for Subclinical Depression Prediction

In this study, we have identified reliable brain biomarkers for SD prediction through the large-scale brain networks driven from resting state fMRI and a machine learning algorithm. Previously we had constructed biomarkers using the degree of centrality of different brain regions. The highest AUC was 0.82 for the right posterior parietal lobule (12). Here, the biomarkers are more reliable, and the highest AUC of 0.957 is achieved while using connections with the cingulate gyrus. Moreover, the arbitrary anatomically adjacent subregions (obtained by the sliding window method) and the anatomically well-defined subregions (obtained by the anatomical-region-based method) produce models with similar performances. These models present significantly higher accuracy than those driven by the randomly selected subregions. These results suggest that anatomical adjacency is important in the

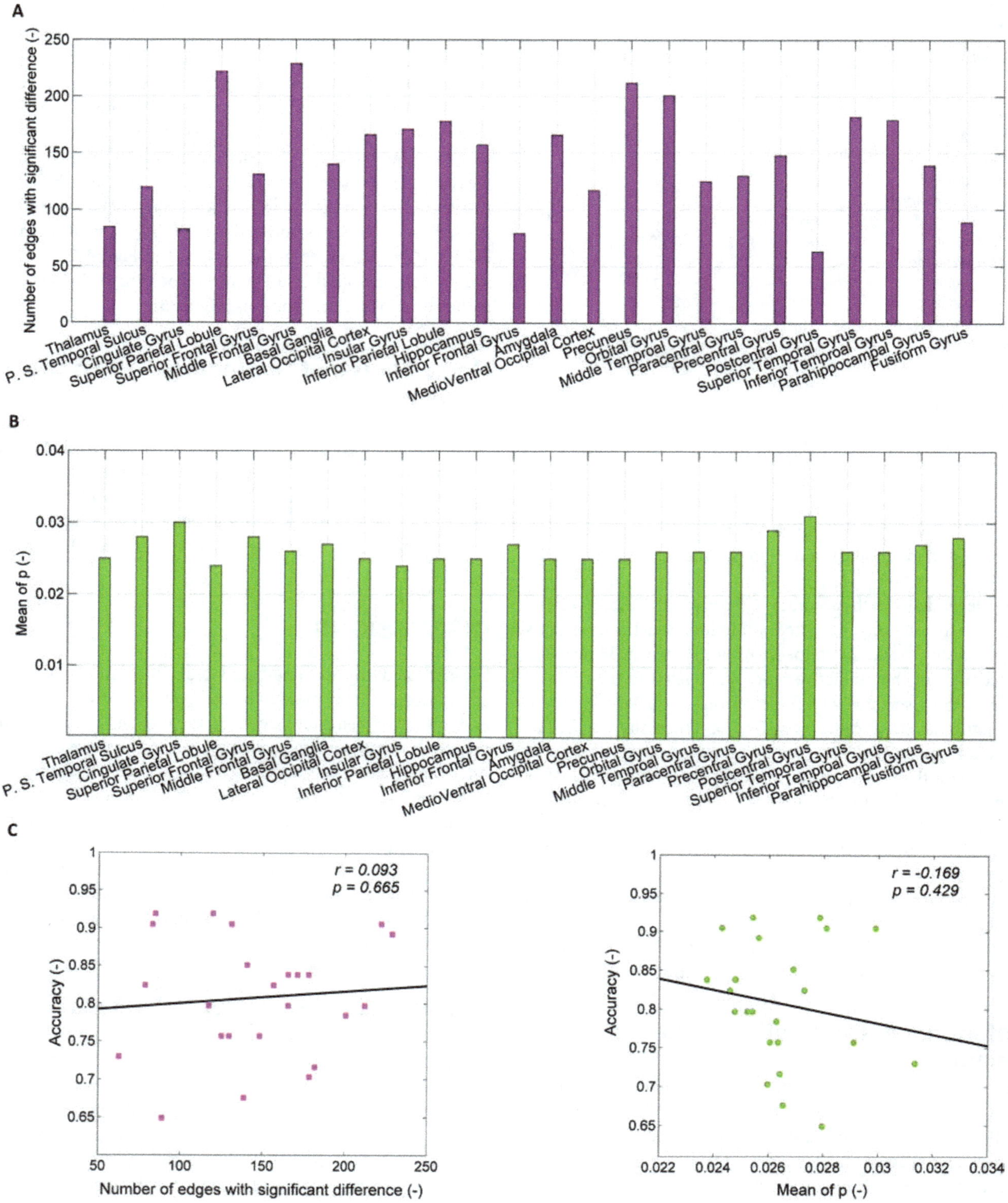

FIGURE 3 | Exclusion of confounders (the number of connections and the mean *p*-value). **(A)** The number of connections with significant difference between healthy controls (HCs) and SDs for each of 24 brain regions; **(B)** the *p*-value for significant difference of connection weight between HCs and SDs for each of 24 regions; **(C)** the relationship between the accuracy of prediction and the number of connections with significant difference (left part), between the accuracy of prediction and the mean of *p*-value for significant difference of connection weight (right part).

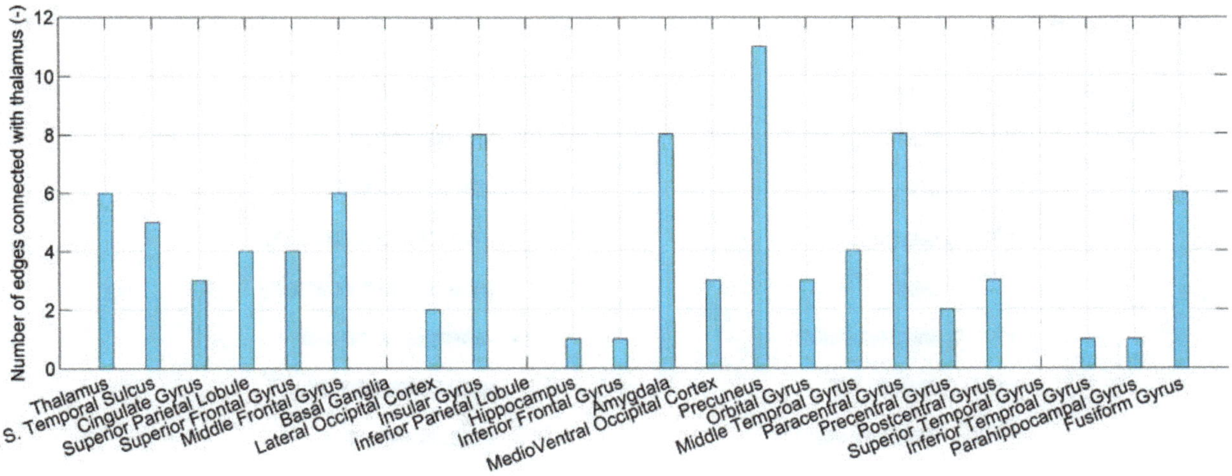

FIGURE 4 | The number of connections that present significant difference and connect the thalamus and each of 24 brain regions.

selection of feature (or connections) while building brain models or biomarkers. However, more sophisticated algorithms of feature selection, such as L_1-regularized sparse canonical correlation analysis (L_1-SCCA), may yield better biomarkers than anatomical adjacency (18, 25).

Dysfunctional Brain Regions in Subclinical Depression

Using the criterion of owing prediction accuracy greater than 0.90, we identified the top five regions associated with dysfunction in SD from 24 cortical and subcortical regions, defined by the human Brainnetome Atlas (44). These regions include the thalamus, posterior superior temporal sulcus, cingulate gyrus, superior parietal lobule, and superior frontal gyrus. Most of these regions had been reported in previous studies of SD. The related findings for each dysfunctional region are described below.

Not unexpectedly, given that the thalamus has multiple functions of relaying information between different subcortical regions and the cerebral cortex, the dysfunctional thalamus is identified in SD. It had been reported that two subtypes of depression had hyperconnectivity between the thalamic and frontostriatal network, resulting in symptoms related to reward processing, adaptive motor control, and action initiation (27, 53). Of particular importance, LHb, a small epithalamic structure, is believed to control reward and aversion processing. The importance of these observations will be discussed in detail below.

Distinct connectivity patterns are observed in subregions of the posterior cingulate cortex for SD (8). The anterior cingulate cortex (ACC) is an important component of reward circuitry, with abnormalities resulting in anhedonia (loss of interest/pleasure), a core symptom in MDD (54). Abnormal ACC is also linked to default model network (DMN, self-related thoughts), hyperconnectivity, and switching between the DMN and the central executive network (CEN, externally-focused cognition) (8, 14, 55, 56).

Previously we had reported that the superior parietal lobule (SPL, Brodmann area 7, BA 7) presented the decreased fractional ALFF (fALFF) (9). The SPL had been proposed to be the key component controlling the executive network and playing a critical role in working memory (57).

The superior frontal gyrus includes the dorsolateral prefrontal cortex (DLPFC) and the medial prefrontal cortex (MPFC). In depression, DLPFC is used for emotion adjustment, with the activity of DLPFC inhibited at rest but increased during symptom remission (58, 59). Our previous work had shown that the functional connectivity between SPL and DLPFC was reduced in SD (9). MPFC is an important component of DMN playing a crucial role in self-referential processing. A lack of DMN inhibition, i.e., self-focus, is a core issue of MDD (60). Most importantly, both regions of the superior frontal gyrus had been the targets for repetitive transcranial magnetic stimulation (rTMS) in depression treatment (61).

Dysfunctional Brain Regions Connected With the Thalamus

We have found that the dysfunctional thalamus in SD is mainly linked with the precuneus, insular gyrus, paracentral lobule, and amygdala. It is not surprising to observe the insula and amygdala because they are the neuroanatomical core of MDD pathology and closely related to anxiety (27). The precuneus is related to anhedonia, and the paracentral lobule (premotor) to anxiety. Positive connectivity between the LHb (an epithalamic structure) and the sensorimotor cortex had been reported by Ely et al. (13).

There is no overlap between the four regions with large number of abnormal connections associated with thalamus and the four regions (except thalamus) of the top five models ranked by accuracy. This is explained by the difference between machine learning and classical statistics which is discussed below.

Lateral Habenula—Beyond a Reasonable Doubt

Only one previous study had investigated the resting state functional connectivity of the LHb in SD (13). Herein, the SD

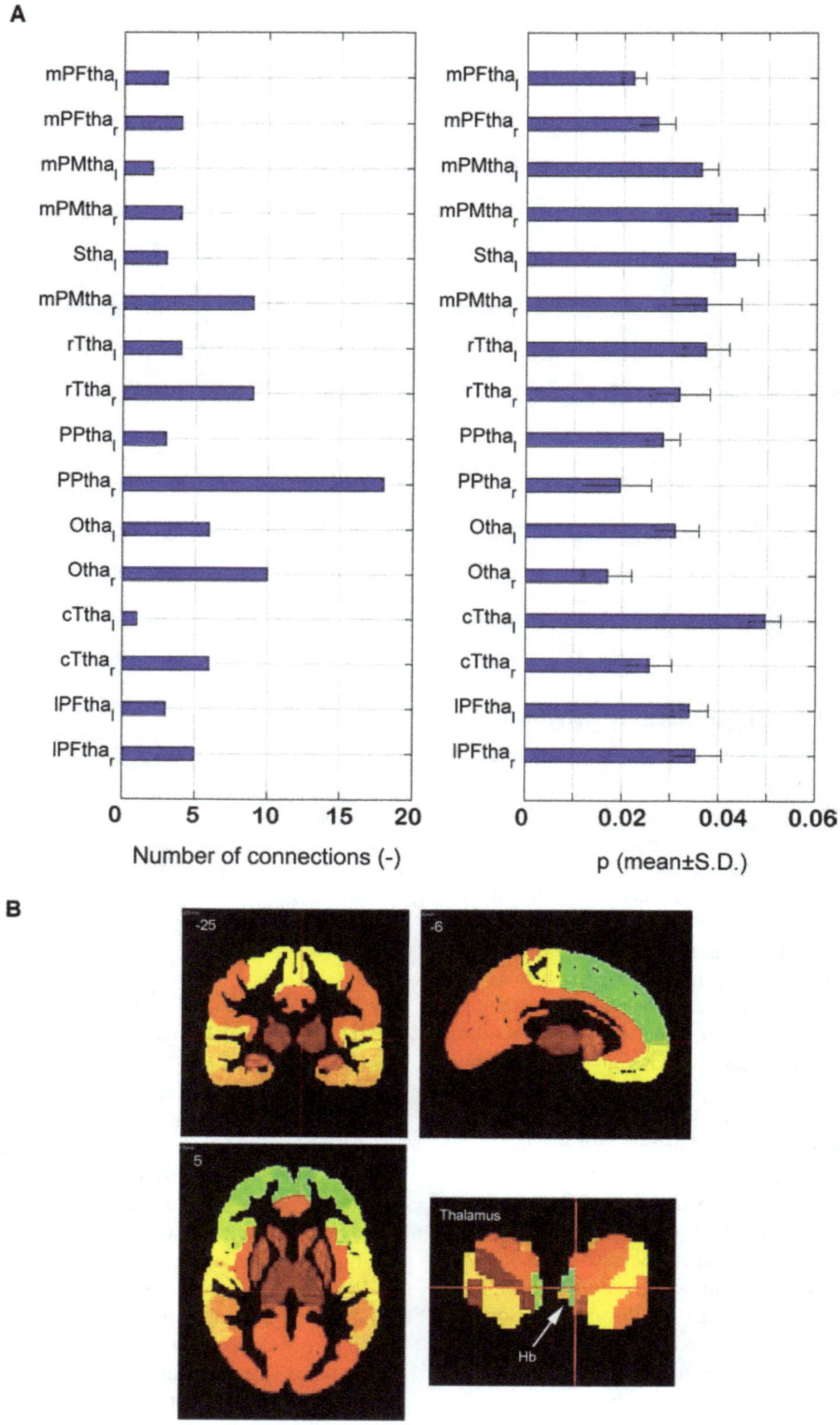

FIGURE 5 | Dysfunctional thalamus and lateral habenula. **(A)** The number of dysfunctional connections for16 subregions of thalamus (the left part) and the *p*-value of the dysfunctional connections with 16 subregions of thalamus (the right part); **(B)** the anatomical atlas of thalamus and LHb.

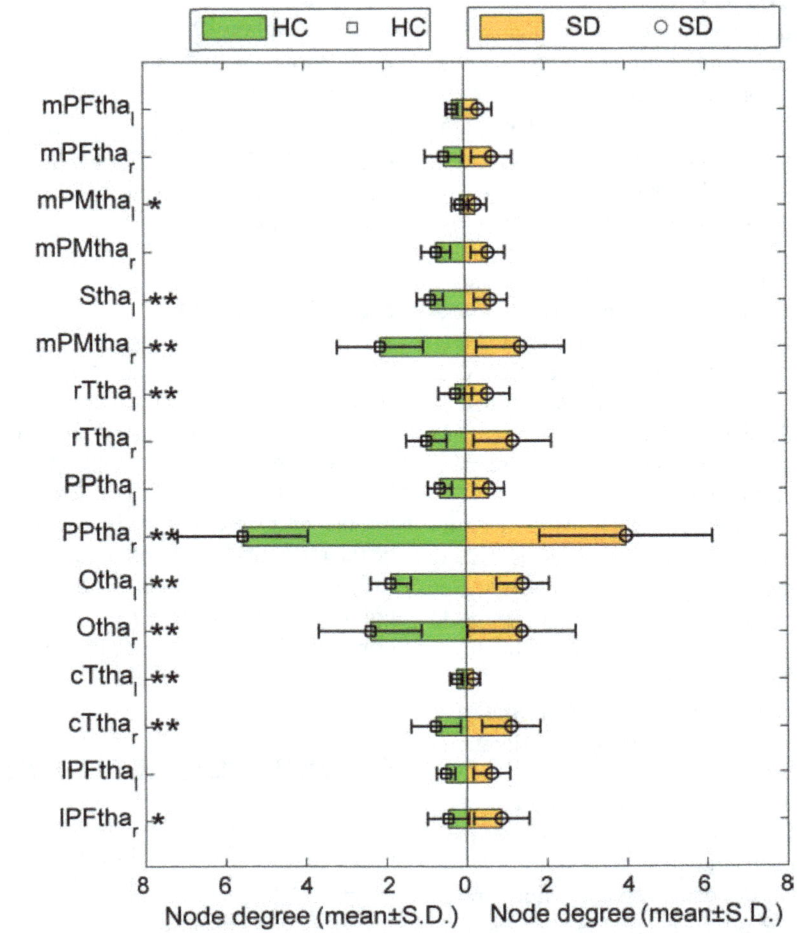

FIGURE 6 | Node degree of 16 subregions in the thalamus of HC and SD.

group shows greater LHb connectivity with DMN and lower connectivity with the salience network, which is consistent with prior finding in MDD. Here we found a lateralized decrease of node degree in the subregion with LHb (at right) in SD. This finding is consistent with our previous finding of decreased subcortical degree centrality (12). We speculate that the decreased node degree of LHb corresponds to its hyperactivity and abnormal bursts. Given that LHb has an inhibitory effect on dopamine neurons, Hikosak (32) proposed that the hyperactivity of LHb results in hypoactivity of dopamine neurons, reducing motor activity in MDD. Hyperactivity of LHb could be the result of bursts. According to Yang et al. (29), LHb burst firing increases in depression and LHb bursts lead to depression in rats. Interestingly, Ely et al. (13) found that LHb connectivity increased in the left and decreased in the right. This may partly explain the decreased node degree of the right LHb.

Among many dysfunctional brain regions, which one is the most likely etiological origin of SD? Is it LHb, as in depression for rats (29)? Given the correlative nature of resting-state fMRI, it is difficult to establish a causal inference (58). Therefore, we do not know which brain region is the cause or consequence of SD. However, based on these evidences given in our study, we believe that LHb may be the origin of SD, beyond a reasonable doubt.

Machine Learning and Classical Statistics

In this study, we have used the classical statistical method, the two-sample t-test, to initially screen the candidate connections with significant difference between SD and HC groups. The selected connections are input into the SVM models as features. The two-sample t-test is actually used as a one feature selection algorithm. The method of using group tests has been proven to yield an inflated bias (62). Thus, we did not carry out strict multiple comparison corrections. More powerful feature selection or dimension reduction algorithms, such as L1-regularized sparse canonical correlation analysis, linear elastic-net, and minimum-redundancy maximum relevancy, can be assessed in the future (25, 63).

Moreover, we found that connections with small p-values do not always lead to high prediction accuracy in machine-learning-based models. This is consistent with previous studies, and originates from the essential difference between group difference and classification (62, 64, 65).

Limitations and Future Works

The sample size is relatively small even though a large population is screened. The prediction accuracy may decrease with the sample size for most disorders (62). The generalizability of these models needs to be validated in independent cohorts. The 50 subjects (25 with high SD scores and 25 with low scores) from the WU-Minn Human Connectome Project (HCP) Consortium's 500 Subjects Release (66), previously used by Ely et al. (13), will be used in the future.

Only the criterion of BDI-II score >13 is relatively simple compared with the complicated clinical evaluation of SD. However, there is no consensus among researchers regarding how to combine different scales to define SD. Besides the widely applied BDI, the National Institutes of Health (NIH) Toolbox Negative Affect Survey Sadness Subscale, and the Achenbach Adult Self-Report (ASR) have been utilized (13, 16). Regression model of BDI-II score may tackle the issue induced by the fixed threshold.

We only distinguished subjects with SD from HC. However, it is probable that SD has several neurophysiological subtypes, as shown in depression (27). With an increased sample size, it may be possible to differentiate these subtypes. Moreover, generalizing our identified biomarkers to distinguish between SD and MDD cannot be done before the specific verification. The study done by Lawson et al. (67) demonstrated that habenula function is also disrupted in MDD. In our group, the data of MDD is being collected so that the verification will be carried out in the near future.

The voxel size of our fMRI images is 3.5 × 3.1 × 3.1 mm, which is larger than the volume of LHb, approximately 18.5 mm^3 per hemisphere (41). As a consequence the precise location of LHb is difficult to determine. The fMRI data with the whole brain coverage and high resolution (2 mm isotropic) is available for 25 subjects with high SD from the HCP (66). Using those high-resolution data, the node degree for LHb and its lateralization may be investigated clearly.

Actually, we have identified the dysfunctional brain regions from the predictive models driven by dysfunctional connections and especially identified LHb as the possible etiological origin of SD. To find the predictive and dysfunctional functional connections is also important. However, there are too many predictive functional connections in the current work to explain one by one. For example, even only for the right posterior parietal thalamus, 18 abnormal functional connections are available. Compared with the connections, the findings on brain regions are more reliable. Once the number of predictive functional connections is reduced to be less than 20 as done by Yahata et al. (25) their explanations will be feasible and valuable.

CONCLUSION

Through integrating functional brain connections and SVM, this study has provided the connectome-based biomarkers for accurate prediction of SD. Abnormal brain connections with the thalamus and LHb are found to be implicated with SD. The right LHb in SD shows the decreased node degree comparing with HC group, but the left LHb does not. This evidence indicates that LHb may be the etiological origin of SD. The generated biomarkers can aid early diagnosis of SD. Furthermore, the identified dysfunctional brain connections and regions may help localize the etiological origin of SD and understand the pathogenesis of SD.

AUTHOR CONTRIBUTIONS

SQ, JH, and XW designed and directed the study. YZ, SQ, BZ, DH, YT, and JH analyzed data. XW recruited participants and acquired data. YZ, SQ, and YT drafted the manuscript. All authors revised and approved the final version of the manuscript.

FUNDING

The Fundamental Research Funds for the Central Universities (N181904003, N172008008), the National Science Foundation of China (81871846), and the Science and Technology Planning Project of Guangzhou (201804010032).

REFERENCES

Lewinsohn PM, Klein DN, Durbin EC, Seeley JR, Rohde P. Family study of subthreshold depressive symptoms: risk factor for MDD? *J Affect Disord* (2003) 77(2):149–57. doi: 10.1016/S0165-0327(02)00106-4

Shankman SA, Lewinsohn PM, Klein DN, Small JW, Seeley JR, Altman SE. Subthreshold conditions as precursors for full syndrome disorders: a 15-year longitudinal study of multiple diagnostic classes. *J Child Psychol Psychiatry* (2009) 50(12):1485–94. doi: 10.1111/j.1469-7610.2009.02117.x

Fergusson DM, Horwood LJ, Ridder EM, Beautrais AL. Subthreshold depression in adolescence and mental health outcomes in adulthood. *Arch Gen Psychiatry* (2005) 62:66–72. doi: 10.1001/archpsyc.62.1.66

Cukrowicz KC, Schlegel EF, Smith PN, Jacobs MP, Van Orden KA, Paukert AP, et al. Suicide ideation among college students evidencing subclinical depression. *J Am Coll Health* (2011) 59(7):575–81. doi: 10.1080/07448481.2010.483710

Lavretsky H, Kumar A. Clinically significant non-major depression: old concepts, new insights. *Am J Geriatr Psychiatry* (2002) 10:239–55. doi: 10.1176/appi.ajgp.10.3.239

VanItallie TB. Subsyndromal depression in the elderly: underdiagnosed and untreated. *Metab Clin Exp* (2005) 54:39–44. doi: 10.1016/j.metabol.2005.01.012

Mikolajczyk RT, Maxwell AE, ElAnsari W, Naydenova V, Stock C, Ilieva S, et al. Prevalence of depressive symptoms in university students from Germany, Denmark, Poland and Bulgaria. *Soc. Epidemiol Psychiatr Sci* (2008) 43:105–12. doi: 10.1007/s00127-007-0282-0

Philippi CL, Motzkin JC, Pujara MS, Koenigs M. Subclinical depression severity is associated with distinct patterns of functional connectivity for subregions of anterior cingulate cortex. *J Psychiatr Res* (2015) 71:103–11. doi: 10.1016/j.jpsychires.2015.10.005

Wei X, Shen H, Ren J, Li X, Xu X, Yang R, et al. Altered resting-state connectivity in college students with nonclinical depressive symptoms. *Plos One* (2014) 9(12):e114603. doi: 10.1371/journal.pone.0114603

Wei X, Shen H, Ren J, Liu W, Yang R, Liu J, et al. Alteration of spontaneous neuronal activity in young adults with non-clinical depressive symptoms. *Psychiat Res Neuroim* (2015) 233(1):36–42. doi: 10.1016/j.pscychresns.2015.04.008

Wei X, Ren J, Liu W, Yang R, Xu X, Liu J, et al. Increased interhemispheric functional connectivity in college students with non-clinical depressive symptoms in resting state. *Neurosci* (2015) 589:67–72. doi: 10.1016/j.neulet.2015.01.034

Gao C, Liu W, Liu Y, Ruan X, Chen X, Liu L, et al. Decreased subcortical and increased cortical degree centrality in a nonclinical college student sample with subclinical depressive symptoms: a resting-state fMRI study. *Front Hum Neurosci* (2016) 10:1–9. doi: 10.3389/fnhum.2016.00617

Ely BA, Xu J, Goodman WK, Lapidus KA, Gabbay V, Stern ER. Resting-state functional connectivity of the human habenula in healthy individuals: associations with subclinical depression. *Hum Brain Mapp* (2016) 37(7):2369–84. doi: 10.1002/hbm.23179

Kaiser RH, Andrews-Hanna JR, Spielberg JM, Warren SL, Sutton BP, Miller GA, et al. Distracted and down: neural mechanisms of affective interference in subclinical depression. *Soc Cogn Affect Neurosci* (2015) 10(5):654–63. doi: 10.1093/scan/nsu100

Dedovic K, Giebl S, Duchesne A, Lue SD, Andrews J, Efanov S, et al. Psychological, endocrine, and neural correlates of attentional bias in subclinical depression. *Anxiety Stress Coping* (2016) 29(5):479–96. doi: 10.1080/10615806.2015.1101457

Petrican R, Saverino C, Rosenbaum RS, Grady C. Inter-individual differences in the experience of negative emotion predict variations in functional brain architecture. *Neuroimage* (2015) 123:80–8. doi: 10.1016/j.neuroimage.2015.08.031

Bassett DS, Sporns O. Network neuroscience. *Nat Neurosci* (2017) 20(3):353. doi: 10.1038/nn.4502

Woo CW, Chang LJ, Lindquist MA, Wager TD. Building better biomarkers: brain models in translational neuroimaging. *Nat Neurosci* (2017) 20(3):365–77. doi: 10.1038/nn.4478

Bzdok D, Meyer-Lindenberg A. Machine learning for precision psychiatry: opportunities and challenges. *Biol Psychiatry Cogn Neurosci Neuroim* (2018) 3(3):223. doi: 10.1016/j.bpsc.2017.11.007

Orru G, Pettersson-Yeo W, Marquand AF, Sartori G, Mechelli A. Using support vector machine to identify imaging biomarkers of neurological and psychiatric disease: a critical review. *Neurosci Biobehav Rev* (2012) 36(4):1140–52. doi: 10.1016/j.neubiorev.2012.01.004

Iniesta R, Stahl D, Mcguffin P. Machine learning, statistical learning and the future of biological research in psychiatry. *Psychol Med* (2016) 46:2455–65. doi: 10.1017/S0033291716001367

Vieira S, Pinaya WHL, Mechelli A. Using deep learning to investigate the neuroimaging correlates of psychiatric and neurological disorders: methods and applications. *Neurosci Biobehav Rev* (2017) 74:58–75. doi: 10.1016/j.neubiorev.2017.01.002

Gao S, Calhoun VD, Shui J. Machine learning in major depression: from classification to treatment outcome prediction. *CNS Neurosci Ther* (2018) 24:1037–52. doi: 10.1111/cns.13048

Dwyer DB, Falkai P, Koutsouleris N. Machine learning approaches for clinical psychology and psychiatry. *Annu Rev Clin Psychol* (2018) 14:91–118. doi: 10.1146/annurev-clinpsy-032816-045037

Yahata N, Morimoto J, Hashimoto R, Lisi G, Shibata K, Kawakubo Y, et al. A small number of abnormal brain connections predicts adult autism spectrum disorder. *Nat Commun* (2016) 7:11254. doi: 10.1038/ncomms11254

Librenzagarcia D, Kotzian BJ, Yang J, Mwangi B, Cao B, Lima LNP, et al. The impact ofmachine learning techniques in thestudy ofbipolar disorder: a systematic review. *Neurosci Biobehav Rev* (2017) 80:538–54. doi: 10.1016/j.neubiorev.2017.07.004

Drysdale AT, Grosenick L, Downar J, Dunlop K, Mansouri F, Meng Y, et al. Resting-state connectivity biomarkers define neurophysiological subtypes of depression. *Nat Med* (2017) 23(1):28–38. doi: 10.1038/nm.4246

Sui J, Qi S, van Erp TGM, Bustillo J, Jiang R, Lin D, et al. Multimodal neuromarkers in schizophrenia via cognition-guided MRI fusion. *Nat Commun* (2018) 9:3028. doi: 10.1038/s41467-018-05432-w

Yang Y, Cui Y, Sang K, Dong Y, Ni Z, Ma S, et al. Ketamine blocks bursting in the lateral habenula to rapidly relieve depression. *Nature* (2018) 554(7692):317–22. doi: 10.1038/nature25509

Matsumoto M, Hikosaka O. Lateral habenula as a source of negative reward signals in dopamine neurons. *Nature* (2007) 447:1111–5. doi: 10.1038/nature05860

Lawson RP, Seymour B, Loh E, Lutti A, Dolan RJ, Dayan P, et al. The habenula encodes negative motivational value associated with primary punishment in humans. *Proc Natl Acad Sci USA* (2014) 111(32):11858–63. doi: 10.1073/pnas.1323586111

Hikosaka O. The habenula: from stress evasion to value-based decision-making. *Nat Rev Neurosci* (2010) 11(7):503–13. doi: 10.1038/nrn2866

Stopper CM, Floresco SB. What's better for me? Fundamental role for lateral habenula in promoting subjective decision biases. *Nat Neurosci* (2014) 17(1):33–5. doi: 10.1038/nn.3587

Li B, Piriz J, Mirrione M, Chung C, Proulx CD, Schulz D, et al. Synaptic potentiation onto habenula neurons in the learned helplessness model of depression. *Nature* (2011) 470:535–9. doi: 10.1038/nature09742

Stamatakis AM, Stuber GD. Activation of lateral habenula inputs to the ventral midbrain promotes behavioral avoidance. *Nat Neurosci* (2012) 15:1105–7. doi: 10.1038/nn.3145

Proulx CD, Hikosaka O, Malinow R. Reward processing by the lateral habenula in normal and depressive behaviors. *Nat Neurosci* (2014) 17:1146– 52. doi: 10.1038/nn.3779

Benarroch EE. Habenula: recently recognized functions and potential clinical relevance. *Neurology* (2015) 85(11):992–1000. doi: 10.1212/WNL.0000000000001937

Boulos LJ, Darcq E, Kieffer BL. Translating the habenula—from rodents to humans. *Biol Psychiatry* (2016) 81(4):296–305. doi: 10.1016/j.biopsych.2016.06.003

Sartorius A, Kiening KL, Kirsch P, von Gall CC, Haberkorn U, Unterberg AW, et al. Remission of major depression under deep brain stimulation of the lateral habenula in a therapy-refractory patient. *Biol Psychiatry* (2010) 67:e9– e11. doi: 10.1016/j.biopsych.2009.08.027

Savitz JB, Nugent AC, Bogers W, Roiser JP, Bain EE, Neumeister A, et al. Habenula volume in bipolar disorder and major depressive disorder: a high-resolution magnetic resonance imaging study. *Biol Psychiatry* (2011) 69(4):336–43. doi: 10.1016/j.biopsych.2010.09.027

Ranft K, Dobrowolny H, Krell D, Bielau H, Bogerts B, Bernstein HG. Evidence for structural abnormalities of the human habenular complex in affective disorders but not in schizophrenia. *Psychol Med* (2010) 40(04):557– 67. doi: 10.1017/S0033291709990821

Salas R, Baldwin P, De Biasi M, Montague R. BOLD responses to negative reward prediction errors in the human habenula. *Front Hum Neurosci* (2010) 36(4). doi: 10.3389/fnhum.2010.00036

Lawson RP, Drevets WC, Roiser JP. Defining the habenula in human neuroimaging studies. *Neuroimage* (2013) 64:722–7. doi: 10.1016/j.neuroimage.2012.08.076

Fan L, Li H, Zhuo J, Zhang Y, Wang J, Chen L, et al. The human brainnetome atlas: a new brain atlas based on connectional architecture. *Cereb Cortex* (2016) 26:3508. doi: 10.1093/cercor/bhw157

Yan C, Zang Y. DPARSF: a MATLAB toolbox for "pipeline" data analysis of resting-state fMRI. *Front Syst Neurosci* (2010) 4:13. doi: 10.3389/fnsys.2010.00013

Cohen JD, Daw N, Engelhardt B, Hasson U, Li K, Niv Y, et al. Computational approaches to fMRI analysis. *Nat Neurosci* (2017) 20:304–13. doi: 10.1038/nn.4499

Weissenbacher A, Kasess C, Gerstl F, Lanzenberger R, Moser E, Windischberger C. Correlations and anticorrelations in resting-state functional connectivity MRI: a quantitative comparison of preprocessing strategies. *Neuroimage* (2009) 47:1408–16. doi: 10.1016/j.neuroimage.2009.05.005

Murphy K, Birn RM, Handwerker DA, Jones TB, Bandettini PA. The impact of global signal regression on resting state correlations: are anti-correlated networks introduced? *Neuroimage* (2009) 44:893–905. doi: 10.1016/j.neuroimage.2008.09.036

Wang J, Zuo X, Gohel S, Milham MP, Biswal BB, He Y. Graph theoretical analysis of functional brain networks: test–retest evaluation on short- and long-term resting-state functional MRI data. *PLoS One* (2011) 6:e21976. doi: 10.1371/journal.pone.0021976

Wang J, Wang X, Xia M, Liao X, Evans A, He Y. GRETNA: a graph theoretical network analysis toolbox for imaging connectomics. *Front Hum Neurosci* (2015) 9:386. doi: 10.3389/fnhum.2015.00458

Benjamini Y, Hochberg Y. Controlling the false discovery rate: a practical and powerful approach to multiple testing. *J R Statist Soc B* (1995) 57:289–300. doi: 10.2307/2346101

Chang CC, Lin CJ. LIBSVM: a library for support vector machines. *ACM Trans Intell Syst Technol* (2011) 2(27):1–27. doi: 10.1145/1961189.1961199

Ferenczi EA, Zalocusky KA , Liston C, Grosenick L, Warden MR, Amatya D, et al. Prefrontal cortical regulation of brainwide circuit dynamics and reward-related behavior. *Science* (2016) 351:aac9698. doi: 10.1126/science.aac9698

Pujara M, Koenigs M. Mechanisms of reward circuit dysfunction in psychiatric illness prefrontalestriatal interactions. *Neuroscience* (2014) 20:82e95. doi: 10.1177/1073858413499407

Whitfield-Gabrieli S, Ford JM. Default mode network activity and connectivity in psychopathology. *Annu Rev Clin Psychol* (2012) 8:49e76. doi: 10.1146/annurev-clinpsy-032511-143049

Hamilton JP, Furman DJ, Chang C, Thomason ME, Dennis E, Gotlib IH. Default-mode and task-positive network activity in major depressive disorder: implications for adaptive and maladaptive rumination. *Biol Psychiatry* (2011) 70:327e333. doi: 10.1016/j.biopsych.2011.02.003

Koenigs M, Barbey AK, Postle BR, Grafman J. Superior parietal cortex is critical for the manipulation of information in working memory. *J Neurosci* (2009) 29(47):14980–6. doi: 10.1523/JNEUROSCI.3706-09.2009

Koenigs M, Grafmanb J. The functional neuroanatomy of depression: distinct roles for ventromedial and dorsolateral prefrontal cortex. *Behav Brain Res* (2009) 201:239–43. doi: 10.1016/j.bbr.2009.03.004

Viviani R. Emotion regulation, attention to emotion, and the ventral attentional network. *Front Hum Neurosci* (2013) 7:746. doi: 10.3389/fnhum.2013.00746

Lemogne C, Delaveau P, Freton M, Guionnet S, Fossati P. Medial prefrontal cortex and the self in major depression. *J Affect Disord* (2012) 136(1–2):e1–e11. doi: 10.1016/j.jad.2010.11.034

Downar J, Daskalakis ZJ. New targets for rTMS in depression: a review of convergent evidence. *Brain Stimul* (2013) 6(3):231–40. doi: 10.1016/j.brs.2012.08.006

Arbabshirani MR, Plis S, Sui J, Calhoun VD. Single subject prediction of brain disorders in neuroimaging: promises and pitfalls. *Neuroimage* (2017) 145:137–65. doi: 10.1016/j.neuroimage.2016.02.079

Brown G, Pocock A, Zhao MJ, Lujan M. Conditional likelihood maximisation: a unifying framework for mutual information feature selection. *J Mach Learn Res* (2012) 13:27–66. doi: 10.1080/00207179.2012.669851

Shmueli G. To explain or to predict? *Stat Sci* (2010) 25:289–310. doi: 10.1214/10-STS330

Bzdok D. Classical statistics and statistical learning in imaging neuroscience. *Front Neurosci* (2017) 11:543. doi: 10.3389/fnins.2017.00543

Van Essen DC, Smith SM, Barch DM, Behrens TE, Yacoub E, Ugurbil K, et al. The WU-Minn Human Connectome Project: an overview. *Neuroimage* (2013) 80:62–79. doi: 10.1016/j.neuroimage.2013.05.041

Lawson RP, Nord CL, Seymour B, Thomas DL, Dayan P, Pilling S, Roiser JP. Disrupted habenula function in major depression. *Mol Psychiatry* (2017) 22:202–8. doi: 10.1038/mp.2016.81

19

Hub Patterns-Based Detection of Dynamic Functional Network Metastates in Resting State: A Test-Retest Analysis

Xin Zhao[1], Qiong Wu[1], Yuanyuan Chen[2], Xizi Song[2], Hongyan Ni[3] and Dong Ming[1,2]**

[1] Department of Biomedical Engineering, College of Precision Instruments and Optoelectronics Engineering, Tianjin University, Tianjin, China, [2] Tianjin International Joint Research Center for Neural Engineering, Academy of Medical Engineering and Translational Medicine, Tianjin University, Tianjin, China, [3] Department of Radiology, Tianjin First Center Hospital, Tianjin, China

***Correspondence:**
Hongyan Ni
nihyan@sina.com
Dong Ming
richardming@tju.edu.cn

The spontaneous dynamic characteristics of resting-state functional networks contain much internal brain physiological or pathological information. The metastate analysis of brain functional networks is an effective technique to quantify the essence of brain functional connectome dynamics. However, the widely used functional connectivity-based metastate analysis ignored the topological structure, which could be locally reflected by node centrality. In this study, 23 healthy young volunteers (21–26 years) were recruited and scanned twice with a 1-week interval. Based on the time sequences of node centrality, we promoted a node centrality-based clustering method to find metastates of functional connectome and conducted a test-retest experiment to assess the stability of those identified metastates using the described method. The hub regions of metastates were further compared with the structural networks' organization to depict its potential relationship with brain structure. Results of extracted metastates showed repeatable dynamic features between repeated scans and high overlapping rate of hub regions with brain intrinsic sub-networks. These identified hub patterns from metastates further highly overlapped with the structural hub regions. These findings indicated that the proposed node centrality-based metastates detection method could reveal reliable and meaningful metastates of spontaneous dynamics and indicate the underlying nature of brain dynamics as well as the potential relationship between these dynamics and the organization of the brain connectome.

Keywords: metastate, dynamic functional connectivity, structural network, clustering analysis, node centrality, hubs

INTRODUCTION

The functional brain connectome, considering the brain as a complex network, indicates the spatial distributions and integrated organizations. Resting-state functional magnetic resonance imaging (rs-fMRI) can provide these kinds of intrinsic information of brain function (Biswal et al., 1995; Cordes et al., 2001) through measuring the synchronization between temporal fluctuations across spatially separated brain regions, which are known as functional connectivity (FC). It is the most basic measure and has been widely used in physiology (Damoiseaux et al., 2008; Betzel et al., 2014; Chen et al., 2017, 2018) and pathology (Bing et al., 2010; Veer, 2010; Widjaja et al., 2013; Ham et al., 2015; Su et al., 2015; Zhuo et al., 2018). More importantly, the brain function in resting state also reveals dynamics or temporal distributions of brain connections, which spontaneously change from seconds to minutes (Chang and Glover, 2010; Calhoun et al., 2014), which is called dynamic FC. Dynamic FC provides a novel insight into brain function which has been proved to contain useful information (Viviano et al., 2017; Xia et al., 2019) and can even be complementary to traditional static FC (Liégeois et al., 2019). It also enables us to better understand the behavior of different subnetworks (Al-Sharoa et al., 2019) and contains the intrinsic neural activities (Hutchison et al., 2013b) associated with the brain functional (Syed et al., 2017; He et al., 2018) or structural organizations (Shen et al., 2015; Cabral et al., 2017). Though dynamic FC presents a promising way to uncover the mysterious activates in human brain function, it is still unclear how brain function dynamically changes.

Metastate in the human brain is an interesting idea with which to describe the spontaneous fluctuation of FC as well as functional networks (Allen et al., 2014; Shakil et al., 2016; Shine et al., 2016; Vidaurre et al., 2017) and originates from a typical concept, "microstates," in electrophysiological studies (Gale, 1983; Lehmann et al., 1987). Metastates are considered as the certain brain FC patterns or brain states that repeatedly appear over and over again in the scanning period and can somehow represent those microstates at mesoscale. Increasing evidence has shown that the occurrence of transition between metastates contains meaningful information about normal aging and schizophrenia (Hansen et al., 2015; Yu et al., 2015; Shakil et al., 2016) and shows great potential regarding intrinsic interactions and complicated organizations (Hutchison et al., 2013a) of brain function (Hutchison et al., 2013a; Andrew and Michael, 2015).

Based on the sliding windowed correlations, plenty of previous studies applied whole brain FC-based clustering to represent and detect brain metastates (Allen et al., 2014; Hansen et al., 2015; Yu et al., 2015; Shakil et al., 2016; Syed et al., 2017; Cheng et al., 2018). It makes sense that the patterns of FC with high similarity represent the same state and the connectivity patterns are the first pictures of the fluctuations of whole brain connection. However, high dimension in connection vectors may limit the findings, and the whole brain FC patterns are not well interpreted. What if using secondary measures of whole brain dynamic FC would yield meaningful representations of metastates? As is common knowledge, brain functional networks exhibit rich-club organization, whereby a small number of nodes tend to be connected densely. In fact, many studies have found that certain nodes or brain regions dynamically participate across different tasks (Schaefer et al., 2014; Bola and Sabel, 2015; Preti et al., 2017) or across different provincial communities (Hansen et al., 2015; Chen et al., 2017; Gordon et al., 2018). These indicated the potential feature of dynamic roles of nodes even in resting state. On the other hand, the node centrality is the secondary measure and can represent the topologic aspects of brain connectivity patterns. The regional activities or the regional signals are the origins of brain connectivity and the node centrality represents the significance of regional activities. Therefore, the patterns of regions/nodes would be reasonably more representative than the patterns of connectivity.

Overall, this paper aims to propose a method to extract the brain metastates using node centrality-based k-means clustering in resting state. Specifically, the node centrality scores were calculated as the degree-based eigenvector centrality (Correa et al., 2012; Meghanathan, 2015a,b) for each windowed FC matrix yielding a dynamic node centrality sequence. The metastates would be defined by the cluster centers after k-means. We expected that the metastates detected by the proposed method can represent meaningful information of brain function or physiological activities in resting state. Because of the lack of mathematical proof of metastates, experimental reliability analysis needs to be verified. Recently, there was a test-retest reliability study (Chao et al., 2018) about dynamic FC, providing the first insight into the reproducibility of dynamic FC but only focusing on the FC not the metastates. Therefore, a test-retest reliability experiment was performed to examine the repeatability of metastates. Furthermore, we further compared the hub distribution between functional metastates and the structural network to explore the potential relationship between them. Through this, we hopefully can verify the reliability of metastates extracted with the proposed method and delineate the potential mechanism of the functional dynamics in resting state.

MATERIALS AND METHODS

Participants and MRI Acquisition

All recruited participants underwent rigorous clinical examinations and psychological evaluations and signed informed written consent. In total, 23 healthy adults (mean age: 23.6 years; range from 21 to 26 years; 12 female), without history of neurological or psychiatric disorders, with current physical and mental health and also with healthy living habits (no drugs, no alcohol addiction, no smoking, normal work and rest, and emotional stability) were included in this study. One week before MRI scanning, participants were told to keep normal emotion, sleeping and food intake (not too heavy, e.g., too hot or too salty). The study was approved by the medical ethics committee for research in humans of Tianjin First Central Hospital.

Magnetic resonance imaging images were acquired on a 3.0T Siemens scanner (Tim Trio, Germany) with a 32-channel head coil at Tianjin First Central Hospital. For each subject, there was a test-retest experiment: scanning twice with 1-week (7 days) interval at the same imaging site and same time (6:00 pm–9:00 pm) of day. Acquisitions included resting-state fMRI with echo-planar imaging (EPI) sequence, high-angular diffusion tensor imaging (DTI) with spin echo-echo planar imaging (SS-SE-EPI) sequence and anatomical T1 images with high-resolution 3-dimensional (3D) magnetization-prepared rapid acquisition with gradient echo (MPRAGE) sequence. Scanning settings for rs-fMRI were as follows: repetition time (TR) = 2.5 s, echo time (TE) = 30 ms, voxel size = 3.0 mm × 3.0 mm × 3.0 mm, flip angle (FA) = 80°, field of view (FOV) = 192 mm × 192 mm, matrix size = 64 × 64, number of slices = 28, slice thickness = 3 mm without interslice gap, scan time = 650 s, timepoints = 260. During scanning, participants were instructed to relax, keep their eyes open, try to keep their head and body still and not think anything special. Scanning settings for high-angular DTI were as follows: TR = 4000 ms, TE = 30 ms, number of slices = 45, slice thickness = 2 mm without interslice gap, voxel size = 2.0 mm × 2.0 mm × 2.0 mm; three unweighted b0 scans and 64 weighted diffusion scans with a weighting of 1000 s/mm^2 were acquired within 12 min. Multiband acceleration sequencing was used with accelerated factor = 4. Scanning parameters for anatomical T1 images were acquired for anatomical reference and definition of the different structural nodes of the network, using the following scanning parameters: TR/TE = 10/4.6 ms, FOV = 240 mm × 240 mm, 176 slices covering the whole brain, 1.0 mm isotropic voxel size, about 5 min.

Image Preprocessing

The fMRI data were preprocessed using the DPABI (V3.0) package[1] (Kevin et al., 2009). Preprocessing steps included removing the first 10 volumes, slice-timing correction, head motion correction, linear trend removal, band-pass filtering with frequency of 0.02–0.1 Hz which depended on the size of sliding window (Hindriks et al., 2016), and spatial smoothing (FWHM = 6 mm full-width at half-maximum Gaussian kernel). Nuisance signals including mean signals from ventricles (CSF), white matter (WM), whole brain (global mean signal) and the 24 motion parameters (six motion parameters, derivative and the quadratic terms) were regressed out (Fox et al., 2005). There has long been controversy regarding global mean signal processing (Kevin et al., 2009 and Fox et al., 2009). Because global mean signal removal brings negative FCs, the global signal contains much non-neural information and is sensitive to head motion. However, researchers from the two perspectives come to a consensus (Murphy and Fox, 2016) about this issue: whether it is essential to do global signal removing really depends on the specific question. In current research, node-degree-based measures were obtained to capture the dynamic networks. It is commonly known that the global mean signal removing can greatly increase the specificity of the fMRI signal. Global mean signal removing will be beneficial for our purpose. In addition, removing the global mean signal can also reduce the impact associated with head motion. To further control head motion effects, we removed the volumes with frame-wise displacement (FD) higher than 0.3 mm and removed the subject remaining with less than 200 volumes. No significant differences were found in terms of mean FD (p = 0.811) or the number of censored volumes (p = 0.723) across all subjects between two scans by using paired t-test.

Diffusion tensor imaging images were preprocessed using DTI-Explore package[2] (Leemans et al., 2009). Preprocessing steps included susceptibility distortions correction (estimating a field distortion map based on the three b0 images), eddy-current distortions and motion corrections (Andersson and Skare, 2002), a robust tensor fitting (Chang et al., 2005) and WM tract reconstruction based on the FACT (fiber assignment by continuous tracking) algorithm (Mori and Van Zijl, 2002; Mori et al., 2010). This procedure resulted in a large sample of all possible (reconstructable) fiber tracts of the brain network. A fiber streamline was stopped when the fiber track reached a voxel with a FA value 0.1 (indicating a low level of preferred diffusion within that particular voxel), when the trajectory of the traced fiber left the brain mask or when the fiber tract made a sharp turn of 45°.

For each subject, T1 images from two sessions were aligned and averaged for better quality. We utilized a two-step non-linear spatial registration method to transform the native functional or diffusional images to MNI space: firstly, native functional image (the first volume) or diffusional image (b0 image) was individually affined to the averaged T1 image; second, this natively averaged T1 image was nonlinearly registered based on the MNI-152 T1 template in FMRIB Software Library (FSL)[3] software package (Linux, United Kingdom). Combining these two steps, we can easily transform all the well preprocessed functional images and diffusional measures into standard MNI space.

Functional Network Construction

In this study, automated atlas labeling (AAL 90) (Tzourio-Mazoyer et al., 2002) was adopted to define the regions of functional networks. Each brain region in the AAL template was used as a regional mask to extract the time signal of BOLD functional data. We excluded the regions from the cerebellum to focus more attention on the brain patterns. Ninety columns of time signals were extracted and a 90 × 90 correlation matrix was calculated using Pearson correlation. Then FC matrixes were obtained by fisher z-transformation. The dynamic sequences of FC matrixes were obtained by the sliding window correlation method. There is still a lack of knowledge regarding what the best window length is and how it influences the results. A large number of previous studies (Hindriks et al., 2016; Chen et al., 2017, 2018) have converged to a short range from 50 to 60 s. Arbitrarily and also empirically, we fixed the length of the rectangle window as 60 s (width = 24 × TR), and the window was shifted with a step of 1 TR = 2.5 s (Hutchison et al., 2013a; Leonardi et al., 2013; Allen et al., 2014). Therefore, for one scan of each subject, a sequence of 232 FC matrixes were obtained.

The meaningless connections in static FC were removed to make the FC matrix to be spared or less redundant. Proportional thresholding on the weighted FC matrix was conducted based on the connection density, which is one of the two thresholding techniques of FC matrixes (the other is deterministic thresholding based on a FC strength). In order to select a proper density thresholding value, one sample t-test was done on the static FC matrixes to find the significant connections which were significantly >0 (FDR $q < 0.05$; focused on positive connections), and two binarized matrixes for each group were presented. A density thresholding value was selected referring to the densities of these group binarized matrixes, which were 0.38 and 0.41. In this paper, 40% of the connections—which had the higher FC strength—were retained (namely, 40% of the connections had higher FC strength and were set to one while the other 60% were set to zeros), yielding binarized connectivity

[1] http://rfmri.org/dpabi

[2] http://www.exploredti.com

[3] https://fsl.fmrib.ox.ac.uk/fsl/fslwiki/

matrixes. Density-based binarization can provide binarized FC matrixes which have the same number of connections. After the density-based thresholding, the FC weights were given back to the remaining connections, yielding weighted matrixes.

Clustering Analysis

The degree-based measure of node centrality is a direct and local topologic measurement including degree centrality and eigenvector centrality. Degree centrality:

$$C_D(i) = \sum_{i \neq j} A_{ij} \tag{1}$$

Eigenvector centrality:

$$C_E(i) = \frac{1}{\lambda_1} \sum_{j=1}^{N} A_{ij} x_j \tag{2}$$

Here, $Ax_j = \lambda x_j$. "A" represents the FC matrix, "x_j" and "λ," respectively, represent the nonzero eigenvector and eigenvalue of "A," "i" and "j" respectively, represent different nodes. Because degree centrality is too local, ignoring the importance of the nodes that the target node connects with, eigenvector centrality is considered here. These node centrality scores were calculated for each spared, weighted and windowed FC matrix, yielding a series of node centrality scores. The yielded node centrality time series represented the node centrality distribution of FC patterns at each windowed time. Then, every node centrality vector was normalized into a standard normal distribution $N(0,1)$. We also compared the difference of this dynamic node centrality with different window length: 20, 30, 50, and 60 s (**Supplementary Figure S1**). The node centrality time series with all kinds of window lengths showed temporally repeated patterns. However, the periods of patterns were shorter, with 20 and 30 s, than that of other two window lengths, which were within the popularly used window length range. The 50 and 60 s patterns were quite similar.

Each node centrality vector of one windowed FC matrix was treated as one sample in clustering analysis. Datasets from scan I and scan II were treated as two independent groups to conduct the clustering analysis separately. Based on the k-means++ algorithm (Arthur and Vassilvitskii, 2007), the clustering results based on all vectors within one group were obtained first with randomized initialization (group-level clustering). And then the resulted cluster centers were used as the initial starts for a second round of clustering within each subject's node centrality vectors in that group (individual clustering). K-means++ was reported to be more independent from the initial points than the original k-means clustering. Within the group-level clustering, an optimization about the number of clusters was conducted with elbow criterion based on the cluster validity index (**Supplementary Figure S2**). Finally, $k = 5$ was outperformed. For the distance measure in k-means, we tried several ones, and arbitrarily selected the correlation distance (1 - Pearson correlation) because of the better clustering and higher stability of the optimal number of clusters. Typical individual results were shown in **Figure 1**. The whole clustering strategies were done for each group separately. Different clusters or centers indicated that the extracted metastates and all the node centrality vectors recognized as the same cluster were averaged to represent the node centrality pattern of that metastate.

When the clustering was done, dwell time and transition time were calculated, which are typically and popularly used features to describe the dynamic of metastates (Allen et al., 2014; Chen et al., 2019). Dwell time was the total time that one metastate appears during the scan period (**Supplementary Figure S3**), which was calculated by the number of windows belonged to one cluster, or the number multiplied by TR (Damaraju et al., 2014; Mennigen et al., 2018; Xia et al., 2019). Transition time represented the times of transitions from one metastate to another during the scan period (Chen et al., 2019; Lee et al., 2019; Xia et al., 2019).

Test-Retest Reliability Analysis

The intra-class correlation coefficient (ICC) (Bartko, 1966) is one of the reliability coefficient indexes to measure test-retest reliability. Bartko (1966) first used it to evaluate the reliability in 1966. Xi-Nian et al. (2010) and Zuo and Xing (2014) used ICC to analyze the test-retest reliability of various fMRI processing methods and indicators, which had important guiding significance for fMRI studies. ICC is equal to the individual variability divided by the total variability, and the value is between 0 and 1. A value of 0 represents completely untrusted, and 1 represents completely trusted. It is generally acknowledged that ICC < 0.4 indicates poor reliability and >0.75 indicates good reliability. ICC is defined as:

$$\mathrm{ICC} = \frac{\sum_{i=1}^{n} (x_{1i} - \bar{x})(x_{2i} - \bar{x})}{(n-1)s_x^2} \tag{3}$$

Here, n represents the total number of subjects; x_{1i} represents the first measurement of the ith subject; x_{2i} represents the second measurement of the ith subject; and $\bar{x}$ and s_x represent the mean value and the standard deviation of all observations, respectively. Before the ICC analysis, the Bartlett and Kolmogorov–Smirnov tests were applied to verify the heteroscedasticity and the normality of the data.

Structural Network Construction

Based on DTI image analysis and fiber tracking, the direct structural connections were calculated. With the AAL-90 parcellation, 90 brain typical regions within individual native space were assigned and used to generate the structural connectivity according to the number of tracts between each pair of regions. Data processing was performed based on the whole brain fiber tracts using TrackVis software[4].

Regional Hub Nodes Analysis

A series of highly connected nodes, having high node degrees or high centralities, are identified as "brain hubs." In this paper, we utilized a typical way to highlight the hub nodes. All nodes were ranked according to node centrality scores, and those higher than the mean up to one standard deviation

[4]http://trackvis.org/

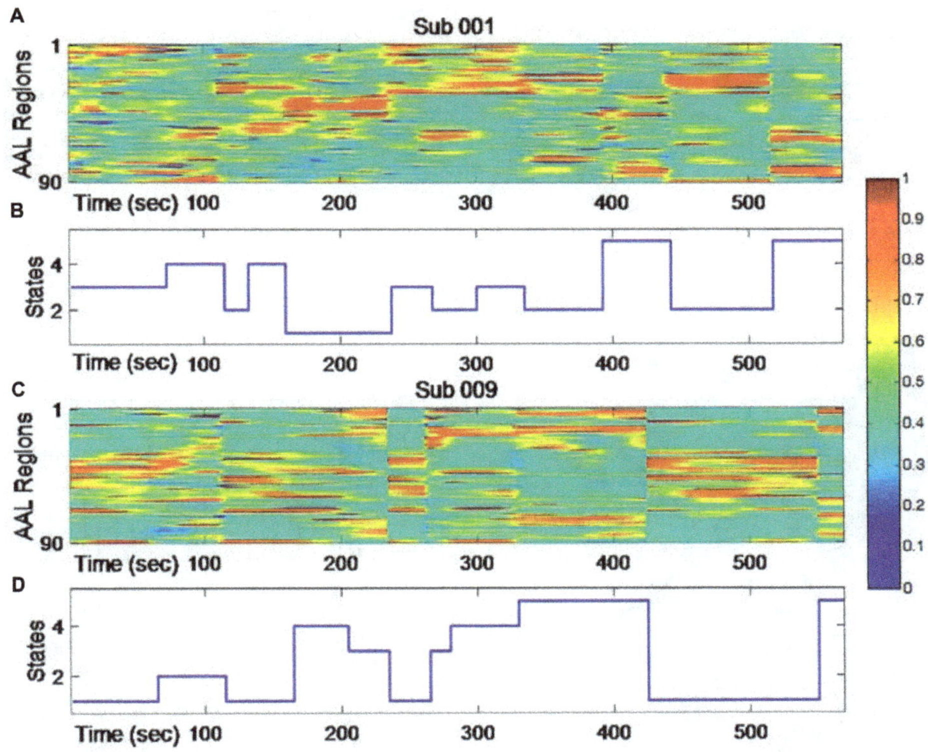

FIGURE 1 | The dynamic changing of node centrality **(A,C)** and changing states of clustering analysis **(B,D)** for two typical subjects. The color represents normalized node centrality score and red means higher centrality.

were recognized as hub nodes (top-ranking nodes based on one standard deviation criteria) (Van Den Heuvel and Sporns, 2013; Dai et al., 2014; Oldham and Fornito, 2018). The node centrality scores representing each metastate were used to define the hub nodes of that metastate. Since the node centrality used here is a kind of degree-based centrality, these hub nodes mainly indicated the provincial hub characteristics. The hub nodes distribution of five metastates were extracted and presented in a 3D view. Also, the transition characteristics between different metastates were analyzed.

For the structural network, rich-club analysis (Heuvel Van Den and Olaf, 2011; Sharaev et al., 2018) was applied to delineate the highly connected sub-network known as rich-club, including all hubs. To define the rich-club, the steps included: (1) ranking nodes according to node centrality scores; (2) applying a threshold to define a subgraph that contains only more than a certain sorted node; (3) calculating the total weight of the connectivity between the reserved subgraph nodes; (4) calculating the weight sum of the same number of edges, which are the highest ranking weights in the complete network; and (5) calculating the ratio of steps 3 and 4. The rich-club coefficient is shown as follows:

$$\emptyset^{w}(r) = \frac{W_{>r}}{\sum_{l=1}^{E_{>r}} w_{l}^{rank}}, \tag{4}$$

where, $W_{>r}$ is the weight sum of the edges in the subgraph with nodal ranking higher than r, $E_{>r}$ is the number of these edges in the subgraph, and w^{rank} is one of the vectors whose weights are ranked from high to low. Due to random networks also showing an increasing function of $\emptyset^{w}(r)$, $\emptyset^{w}(r)$ is typically normalized by a set of comparable random networks of equal size and similar connectivity distribution, resulting in a normalized rich-club coefficient $\emptyset^{w}_{norm}(r)$, which was computed as:

$$\emptyset^{w}_{norm}(r) = \frac{\emptyset^{w}(r)}{\emptyset^{w}_{rand}(r)}, \tag{5}$$

Where, $\emptyset^{w}_{rand}(r)$ w rand is computed as the averaged rich-club coefficient from 1000 random networks preserving the same degree. This normalized rich-club coefficient gives a better indicator of the significance of the rich-club effect. For this metric, if for certain values of r then we have $\emptyset^{w}_{norm}(r) > 1$, which denotes the presence of the rich-club effect.

RESULTS

Clustering Results

As shown in **Figure 1**, individual node centrality vectors and the corresponding time series of clusters' labels from two typical subjects were presented. It could be found that the clustering results were well in accordance with the temporal changes of node centrality distributions. For two scans and the average group, the cluster centers were shown in **Figure 2**, including state 1

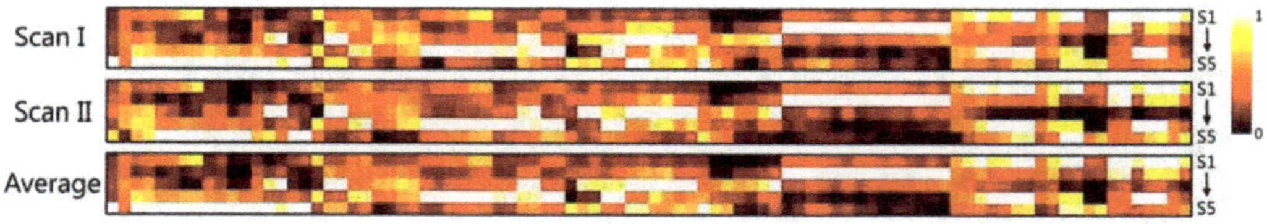

FIGURE 2 | The clustering results for scan I, scan II and the averaged centers from two scans. The hotter regions represent a higher level of node centrality.

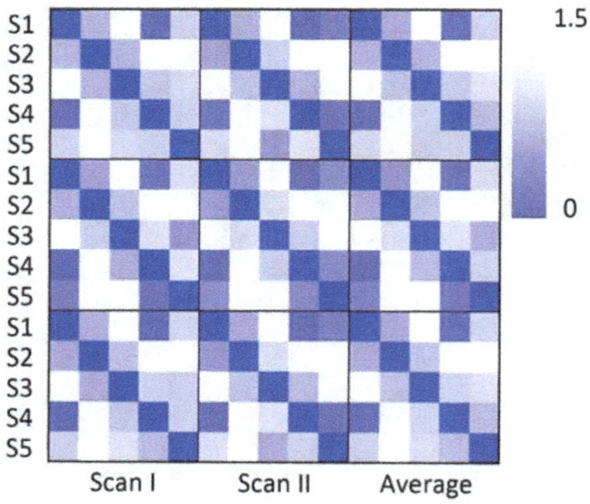

FIGURE 3 | The correlation distance of the cluster center for scan I, scan II and the averaged centers from two scans. The dark color indicates the close correlation distance and high correlation, which represents that the two states can be considered to be the same state.

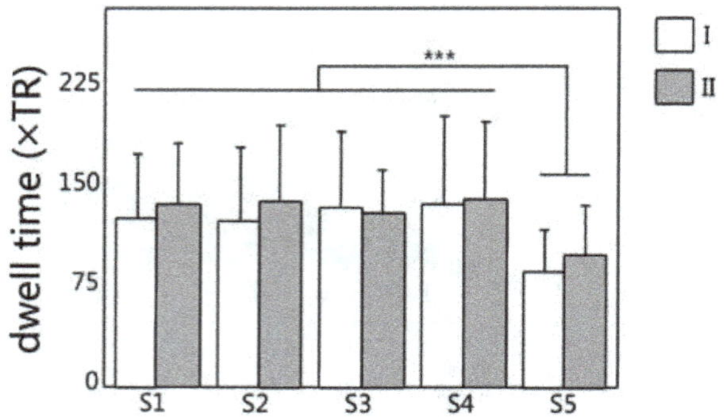

FIGURE 4 | The dwell time of metastates under clustering, for all five metastates of two scans. White represents the dwell time of scan I, and gray represents the dwell time of scan II. ***Represents significant difference.

(S1), state 2 (S2), state 3 (S3), state 4 (S4), and state 5 (S5). The **Figure 3** indicated distances between each of the two cluster centers. The dark color indicated low distance, which represented that the two clusters were closed metastates. On the contrary, the two states were quite different, which should be considered as two different metastates. There was high consistency between the clustering results from two scans, and the cluster centers from one group could exactly correspond to the similar one from the other group.

Test-Retest Results

The dwell time and transition time were illustrated in **Figures 4, 5A**. In **Figure 4**, there was no significant difference between two scans in these two features, under FDR corrected $p < 0.05$. However, for both scans, after one-way ANOVA and t-test analysis, the dwell time of S5 was significantly lower than that of the other four ($p < 0.001$). The transition time matrixes, depicted in **Figure 5A**, also showed similar patterns between two scans. In the transition time matrix, the columns of a state represented that the time switched from other states to that state, and the rows of a state represented that the time moved from that state to other states. The ICC matrix (**Figure 5B**) of these two features (diagonal for dwell time and non-diagonal for transition time) revealed the reliability of the appearances of the observed metastates across 1-week interval scans. Results showed that there was high degree of reliability (ICC $>$ 0.4) for dwell time of states 1–4 and most transition time between states. S5 showed relatively low reliability in its dwell time and high reliability only in transition from S1 to S5.

Hub Nodes of Networks

The node centrality distributions for different groups were showed in **Figure 6A**, for Scan I, Scan II and the average separately. Thresholding (mean + 1 standard deviation) the hub nodes on the averaged node centrality scores provided the binarized map indicating the hub nodes for each metastate, as well as the corresponding spatial visualization with glass brain in **Figure 6B**. The **Figure 6B** showed the hub node distribution of each metastate, including S1, S2, S3, S4, and S5. Moreover, the transition characteristics between different metastates (the thicker line represented the higher transition time) were described. Also, the overlapping rates of the hub regions with brain intrinsic sub-networks were shown. The detailed information of these hub nodes for each metastate is listed in **Table 1** along with one of the previously well-established brain intrinsic sub-networks: the frontoparietal network (FPN), occipital network (OCC), sensorimotor network (SMN), default mode network (DMN) and cingulo-opercular network (CON, mainly includes the subcortical nucleus). Segmented based on AAL, these hub patterns of each metastate could be uniquely assigned as

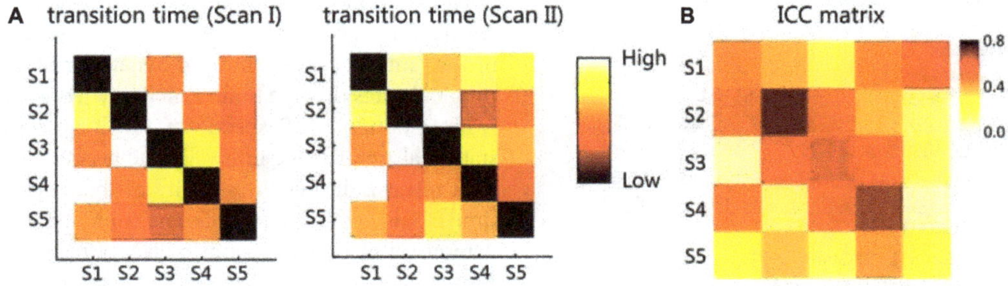

FIGURE 5 | (A) The transition time matrix between different metastates for two scans. **(B)** The ICC matrix of two features (diagonal for dwell time and non-diagonal for transition time). Red to yellow indicates the time from high to low.

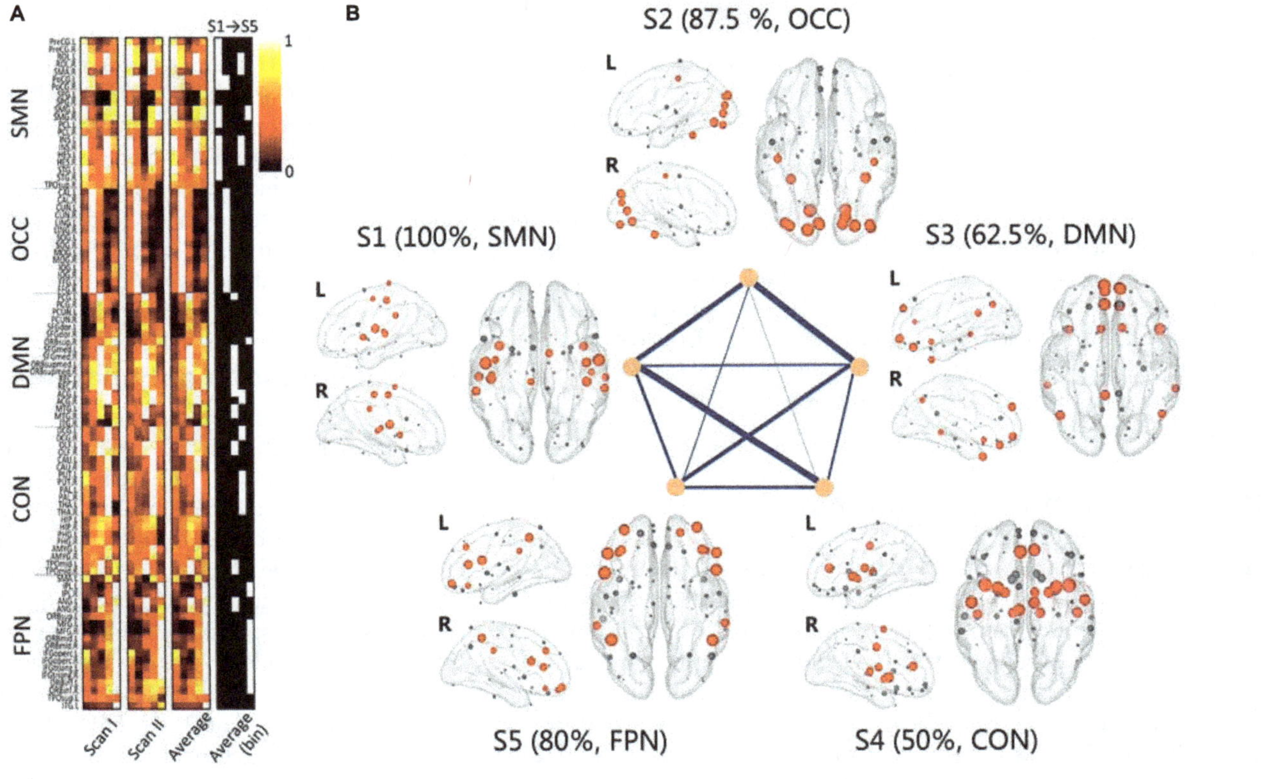

FIGURE 6 | The group averaging results of the clustering. **(A)** The node centrality distribution for different groups, for Scan I, Scan II and the average separately; the binary one represents the hub regions for each metastate; **(B)** the 3D view of the hub regions for each metastate, red nodes represent the hub nodes; gray nodes represent the non-hub nodes. Transitions between different metastates are connected by straight lines, and thicker line represent the higher transition time. Each metastate shows the corresponding brain sub-networks and overlapping rate of hub regions with brain sub-networks.

one of these intrinsic networks, according to the overlapping rate between hub nodes and intrinsic sub-network regions. In **Table 1**, the underlined regions are the most overlapping regions between hub nodes and intrinsic network (state 1: 17/17 with SMN; state 2: 14/16 with OCC; state 3: 10/16 with DMN; state 4: 9/18 with CON; state 5: 12/15 with FPN). The hub nodes of the structural network are also listed in **Table 1** and visualized in **Figure 7**, which resulted from rich-club analysis. The hub regions shared with the structural network for each metastate are boldfaced in **Table 1**.

DISCUSSION

In this paper, we proposed a method to extract metastates based on the node centrality of the dynamic functional networks and assessed the appearance of these metastates with test-retest across a 1-week interval. To our knowledge, this is the first study to analyze the repeatability of metastates of dynamic functional networks with time interval in the resting state. Furthermore, we also found the coupling relationship between dynamic functional networks and the structural network at the hub regions level. Several main findings are as follows: (1) the

TABLE 1 | Hub regions of both metastate and structural network.

Network	Hub Regions
State 1 (SMN)	PreCG.L, PreCG.R, ROL.L, ROL.R, **SMA.L**, **SMA.R**, INS.L, INS.R, PoCG.L, PoCG.R, SMG.L, SMG.R, PCL.L, HES.L, HES.R, STG.L, STG.R
State 2 (OCC)	CAL.L, CAL.R, CUN.L, CUN.R, LING.L, LING.R, **SOG.L**, **SOG.R**, MOG.L, MOG.R, IOG.L, IOG.R, FFG.L, FFG.R, PoCG.L, PoCG.R
State 3 (DMN)	PCG.L, **SFGmed.L**, **SFGmed.R**, ORBsupmed.L, ORBsupmed.R, REC.L, REC.R, ACG.L, MTG.L, MTG.R, OLF.L, OLF.R, TPOmid.L, TPOmid.R, ANG.L, ANG.R
State 4 (CON)	ROL.L, ROL.R, **SMA.R**, INS.L, INS.R, HES.L, HES.R, ACG.L, ACG.R, DCG.L, **DCG.R**, CAU.L, PUT.L, PUT.R, PAL.L, PAL.R, THA.L, THA.R
State 5 (FPN)	SMG.L, SMG.R, ORBsup.R, IPL.L, IPL.R, MFG.L, MFG.R, ORBmid.L, ORBmid.R, FGoperc. L, IIFGoperc.R, IFGtriang. L, IFGtriang.R, ORBinf.L, ORBinf.R
Structural	SFGdor.L, SFGdor.R, **SMA.L**, **SMA.R, SFGmed.L**, **DCG.R**, **SOG.L**, **SOG.R**, MOG.L, PCUN.L, PCUN.R, **PUT.L**, **PUT.R**, **THA.L**, **THA.R**,

proposed method showed high reliability in individual metastates extracted across a 1-week interval; (2) the hub regions of each metastate highly overlapped with the intrinsic functional brain subnetworks; (3) the hubs of metastates were highly overlapped with the structural core network. It can be speculated that the dynamic transitions between metastates are potentially associated with the core structure of the structural network, indicating structural constraint.

Repeatability of Proposed Method

Previous studies suggested that a high frequency of FC state transitions existed in the brain (Damaraju et al., 2014; Li et al., 2017; Marusak et al., 2017), but the stability of these states as well as their transitions have not been proved. In our study, the changes of dwell time and transition time can reflect the temporal characteristics of functional metastates, which indicates that metastates show a process of stable dynamic changes over time. As shown in **Figures 4**, **5**, according to the metastate results of the same group of subjects at two scans in different time, the repeatability of the metastate time series can be detected. Dwell time can demonstrate the importance of a certain state in the temporal series of brain dynamic function. Longer dwell time indicates that the brain function corresponding to this state is more dominant. Respectively, for five metastates, there is no statistical significance in dwell time between scan I and scan II. This result indicates the stability of the metastate. At the same time, S5 is significantly different from the other states, which demonstrates that S5 is not active at resting state (**Figure 4**). The transition time indicates the information exchange and cooperation mechanism between metastates (Chen et al., 2019). In the brain dynamic functional network time series during resting state, the more frequently the state is transiting indicates that there is more information exchange in this state, which may involve an internally close collaboration or interaction mechanism. It is observed that the average number of metastate transitions is highly consistent (**Figure 5A**). Moreover, a majority of ICCs are higher than 0.4, which illustrates good reliability (**Figure 5B**). Interestingly, compared with other states, the transitions of S5 shows a low reliability, which may be related to the instability of S5. It is concluded that the dynamic transition rules of the metastates obtained by the two scans are almost the same, which indicates that the time series of brain metastate transitions in the same individual have good repeatability in different time periods.

Specific Representations of Functional Metastates

The hub nodes of each FC network metastate show the particularity in spatial distribution. Considering the hub node distribution of each metastate and functional subnetwork, it is found that the hub node distribution is highly consistent with the functional subnetwork nodes. Hub nodes for each metastate are mainly located in the corresponding subnetwork. Specifically, five metastates correspond to specific networks with FC, such as the FPN (Emerson and Cantlon, 2012; Di and Biswal, 2015; Lee and Telzer, 2016), OCC (Yan et al., 2011; Damoiseaux et al., 2016; Chen et al., 2017; Zhang et al., 2017), SMN (Jolles et al., 2011; Pujol et al., 2014; He et al., 2016; Syed et al., 2017), DMN (Betzel et al., 2014; Wu et al., 2014; Jiao et al., 2016, 2017) and

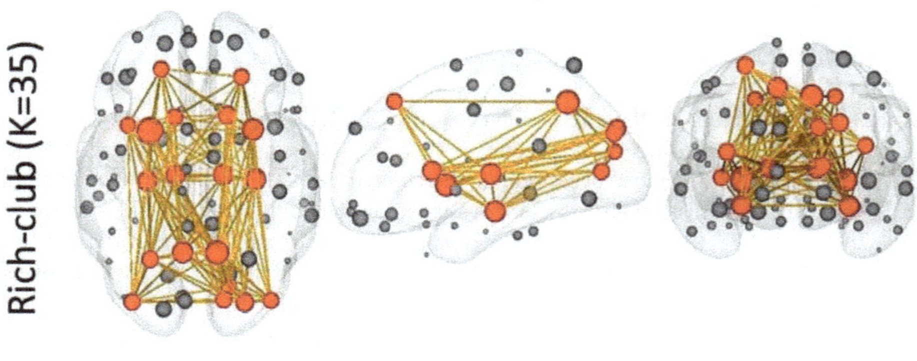

FIGURE 7 | The rich-club results of the structural network. Red nodes represent the hub nodes of the structural network; gray nodes represent the non-hub nodes. The yellow lines depict the connectivity.

(CON, mainly includes the subcortical nucleus) (Betzel et al., 2014; Luca et al., 2014; Raichlen et al., 2016; Long et al., 2017), respectively (**Figure 6**). Accordingly, the dynamic changes of the brain functional network reflect the characteristics whereby different functional modules are "activated" alternately in a certain time series.

It is found that the hub node distributions of five metastates respectively, correspond with five intrinsic functional networks, which reveals the physiological significance of metastates. Among them, S5 corresponds to the FPN, which has a low repeatability. As the main network in higher the cognitive and thinking consciousness processes, the FPN is susceptible to brain activity at resting state (Zanto and Adam, 2013; Gulbinaite et al., 2014; Alarcón et al., 2018). A low repeatability of S5 can be explained in that the resting state is an ambiguous and imprecise state of brain function. Furthermore, S5 is relatively less active in resting state with a lower dwell time, which further indicates that the FPN is a brain network involved in higher cognitive processes. The changes of dynamic network time series seem to imply that the brain shows dynamic "activation" characteristics of different intrinsic networks or cognitive resources. On the other hand, the intrinsic networks or network modularization structure are closely related to the rotational activity of the dynamic local brain regions. Therefore, it is speculated that compared with the traditional network modularization organization of static FC, the single spatial integration and separation characteristics reveal the internal mechanism. This particular pattern of temporal and spatial organization may better reflect the organization and operation mechanism of brain networks. It is interesting to find that the hub nodes of metastate are not fully consistent with the intrinsic network of brain regions. Further analyzing the distribution of hub nodes, we can find that the hub nodes of each metastate respectively, belong to local hubs and global hubs. The local hub is responsible for information integration within the network, and the global hub is responsible for information integration between networks. Thus, we can speculate that the changes of hub nodes reflect the integration ability of local brain functional resources, and it is simultaneously constrained by the global network structure.

Coupling With the Structural Network

Through the rich-club analysis, we extracted the structural core of the structural network (**Figure 7**). The most important nodes were obtained in the structural network, which are highly overlapped with hub nodes. In addition, a small number of hub nodes in each metastate belonged to the rich-club. It is indicated that the dynamic changes of functional metastates are the spontaneous transition of the intrinsic function resources, which are captured based on the node centrality. This transition mechanism relies on the structural core of the structural network, which plays an important connector role in the metastate transition process (Hagmann et al., 2008; Yong et al., 2009; Heuvel Van Den and Olaf, 2011). At the same time, the constant changes of metastates reflect the feeder effect of local intrinsic networks. The connect-feed theory simplifies brain network connectivity from an information-processing perspective (Bullmore and Sporns, 2009). Connective core nodes and hub nodes are defined as the connectors, which have the effect of globally connecting different modules. Connectivity that connects edge nodes or local network nodes to core nodes or hub nodes is known as feeder, which can transfer local information to advanced network structure.

LIMITATIONS

We have designed a test-retest study to assess the reliability of functional metastates, but there are still several aspects that need further improvements. First, strictly inclusive participants are of a relatively small size. Although we have some potential influential factors that may affect the results, it is still hard to be sure because of the small sample size. Specially, it is more focused on the age at about 20 s and may not be represented. To further corroborate our results and elucidate the spontaneous fluctuations of the FC through metastates transitions, a better study should be performed to follow subjects from wide ages. A study a with large sample will also improve estimates of FC variability and permit patterns of connectivity, which may be critical for future investigations. Second, as mentioned in the discussion section, the brain parcellation atlas used is a commonly used one, and there are many finer templates with higher spatial resolution and more detailed or specific divisions of brain regions. With finer parcellation, it is probable to obtain more spatially dependent patterns represented as metastates and provide more information about coupling between dynamic function in resting state and intrinsic structure. It is also another powerful way to verify the reliability of the proposed method at different spatial levels of brain parcellation. Third, how the hub regions are identified here is not rigorous, but relatively comparable. With that said, we used the normalized rich-club coefficient to find the hubs of the structural network, and spurious hubs nodes will probably be found. At the same time, there were many details that were arbitrary and tricky from the perspective of more rigorous thinking, for example the functional network thresholding, the sliding window size and the fMRI preprocessing. This makes it difficult to draw a strong conclusion. However, the methods here provide a general method and insight view of the dynamic hub nodes of functional networks. Future work should use stricter methods to identify the hub nodes, for example using non-parametrical testing and multiple comparison correction. Fourth, the exact sliding window size is important and should be carefully considered in dynamic FC research. In this work, we arbitrarily chose an empirically used window length in previous literatures without further exploring the potential effects for varied window lengths. Future work on the effect of window size on metastate extraction is needed. What is more important about this is whether the sliding window correlation method reflects the dynamic FC, which has been the focus of several studies (Leonardi and Van De Ville, 2015; Hindriks et al., 2016) and resulted in two sides. For example, with surrogate data, Hindriks et al. (2016) concluded that with the sliding window-based method it was hard to reflect the dynamic FC, and Leonardi suggested that an extra 0~1/w low frequent pass filtering on the sequence of dynamic FC can reduce spurious information about dynamic FC, even though plenty of studies have found meaningful things about dynamic FC. In our thoughts, what really mattered is to know what kind of or how to describe the characteristics of dynamic FC in resting state. In any case, a surrogate can never represent real fMRI data and we also never know the exact information underlying our brain function. However, with careful thinking, we might still explore the nature of dynamic FC in practice.

CONCLUSION

In conclusion, we proposed a clustering method to extract metastates based on the node centrality of the dynamic functional networks, assessed the dynamic features of these metastates in resting state across a 1-week interval and further explored the possible meanings of these metastates. These metastates were repeatable and highly related to the intrinsic subsystems of brain function in resting state. Considering the overlapping of the hub nodes between metastates and the structural network, we also speculated that dynamic functional network metastates were coupled with or constrained by the structural network. We might further conclude that the metastates, or possible sub-systems, interacted with each other in an alternate provincial centralization under the core frame of the structural network. In additional, node-based representation of dynamic function networks, as well as metastates, might provide a new useful insight into the underlying information of spontaneous dynamics in resting state networks.

AUTHOR CONTRIBUTIONS

XZ and QW were in charge of the analysis work and wrote the manuscript. YC and QW processed all the image data and conducted the main analysis work. YC and HN collected the MRI data. XS and HN provided some useful guidance and ideas. YC, XZ, and DM designed and provided the original idea. HN, XZ, and DM sponsored the whole research.

FUNDING

This research was supported by the National Key Research and Development Program of China (grant number 2017YFB1002504), National Natural Science Foundation of China (Nos. 81571762, 81630051, 81801787, and 30870713), Tianjin Natural Science Foundation Project (grant number 16JCYBJC25900), and China Postdoctoral Science Foundation (2018M640238).

REFERENCES

Alarcón, G., Pfeifer, J. H., Fair, D. A., and Nagel, B. J. (2018). Adolescent ext. *Front. Behav. Neurosci.* 12:73. doi: 10.3389/fnbeh.2018.00073

Allen, E. A., Damaraju, E., Plis, S. M., Erhardt, E. B., Eichele, T., and Calhoun, V. D. (2014). Tracking whole-brain connectivity dynamics in the resting state. *Cereb. Cortex* 24, 663–676. doi: 10.1093/cercor/bhs352

Al-Sharoa, E., Al-Khassaweneh, M., and Aviyente, S. (2019). Tensor based temporal and multi-layer community detection for studying brain dynamics during resting state fMRI. *IEEE Trans. Biomed. Eng.* 66, 695–709. doi: 10.1109/TBME.2018.2854676

Andersson, J. L. R., and Skare, S. (2002). A model-based method for retrospective correction of geometric distortions in diffusion-weighted EPI. *Neuroimage* 16, 177–199. doi: 10.1006/nimg.2001.1039

Andrew, Z., and Michael, B. (2015). Towards a statistical test for functional connectivity dynamics. *Neuroimage* 114, 466–470. doi: 10.1016/j.neuroimage.2015.03.047

Arthur, D., and Vassilvitskii, S. (2007). "k-means++: The advantages of careful seeding," in *Proceedings of the Eighteenth annual ACM-SIAM Symposium on Discrete Algorithms* (Philadelphia, PA: Society for Industrial and Applied Mathematics), 1027–1035. doi: 10.1145/1283383.1283494

Bartko, J. J. (1966). The intraclass correlation coefficient as a measure of reliability. *Psychol. Rep.* 19, 3–11. doi: 10.2466/pr0.1966.19.1.3

Betzel, R. F., Byrge, L., He, Y., Goñi, J., Zuo, X. N., and Sporns, O. (2014). Changes in structural and functional connectivity among resting-state networks across the human lifespan. *Neuroimage* 102, 345–357. doi: 10.1016/j.neuroimage.2014.07.067

Bing, Z., Tan, C., Tang, J., and Chen, X. (2010). Brain functional connectivity of functional magnetic resonance imaging of patients with early-onset schizophrenia. *J. Cent. South Univ.* 35, 17–24. doi: 10.3969/j.issn.1672-7347.2010.01.003

Biswal, B., Yetkin, F. Z., Haughton, V. M., and Hyde, J. S. (1995). Functional connectivity in the motor cortex of resting. *MRM* 34, 537–541.

Bola, M., and Sabel, B. A. (2015). Dynamic reorganization of brain functional networks during cognition. *Neuroimage* 114, 398–413. doi: 10.1016/j.neuroimage.2015.03.057

Bullmore, E., and Sporns, O. (2009). Complex brain networks: graph theoretical analysis of structural and functional systems. *Nat. Rev. Neurosci.* 10, 186–198. doi: 10.1038/nrn2575

Cabral, J., Kringelbach, M. L., and Deco, G. (2017). Functional connectivity dynamically evolves on multiple time-scales over a static structural connectome: models and mechanisms. *Neuroimage* 160, 84–96. doi: 10.1016/j.neuroimage.2017.03.045

Calhoun, V. D., Miller, R., Pearlson, G., and Adali, T. (2014). The chronnectome: time-varying connectivity networks as the next frontier in fmri data discovery. *Neuron* 84, 262–274. doi: 10.1016/j.neuron.2014.10.015

Chang, C., and Glover, G. H. (2010). Time-frequency dynamics of resting-state brain connectivity measured with fMRI. *Neuroimage* 50, 81–98. doi: 10.1016/j.neuroimage.2009.12.011

Chang, L. C., Jones, D. K., and Pierpaoli, C. (2005). RESTORE: robust estimation of tensors by outlier rejection. *Magn. Reson. Med.* 53, 1088–1095. doi: 10.1002/mrm.20426

Chao, Z., Baum, S. A., Adduru, V. R., Biswal, B. B., and Michael, A. M. (2018). Test-retest reliability of dynamic functional connectivity in resting state fMRI. *Neuroimage* 183, 907–918. doi: 10.1016/j.neuroimage.2018.08.021

Chen, Y., Liu, Y., Zhou, P., Zhang, X., Wu, Q., Zhao, X., et al. (2019). The transitions between dynamic micro-states reveal age-related functional network reorganization. *Front. Physiol.* 9:1852. doi: 10.3389/fphys.2018.01852

Chen, Y., Wang, W., Zhao, X., Sha, M., Liu, Y., Zhang, X., et al. (2017). Age-related decline in the variation of dynamic functional connectivity: a resting state analysis. *Front. Aging Neurosci.* 9:203. doi: 10.3389/fnagi.2017.00203

Chen, Y., Zhao, X., Zhang, X., Liu, Y., Zhou, P., Ni, H., et al. (2018). Age-related early/late variations of functional connectivity across the human lifespan. *Neuroradiology* 60, 403–412. doi: 10.1007/s00234-017-1973-1

Cheng, L., Zhu, Y., Sun, J., Deng, L., He, N., Yang, Y., et al. (2018). Principal States of dynamic functional connectivity reveal the link between resting-state and task-state brain: an fMRI study. *Int. J. Neural Syst.* 28:1850002. doi: 10.1142/s0129065718500028

Cordes, D., Haughton, V. M., Arfanakis, K., Carew, J. D., Turski, P. A., Moritz, C. H., et al. (2001). Frequencies contributing to functional connectivity in the cerebral cortex in "resting-state" data. *Ajnr Am. J. Neuroradiol.* 22, 1326–1333.

Correa, C. D., Tarik, C., and Kwan-Liu, M. (2012). Visual reasoning about social networks using centrality sensitivity. *IEEE Trans. Vis. Comput. Graph.* 18, 106–120. doi: 10.1109/tvcg.2010.260

Dai, Z., Yan, C., Li, K., Wang, Z., Wang, J., Cao, M., et al. (2014). Identifying and mapping connectivity patterns of brain network hubs in Alzheimer's Disease. *Cereb. Cortex* 25, 3723–3742. doi: 10.1093/cercor/bhu246

Damaraju, E., Allen, E. A., Belger, A., Ford, J. M., Mcewen, S., Mathalon, D. H., et al. (2014). Dynamic functional connectivity analysis reveals transient states of dysconnectivity in schizophrenia. *Neuroimage Clin.* 5, 298–308. doi: 10.1016/j.nicl.2014.07.003

Damoiseaux, J. S., Beckmann, C. F., Arigita, E. J. S., Barkhof, F., Scheltens, P., Stam, C. J., et al. (2008). Reduced resting-state brain activity in the "default network" in normal aging. *Cereb. Cortex* 18, 1856–1864. doi: 10.1093/cercor/bhm207

Damoiseaux, J. S., Viviano, R. P., Yuan, P., and Raz, N. (2016). Differential effect of age on posterior and anterior hippocampal functional connectivity. *Neuroimage* 133, 468–476. doi: 10.1016/j.neuroimage.2016.03.047

Di, X., and Biswal, B. B. (2015). Dynamic brain functional connectivity modulated by resting-state networks. *Brain Struct. Funct.* 220, 37–46. doi: 10.1007/s00429-013-0634-3

Emerson, R. W., and Cantlon, J. F. (2012). Early math achievement and functional connectivity in the fronto-parietal network. *Dev. Cogn. Neurosci.* 2, S139–S151. doi: 10.1016/j.dcn.2011.11.003

Fox, M. D., Dongyang, Z., Snyder, A. Z., and Raichle, M. E. (2009). The global signal and observed anticorrelated resting state brain networks. *J. Neurophysiol.* 101, 3270–3283. doi: 10.1152/jn.90777.2008

Fox, M. D., Snyder, A. Z., Vincent, J. L., Maurizio, C., Essen Van, D. C., and Raichle, M. E. (2005). The human brain is intrinsically organized into dynamic, anticorrelated functional networks. *Proc. Natl. Acad. Sci. U.S.A.* 102, 9673–9678. doi: 10.1073/pnas.0504136102

Gale, A. (1983). "Functional states of the brain: their determinants," in *Biological Psychology*, eds M. Koukkou, D. Lehmann and J. Angst (Amsterdam: Elsevier/North-Holland Biomedical Press), 79–80. doi: 10.1016/0301-0511(83)90068-6

Gordon, E. M., Lynch, C. J., Gratton, C., Laumann, T. O., Gilmore, A. W., Greene, D. J., et al. (2018). Three distinct sets of connector hubs integrate human brain function. *Cell Rep.* 24, 1687.e4–1695.e4. doi: 10.1016/j.celrep.2018.07.050

Gulbinaite, R., van Rijn, H., and Cohen, M. X. (2014). Fronto-parietal network oscillations reveal relationship between working memory capacity and cognitive control. *Front. Hum. Neurosci.* 8:761. doi: 10.3389/fnhum.2014.00761

Hagmann, P., Cammoun, L., Gigandet, X., Meuli, R., Honey, C. J., Van Wedeen, J., et al. (2008). Mapping the structural core of human cerebral cortex. *PLoS Biol.* 6:e159. doi: 10.1371/journal.pbio.0060159

Ham, J. H., Cha, J., Lee, J. J., Baek, G. M., Sunwoo, M. K., Hong, J. Y., et al. (2015). Nigrostriatal dopamine-independent resting-state functional networks in Parkinson's disease. *Neuroimage* 119, 296–304. doi: 10.1016/j.neuroimage.2015.06.077

Hansen, E. C. A., Battaglia, D., Spiegler, A., Deco, G., and Jirsa, V. K. (2015). Functional connectivity dynamics: modeling the switching behavior of the resting state. *Neuroimage* 105, 525–535. doi: 10.1016/j.neuroimage.2014.11.001

He, C. C., Chen, Y. C., Jian, T. R., Chen, H., Guo, X., Wang, J., et al. (2018). Dynamic functional connectivity analysis reveals decreased variability of the default-mode network in developing autistic brain. *Autism Res.* 11, 1479–1493. doi: 10.1002/aur.2020

He, H., Luo, C., Chang, X., Shan, Y., Cao, W., Gong, J., et al. (2016). The Functional integration in the sensory-motor system predicts aging in healthy older adults. *Front. Aging Neurosci.* 8:306. doi: 10.3389/fnagi.2016.00306

Heuvel Van Den, M. P., and Olaf, S. (2011). Rich-club organization of the human connectome. *J. Neurosci. Off. J. Soc. Neurosci.* 31, 15775–15786. doi: 10.1523/JNEUROSCI.3539-11.2011

Hindriks, R., Adhikari, M. H., Murayama, Y., Ganzetti, M., Mantini, D., Logothetis, N. K., et al. (2016). Corrigendum to "Can sliding-window correlations reveal dynamic functional connectivity in resting-state fMRI?". *Neuroimage* 132:115. doi: 10.1016/j.neuroimage.2016.02.007

Hutchison, R. M., Womelsdorf, T., Allen, E. A., Bandettini, P. A., Calhoun, V. D., Corbetta, M., et al. (2013a). Dynamic functional connectivity: promise, issues, and interpretations. *Neuroimage* 80, 360–378. doi: 10.1016/j.neuroimage.2013.05.079

Hutchison, R. M., Womelsdorf, T., Gati, J. S., Everling, S., and Menon, R. S. (2013b). Resting-state networks show dynamic functional connectivity in awake humans and anesthetized macaques. *Hum. Brain Mapp.* 34, 2154–2177. doi: 10.1002/hbm.22058

Jiao, Z., Ma, K., Wang, H., Zou, L., and Xiang, J. (2016). Functional connectivity analysis of brain default mode networks using hamiltonian path. *CNS Neurol. Disord. Drug Targets* 16, 44–50. doi: 10.2174/1871527314666161124120040

Jiao, Z., Wang, H., Ma, K., Zou, L., and Xiang, J. (2017). Directed connectivity of brain default networks in resting state using GCA and motif. *Front. Biosci.* 22:1634–1643. doi: 10.2741/4562

Jolles, D. D., Buchem Van, M. A., Crone, E. A., and Rombouts, S. A. (2011). A comprehensive study of whole-brain functional connectivity in children and young adults. *Cereb. Cortex* 21, 385–391. doi: 10.1093/cercor/bhq104

Kevin, M., Birn, R. M., Handwerker, D. A., Jones, T. B., and Bandettini, P. A. (2009). The impact of global signal regression on resting state correlations: are anti-correlated networks introduced? *Neuroimage* 44, 893–905. doi: 10.1016/j.neuroimage.2008.09.036

Lee, T. H., and Telzer, E. H. (2016). Negative functional coupling between the right fronto-parietal and limbic resting state networks predicts increased self-control and later substance use onset in adolescence. *Dev. Cogn. Neurosci.* 20, 35–42. doi: 10.1016/j.dcn.2016.06.002

Lee, Y.-B., Yoo, K., Roh, J. H., Moon, W.-J., and Jeong, Y. (2019). Brain-state extraction algorithm based on the state transition (BEST): a dynamic functional brain network analysis in fMRI study. *Brain Topogr.* 32, 897–913. doi: 10.1007/s10548-019-00719-7

Leemans, A., Jeurissen, B., and Sijbers, J. (2009). Explore DTI: a graphical toolbox for processing, analyzing, and visualizing diffusion MR data. *Proc. Int. Soc. Magn. Reson. Med. Sci. Meet* 2009:3537.

Lehmann, D., Ozaki, H., and Pal, I. (1987). EEG alpha map series: brain micro-states by space-oriented adaptive segmentation ?. *Electroencephalogr. Clin. Neurophysiol.* 67, 271–288. doi: 10.1016/0013-4694(87)90025-3

Leonardi, N., Richiardi, J., Gschwind, M., Simioni, S., Annoni, J. M., Schluep, M., et al. (2013). Principal components of functional connectivity: a new approach to study dynamic brain connectivity during rest. *Neuroimage* 83, 937–950. doi: 10.1016/j.neuroimage.2013.07.019

Leonardi, N., and Van De Ville, D. (2015). Erratum to "On spurious and real fluctuations of dynamic functional connectivity during rest.". *Neuroimage* 104, 430–436. doi: 10.1016/j.neuroimage.2014.09.007

Li, J., Zhang, D., Liang, A., Liang, B., Wang, Z., Cai, Y., et al. (2017). High transition frequencies of dynamic functional connectivity states in the creative brain. *Sci. Rep.* 7:46072. doi: 10.1038/srep46072

Liégeois, R., Li, J., Kong, R., Orban, C., Van De Ville, D., Ge, T., et al. (2019). Resting brain dynamics at different timescales capture distinct aspects of human behavior. *Nat. Commun.* 10:2317. doi: 10.1038/s41467-019-10317-7

Long, X., Benischek, A., Dewey, D., and Lebel, C. (2017). Age-related functional brain changes in young children. *Neuroimage* 155, 322–330. doi: 10.1016/j.neuroimage.2017.04.059

Luca, C., Halford, G. S., Andrew, Z., Harding, I. H., Ramm, B. J., Tim, C., et al. (2014). Complexity in relational processing predicts changes in functional brain network dynamics. *Cereb. Cortex* 24, 2283–2296. doi: 10.1093/cercor/bht075

Marusak, H. A., Elrahal, F., Peters, C. A., Kundu, P., Lombardo, M. V., Calhoun, V. D., et al. (2017). Mindfulness and dynamic functional neural connectivity in children and adolescents. *Behav. Brain Res.* 336, 211–218. doi: 10.1016/j.bbr.2017.09.010

Meghanathan, N. (2015a). Correlation Coefficient Analysis of Centrality Metrics for Complex Network Graphs. 4th Comput. *Sci. On line Conf.* 348, 11–20. doi: 10.1007/978-3-319-18503-3_2

Meghanathan, N. (2015b). "Use of Centrality Metrics to Determine Connected Dominating Sets for Real-World Network Graphs," in *proceedings of the 12th International Conference on Information Technology - New Generations*, (Las Vegas, NV), 243–248.

Mennigen, E., Fryer, S. L., Rashid, B., Damaraju, E., Du, Y., Loewy, R. L., et al. (2018). Transient patterns of functional dysconnectivity in clinical high risk and early illness schizophrenia individuals compared with healthy controls. *Brain Connect.* 9, 60–76. doi: 10.1089/brain.2018.0579

Mori, S., Crain, B. J., Chacko, V. P., and Zijl Van, P. C. (2010). Three-dimensional tracking of axonal projections in the brain by magnetic resonance imaging. *Ann. Neurol.* 45, 265–269. doi: 10.1002/1531-8249(199902)45:2<265::aid-ana21>3.0.co;2-3

Mori, S., and Van Zijl, P. C. M. (2002). Fiber tracking: principles and strategies - A technical review. *NMR Biomed* 15, 468–480. doi: 10.1002/nbm.781

Murphy, K., and Fox, M. D. (2016). Towards a consensus regarding global signal regression for resting state functional connectivity MRI. *Neuroimage* 154, S1053811916306711. doi: 10.1016/j.neuroimage.2016.11.052

Oldham, S., and Fornito, A. (2018). The development of brain network hubs. *Dev. Cogn. Neurosci.* doi: 10.1016/j.dcn.2018.12.005 Epub 2018 Dec 13.

Preti, M. G., Bolton, T. A. W., and Van De Ville, D. (2017). The dynamic functional connectome: state-of-the-art and perspectives. *Neuroimage* 160, 41–54. doi: 10.1016/j.neuroimage.2016.12.061

Pujol, J., Macià, D., Blanco-Hinojo, L., Martínez-Vilavella, G., Sunyer, J., Torre, R. D., et al. (2014). Does motion-related brain functional connectivity reflect both artifacts and genuine neural activity? *Neuroimage* 101, 87–95. doi: 10.1016/j.neuroimage.2014.06.065

Raichlen, D. A., Bharadwaj, P. K., Fitzhugh, M. C., Haws, K. A., Torre, G. A., Trouard, T. P., et al. (2016). Differences in resting state functional connectivity between young adult endurance athletes and healthy controls. *Front. Hum. Neurosci.* 10:610. doi: 10.3389/fnhum.2016.00610

Schaefer, A., Margulies, D. S., Lohmann, G., Gorgolewski, K. J., Smallwood, J., Kiebel, S. J., et al. (2014). Dynamic network participation of functional connectivity hubs assessed by resting-state fMRI. *Front. Hum. Neurosci.* 8:195. doi: 10.3389/fnhum.2014.00195

Shakil, S., Lee, C. H., and Keilholz, S. D. (2016). Evaluation of sliding window correlation performance for characterizing dynamic functional connectivity and brain states. *Neuroimage* 133, 111–128. doi: 10.1016/j.neuroimage.2016.02.074

Sharaev, M., Orlov, V., Ushakov, V., and Velichkovsky, B. (2018). Information transfer between rich-club structures in the human brain. *Procedia Comput. Sci.* 123, 440–445. doi: 10.1016/j.procs.2018.01.067

Shen, K., Hutchison, R. M., Bezgin, G., Everling, S., and McIntosh, A. R. (2015). Network structure shapes spontaneous functional connectivity dynamics. *J. Neurosci.* 35, 5579–5588. doi: 10.1523/JNEUROSCI.4903-14.2015

Shine, J. M., Koyejo, O., and Poldrack, R. A. (2016). Temporal metastates are associated with differential patterns of time-resolved connectivity, network topology, and attention. *Proc. Natl. Acad. Sci. U.S.A.* 113, 9888–98891. doi: 10.1073/pnas.1604898113

Su, L., An, J., Ma, Q., Qiu, S., and Hu, D. (2015). Influence of resting-state network on lateralization of functional connectivity in mesial temporal lobe epilepsy. *Am. J. Neuroradiol.* 36, 1479–1487. doi: 10.3174/ajnr.A4346

Syed, M. F., Lindquist, M. A., Pillai, J. J., Agarwal, S., Gujar, S. K., Choe, A. S., et al. (2017). Dynamic functional connectivity states between the dorsal and ventral sensorimotor networks revealed by dynamic conditional correlation analysis of resting-state functional magnetic resonance imaging. *Brain Connect.* 7, 635–642. doi: 10.1089/brain.2017.0533

Tzourio-Mazoyer, N., Landeau, B., Papathanassiou, D., Crivello, F., Etard, O., Delcroix, N., et al. (2002). Automated anatomical labeling of activations in SPM using a macroscopic anatomical parcellation of the MNI MRI single-subject brain. *Neuroimage* 15, 273–289. doi: 10.1006/nimg.2001.0978

Van Den Heuvel, M. P., and Sporns, O. (2013). Network hubs in the human brain. *Trends Cogn. Sci.* 17, 683–696. doi: 10.1016/j.tics.2013.09.012

Veer, I. M. (2010). Whole brain resting-state analysis reveals decreased functional connectivity in major depression. *Front. Syst. Neurosci.* 4:41. doi: 10.3389/fnsys.2010.00041

Vidaurre, D., Smith, S. M., and Woolrich, M. W. (2017). Brain network dynamics are hierarchically organized in time. *Proc. Natl. Acad. Sci. U.S.A.* 114, 12827–12832. doi: 10.1073/pnas.1705120114

Viviano, R. P., Raz, N., Yuan, P., and Damoiseaux, J. S. (2017). Associations between dynamic functional connectivity and age, metabolic risk, and cognitive performance. *Neurobiol. Aging* 59,135–143. doi: 10.1016/j.neurobiolaging.2017.08.003

Widjaja, E., Zamyadi, M., Raybaud, C., Snead, O. C., and Smith, M. L. (2013). Abnormal functional network connectivity among resting-state networks in children with frontal lobe epilepsy. *Am. J. Neuroradiol.* 34, 2386–2392. doi: 10.3174/ajnr.A3608

Wu, X., Yu, X., Yao, L., and Li, R. (2014). Bayesian network analysis revealed the connectivity difference of the default mode network from the resting-state to task-state. *Front. Comput. Neurosci.* 8:118. doi: 10.3389/fncom.2014.00118

Xia, Y., Chen, Q., Li, M., and Jiang, Q. (2019). Tracking the dynamic functional connectivity structure of the human brain across the adult lifespan. *bioRxiv* 40, 717–728. doi: 10.1002/hbm.24385

Xi-Nian, Z., Clare, K., Adelstein, J. S., Klein, D. F., Castellanos, F. X., and Milham, M. P. (2010). Reliable intrinsic connectivity networks: test-retest evaluation using ICA and dual regression approach. *Neuroimage* 49, 2163–2177. doi: 10.1016/j.neuroimage.2009.10.080

Yan, L., Yan, Z., Bo, W., and Wang, D. J. J. (2011). Loss of coherence of low frequency fluctuations of BOLD FMRI in visual cortex of healthy aged subjects. *Open Neuroimag. J.* 5, 105–111. doi: 10.2174/1874440001105010105

Yong, H., Jinhui, W., Liang, W., Chen, Z. J., Chaogan, Y., Hong, Y., et al. (2009). Uncovering intrinsic modular organization of spontaneous brain activity in humans. *PLoS One* 4:e5226. doi: 10.1371/journal.pone.0005226

Yu, Q., Erhardt, E. B., Sui, J., Du, Y., He, H., Hjelm, D., et al. (2015). Assessing dynamic brain graphs of time-varying connectivity in fMRI data: application to healthy controls and patients with schizophrenia. *Neuroimage* 107, 345–355. doi: 10.1016/j.neuroimage.2014.12.020

Zanto, T. P., and Adam, G. (2013). Fronto-parietal network: flexible hub of cognitive control. *Trends Cogn. Sci.* 17, 602–603. doi: 10.1016/j.tics.2013.10.001

Zhang, H., Lee, A., and Qiu, A. (2017). A posterior-to-anterior shift of brain functional dynamics in aging. *Brain Struct. Funct* 222, 3665–3676. doi: 10.1007/s00429-017-1425-z

Zhuo, C., Wang, C., Wang, L., Guo, X., Xu, Q., Liu, Y., et al. (2018). Altered resting-state functional connectivity of the cerebellum in schizophrenia. *Brain Imaging Behav.* 12, 383–389. doi: 10.1007/s11682-017-9704-0

Zuo, X. N., and Xing, X. X. (2014). Test-retest reliabilities of resting-state FMRI measurements in human brain functional connectomics: a systems neuroscience perspective. *Neurosci. Biobehav. Rev.* 45, 100–118. doi: 10.1016/j.neubiorev.2014.05.009

Permissions

All chapters in this book were first published by Frontiers; hereby published with permission under the Creative Commons Attribution License or equivalent. Every chapter published in this book has been scrutinized by our experts. Their significance has been extensively debated. The topics covered herein carry significant findings which will fuel the growth of the discipline. They may even be implemented as practical applications or may be referred to as a beginning point for another development.

The contributors of this book come from diverse backgrounds, making this book a truly international effort. This book will bring forth new frontiers with its revolutionizing research information and detailed analysis of the nascent developments around the world.

We would like to thank all the contributing authors for lending their expertise to make the book truly unique. They have played a crucial role in the development of this book. Without their invaluable contributions this book wouldn't have been possible. They have made vital efforts to compile up to date information on the varied aspects of this subject to make this book a valuable addition to the collection of many professionals and students.

This book was conceptualized with the vision of imparting up-to-date information and advanced data in this field. To ensure the same, a matchless editorial board was set up. Every individual on the board went through rigorous rounds of assessment to prove their worth. After which they invested a large part of their time researching and compiling the most relevant data for our readers.

The editorial board has been involved in producing this book since its inception. They have spent rigorous hours researching and exploring the diverse topics which have resulted in the successful publishing of this book. They have passed on their knowledge of decades through this book. To expedite this challenging task, the publisher supported the team at every step. A small team of assistant editors was also appointed to further simplify the editing procedure and attain best results for the readers.

Apart from the editorial board, the designing team has also invested a significant amount of their time in understanding the subject and creating the most relevant covers. They scrutinized every image to scout for the most suitable representation of the subject and create an appropriate cover for the book.

The publishing team has been an ardent support to the editorial, designing and production team. Their endless efforts to recruit the best for this project, has resulted in the accomplishment of this book. They are a veteran in the field of academics and their pool of knowledge is as vast as their experience in printing. Their expertise and guidance has proved useful at every step. Their uncompromising quality standards have made this book an exceptional effort. Their encouragement from time to time has been an inspiration for everyone.

The publisher and the editorial board hope that this book will prove to be a valuable piece of knowledge for researchers, students, practitioners and scholars across the globe.

List of Contributors

Yegang Hu and Jicong Zhang
School of Biological Science and Medical Engineering, Beihang University, Beijing, China
Beijing Advanced Innovation Centre for Big Data-Based Precision Medicine, Beihang University, Beijing, China
Beijing Advanced Innovation Centre for Biomedical Engineering, Beihang University, Beijing, China
Hefei Innovation Research Institute, Beihang University, Hefei, China

Chunli Yin and Yuping Wang
Department of Neurology, Xuanwu Hospital, Capital Medical University, Beijing, China
Beijing Key Laboratory of Brain Functional Disease and Neuromodulation, Beijing, China

Bo-yong Park and Mansu Kim
Department of Electrical and Computer Engineering, Sungkyunkwan University, Suwon, South Korea
Center for Neuroscience Imaging Research, Institute for Basic Science, Suwon, South Korea

Mi Ji Lee
Departments of Neurology, Samsung Medical Center, Sungkyunkwan University School of Medicine, Seoul, South Korea

Se-Hong Kim
Department of Family Medicine, St. Vincent's Hospital, Catholic University College of Medicine, Suwon, South Korea

Hyunjin Park
Center for Neuroscience Imaging Research, Institute for Basic Science, Suwon, South Korea
School of Electronic and Electrical Engineering, Sungkyunkwan University, Suwon, South Korea

Daihong Liu
Department of Radiology, Southwest Hospital, Third Military Medical University (Army Medical University), Chongqing, China
Department of Imaging Diagnosis, Lanzhou General Hospital of Chinese PLA Lanzhou Command (PLA No. 940 Hospital), Lanzhou, China

Lihua Chen
Department of Radiology, PLA No. 904 Hospital, Wuxi, China

Wu Yang
Medical Company, The Chinese People's Liberation Army No.31610 Troop, Zhoushan, China

Shanshan Duan
Department of Endocrinology, Southwest Hospital, Third Military Medical University (Army Medical University), Chongqing, China

Xuntao Yin, Yanshu Shi and Jian Wang
Department of Radiology, Southwest Hospital, Third Military Medical University (Army Medical University), Chongqing, China

Jiuquan Zhang
Department of Radiology, Chongqing University Cancer Hospital & Chongqing Cancer Institute & Chongqing Cancer Hospital, Chongqing, China
Key Laboratory for Biorheological Science and Technology of Ministry of Education (Chongqing University), Chongqing University Cancer Hospital & Chongqing Cancer Institute & Chongqing Cancer Hospital, Chongqing, China

Lizhu Luo, Xiangchao Kong, Fengmei Lu and Jiaojian Wang
The Clinical Hospital of Chengdu Brain Science Institute, MOE Key Laboratory for Neuroinformation, University of Electronic Science and Technology of China, Chengdu, China

Kunhua Wu
Department of MRI, The First People's Hospital of Yunnan Province, The Affiliated Hospital of Kunming University of Science and Technology, Kunming, China

Yi Lu
The Department of Medical Imaging, The First Affiliated Hospital of Kunming Medical University, Kunming, China

Shan Gao
The Clinical Hospital of Chengdu Brain Science Institute, MOE Key Laboratory for Neuroinformation, University of Electronic Science and Technology of China, Chengdu, China
School of Foreign Languages, University of Electronic Science and Technology of China, Chengdu, China

Fengchun Wu and Huawang Wu
The Affiliated Brain Hospital of Guangzhou Medical University (Guangzhou Huiai Hospital), Guangzhou, China
Guangdong Engineering Technology Research Center for Translational Medicine of Mental Disorders, Guangzhou, China

Bin Wang, Ting Li, Mengni Zhou, Yan Niu, Xin Wang, Rui Cao, Jie Xiang, Xiaohong Cui, Junjie Chen and Dandan Li
College of Information and Computer, Taiyuan University of Technology, Taiyuan, China

Shuo Zhao
Faculty of Human Health Science, Graduate School of Medicine, Kyoto University, Kyoto, Japan

Ting Yan
Translational Medicine Research Center, Shanxi Medical University, Taiyuan, China

Liu Yang
Department of Neurology, Xuanwu Hospital, Capital Medical University, Beijing, China

Yan Yan, Yonghao Wang and Tianyi Yan
School of Life Science, Beijing Institute of Technology, Beijing, China

Xiaochen Hu
Department of Psychiatry and Psychotherapy, Medical Faculty, University of Cologne, Cologne, Germany

Piu Chan
Department of Neurology, Xuanwu Hospital, Capital Medical University, Beijing, China
Beijing Institute of Geriatrics, Beijing, China
National Clinical Research Center for Geriatric Disorders, Beijing, China

Ying Han
Department of Neurology, Xuanwu Hospital, Capital Medical University, Beijing, China
Beijing Institute of Geriatrics, Beijing, China
National Clinical Research Center for Geriatric Disorders, Beijing, China
Center of Alzheimer's Disease, Beijing Institute for Brain Disorders, Beijing, China

Jian Xu
Department of Medical Information Engineering, School of Electrical Engineering and Information, Sichuan University, Chengdu, China
School of Information Engineering, Hubei University for Nationalities, Enshi, China

Jessica A. Turner
Department of Psychology and the Neuroscience Institute, Georgia State University, Atlanta, GA, United States
Mind Research Network, Albuquerque, NM, United States

Fuqin Chen and Junran Zhang
Department of Medical Information Engineering, School of Electrical Engineering and Information, Sichuan University, Chengdu, China

Taiyuan Liu and Meiyun Wang
Department of Medical Imaging, Henan Provincial People's Hospital, Zhengzhou, China

Ting Wang
Department of Computer Science, Chengdu University of Information Technology, Chengdu, China

Huijuan Yuan
Department of Endocrinology, Henan Provincial People's Hospital, Zhengzhou, China

Jie Lu
Department of Radiology, Xuanwu Hospital, Capital Medical University, Beijing, China

Jihai Xiao
Center of Information Management and Development, Taiyuan University of Technology, Taiyuan, China

Hui Xu
Department of Medical Imaging, The First Affiliated Hospital of Xi'an Jiaotong University, Xi'an, China
Key Laboratory of Biomedical Information Engineering of Education Ministry, Institute of Biomedical Engineering, Xi'an Jiaotong University, Xi'an, China
Faculty of Dentistry, University of Toronto, Toronto, ON, Canada

Chenguang Guo, Haining Li, Ming Zhang and Yuan Wang
Department of Medical Imaging, The First Affiliated Hospital of Xi'an Jiaotong University, Xi'an, China

Lin Gao
Key Laboratory of Biomedical Information Engineering of Education Ministry, Institute of Biomedical Engineering, Xi'an Jiaotong University, Xi'an, China

Wenhao Jiang and Tricia Z. King
Department of Psychology and the Neuroscience Institute, Georgia State University, Atlanta, GA, United States

Raquel Monteiro and Miguel Castelo-Branco
Coimbra Institute for Biomedical Imaging and Translational Research, Instituto de Ciências Nucleares Aplicadas à Saúde, University of Coimbra, Coimbra, Portugal
Faculty of Medicine, University of Coimbra, Coimbra, Portugal

Marco Simões
Coimbra Institute for Biomedical Imaging and Translational Research, Instituto de Ciências Nucleares Aplicadas à Saúde, University of Coimbra, Coimbra, Portugal
Faculty of Medicine, University of Coimbra, Coimbra, Portugal
Center for Informatics and Systems, University of Coimbra, Coimbra, Portugal

João Andrade
Faculty of Medicine, University of Coimbra, Coimbra, Portugal

Susana Mouga
Coimbra Institute for Biomedical Imaging and Translational Research, Instituto de Ciências Nucleares Aplicadas à Saúde, University of Coimbra, Coimbra, Portugal
Faculty of Medicine, University of Coimbra, Coimbra, Portugal
Neurodevelopmental and Autism Unit from Child Developmental Center, Hospital Pediátrico, Centro Hospitalar e Universitário de Coimbra, Coimbra, Portugal

Felipe França
PESC-COPPE, Universidade Federal do Rio de Janeiro, Rio de Janeiro, Brazil

Guiomar Oliveira
Coimbra Institute for Biomedical Imaging and Translational Research, Instituto de Ciências Nucleares Aplicadas à Saúde, University of Coimbra, Coimbra, Portugal
Faculty of Medicine, University of Coimbra, Coimbra, Portugal
Neurodevelopmental and Autism Unit from Child Developmental Center, Hospital Pediátrico, Centro Hospitalar e Universitário de Coimbra, Coimbra, Portugal
University Clinic of Pediatrics, Faculty of Medicine of the University of Coimbra, Coimbra, Portugal
Centro de Investigação e Formação Clínica, Hospital Pediátrico, Centro Hospitalar e Universitário de Coimbra, Coimbra, Portugal

Paulo Carvalho
Center for Informatics and Systems, University of Coimbra, Coimbra, Portugal

Ziliang Xu, Xuejuan Yang, Lin Liu, Jinbo Sun, Peng Liu and Wei Qin
Engineering Research Center of Molecular and Neuro Imaging of Ministry of Education, School of Life Science and Technology, Xidian University, Xi'an, China

Ming Gao
Assisted Reproduction Center, Northwest Women's and Children's Hospital, Xi'an, China
Department of Urology, Xijing Hospital, Fourth Military Medical University, Xi'an, China
Department of Andrology, Xiyuan Hospital, China Academy of Chinese Medical Sciences, Beijing, China

Swati Shah, Sanhita Sinharay, William Schreiber-Stainthorp, Siva Muthusamy, Dianne Lee and Dima A. Hammoud
Center for Infectious Disease Imaging (CIDI), Radiology and Imaging Sciences, Clinical Center, National Institutes of Health (NIH), Bethesda, MD, United States

Kenta Matsuda and Vanessa Hirsch
Laboratory of Molecular Microbiology, National Institute of Allergy and Infectious Diseases (NIAID), NIH, Bethesda, MD, United States

Paul Wakim
Biostatistics and Clinical Epidemiology Service, Clinical Center, NIH, Bethesda, MD, United States

Avindra Nath
National Institute of Neurological Disorder and Stroke (NINDS), NIH, Bethesda, MD, United States

Michele Di Mascio
AIDS Imaging Research Section, Division of Clinical Research, NIAID, NIH, Rockville, MD, United States

Flor A. Espinoza, Victor M. Vergara and Eswar Damaraju
Mind Research Network, Albuquerque, NM, United States
Tri-Institutional Center for Translational Research in Neuroimaging and Data Science (TReNDS), Georgia State University, Georgia Institute of Technology, Emory University, Atlanta, GA, United States

Kyle G. Henke
Mind Research Network, Albuquerque, NM, United States
Department of Mathematics and Statistics, The University of New Mexico, Albuquerque, NM, United States

Ashkan Faghiri
Mind Research Network, Albuquerque, NM, United States
Tri-Institutional Center for Translational Research in Neuroimaging and Data Science (TReNDS), Georgia State University, Georgia Institute of Technology, Emory University, Atlanta, GA, United States
Department of Electrical and Computer Engineering, The University of New Mexico, Albuquerque, NM, United States

Jessica A. Turner
Tri-Institutional Center for Translational Research in Neuroimaging and Data Science (TReNDS), Georgia State University, Georgia Institute of Technology, Emory University, Atlanta, GA, United States
Department of Psychology and Neuroscience, Georgia State University, Atlanta, GA, United States

Aysenil A. Belger
Department of Psychiatry, University of North Carolina at Chapel Hill, Chapel Hill, NC, United States

Judith M. Ford and Daniel H. Mathalon
Departmentof Psychiatry, University of California, San Francisco, San Francisco, CA, United States
San Francisco VA Medical Center, San Francisco, CA, United States

Sarah C. McEwen
Pacific Neuroscience Institute, Santa Monica, CA, United States
John Wayne Cancer Institute, Department of Translational Neurosciences and Neurotherapeutics, Santa Monica, CA, United States

Bryon A. Mueller
Department of Psychiatry, University of Minnesota, Minneapolis, MN, United States

Steven G. Potkin and Adrian Preda
Department of Psychiatry and Human Behavior, University of California, Irvine, Irvine, CA, United States

Jatin G. Vaidya
Department of Psychiatry, The University of Iowa, Iowa City, IA, United States

Theo G. M. van Erp
Clinical Translational Neuroscience Laboratory, Department of Psychiatry and Human Behavior, University of California, Irvine, Irvine, CA, United States
Center for the Neurobiology of Learning and Memory, University of California, Irvine, Irvine, CA, United States

Vince D. Calhoun
Mind Research Network, Albuquerque, NM, United States
Tri-Institutional Center for Translational Research in Neuroimaging and Data Science (TReNDS), Georgia State University, Georgia Institute of Technology, Emory University, Atlanta, GA, United States
Department of Electrical and Computer Engineering, The University of New Mexico, Albuquerque, NM, United States
Department of Psychology and Neuroscience, Georgia State University, Atlanta, GA, United States

Zhuqing Long
Medical Apparatus and Equipment Deployment, Nanfang Hospital, Southern Medical University, Guangzhou, China
School of Biomedical Engineering, Capital Medical University, Beijing, China

Jinchang Huang
Department of Acupuncture and Minimally Invasive Oncology, Beijing University of Chinese Medicine Third Affiliated Hospital, Beijing, China

Bo Li
Department of Traditional Chinese Medicine, Beijing Chest Hospital, Capital Medical University, Beijing, China
Beijing Tuberculosis and Thoracic Tumor Research Institute, Beijing, China

Zuojia Li, Zihao Li and Hongwen Chen
Medical Apparatus and Equipment Deployment, Nanfang Hospital, Southern Medical University, Guangzhou, China

Bin Jing
School of Biomedical Engineering, Capital Medical University, Beijing, China

Evrim Acar and Carla Schenker
Machine Intelligence Department, Simula Metropolitan Center for Digital Engineering, Oslo, Norway

Yuri Levin-Schwartz
Department of Environmental Medicine and Public Health, Icahn School of Medicine at Mount Sinai, New York, United States

Vince D. Calhoun
The Mind Research Network, Albuquerque, NM, United States
Department of Electrical and Computer Engineering, University of New Mexico, Albuquerque, NM, United States

Suchita Bhinge, Qunfang Long and Tülay Adali
Department of Computer Science and Electrical Engineering, University of Maryland Baltimore County, Baltimore, MD, United States

Xinhua Wei
Department of Radiology, Guangzhou First People's Hospital, School of Medicine, South China University of Technology, Guangzhou, China

Vince D. Calhoun
The Mind Research Network, Albuquerque, NM, United States
Department of Electrical and Computer Engineering, University of New Mexico, Albuquerque, NM, United States

Yunkai Zhu, Bo Zhang and Dianning He
Sino-Dutch Biomedical and Information Engineering School, Northeastern University, Shenyang, China

Shouliang Qi and Yueyang Teng
Sino-Dutch Biomedical and Information Engineering School, Northeastern University, Shenyang, China
Key Laboratory of Medical Image Computing of Northeastern University (Ministry of Education), Shenyang, China

Jiani Hu
Department of Radiology, Wayne State University, Detroit, United States

Xin Zhao and Qiong Wu
Department of Biomedical Engineering, College of Precision Instruments and Optoelectronics Engineering, Tianjin University, Tianjin, China

Yuanyuan Chen and Xizi Song
Tianjin International Joint Research Center for Neural Engineering, Academy of Medical Engineering and Translational Medicine, Tianjin University, Tianjin, China

Hongyan Ni
Department of Radiology, Tianjin First Center Hospital, Tianjin, China

Dong Ming
Department of Biomedical Engineering, College of Precision Instruments and Optoelectronics Engineering, Tianjin University, Tianjin, China
Tianjin International Joint Research Center for Neural Engineering, Academy of Medical Engineering and Translational Medicine, Tianjin University, Tianjin, China

Index

www.ingramcontent.com/pod-product-compliance
Lightning Source LLC
LaVergne TN
LVHW082215200926
848484LV00008B/2262